A Concise Guide to Differential Diagnosis in Palaeopathology

A Concise Guide to Differential Diagnosis in Palaeopathology is a practical guide to the identification of pathological conditions in human skeletal remains.

This guide serves as an essential first step in differential diagnosis, helping readers identify potential conditions that may have caused observed lesions, enabling them to conduct more targeted and effective research in palaeopathological and clinical literature. The book features an intuitive organisation with chapters arranged by disease aetiology, complemented by clear graphs, detailed figures, and concise bulleted lists highlighting key manifestations for each anatomical area. This format enables readers to access information easily and efficiently, facilitating an initial narrowing down of potential diseases, which can be overwhelming for newcomers to the field of palaeopathology, especially when working with limited resources and under pressing deadlines. By boiling the information down to the key elements, this guide acts as a quick reference and forms a helpful, practical, concise resource for students, teachers, and professionals, for teaching and data collection in the field and in the lab.

A Concise Guide to Differential Diagnosis in Palaeopathology is going to be essential for students in palaeopathology, bioarchaeology, and biological anthropology courses, and for practising anthropologists with varying experience levels seeking to identify unfamiliar pathological conditions in human skeletal remains.

Efthymia Nikita is Associate Professor of Bioarchaeology at the Science and Technology in Archaeology and Culture Research Center (STARC) of the Cyprus Institute. She studies human skeletal remains in the Mediterranean from prehistoric to medieval contexts, examining health, diet, demography, and other important aspects of life in the past. She has published over 120 scientific articles and book chapters, including the textbook *Osteoarchaeology* (Elsevier 2017), which received an honourable mention at the Association of American Publishers Awards for Professional and Scholarly Excellence. She is co-editor-in-chief of the second edition of Elsevier's *Encyclopedia of Archaeology* and of the *Journal of Archaeological Science*. In 2022, she was awarded the Dan David Prize for her contribution to the study of the past.

Mahmoud Mardini is Project Manager for Cultural Heritage at the Eratosthenes Centre of Excellence, Cyprus University of Technology. He completed an MSc in Osteoarchaeology at the University of Sheffield and a PhD in Science and Technology in Archaeology and Culture at the Cyprus Institute. He has participated in several excavations in the Eastern Mediterranean and has published 14 research papers on osteoarchaeology and Lebanese archaeology. Moreover, he was Associate Editor for Bioarchaeology at the Society for Archaeological Sciences Bulletin, and contributed to the development of several open-access resources for the promotion of the archaeological sciences in the Eastern Mediterranean.

A Concise Guide to Differential Diagnosis in Palaeopathology

Navigating the First Steps of Disease Identification in Human Skeletal Remains

Efthymia Nikita and Mahmoud Mardini

Routledge
Taylor & Francis Group
LONDON AND NEW YORK

Designed cover image: A case of scaphocephaly; drawing based on skull from the Duckworth Collection, University of Cambridge.

First published 2026
by Routledge
4 Park Square, Milton Park, Abingdon, Oxon OX14 4RN

and by Routledge
605 Third Avenue, New York, NY 10158

Routledge is an imprint of the Taylor & Francis Group, an informa business

British Library Cataloguing-in-Publication Data
A catalogue record for this book is available from the British Library

ISBN: 978-1-032-75647-9 (hbk)
ISBN: 978-1-032-72492-8 (pbk)
ISBN: 978-1-003-47502-6 (ebk)

DOI: 10.4324/9781003475026

Typeset in Times New Roman
by SPi Technologies India Pvt Ltd (Straive)

MIX
Paper | Supporting responsible forestry
FSC® C013056

Printed and bound in Great Britain by
TJ Books, Padstow, Cornwall

E.N. dedicates this book to Dimitris and Panos for their support—and their patience, most of the time.

M.M. dedicates this book to Christina for her constant encouragement and support.

Contents

Figures

Tables

Boxes

Preface

As a graduate student (many years ago…), the first author had to write an essay on palaeopathology. She thought, "That's easy; I'll simply list the pathological conditions one can identify on human bones." After a couple of hours into the literature review, it became clear that the topic is far more complicated than that. Palaeopathology is a fascinating field that can offer insights into highly diverse aspects of past life. Nonetheless, differential diagnosis, the process of narrowing down the diseases that could have caused the lesions observed on a skeleton, can be a daunting task. Dozens of excellent textbooks have been written on the topic, and hundreds of case studies on specific diseases have been published from around the world. Yet, formal training in palaeopathology is lacking in many countries, while most graduate programs in bioarchaeology cover palaeopathology within a single module. This may be enough to offer a basic understanding of different pathological processes and how they may appear skeletally, but it is often not sufficient to give students the confidence to engage in differential diagnosis unless they handle common or very distinct conditions.

Taphonomic damage, lack of reference collections (though see the Introduction regarding the importance of not relying exclusively on a comparative approach), and limited resources to complete the bioarchaeological analysis (of which palaeopathology is only part) can result in several conditions being misdiagnosed or ignored altogether. Thus, we felt it was important to create a resource that can help bioarchaeologists engage in the first steps of differential diagnosis, that is, the steps where scholars make an initial list of potential diseases before they start narrowing it down using more specialised resources. In creating this book, we had in mind primarily scholars with limited formal training in palaeopathology, little practical experience working with different diseases, and access to restricted resources, in terms of both medical collections but also time and money to complete their analysis. We did not aim to create a resource to oversimplify the complex process of differential diagnosis, and we strongly discourage scholars to base their diagnosis on superficial similarities between the lesions they record and those presented in this book. This book was created as a supplement to the current literature, aimed to be used as an initial resource before more authoritative texts are consulted. We describe in more detail our recommended use of the book in the Introduction.

We are deeply grateful to the many people who made the completion of this work possible. First of all, we are indebted to the hundreds of scholars who have contributed to the field of palaeopathology and on whose work we had the privilege to base ours. These scholars include seminal figures like Donald Ortner, Jane Buikstra, Anne Grauer, Simon Mays, Mary Lewis, Tony Waldron, Charlotte Roberts, Keith Manchester, Arthur Aufderheide, Megan Brickley, but also the hundreds of authors who have published research papers and case studies on the topic. Moreover, this book would not have been possible without the kind permission of several colleagues to access skeletal collections and take photographs to illustrate this work. The following colleagues not only allowed access to the collections but also spent considerable time taking out boxes for us and helping throughout the photography process: Elizabeth Craig-Atkins and Nina Maaranen from the Department of Archaeology, University of Sheffield, Emma Pomeroy and Trish Biers from The Duckworth Laboratory, University of Cambridge, Ahmet İhsan Aytek from Burdur Mehmet Akif Ersoy Üniversitesi, Dion Stoop and Suzan ten zijthoff from Noordelijk Archeologisch Depot at Provincie Groningen, Martijn van Haasteren and Inge van der Jagt from the Rijksdienst voor het Cultureel Erfgoed, Maria-Eleni Chovalopoulou, Christina Christodoulou, and Nefeli Garoufi from the National and Kapodistrian University of Athens. There are no words to express how grateful we feel for their support. We are also thankful to the Department of Antiquities in Cyprus for the permission to use photographs that we had obtained during the study of selected materials, but also to Anna Moles, University of Groningen, for bringing us in contact with the Noordelijk Archeologisch Depot and Rijksdienst voor het Cultureel Erfgoed. Moreover, we are deeply grateful to Lucie Biehler-Gomez, Kathryn Marklein, Paraskevi Tritsaroli, and Gkampriella Selempa for reading the entire book and sharing with us valuable comments for its improvement. Any omissions are clearly the authors' exclusive responsibility. This book has been made open access through the generous support of the Dan David prize, awarded to E.N., and the A. G. Leventis Chair in Archaeological Sciences at the Cyprus Institute. Last but certainly not least, we are indebted to our families for their love, patience, and support throughout the years.

A lot of hard work went into preparing this book, far more than we had anticipated when we started working on it! Despite our best efforts, mistakes are unavoidable; please bring to our attention any errors, and we will amend them in the future. Until then, we hope that you will find our small contribution to the challenging and exciting field of palaeopathology useful.

Chapter 1

Introduction

How to use and how not to use this book

This book stemmed out of our realisation that many diseases go unrecorded or unpublished in bioarchaeology due to the challenging task of differential diagnosis, a phenomenon that can result in severe biases in our understanding of past disease patterns. Palaeopathology, the study of diseases that afflicted individuals in the past, as explored through the analysis of human remains, as well as animal remains, textual sources, artwork, and other lines of evidence, can elucidate several critical aspects of past disease and its biocultural implications across time and space. This is exemplified in the ONE Paleopathology approach, which has emerged over the past years as an integrated approach aimed at understanding health diachronically, drawing from One Health's emphasis on the interconnectedness of humans, animals, and the environment.

Palaeopathology's contribution to a better understanding of past life is founded on the accurate identification of different diseases in skeletal remains. However, differential diagnosis is a challenging task, and for many scholars, it can even be daunting. First, as highlighted by the osteological paradox, many conditions (e.g. many infectious diseases) do not present on the skeleton by the time of death, so there may be no skeletal evidence at all to allow the identification of the disease(s) that affected the individuals. Even when pathological lesions are visible, the human skeleton can only respond to different insults through abnormal bone formation, abnormal bone loss/absence, abnormal size, and/or abnormal shape. As a result, several diseases with different aetiologies can cause similar lesions, and many pathological conditions only produce non-specific skeletal changes. Of relevance here, particularly when past diseases are studied at the population level (palaeoepidemiological studies), are the concepts of sensitivity and specificity. The former expresses the probability that individuals with a specific disease will show skeletal markers of that disease, while the latter is the probability that individuals without a specific disease will show no skeletal markers of that disease. In palaeopathological contexts, both sensitivity and specificity tend to be low, especially for certain disease groups, like infectious or neoplastic conditions. Adding further to the above limitations, in most archaeological contexts, the entire skeleton is not available for study, while diverse taphonomic factors can inhibit the recording of lesions and/or resemble pathological changes (pseudopathology).

Diagnosis in palaeopathology is primarily based on the morphology and distribution of lesions throughout the skeleton. These characteristics are compared against reference samples, such as skeletons in medical pathology museums or imaging data (e.g. radiographs) of living individuals. The former were mostly collected before modern medical treatments (e.g. antibiotics) became available, so they are likely to represent the course of diseases in archaeological populations. Having said that, even in the past, different communities used treatments

DOI: 10.4324/9781003475026-1

that may have influenced disease progression and manifestations (e.g. the use of mercury to treat syphilis), while modern patients may not comply with the prescribed treatments, which will also affect disease progression. Moreover, reference collections in medical pathology museums usually include only severe expressions of the pathological conditions, and the accompanying documentation varies; thus, it is often unclear how the diagnosis was performed and how accurate it is. Furthermore, even when medical pathological museums have documented diagnoses, clinical classifications change over time, and this may impact comparative diagnoses if not considered. On the other hand, imaging data from living patients capture a range of the expression of different conditions, but they often do not capture lesions visible on dry bones, especially subtle lesions. In addition, clinical imaging tends to be limited to certain areas, which does not allow the effective study of the distribution of lesions across the body, while an additional issue is the fact that imaging parameters and fields of view are often not focused on the bone, but on other tissues.

Due to these limitations of the so-called "comparative approach," but also the fact that this approach does not promote an understanding of the biological processes that may have caused the observed skeletal lesions, emphasis has been growing towards the so-called "biological approach." This approach is based on understanding the pathophysiology of different diseases; thus, it allows for the identification of lesions that can be anticipated based on a certain disease process, even if they have not been reported in the clinical and palaeopathological record.

Adopting the above approaches, several seminal works have been written for the identification of diseases in skeletal remains. Moreover, ample palaeopathological case studies are also critical resources for differential diagnosis. Nonetheless, for many scholars, narrowing down the potential pool of diseases to a manageable number that allows a more systematic engagement with the palaeopathological and clinical literature can be a daunting task. This is due to the fact that many diseases affect the human skeleton in similar ways, but also due to the lack of formal training in palaeopathology in many parts of the world. The available palaeopathological literature is vast, and there are too many parameters to consider, particularly when one has no solid starting point. Pressing deadlines and limited resources add further constraints to a proper engagement with differential diagnosis. As a result, in our experience, many pathological conditions will either be misdiagnosed, or a note and a few photos of the pathological lesions will be taken during data collection with the intention to engage in differential diagnosis at a later point, which never comes due to other pressing tasks. Both the misdiagnosis and overlooking of disease in past skeletons can have serious effects on our understanding of disease and its biocultural implications across time.

We wrote this book in an attempt to contribute towards amending this issue. Specifically, this book was written to help scholars with the first steps of differential diagnosis, that is, with an initial narrowing down of the diseases that could have produced the observed lesions, before they engage more systematically with the palaeopathological and clinical literature. This book is <u>not</u> a substitute for formal palaeopathological training, but we hope it serves to invite more researchers into a field that can be intimidating and provide educators with an open access resource to teach from. Below, we describe in more detail how we recommend readers to use this work.

How to use and how NOT to use this book

This book outlines how different diseases appear macroscopically on the human skeleton. It does not cover microscopy or molecular analyses, and minimally touches on medical imaging, although these are very important in palaeopathology. The reason for focusing on macroscopic methods is that the book aims to facilitate one of the initial steps of palaeopathological diagnosis, where scholars attempt an initial narrowing down of the conditions that could have caused the lesions observed in a skeleton. This initial step is based on macroscopic observation, whereas more advanced approaches are employed in the following steps of attempting to narrow down the diagnosis further.

This book should not be used as a shortcut to differential diagnosis! Differential diagnosis is challenging, and scholars will need to consider several variables when engaging with it. This book is meant to be a useful tool during the initial steps of differential diagnosis, specifically aimed at an initial narrowing down of the diseases that could have produced the observed lesions, before delving into more authoritative texts. We believe that this step is often the most demotivating, especially for scholars with limited training and experience; thus, we hope that this book will serve as an important building block, but in the context of a broader and integrated approach. Specifically, we recommend the following steps in diagnosing diseases on skeletal remains:

1 Carefully observe and record the morphology of each lesion using detailed notes and photographs. Be careful to differentiate pathological lesions from normal anatomical variation and taphonomic damage.
2 Record the anatomical distribution of lesions, preferably using a skeletal diagram to easily visualise this distribution. Make sure to also note which parts of the skeleton are not preserved for examination (e.g. due to taphonomic damage) as this can affect the observed distribution patterns.
3 Use this book to create an initial list of diseases that could have caused the observed lesions.

   a Do not overdiagnose! At this stage, it is best to list all diseases that could have caused the lesions you observe in the skeleton under study, rather than narrow down too much and miss important conditions. Remember also that this book could not cover every disease that may affect the human skeleton; instead, we focused on conditions commonly seen in the palaeopathological record and/or often covered in palaeopathology textbooks. Thus, be aware that the condition seen in the remains you examine may not be among the ones presented here (or in similar works).
   b Use the information given in this book regarding the distribution and morphology of the lesions as a broad guideline. Do not expect to find this exact distribution and/or the full list of lesions in the skeleton of an individual who suffered from a certain disease. The same disease can affect different individuals very differently depending on their immune system, nutritional status, access to care, and other parameters. Also, disease expression will depend on the time for which a disease afflicted an individual, whether the condition was active or healing/healed at the time of death, and other factors.
   c When working with commingled remains, it is difficult or even impossible to assess the distribution of lesions in different parts of the skeleton, and this poses additional serious challenges in differential diagnosis. Use the information given in the skeletal diagrams, focusing on the anatomical area where you have identified pathological lesions and make a list of the conditions that match the pattern you observe. Then check how the rest of the skeleton is anticipated to be affected by each of these conditions, and examine the rest of the commingled assemblage to see whether any elements show signs of the anticipated lesions. At this point, it is critical to determine whether these different elements could indeed belong to the same individual based on sex, age, robusticity/size, and any other available data.

d Beware of terminology. An issue we faced in the preparation of this book has been the non-standard and often ambiguous terminology used to describe pathological lesions in the literature. The importance of using precise and standardised terminology in differential diagnosis has been repeatedly flagged and culminated in the document Nomenclature in Palaeopathology (Manchester et al. 2016). Nonetheless, non-standard terms are still used frequently in publications, oftentimes because of training and translation, given the great diversity of global scholars who engage in palaeopathology. Here, we made sure to avoid common pitfalls, e.g. we do not use the term periostitis to refer to periosteal new bone formation unless it is associated with inflammation. However, several terms, such as porosity, bone loss, and pitting, are often used interchangeably in the literature, and this is the approach we had to follow here due to the lack of clarification of how each of these terms is used in different papers.

4 Now that a more concise list of diseases that could have afflicted the individual under study has been reached, narrow further the diagnosis using more authoritative palaeopathological and clinical texts.

a At the end of each chapter, we provide References and Suggested Readings where you can find important additional resources to consult. These should, however, be treated as a starting point since the relevant literature is vast.
b Start with the seminal palaeopathology works of Buikstra (2019) – an excellent update of the work by Ortner and Putschar (1981) and then Ortner (2003) –, Waldron (2020), Steinbock (1976), and Aufderheide and Rodríguez-Martín (1998). For juvenile remains, make sure to consult Lewis (2017), while for more specific disease groups, consult the appropriate textbooks (e.g. for metabolic disorders, see Brickley et al. 2020; for joint disease, see Burt et al. 2013 and Rogers and Waldron 1995). In these books, do not simply check the images and try to pattern match with your lesions, but pay careful attention to the information regarding the pathogenesis and pathophysiology of the conditions, as well as parameters such as their geographic distribution, age and sex predilection, etc.
c Consult the numerous case studies and more synthetic papers published at the key journals of the field (International Journal of Paleopathology, International Journal of Osteoarchaeology) but also more broadly (e.g. Journal of Archaeological Science, Archaeological and Anthropological Sciences, American Journal of Biological Anthropology). Again, do not simply pattern-match but place emphasis on the differential diagnosis provided by the authors.
d Review the clinical literature. Keep in mind that modern patients may have received treatment; thus, the expression of different diseases would be different in them compared to individuals in the past, who had different medical means available. In addition, keep in mind that certain diseases have evolved over time, so their modern manifestation may not match that seen in the past. Despite these potential complications, consulting modern cases is essential; otherwise, one ends up diagnosing diseases on unknown cases from other unknown cases. Pay attention, though, to the description of the treatments that were used in each clinical study you consult, which are typically disclosed.

5 Systematically evaluate the data gathered in steps 3 and 4 to determine the pathological conditions that match the patterns observed in the skeleton you study and cannot be excluded. Also assess how confident your diagnosis is using the modified Istanbul Terminological Protocol (Appleby et al. 2015). In this step, remember again that the same pathological condition can affect different individuals in various ways. Remember also that

multiple diseases could have affected an individual simultaneously, thus the lesions you see may reflect more than one condition. Finally, do not restrict the potential pathologies to a single group of diseases (e.g. infectious, metabolic); instead, keep in mind that conditions with different aetiologies can manifest similarly in the skeleton, and a definitive diagnosis may often not be possible to reach.

As highlighted by Mays (2020), upon initial observation of the skeleton, a researcher intuitively makes a list of conditions that could have produced the observed lesions based on prior experience. Nonetheless, this intuitive step may cause issues for inexperienced scholars. In some cases, one may formulate a diagnostic hypothesis based on insufficient data and spend the remaining steps of the diagnostic process trying to support this initial false hypothesis. In other cases, scholars may not be able to pose any initial hypotheses due to a lack of prior experience, which can make the subsequent steps of differential diagnosis overwhelming. This is where we feel the current book can make a contribution. We emphasise again, however, that it is imperative for scholars to use it critically and to employ additional resources to corroborate their diagnosis and/or narrow it down further. It is also important to be open to consulting other specialists, whether fellow palaeopathologists, clinical pathologists, or scholars from other fields.

To cite or not to cite?

In this book, we decided to avoid in-text citations, following a practice seen in several medical reference books (e.g. Callan 2012, Pelechas et al. 2019) or even in earlier palaeopathology books (e.g. Rogers and Waldron 1995) and other reference works, such as encyclopaedias. This decision was based on the fact that the information we give in the main text of the chapters is mostly introductory and can be easily found in several palaeopathology or clinical books and papers. Moreover, citations would break the flow of the text and increase the length of the book unnecessarily, whereas we tried to keep it as concise as possible. Instead, we opted to provide extensive suggested reading lists at the end of each chapter. These lists do not include all the resources we have used, but we tried to include the key ones that readers can consult to gain a deeper understanding of the topics covered in each chapter. We did include very few in-text citations when we needed to make reference to a very specific study (though we have kept these to a minimum), as well as in the legends of the figures and/or boxes presenting the key manifestations of different conditions. The citations given for the skeletal manifestations of each condition are selected and not exhaustive of the sources we consulted. We tried to include seminal works from the palaeopathological and medical literature, and a selection of additional key publications. Often, the same manifestations of a pathological condition were presented in different publications. For this reason, we placed emphasis on citing a variety of authors to enhance inclusivity in this work and show younger readers the multitude of sources one may consult to reach differential diagnosis. Before closing the topic of citing, we would like to emphasise, particularly to younger readers, the need to cite in their own research the original clinical and palaeopathological works, in addition to (or instead of) the current volume.

How to use the book figures

The figures included in this book fall under three broad categories: (1) Skeletal diagrams outlining some of the most common or likely to be encountered manifestations of different diseases in human skeletal remains, (2) Photographs of skeletal elements with representative lesions, and (3) Radiographs (or other imaging data) from living patients.

When using the skeletal diagrams, as well as the boxes presenting the manifestation of different conditions, remember that both the distribution and the morphology of the lesions will vary in different individuals based on the severity of the disease, the individual's immune status, the availability of medical treatment, and other factors. Indeed, while searching the literature in order to create these images, we found great variability in the information given in different clinical studies regarding which parts of the skeleton may be more afflicted by each disease and how. Moreover, in the list of potential lesions per condition, we provide lesions that correspond to different stages of the disease, with some being much more common than others. Therefore, you must treat the information provided only as a broad outline to help you narrow down, at an initial level, the potential diseases that afflicted the individual you study. Do not expect to find this exact lesion distribution or the exact same manifestation of lesions in the skeleton. Note also that in these diagrams we provide either a juvenile or an adult skeleton depending on the earliest most common age of onset of each condition; however, most diseases affect individuals belonging to different age groups. Thus, do not assume that because we use a juvenile skeleton to depict the distribution of lesions, the condition cannot be found in adults, and vice versa. Finally, in each of these diagrams, we have used very dark grey to denote the areas more often or more distinctly affected by each condition, and different shades of grey for the anatomical areas affected less frequently. In each case, we started from darker hues and moved to increasingly lighter ones, depending on how detailed the available information was regarding the distribution of lesions in the skeleton. For example, in cases where all we could find in the literature was a note that any bone may exhibit lesions, but skeletal elements X and Y are most often affected, we used very dark grey for elements X and Y, and dark grey for the rest of the skeleton. In cases where we found in the literature that skeletal element X is the most often affected, element Y often also shows lesions, but the entire skeleton may be involved in a disease, we used very dark grey for X, dark grey for Y, and lighter grey for the rest of the skeleton. Thus, the shades are relative and, as stressed above, they can vary considerably depending on which study one consults.

With regard to the photographs of pathological cases, the majority of the skeletons available for photography came from archaeological contexts; thus, there were no medical records available to allow a secure diagnosis. In many cases, only single elements of these skeletons were available to examine, preventing proper differential diagnosis on our part. Nonetheless, we selected cases that we believe represent classical examples of the manifestation of the different conditions. An associated limitation is that we could not capture the broad spectrum of expression of these conditions, which is a well-known issue in the palaeopathological literature. Therefore, as with the skeletal diagrams, these photographs should be used as a general guide. Finally, radiographs and visuals using other medical imaging techniques were used for diseases where we could not obtain dry bone photographs. We tried to use images that depict lesions that would be identifiable on dry bones, but a direct correspondence between the two is impossible. It is important to use all types of visuals simultaneously; do not simply try to identify which photograph matches best the lesions you observe in your case.

A few concluding words

Palaeopathology would take a lifetime to master, and, even then, it would require a constant reassessment of our knowledge and diagnoses given the continuous emergence of new information and technologies. We know first-hand how overwhelming differential diagnosis can be. There are too many possibilities to consider, too many books and papers to consult, and many obscure terms to understand. However, it is essential that all bioarchaeologists engage with palaeopathology (and by extension with differential diagnosis) more systematically. There is no question that the currently published accounts of various diseases give a biased impression of past disease patterns, largely because they tend to be focused in geographical areas where there is a stronger tradition in palaeopathological training. Although the situation is improving, with an increasing number of papers covering different conditions in several parts of the world, it is imperative to promote such initiatives further. We hope that this book will give you a useful starting point and the confidence to engage more systematically with differential diagnosis, for a better understanding of past disease and its broader implications.

References and suggested readings

Appleby, J., Thomas, R., Buikstra, J. (2015). Increasing confidence in paleopathological diagnosis–Application of the Istanbul terminological framework. *International Journal of Paleopathology* 8:19–21. https://doi.org/10.1016/j.ijpp.2014.07.003

Aufderheide, A., Rodríguez-Martín, C. (1998). *The Cambridge Encyclopedia of Human Paleopathology*. Cambridge: Cambridge University Press.

Biehler-Gomez, L., Cattaneo, C. (2020). *Interpreting Bone Lesions and Pathology for Forensic Practice*. San Diego: Academic Press.

Brickley, M.B., Ives, R., Mays, S. (2020). *The Bioarchaeology of Metabolic Bone Disease*. San Diego: Academic Press.

Buikstra, J.E. (2019). *Ortner's Identification of Pathological Conditions in Human Skeletal Remains*. San Diego: Academic Press.

Buikstra, J.E., Cook, D.C., Bolhofner, K.L. (2017). Introduction: Scientific rigor in paleopathology. *International Journal of Paleopathology* 19:80–87. https://doi.org/10.1016/j.ijpp.2017.08.005

Buikstra, J.E., Uhl, E.W., Wissler, A. (2023). Big pictures in 21st-century Paleopathology: Interdisciplinarity and transdisciplinarity. In *The Routledge Handbook of Paleopathology*, edited by Grauer, A.L., pp. 625–636. London: Routledge.

Burt, N.M., Semple, D., Waterhouse, K., Lovell, N.C. (2013). *Identification and Interpretation of Joint Disease in Paleopathology and Forensic Anthropology*. Springfield, IL: Charles C. Thomas.

Callan, M. (2012). *The Rheumatology Handbook*. London: Imperial College Press.

Grauer, A.L. (2008). Macroscopic analysis and data collection in palaeopathology. In *Advances in Human Palaeopathology*, edited by Pinhasi, R., May, S., pp. 57–76. Hoboken, NJ: John Wiley & Sons.

Grauer, A.L. (2012). *A Companion to Paleopathology*. Hoboken, NJ: John Wiley & Sons.

Grauer, A.L. (2023). *The Routledge Handbook of Paleopathology*. London: Routledge.

Grauer, A.L., Buikstra, J.E. (2019). Themes in paleopathology. In *Ortner's Identification of Pathological Conditions in Human Skeletal Remains*, edited by Buikstra, J., pp. 21–33. San Diego: Academic Press.

Klaus, H.D. (2017). Paleopathological rigor and differential diagnosis: Case studies involving terminology, description, and diagnostic frameworks for scurvy in skeletal remains. *International Journal of Paleopathology* 19:96–110. https://doi.org/10.1016/j.ijpp.2015.10.002

Klaus, H.D., Lynnerup, N. (2019). Abnormal bone: Considerations for documentation, disease process identification, and differential diagnosis. In *Ortner's Identification of Pathological Conditions in Human Skeletal Remains*, edited by Buikstra, J., pp. 59–89. San Diego: Academic Press.

Lewis, M. (2017). *Paleopathology of Children. Identification of Pathological Conditions in the Human Skeletal Remains of Non-Adults*. San Diego: Academic Press.

Manchester, K., Ogden, A., Storm, R. (2016). *Nomenclature in Palaeopathology*. Available at the Paleopathology Association website https://paleopathology-association.wildapricot.org/ (last accessed: April 2025)

Mann, R.W., Hunt, D.R. (2005). *Photographic Regional Atlas of Bone Disease. A Guide to Pathologic and Normal Variation in the Human Skeleton*, 3rd edition. Springfield, IL: Charles C. Thomas.
Mays, S. (2012). The relationship between paleopathology and the clinical sciences. In *A Companion to Paleopathology*, edited by Grauer, A.L., pp. 285–309. Hoboken, NJ: John Wiley & Sons.
Mays, S. (2018). How should we diagnose disease in palaeopathology? Some epistemological considerations. *International Journal of Paleopathology* 20:12–19. https://doi.org/10.1016/j.ijpp.2017.10.006
Mays, S. (2020). A dual process model for paleopathological diagnosis. *International Journal of Paleopathology* 31:89–96. https://doi.org/10.1016/j.ijpp.2020.10.001
Mays, S. (2023). The macroscopic study of human skeletal paleopathology. In *The Routledge Handbook of Paleopathology*, edited by Grauer, A.L., pp. 19–42. London: Routledge.
Milner, G.R., Boldsen, J.L. (2017). Life not death: Epidemiology from skeletons. *International Journal of Paleopathology* 17:26–39. https://doi.org/10.1016/j.ijpp.2017.03.007
Ortner, D.J. (2003). *Identification of Pathological Conditions in Human Skeletal Remains*, 2nd edition. San Diego: Academic Press.
Ortner, D.J. (2009). Issues in paleopathology and possible strategies for dealing with them. *Anthropologischer Anzeiger* 67:323–340.
Ortner, D.J. (2011). Human skeletal paleopathology. *International Journal of Paleopathology* 1:4–11. https://doi.org/10.1016/j.ijpp.2011.01.002
Ortner, D.J. (2012). Differential diagnosis and issues in disease classification. In *A Companion to Paleopathology*, edited by Grauer, A.L., pp. 250–267. Hoboken, NJ: John Wiley & Sons.
Ortner, D.J., Putschar, W.G.J. (1981). *Identification of Pathological Conditions in Human Skeletal Remains*, 1st edition. Washington, DC: Smithsonian Institution Press.
Pelechas, E., Kaltsonoudis, E., Voulgari, P.V., Drosos, A.A. (2019). *Illustrated Handbook of Rheumatic and Musculo-Skeletal Diseases*. Berlin: Springer International Publishing.
Pinhasi, R., Mays, S. (2008). *Advances in Human Palaeopathology*. Hoboken, NJ: John Wiley & Sons.
Resnick, D. (2002). *Diagnosis of Bone and Joint Disorders*, 4th edition. Philadelphia: W.B. Saunders.
Robbins Schug, G., Buikstra, J.E. (2025). From ONE Health to ONE Paleopathology: Deep-time perspectives on health in the face of climate and environmental change. *Encyclopedia* 5:13. https://doi.org/10.3390/encyclopedia5010013
Roberts, C.A., Manchester, K. (2005). *The Archaeology of Disease*, 3rd edition. Cheltenham: The History Press.
Rogers, J., Waldron, T. (1995). *A Field Guide to Joint Disease in Archaeology*. Hoboken, NJ: John Wiley & Sons.
Steinbock, R. (1976). *Paleopathological Diagnosis and Interpretation: Bone Disease in Ancient Human Populations*. Springfield, IL: Charles Thomas Publisher.
Vlok, M. (2023). Technical note: The use and misuse of threshold diagnostic criteria in paleopathology. *American Journal of Biological Anthropology* 181:326–335. https://doi.org/10.1002/ajpa.24721
Waldron, T. (2020). *Palaeopathology*, 2nd edition. Cambridge: Cambridge University Press.
Walker, D. (2012). *Disease in London, 1st to 19th Centuries: An Illustrated Guide to Diagnosis*. Museum of London Archaeology Monograph 56. London: Museum of London Archaeology.
World Health Organization. (2023). *One Health*. https://www.who.int/news-room/fact-sheets/detail/one-health (last accessed 3 June 2025).

Chapter 2

Developmental anomalies

Developmental anomalies are abnormalities in an individual's development that may appear at birth or later in life (Box 2.1). They are caused by genetic and environmental factors. With regard to genetic factors, gene mutations and chromosomal abnormalities have been linked to various developmental conditions. Regarding environmental impacts, teratogenic agents such as infections, exposure to radiation, environmental chemicals, drugs, maternal diabetes, malnutrition, as well as alcohol consumption, smoking, and others, can affect the embryo or fetus, potentially producing such anomalies.

Many developmental anomalies are classified as skeletal dysplasias. Such dysplasias are characterised by abnormal skeletal morphology or size, the presence of more or fewer bones than usual, and/or irregularities in bone texture resulting from disturbed ossification. Skeletal dysplasias include osteodysplasias, chondrodysplasias, and dysostoses. Osteodysplasias are characterised by irregular bone mineralisation or density. Chondrodysplasias arise from genetic anomalies that affect cartilage formation and often result in reduced stature. Finally, dysostoses refer to the malformation of single bones or groups of bones.

Developmental anomalies range from minor to severe. The latter may cause death in early life; thus, the study of such anomalies in palaeopathological contexts is often restricted to less severe conditions. In this chapter, developmental anomalies are organised according to the anatomical area primarily affected, while conditions involving multiple anatomical areas or even the entire skeleton are presented at the end.

Box 2.1 Developmental or congenital?

Although the terms "developmental" and "congenital" are often considered to have the same meaning, they do not. A congenital condition originates prenatally and is observable at or shortly after birth. In contrast, developmental anomalies include congenital ones but also disorders that appear postnatally. Thus, the term "developmental" has been preferred in this chapter because it has a broader meaning.

DOI: 10.4324/9781003475026-2

Skull

Craniosynostosis

Craniosynostosis is the premature closure of specific cranial sutures; it restricts the expansion of the skull in certain directions and promotes compensatory growth in others. The resulting skull morphology depends upon the sutures affected, and the sequence and timing of their fusion (Table 2.1, Figures 2.1–2.3). Craniosynostosis can affect a single suture (simple) or more (compound). The sagittal suture is the one affected most commonly. The condition is classified as primary, when it appears in isolation, or secondary, when it is linked to other disorders, such as hyperthyroidism.

Microcephaly

Microcephaly is characterised by an abnormally small cranium due to inadequate development of the brain (Box 2.2, Figure 2.4). The condition may be congenital or appear during the first years of life; in the latter case, infants have a normal head circumference at birth, but the cranium does not grow as expected later on. The aetiology of microcephaly is multifactorial and includes genetic mutations, metabolic disorders, infections, postnatal trauma, and other factors.

Table 2.1 Skeletal manifestation of craniosynostosis

Type and suture affected	*Skeletal manifestation*
Scaphocephaly/dolichocephaly *Affected suture*: sagittal	• elongated cranium • small biparietal diameter • frontal and occipital bossing • raised keel of bone across sagittal suture
Trigonocephaly *Affected suture*: metopic	• cranium narrow anteriorly and broad posteriorly (triangularly shaped when viewed from the top) • parietal and occipital bossing • small inter-orbital distance (hypotelorism) • pointed forehead • osseous ridge between glabella and bregma
Frontal plagiocephaly *Affected sutures*: unilateral involvement of coronal suture	• flattened frontal bone on affected side • contralateral frontal bossing
Occipital plagiocephaly *Affected sutures*: unilateral involvement of lambdoid suture	• flattened occipital and parietal bones on affected side • contralateral parietal and frontal bossing
Brachycephaly *Affected sutures*: bilateral involvement of coronal suture	• almost circular skull • frontal bossing • flattened occipital bone
Oxycephaly *Affected sutures*: coronal and lambdoid, or coronal and sagittal, or all sutures	• tall, cone-shaped head • great inter-orbital distance (hypertelorism) • digital impressions resulting from elevated intracranial pressure
Cloverleaf deformity *Affected sutures*: bilateral involvement of multiple or all sutures	• three-lobed-looking skull from the front • bulging frontal eminences • bulging at parieto-squamosal sutures • constricted and upright parietals

(Data from Cohen 2000; Lewis 2017; Mann and Hunt 2012)

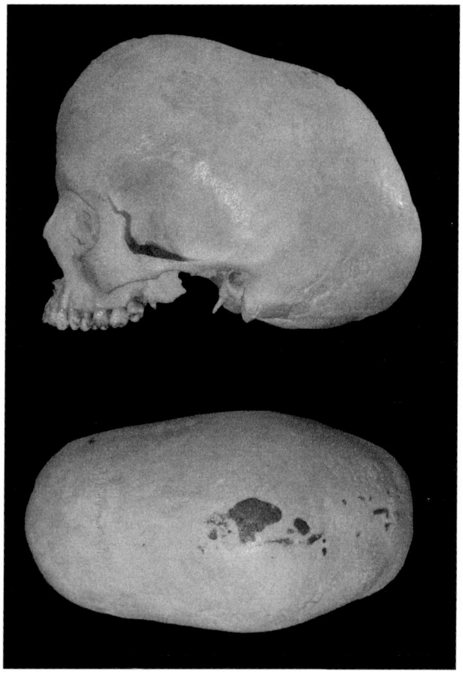

Figure 2.1 Scaphocephaly. Note the pronounced elongation of the cranium and the closure of the sagittal suture, whereas the remaining sutures are still open. (Photos by Efthymia Nikita; copyright: Duckworth Laboratory, University of Cambridge)

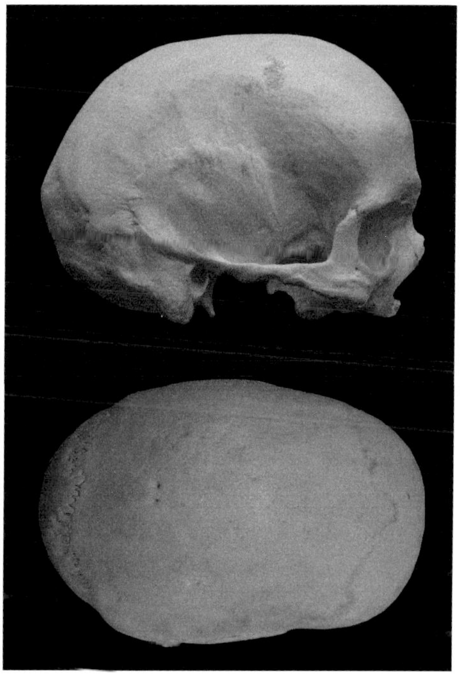

Figure 2.2 Scaphocephaly. Note the elongation of the cranium and the closure of the sagittal suture, whereas the remaining sutures are still open. (Photos by Efthymia Nikita; copyright: Duckworth Laboratory, University of Cambridge)

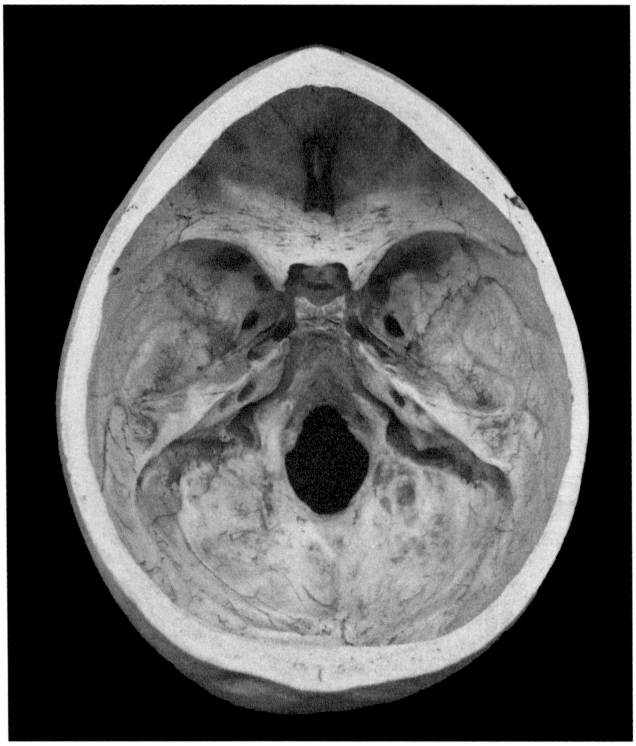

Figure 2.3 Trigonocephaly. Note the anterior narrowing of the cranium and its overall triangular shape when viewed from the top. (O.O.54 No 2232, No 2229; photo by Efthymia Nikita; copyright: Duckworth Laboratory, University of Cambridge)

Box 2.2 Skeletal manifestation of microcephaly

- small skull (occipito-frontal circumference over two or three standard deviations below mean)
- cranial capacity < 1000cc
- large-looking face compared with small vault
- narrow, receding frontal bone
- flattened occipital bone
- prominent nose
- micrognathia
- small stature

(Data from Aufderheide and Rodríguez-Martín 1998; Barnes 2012a; Lewis 2017; Morris et al. 2016)

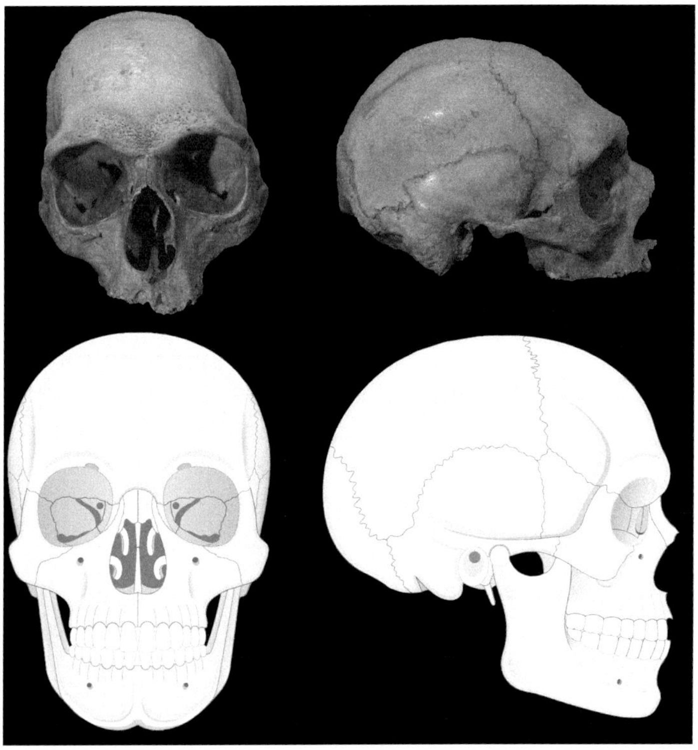

Figure 2.4 Microcephaly. Note the abnormally small cranium (top) compared to the drawing of normal cranium (bottom), the large-looking face compared with the small vault, the narrow and receding frontal bone, and the prominent nose. (Human cranium: Bedford 2286 1; photos by Efthymia Nikita; copyright: Duckworth Laboratory, University of Cambridge; drawings from https://www.humanbiomedia.org/ available under a Creative Commons Attribution 4.0 License)

Macrocephaly

Macrocephaly is an abnormal increase in head circumference; it is often linked to megalencephaly, that is, an abnormal increase in brain size, as well as hydrocephalus (see below).

Hydrocephalus

In cases of hydrocephalus, an abnormal enlargement of the cranium results from excessive accumulation of cerebrospinal fluid due to the abnormal production, defective absorption, or obstructed circulation of this fluid. Hydrocephalus may be congenital or acquired. If it is acquired, potential etiological factors include infections of the central nervous system, brain tumours, cranial trauma, and intracranial haemorrhage. This condition may appear in isolation or as part of a disease syndrome.

Hydrocephalus usually appears within the first six months of life; however, it can arise at any point, from in utero to adulthood. The appearance of this condition depends on the affected individual's age of onset. In infants, the cranial sutures are still open; thus, increased intracranial volume can lead to the separation of the cranial vault bones, affecting the morphology and dimensions of the cranium greatly (Box 2.3, Figure 2.5). In contrast, in older

Box 2.3 Skeletal manifestation of hydrocephalus

- enlarged cranial vault
- globular cranium
- frontal bossing
- rather normal face
- thin cranial bones
- flat cranial base
- enlarged foramen magnum
- widened/enlarged sutures and fontanelles, open through adult life
- wormian bones
- pronounced intracranial vascular sulci markings

(Data from Aufderheide and Rodríguez-Martín 1998; Dewan et al. 2018; Richards and Anton 1991)

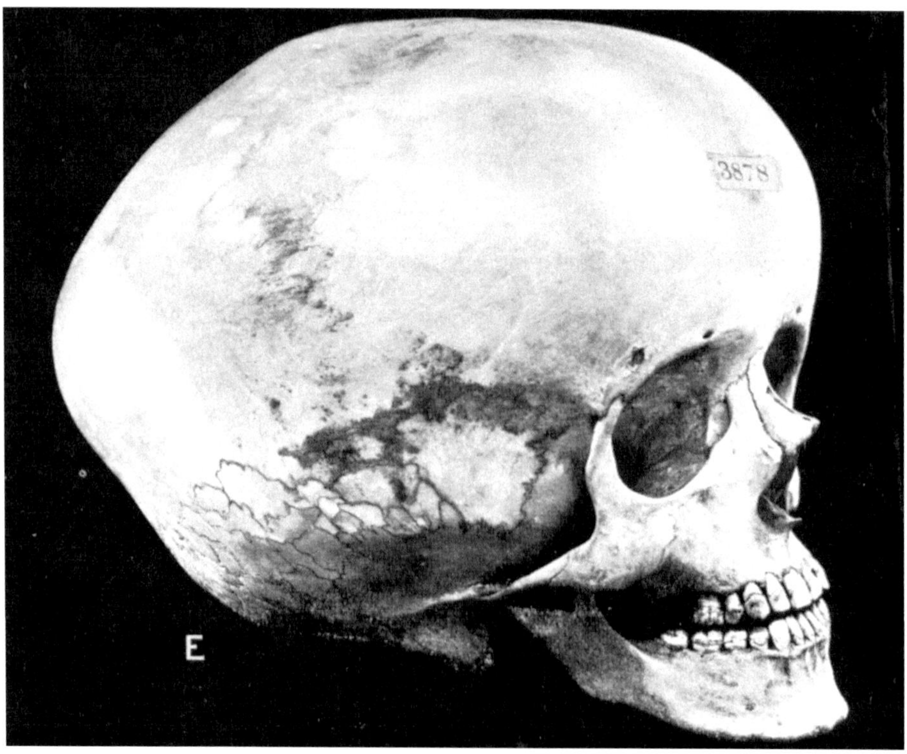

Figure 2.5 Skull of 25-year-old male with hydrocephalus, Hunterian Museum of the Royal College of Surgeons. Note the enlarged globular cranium, with frontal bossing and multiple wormian bones. (From Gladstone, R.J. (1905). A study of the relations of the brain to the size of the head. *Biometrika* 4:105–123; this work is in the public domain and can be accessed through Wikimedia Commons: https://commons.wikimedia.org/wiki/File:Hydrocephalic_skull.jpg)

individuals, where the sutures have fused, hydrocephalus causes expansion of the ventricles and elevated intracranial pressure, but it does not alter the head circumference.

Anencephaly

Anencephaly is the lack of a large part of the brain and skull, when the rostral neuropore fails to close during embryonic development (Box 2.4). It is classified as a neural tube defect, that is, part of a group of serious congenital anomalies. Infants with anencephaly usually die within hours or days after birth. Regarding its aetiology, this condition has been associated with infections during pregnancy (e.g. rubella, varicella-zoster virus), exposure to teratogenic chemicals, maternal health problems (e.g. diabetes), hyperthermia, maternal nutrient deficiencies (especially folic acid), as well as genetics (e.g. association with Meckel–Gruber syndrome).

Aural atresia

Aural atresia appears as a malformed or altogether absent external auditory meatus (Box 2.5). It is associated with an abnormal development of the first and second branchial arches or the first branchial cleft.

Oral clefts

Oral clefts are congenital anomalies whose expression depends on the affected anatomical structures, the involved side, and the degree of severity. They can occur in isolation or be associated with various syndromes. Individuals with oral clefts often have difficulties with feeding, hearing, and speech development, and infants with oral clefts, especially when associated with genetic syndromes, exhibit a higher mortality compared to healthy ones.

Box 2.4 Skeletal manifestation of anencephaly

- minimally formed cranial vault
- deformed skull base
- rudimentary orbits

(Data from Alghamdi et al. 2017; Irurita et al. 2015)

Box 2.5 Skeletal manifestation of aural atresia

- spectrum of expression, from narrowed to obliterated external auditory canal (with different degrees of involvement of the middle and inner ear structures)
- mostly unilateral (especially on right side)

(Data from De la Cruz et al. 1985; Keenleyside 2011; Kösling et al. 2009)

Box 2.6 Skeletal manifestation of cleft lip

- mostly unilateral
- notches/indentations between central incisors or between lateral incisors and canines; severe bilateral forms result in rounded premaxillary process
- often linked to developmental dental anomalies (e.g. hypodontia, microdontia) in the region of the cleft and beyond

(Data from Barnes 2008; Haque and Alam 2015; Latief et al. 2010; Menezes and Vieira 2008)

Box 2.7 Skeletal manifestation of cleft palate

- bilateral or unilateral
- ranging from minor cleft to full cleft (U-shaped hard palate)
- may occur alone or together with cleft lip
- often associated to hypodontia or supernumerary teeth

(Data from Haque and Alam 2015; Kosowski et al. 2012; Lewis 2017; Menezes and Vieira 2008)

Cleft lip results from the complete or partial failure of union between the maxillary process and the medial nasal process (Box 2.6). In cases of cleft palate, there is an open connection between the oral and nasal cavities (Box 2.7, Figure 2.6). It results from the incomplete fusion of the palatal shelves during early embryonic development.

Stafne's defects

Stafne's defects are concavities on the lingual surface of the mandible (Box 2.8, Figure 2.7). They may arise from several processes, such as: (1) the entrapment or aberrant development of salivary gland tissue during embryonic development; (2) erosion caused by pressure from the facial artery; (3) the enlargement of the submandibular salivary gland or other soft tissues; or (4) localised failed ossification. Stafne's defects are usually asymptomatic; thus, they may be classified as normal anatomical variations rather than pathological conditions. Other developmental anomalies seen in the mandible are listed in Box 2.9.

Spine

Supernumerary vertebrae

An extra vertebra may develop if there is an extra pair of somites (embryological precursors to vertebrae) during embryonic development. It is important to distinguish such vertebrae from anatomical changes occurring as a result of vertebral border shifting (see below).

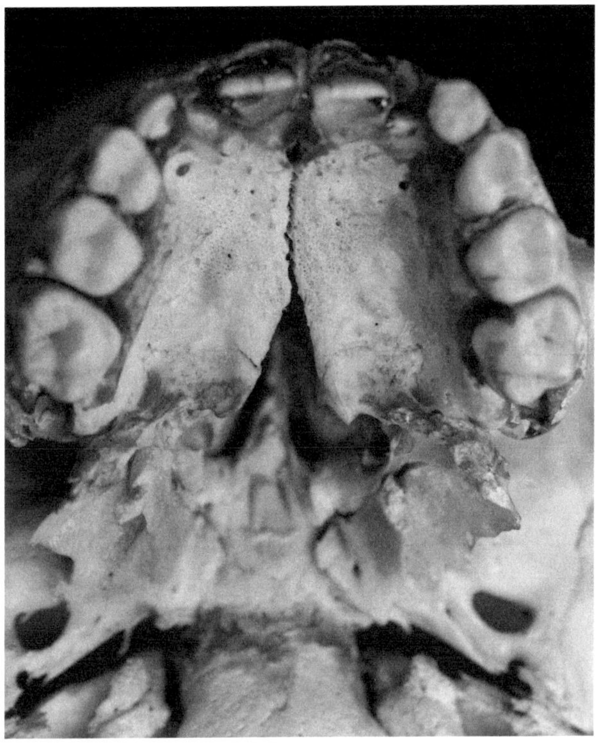

Figure 2.6 Juvenile with bilateral cleft palate. (Photo by Efthymia Nikita; copyright: Duckworth Laboratory, University of Cambridge)

Box 2.8 Skeletal manifestation of Stafne's defects

- circular or oval concavities on the lingual mandibular surface (mostly near molar area or anterior to mandibular angle; rarely located anteriorly, between incisor and premolar areas; very rarely located on ascending ramus)
- size varies, but usually 10–30 mm in length and less than 10 mm in depth
- concavity margins clearly defined or continuous with the cortical bone
- concavity floor rough or smooth
- mostly unilateral

(Data from Katz et al. 2001; Mann 2001; Philipsen et al. 2002; Stafne 1942)

Vertebral border shifting

A vertebral border shift may occur during the development of the vertebrae, when the sclerotomes are separated into cranial and caudal parts, with each part subsequently fusing with its adjacent counterpart (Box 2.10). Vertebrae may shift to either side of a border (cervical-thoracic, thoracic-lumbar, lumbar-sacrum, sacrum-coccyx); these shifts are characterised as cranial or caudal. When such shifts occur, the vertebrae positioned at the ends of a vertebral

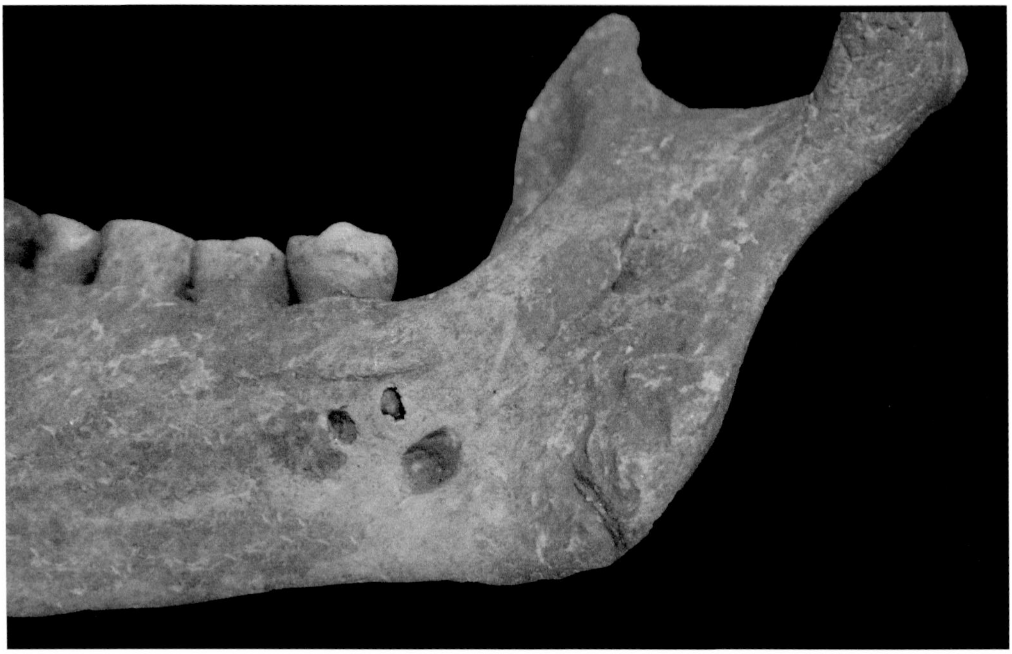

Figure 2.7 Stafne's defect in the lingual surface of the right mandibular corpus. (Iron Age Wandlebury, Cambs, Eu.1.3.379; photo by Efthymia Nikita; copyright: Duckworth Laboratory, University of Cambridge)

Box 2.9 Other mandibular developmental anomalies

- hypoplasia
  - affecting ascending ramus and dorsal part of mandibular body
  - mild to severe expressions
- bifid condyle
  - mostly unilateral
  - bifid corresponding temporal articular joint
- cleft mandible
  - unmerged two halves of the mandible
  - variable degrees of expression
- coronoid hyperplasia
  - enlarged mandibular coronoid processes
  - usually bilateral

(Data from Barnes 2012a)

Box 2.10 Skeletal manifestation of vertebral border shifting

Cervical-thoracic border

- cranial border shift
    - cervical ribs (cervical vertebral costal processes develop into ribs)
        - small tubercles to rib-like extensions
        - mostly in C7; rarely in C6, C5, or C4
        - may terminate in free end, connect with manubrium, or articulate/fuse with first rib
- caudal border shift
    - rudimentary T1 transverse processes
    - rudimentary first rib (variable in size, abnormal in shape, may articulate/fuse to second rib or connect with manubrium)
    - rudimentary cervical-like transverse foramina on T1

Thoracic-lumbar border

- caudal border shift
    - lumbar ribs (lumbar vertebral transverse processes develop into ribs)
        - mostly bilateral and asymmetric
        - small tubercles to separate articulating ribs
- cranial border shift
    - rudimentary or absent twelfth thoracic ribs
    - hypoplasia/aplasia of rib facets on T12
    - transitional apophyseal facets on T12 (inferior facets exhibit curvature resembling that of the lumbar region, superior facets present flat morphology akin to thoracic facets)

Lumbar-sacral border

- sacralisation of fifth lumbar vertebra (cranial border shift)
    - partial or complete L5-sacrum fusion:
        - type I: unilateral or bilateral hypertrophy of L5 transverse processes
        - type II: widened (and possibly bifurcated) L5 transverse processes articulate with sacral alae (contact facets visible on alae and/or transverse processes)
        - type III: unilateral or bilateral L5 transverse processes-alae fusion; sacrum appears to have six segments and five foramina
        - type IV: mixed expressions (different types manifesting on each side)
    - hemisacralisation: lumbar vertebra morphology on one side and sacral morphology on the other

- lumbarisation of first sacral vertebra (caudal border shift)
    - partial or complete
    - unilateral or bilateral
    - S1 assumes lumbar characteristics and may separate from the rest of the sacrum
    - it appears that there are six lumbar vertebrae and four sacral segments

(Data from Barnes 1994, 2008, 2012a; Drew and Kjellström 2021; Tini et al. 1977)

region will show morphological changes as they acquire characteristics typical of the adjacent region. For example, when a cranial shift occurs at the lumbosacral border, the fifth lumbar vertebra may become partially or fully fused with the first sacral vertebra (it is "sacralised") (Figures 2.8–2.10). In contrast, in the case of a lumbosacral caudal shift, the first sacral vertebra exhibits features characteristic of lumbar vertebrae, becoming partially or fully "lumbarised" (Figure 2.11).

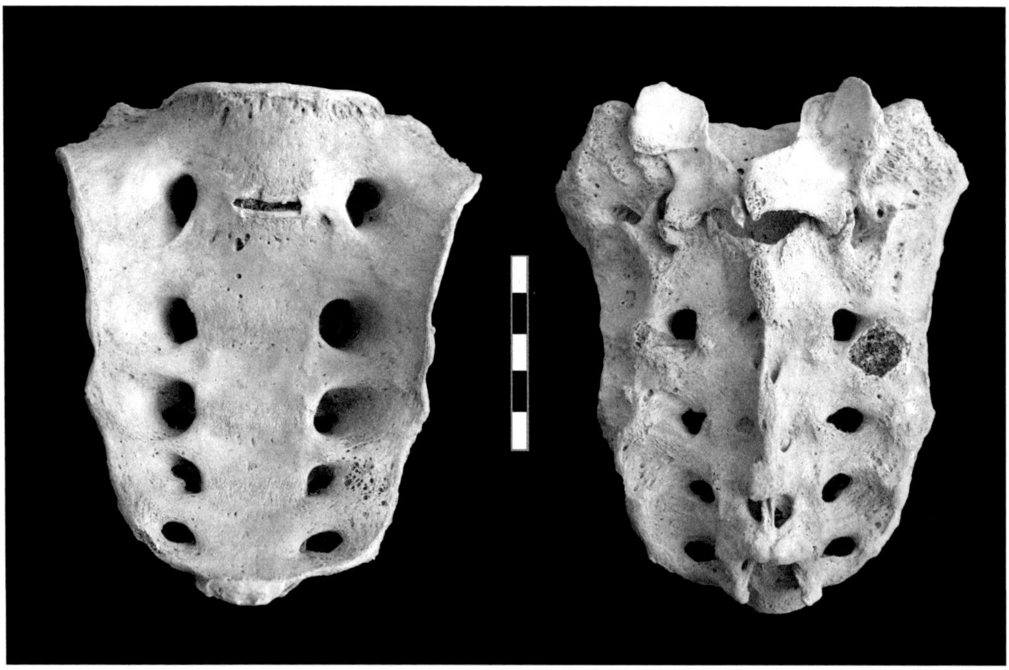

Figure 2.8 Partial sacralisation of a fifth lumbar vertebra. Note that the L5 transverse processes are fully fused with the sacral alae, osseous bridges have partly fused the L5 body with the sacrum anteriorly, while the L5 inferior articular facets are not fused with the sacrum. Note also that the two halves of the L5 neural arch have not fused. The sacrum appears to have six segments and five foramina. (Sbide, Roman/Byzantine; photos by Efthymia Nikita, with the kind permission of Dr. Ahmet Ihsan Aytek, Burdur Mehmet Akif Ersoy University)

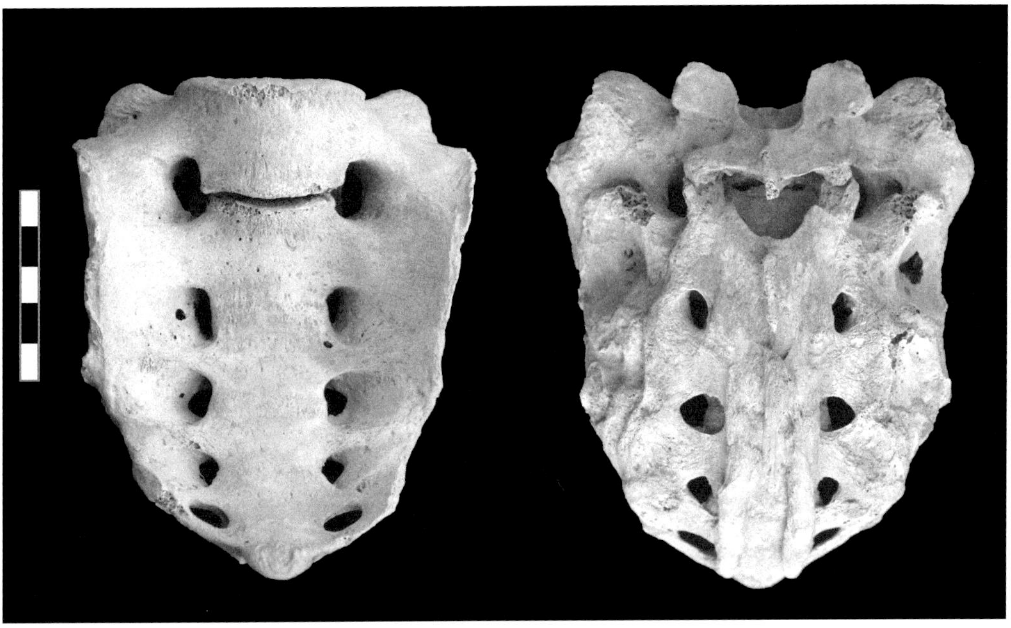

Figure 2.9 Partial sacralisation of a fifth lumbar vertebra. Note that the L5 transverse processes are fully fused with the sacral alae, but the L5 body and inferior articular facets are not fused with the sacrum. (Sbide, Roman/Byzantine; photos by Efthymia Nikita, with the kind permission of Dr. Ahmet Ihsan Aytek, Burdur Mehmet Akif Ersoy University)

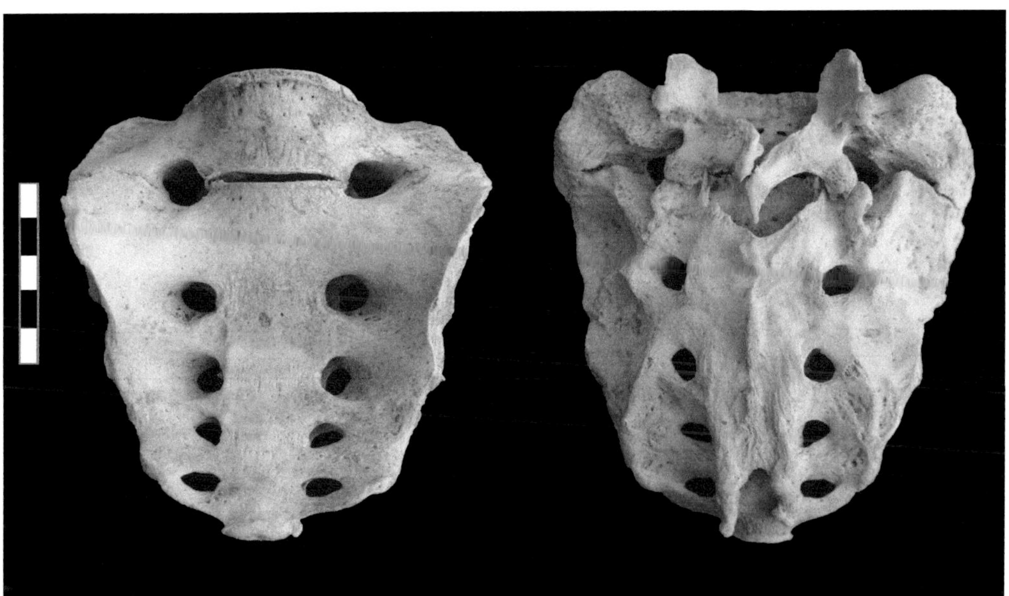

Figure 2.10 Partial sacralisation of a fifth lumbar vertebra. Note that the L5 transverse processes are partially fused with the sacral alae. Neither the body nor the inferior articular facets are fused with the sacrum. Note also that the two halves of the L5 neural arch have not fused. (Sbide, Roman/Byzantine; photos by Efthymia Nikita, with the kind permission of Dr. Ahmet Ihsan Aytek, Burdur Mehmet Akif Ersoy University)

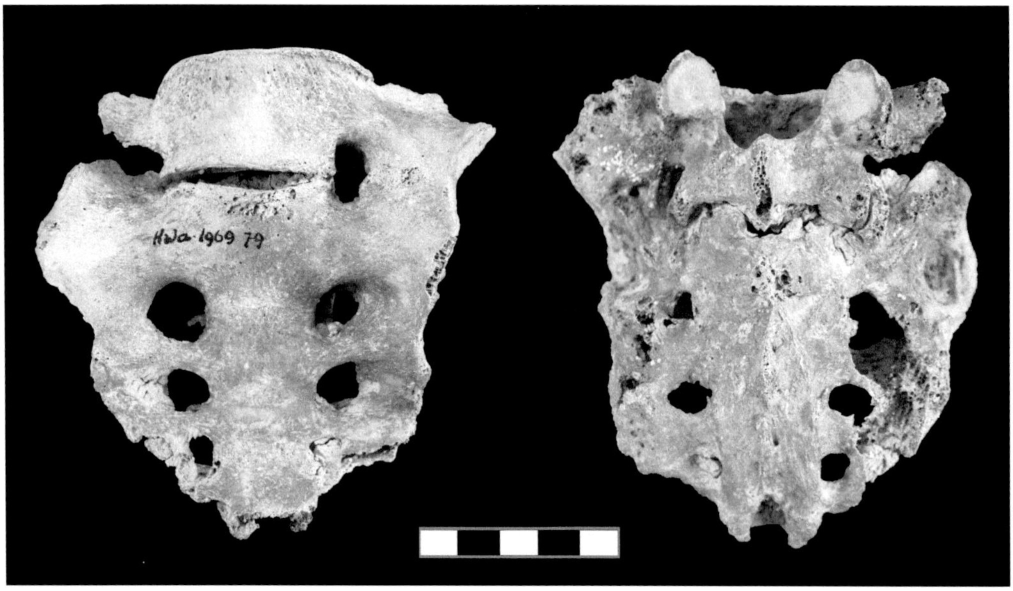

Figure 2.11 Partial lumbarisation of a first sacral vertebra. Note that the S1 is partially separated from the rest of the sacrum, as visible on the right side of this element but also in the separation of the S1 body and neural arch from S2. The remaining sacrum appears to have four sacral segments. (Female, Young/Middle adult, Eemsdelta-Hoogwatum, Collection NAD Nuis inv. Nr. G 2018-IX.232; photos by Efthymia Nikita, with permission from the Noordelijk Archeologisch Depot)

Os odontoideum

This is a rare condition where the dens has not fused with the rest of the axis, resulting in the formation of a hypoplastic ossicle (Box 2.11). In less severe developmental disorders of the dens, the apical tip may fail to unite with the base, leading to the formation of an ossicle that can attach to the atlas or foramen magnum. In some cases, there may be agenesis of the apical tip, which makes the dens appear short and blunt. These anomalies are associated with segmental defects and cranial shifting at the occipital-cervical border. However, they may also be acquired in cases where an odontoid fracture causes avascular necrosis.

Os odontoideum may cause no symptoms, but it has also been associated with headache, neck pain, and torticollis. Additionally, the atlanto-axial joint may dislocate even with

Box 2.11 Skeletal manifestation of os odontoideum

- dens detached and forming a separate ossicle
- roughened, rounded, and/or mound-shaped C2 surface where the odontoid process normally attaches
- further abnormalities in C2 morphology
- possible dislocation of atlantoaxial articulation

(Data from Clements et al. 1995; Mann et al. 2013)

minimal trauma, leading to vertebral artery occlusion and infarction of the brainstem. Note that os odontoideum can be found in association with Klippel–Feil syndrome, Down syndrome, epiphyseal dysplasia, and other disorders.

Block vertebra

The term "block vertebra" expresses the congenital fusion of at least two vertebrae (Box 2.12). This condition results when a fissure between precursor developing units of the resegmented sclerotome does not form, and as a result, adjacent vertebral segments do not separate. The fusion of the vertebrae may be complete or partial. Although gene mutations may contribute to the formation of block vertebrae, segmentation errors may also arise from disruptions in the blood supply to the vertebrae, as well as from environmental factors, such as hypoxia, exposure to carbon monoxide, maternal diabetes, and certain drugs.

A rather common case of block vertebra in palaeopathological contexts is the Klippel–Feil syndrome (Box 2.13, Figures 2.12 and 2.13). Beyond the spine, individuals with this syndrome may show skeletal abnormalities such as cleft palate, limb length discrepancies, or Sprengel's deformity. In some cases, the Klippel–Feil syndrome may be part of more complex disorders, such as the Wildervanck syndrome.

Hemivertebrae

Hemivertebrae are characterised by the lack of half of the vertebra and are a major aetiology of congenital scoliosis (Box 2.14). They form when one of the paired somites fails to move to the midline in time, and thus it does not fuse with its partner to form a sclerotome.

Box 2.12 Skeletal manifestation of block vertebra

- partially or fully fused successive vertebrae
- fusion involves vertebral bodies and posterior elements
- mostly in cervical spine, occasionally in thoracic, rarely in lumbar vertebrae

(Data from Barnes 1994, 2012a)

Box 2.13 Skeletal manifestation of Klippel–Feil syndrome

- type I: multiple cervical and upper thoracic vertebrae fused; linked to other developmental abnormalities
- type II: two or three vertebrae fused (mostly C2–C3, followed by C5–C6, occasionally T2–T5); it is the most common type; may be associated with other anomalies (e.g. hemivertebrae)
- type III: block of fused cervical vertebrae, with the thoracic and lumbar vertebrae also showing segmental errors

(Data from Barnes 1994; Gunderson et al. 1967)

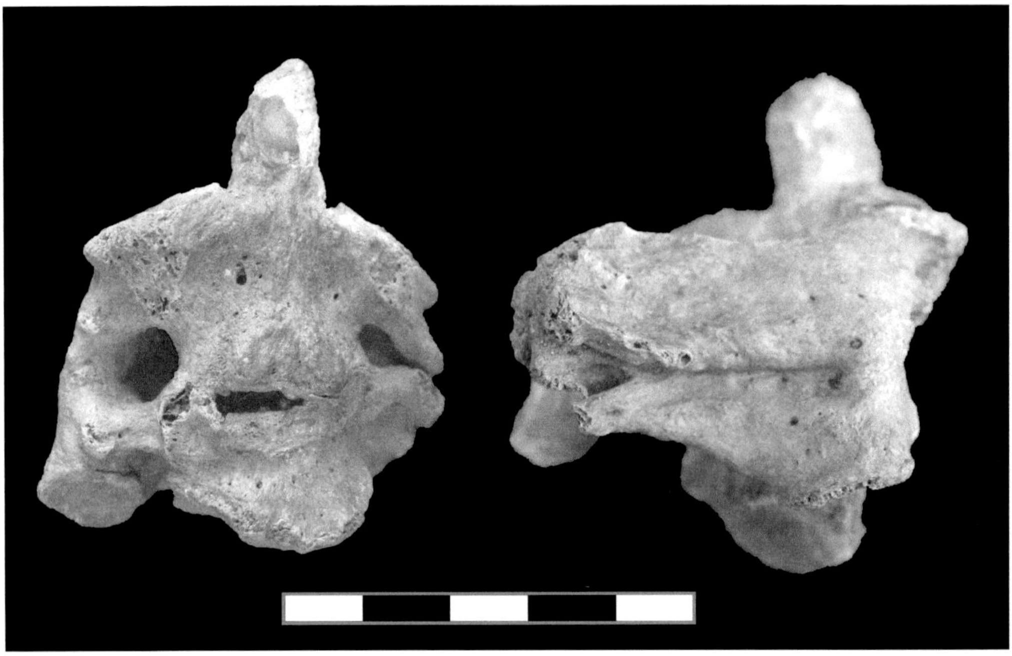

Figure 2.12 Klippel–Feil syndrome type II (congenitally fused C2 and C3). Note that the vertebral bodies are partially fused while the neural arches are fully fused. (Sbide, Roman/Byzantine; photos by Efthymia Nikita, with the kind permission of Dr. Ahmet Ihsan Aytek, Burdur Mehmet Akif Ersoy University)

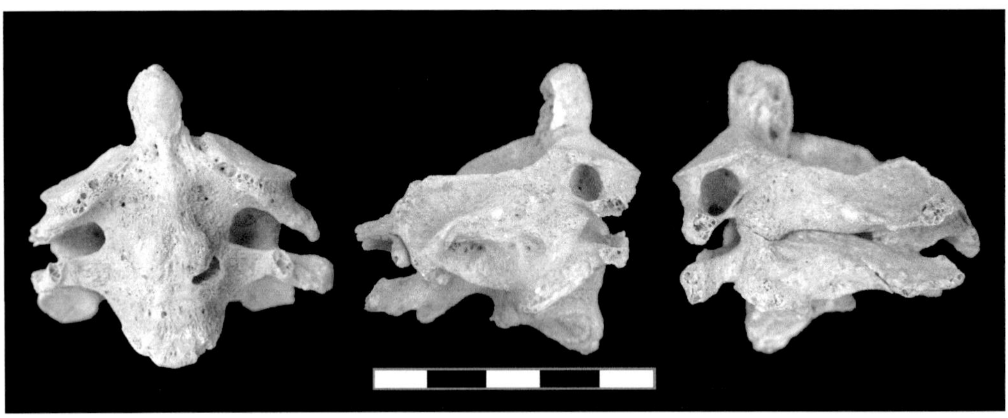

Figure 2.13 Klippel–Feil syndrome type II (congenitally fused C2 and C3). Note that the vertebral bodies are almost fully fused, while the neural arches are fully fused on the right side but unfused on the left. (Kibyra, Byzantine; photos by Efthymia Nikita, with the kind permission of Dr. Ahmet Ihsan Aytek, Burdur Mehmet Akif Ersoy University)

Box 2.14 Skeletal manifestation of hemivertebrae

- lack of half of the vertebra
- often coexisting with other vertebral defects
- unilateral (causing scoliosis) or contralateral (having limited effects)
- may unite with adjacent vertebrae or remain separated

(Data from Barnes 2012a, 2012b)

Hemivertebrae have been associated with spondylothoracic dysostosis, cleidocranial dysostosis, mucopolysaccharidoses, and other disorders.

Sagittal cleft vertebrae ("Butterfly vertebrae")

Sagittal clefts occur on vertebral bodies due to the persistence of a foetal notochord segment, which did not completely recede (Box 2.15). While sagittal cleft vertebrae may have no symptoms, they can also cause lower back pain. Moreover, they may coexist with supernumerary vertebrae and spina bifida, and they have been linked to several syndromes, such as craniofacial synostosis, spondylothoracic dysostosis, and Klippel–Feil syndrome.

Cleft neural arch

Hypoplasia or aplasia of the neural arch may lead to the lack of union between the two halves of the arch (Box 2.16). As a result, there is an osseous cleft of varying size, with fibrocartilage keeping the two halves together.

Box 2.15 Skeletal manifestation of sagittal cleft vertebrae

- vertebral body separated into two lateral halves
- slight to complete separation
- two halves of equal size, but bilateral or unilateral hypoplasia is possible
- may manifest as large area of missing bone from vertebral body, sparing vertebral border
- mostly in thoracic or lumbar spine
- mostly in one vertebra but two adjacent vertebrae may be affected
- compensatory changes to adjacent vertebrae
- kyphosis or scoliosis
- normal neural arch (fissure of vertebral arch is rare)

(Data from Aufderheide and Rodríguez-Martín 1998; Barnes 1994; Brasili et al. 2002; Müller et al. 1986)

Box 2.16 Skeletal manifestation of cleft neural arch

- mostly in lower lumbar/first sacral vertebrae; thoracic spine rarely involved; among cervical vertebrae, usually only atlas affected
- mostly involving one or two vertebrae
- expression ranging from minimal laminar and spinous process bifurcation to cleft laminae; unilateral aplasia of the neural arch → asymmetric cleft, bilateral aplasia → absence of entire neural arch

(Data from Barnes 2012a)

Spina bifida

Spina bifida is characterised by the incomplete closure of the neural arches of the sacral and/or lumbar vertebrae as a result of the failure of the caudal neuropore to close (Box 2.17, Figures 2.14–2.16). This condition is classified as a neural tube defect and is linked to abnormal spinal cord development. It may be asymptomatic, but it can also cause severe complications. Its aetiology is multifactorial. The main environmental factor linked to the development of spina bifida is insufficient maternal intake of folic acid during the preconception and

Box 2.17 Skeletal manifestation of spina bifida

- incomplete closure of vertebral neural arches
- partial (affecting one or few sacral vertebrae) or complete (affecting all sacral vertebrae)
- symmetric or asymmetric
- two degrees of severity:
  - spina bifida occulta
    - incompletely fused posterior neural arches
    - meningeal and/or neural tissues covered by skin, and hypostotic area protected by fibrous tissue
    - linked to other disorders, e.g. hydrocephalus, clubfoot deformity, cardiac defects; alternatively, it may be asymptomatic or lead to gradual nervous system deterioration
  - spina bifida cystica
    - more severe
    - exposed meninges and/or neural tissue (meningocele if only the meninges herniate, myelomeningocele if neural tissue also herniates, myelocele if skin and meninges fail to close at the defect, in which case infection is lethal)
    - linked to other disorders, e.g. hemivertebrae, block vertebra

(Data from Aufderheide and Rodríguez-Martín 1998; Barnes 1994; Graham and Parsch 2009; Kumar and Tubbs 2011)

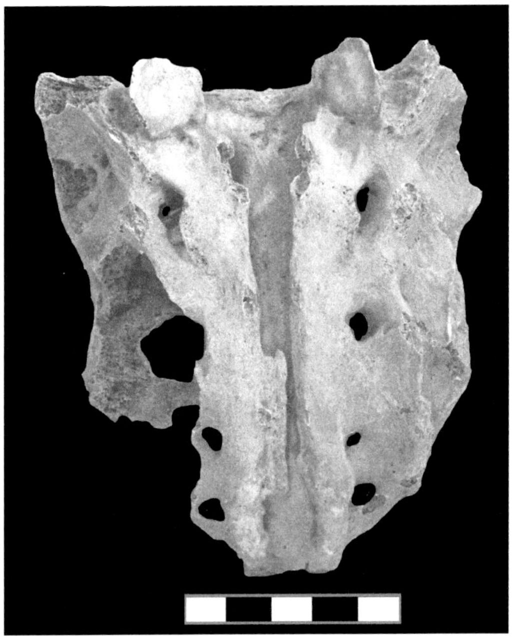

Figure 2.14 Complete sacral spina bifida. Note that all sacral vertebrae show incomplete closure of the neural arches, though in S3 and S4 there is partial closure. (Diever, Reformed Church graveyard, Collection NAD Nuis inv. Nr. D 2019-III.468; photo by Efthymia Nikita, with permission from the Noordelijk Archeologisch Depot)

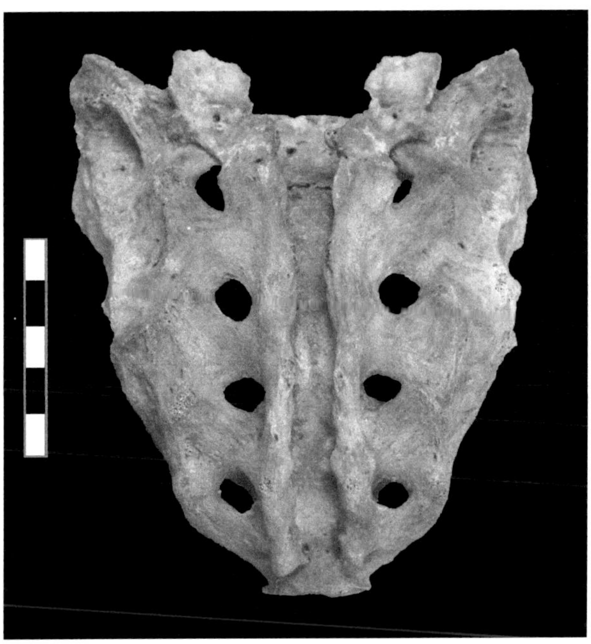

Figure 2.15 Complete sacral spina bifida, whereby all sacral vertebrae show incomplete closure of the neural arches. (Male, Young adult, Diever, Reformed Church graveyard, Collection NAD Nuis inv. Nr. D 2019-III.471; photo by Efthymia Nikita, with permission from the Noordelijk Archeologisch Depot)

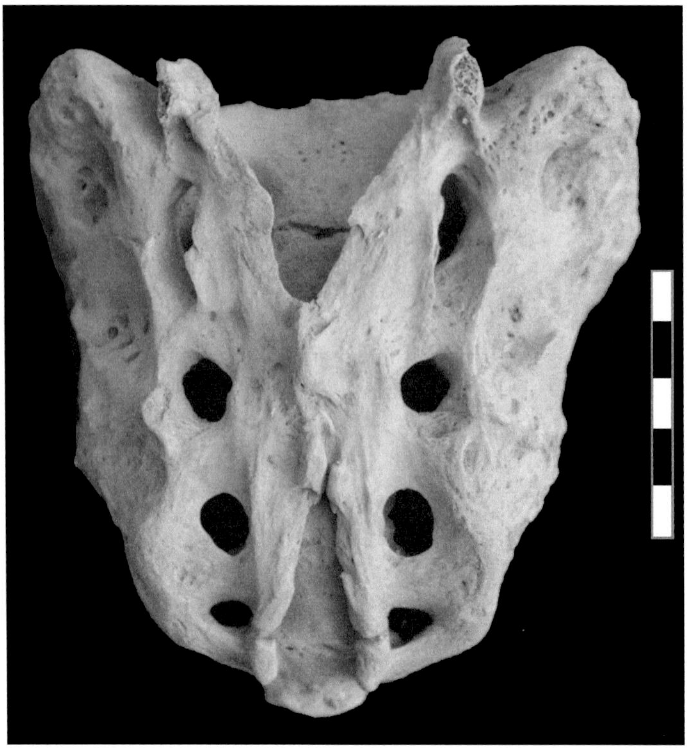

Figure 2.16 Partial sacral spina bifida, where the neural arches of S2 and S3 have closed. (Sbide, Roman/Byzantine; photo by Efthymia Nikita, with the kind permission of Dr. Ahmet Ihsan Aytek, Burdur Mehmet Akif Ersoy University)

periconception periods. Folic acid, also known as vitamin B9, can be found in various foods. Thus, folate deficiency is often the result of an overall inadequate diet rather than the insufficient consumption of specific foods.

Thorax

Selected developmental anomalies that may be found in the ribs are listed in Box 2.18, while anomalies affecting the sternum are given in Box 2.19.

Box 2.18 Developmental anomalies of the ribs

- supernumerary ribs
  - associated with vertebral border shifting
  - bilateral or unilateral
  - intrathoracic ribs

- emergence from inferior-posterior part of parent rib
- growing parallel to parent rib or projecting inferiorly
- mostly unilateral

- rib hypoplasia/aplasia
  - associated with vertebral border shifting
  - mostly in ribs 1 and 12
- bifurcation (Figure 2.17)
  - single head but body forks at sternal end
  - mostly on right side
  - mostly on ribs 3, 4, and 5
- rib fusion (Figures 2.18 and 2.19)
- abnormal width (hyperplasia)
- bridging
  - osseous bridge between adjacent ribs

(Data from Barnes 1994, 2012a, Lewis 2017)

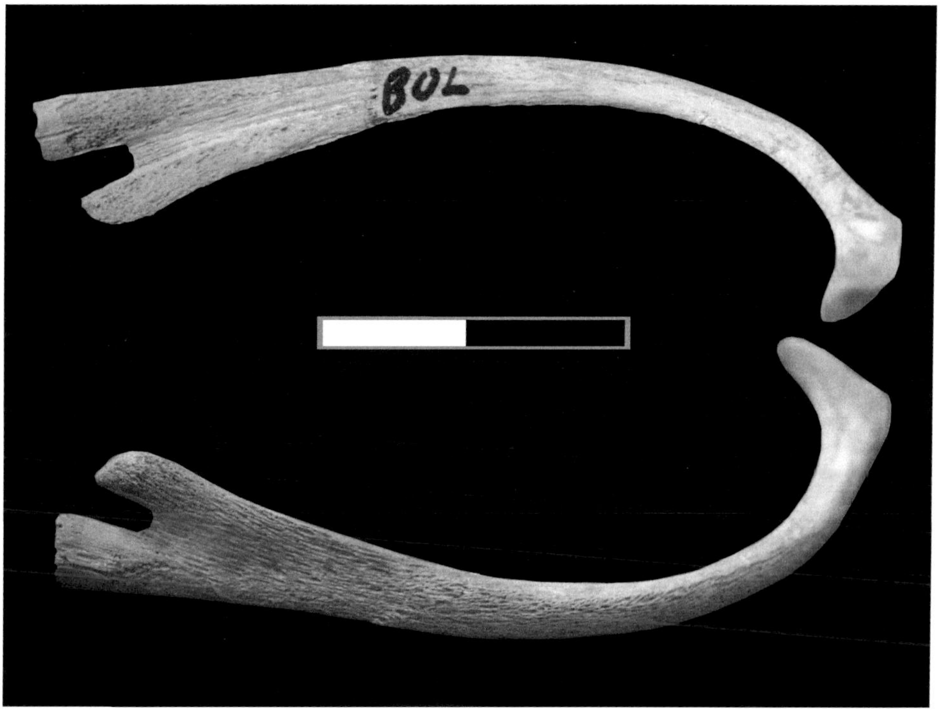

Figure 2.17 Bifurcated rib. Note that there is a single head but the body forks at the sternal end. (Foetus, Parish Church of St Mary and St Lawrence, Bolsover, 13th c CE, BOL 014; photos by Efthymia Nikita; copyright: Human Skeletal Collection, University of Sheffield)

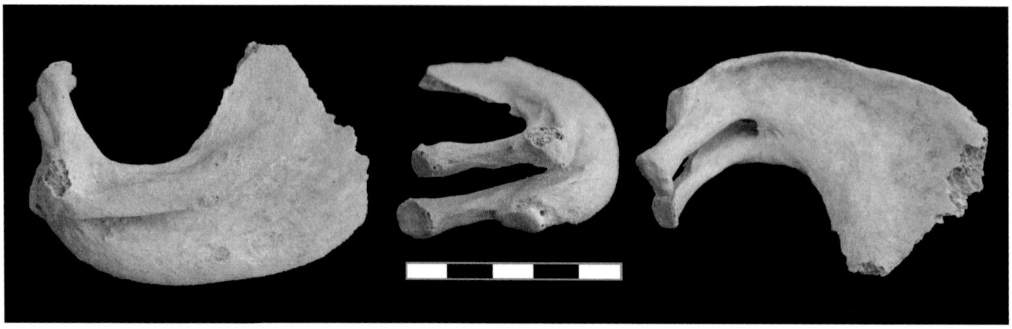

Figure 2.18 Fused ribs. Note that the head and neck are distinct, while the shafts are fused. (Philadelphia, Roman/Byzantine; photos by Efthymia Nikita, with the kind permission of Dr. Ahmet Ihsan Aytek, Burdur Mehmet Akif Ersoy University)

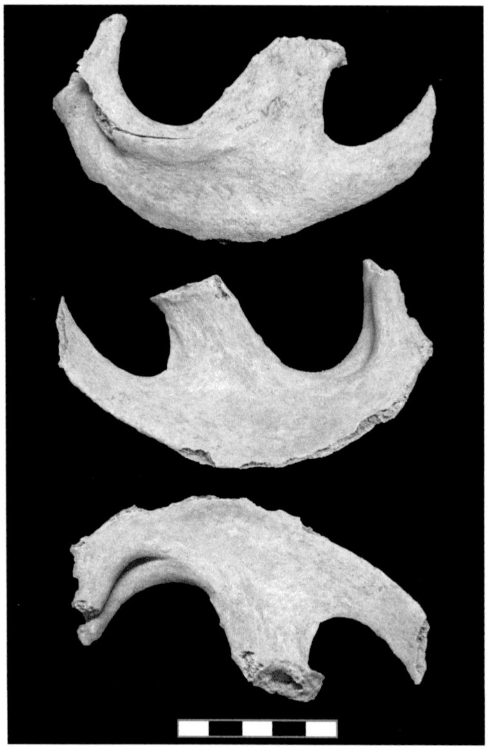

Figure 2.19 Fused first and second ribs. (Probable male, Adult, Aduard, Cistersian Monastery of St. Bernardus, Collection NAD Nuis inv. Nr. G 2013-IV.121; photos by Efthymia Nikita, with permission from the Noordelijk Archeologisch Depot)

Box 2.19 Developmental anomalies of the sternum

- bifid sternum
- cleft, fissure, or aperture in manubrium
- cleft, fissure, or aperture in corpus sterni
- abnormally wide or narrow sternebrae
- bilateral or unilateral hypoplasia or aplasia of sternebrae
- fused manubrium-corpus sterni
- misplaced manubrium-corpus sterni joint
- fused xiphoid process-corpus sterni
- sternal hyperplasia → overelongated corpus sterni or xiphoid process

(Data from Barnes 1994, 2012a)

Long bones

Developmental anomalies that may be encountered in the long bones are listed in Box 2.20.

Box 2.20 Developmental anomalies of the long bones

- asymmetric limb lengths
- abnormal shortening of entire limb (micromelia)
- abnormal shortening of proximal limb (humerus, femur) (rhizomelia)
- abnormal shortening of middle limb (radius-ulna, tibia-fibula) (mesomelia)
- complete absence of limb (amelia)
- absence of parts of a limb (meromelia)
- radial (preaxial) or ulnar (postaxial) side agenesis (hemimelia)
- limb underdevelopment (hypoplasia)
- underdeveloped hands or feet connected to trunk via small and irregular bones (phocomelia)
- proximal radius and ulna congenital synostosis:
  - unilateral or bilateral
  - different aetiologies:
    - segmentation defect (Type I)
    - radial head congenital dislocation (Type II)
- tibia and fibula congenital synostosis
- other long bones congenitally fused (e.g. humerus-ulna or humerus-radius)

(Data from Antón and Polidoro 2000; Barnes 2012a; Frantz and O'Rahilly 1961; McIntyre and Benson 2002; Taneja et al. 2021; Waldron 2020)

Box 2.21 Developmental anomalies of the shoulder girdle

- clavicular hypoplasia or aplasia
    - unilateral or bilateral
    - often linked to cleidocranial dysostosis
    - may affect acromial, sternal or central sections
- separation of os acromiale from scapular spine
- scapular neck hypoplasia or dysplasia
- Sprengel's deformity
    - elevated, hypoplastic scapula
    - rotated axillary and vertebral borders

(Data from Barnes 2012a)

Shoulder girdle

Box 2.21 lists some of the developmental anomalies found in the clavicle and scapula.

Hand and foot bones

Clubfoot deformity

Clubfoot deformity (Box 2.22, Figure 2.20) is a congenital anomaly with two main types, idiopathic and secondary. Idiopathic clubfoot is associated with genetic predisposition and environmental factors (e.g. maternal smoking during pregnancy). Secondary clubfoot is

Box 2.22 Skeletal manifestation of clubfoot deformity

- many expressions:
    - talipes equinovarus (the most common)
    - talipes equinovalgus
    - talipes varus
    - talipes valgus
    - talipes calcaneus
    - talipes calcaneovalgus
    - talipes planovalgus
- unilateral or bilateral
- distorted shape of affected foot bones
- disuse atrophy of leg bones as a secondary effect

(Data from Aufderheide and Rodríguez-Martín 1998; Barnes 2008)

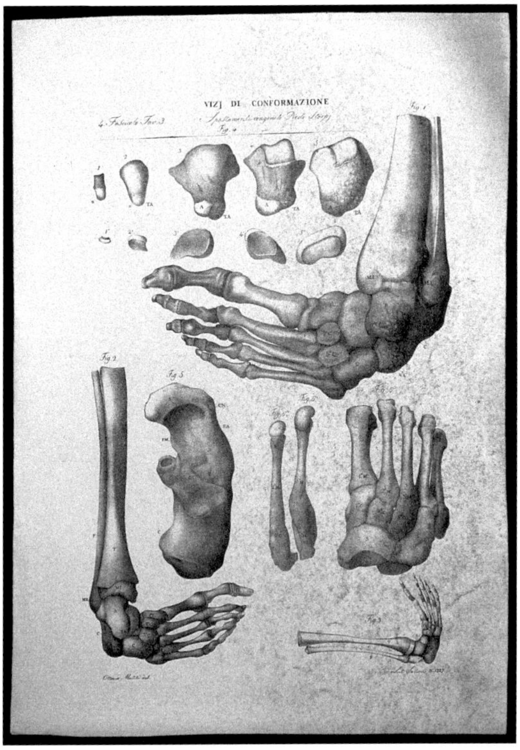

Figure 2.20 Clubfoot deformity and other foot bone deformities. (Lithograph by Salucci after Ottavio Muzzi, c. 1843. Source: Wellcome Collection; licensed under a Public Domain Mark License)

associated with other medical conditions, such as arthrogryposis multiplex congenita. Note that positional clubfoot, which can result from foetal positioning in utero, is not true clubfoot. Rarely, the hand manifests club deformity known as talipomanus. Other developmental anomalies found in the hand and foot bones are given in Box 2.23.

Box 2.23 Other developmental anomalies of the hand and foot bones

- aplasia, hypoplasia, or hyperplasia of hand/foot bones
- partial or complete union between digits (syndactyly)
- shortened digits (brachydactyly)
- agenesis of all or part of the digital ray (ectrodactyly)
- extra digits (polydactyly)
    - expression ranging from bifurcation and duplication of metacarpal or phalangeal bones to duplication of entire digit
    - mostly in medial or lateral digit (but may affect central digits)

- unification (coalition) between carpals or tarsals, carpals-metacarpals, tarsals-metatarsals, metatarsals-phalanges, metacarpals-phalanges, manual or pedal phalanges
  - bilateral or unilateral
  - bones may be united with bony bridges (osseous coalition), fibrous tissue, cartilage, or combination of both (non-osseous coalition); in dry bone non-osseous coalition appears as matching lytic-like lesions between the two bones
- bipartite carpals or tarsals
  - bipartite bone segments held together by cartilage, fibrous tissue, or a combination of both
  - partial or complete expressions
- separate marginal elements
  - may fuse with parent bone or form separate ossicles (e.g. os naviculare, os trigonum)
- congenital absence of joint between phalanges within a digit (symphalangism)
- supernumerary hand or foot bones (independent ossicles or attached to regular elements)

(Data from Anderson 1987; Barnes 1994, 2012a; Case and Burnett 2012; Meltzer 1987; O'Rahilly 1953; Silva 2011; Solomon et al. 2003; Venning 1956)

Multiple anatomical areas

Occipitalisation of the atlas

Occipitalisation of the atlas (or atlanto-occipital assimilation) is the fusion of the atlas with the occipital bone when the fourth occipital sclerotome and the first cervical sclerotome fail to segment in the developing embryo (Box 2.24, Figure 2.21). The fusion may be partial or complete. While atlas occipitalisation can be asymptomatic in some individuals, it often results in various symptoms, such as head, neck, and upper limb pain, sensory disturbances, muscle weakness, restricted head and neck mobility, and torticollis. Furthermore, complete fusion may cause vertebral artery compression, which can result in various symptoms due to diminished cerebral blood flow.

Box 2.24 Skeletal manifestation of occipitalisation of the atlas

- fusion of atlas with occipital bone around foramen magnum
- partial or complete
- unilateral or bilateral
- premature degeneration of atlantoaxial joint

(Data from Al-Motabagani and Surendra 2006; Gholve et al. 2007; Lewis 2017)

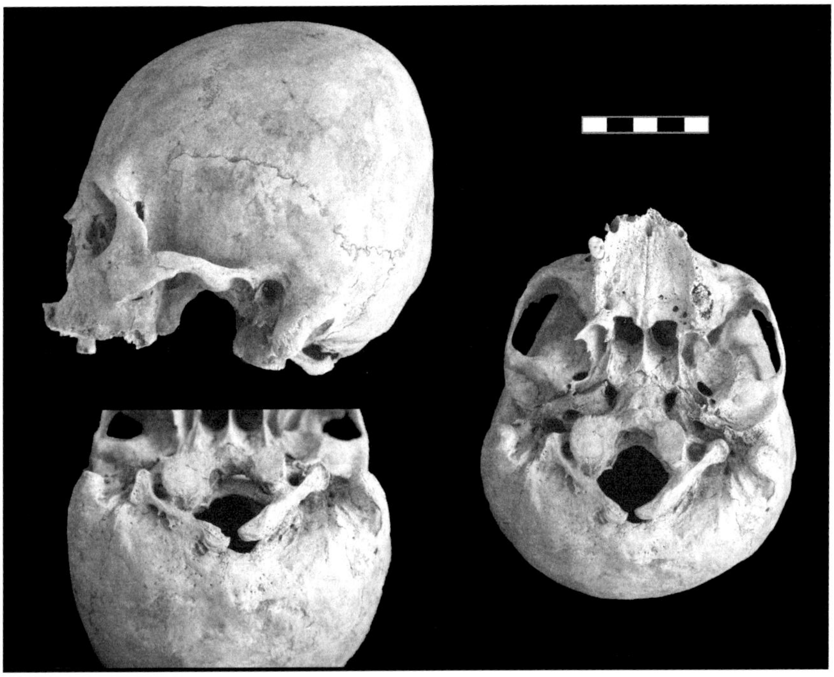

Figure 2.21 Occipitalisation of the atlas; the atlas is fused with the occipital bone, and there is no posterior midline fusion of its two hemiarches. The skull is brachycephalic, but the coronal and lambdoid sutures are still open, so this cranial shape anomaly cannot be associated with craniosynostosis. (Alanya Castle, Ottoman; photos by Efthymia Nikita, with the kind permission of Dr. Ahmet Ihsan Aytek, Burdur Mehmet Akif Ersoy University)

Developmental dysplasia of the hip

Developmental dysplasia of the hip (DDH) is the abnormal formation of the hip joint and can have different degrees of severity: dysplasia, subluxation, and dislocation (Box 2.25, Figures 2.22–2.26). It arises from genetic predisposition and mechanical stress factors that act before and after birth. Various parameters related to gestation and delivery are important risk factors, and include breech presentation, primiparity, and low amniotic fluid. The risk of

Box 2.25 Skeletal manifestation of developmental dysplasia of the hip*

- false acetabulum formation
- oval or triangular true acetabulum, shallow with porous floor, and cysts along the margin
- false acetabulum superior or postero-superior to true one
- small, flat, or mushroom-shaped femoral head or normally sized but antero-posteriorly oval-shaped head

- short and thin neck; often anteverted
- lesser trochanter mispositioned (superiorly, inferiorly, or laterally); normal-shaped, elongated, or mushroom-shaped
- small greater trochanter
- small intertrochanteric distance
- reduced distal femoral articular surface
- reduced femoral and tibial dimensions (length and diaphyseal circumference)
- valgus knee
- small proximal tibial articular surface
- compensatory external tibial torsion
- wide greater sciatic notch
- more triangular-shaped obturator foramen
- shorter and wider ilium, sloping posteriorly

(Data from Blatt 2015; Dunn 1976; Mitchell and Redfern 2008, 2011)

* Depending on severity, developmental dysplasia of the hip may manifest as acetabular dysplasia, subluxation, or dislocation; acetabular dysplasia and subluxation are less likely to be identified bioarchaeologically; thus, this list includes only cases of dislocation.

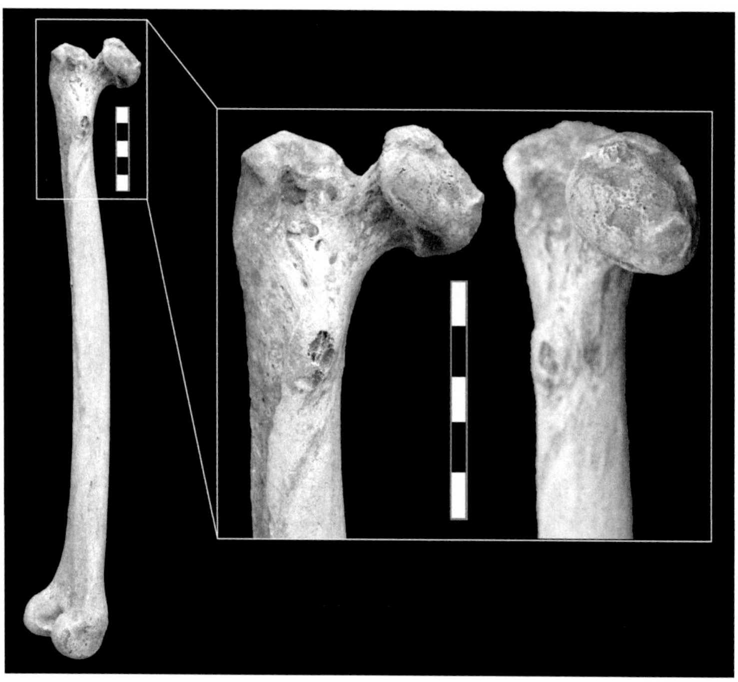

Figure 2.22 Developmental dysplasia of the hip of the most severe form, hip dislocation (see also Figure 2.23). Note the abnormal morphology of the proximal left femur and particularly the deformed head, thinned neck, mispositioned lesser trochanter, and greater trochanter of reduced size. (Samantaş, Byzantine; photos by Efthymia Nikita, with the kind permission of Dr. Ahmet Ihsan Aytek, Burdur Mehmet Akif Ersoy University)

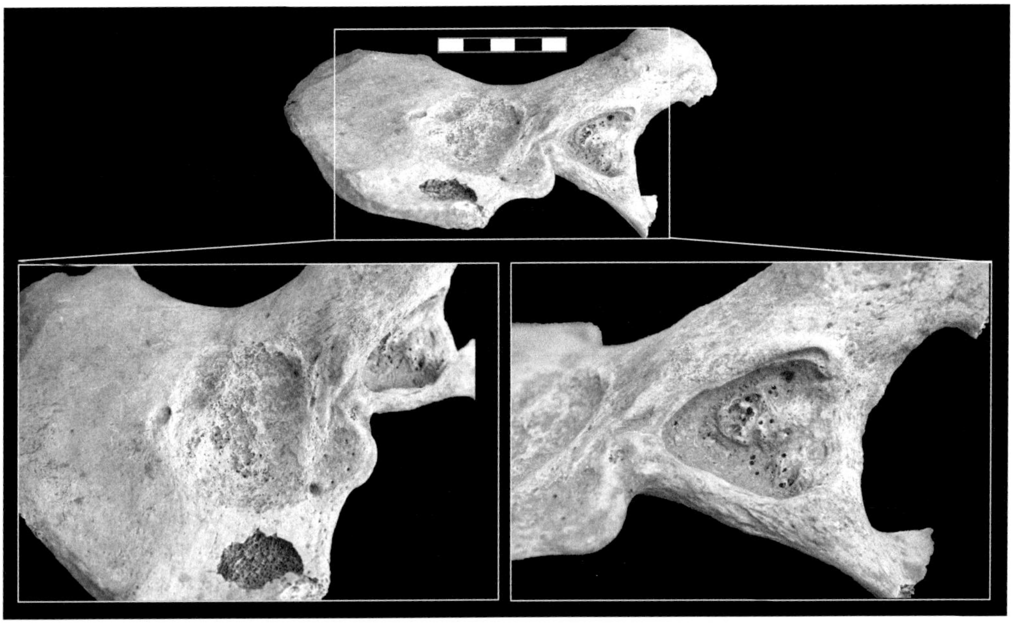

Figure 2.23 Developmental dysplasia of the hip seen in a left os coxa. Note the triangular true acetabulum with porous floor, as well as the false acetabulum superior to the true one. (Same individual as in Figure 2.22; photos by Efthymia Nikita, with the kind permission of Dr. Ahmet Ihsan Aytek, Burdur Mehmet Akif Ersoy University)

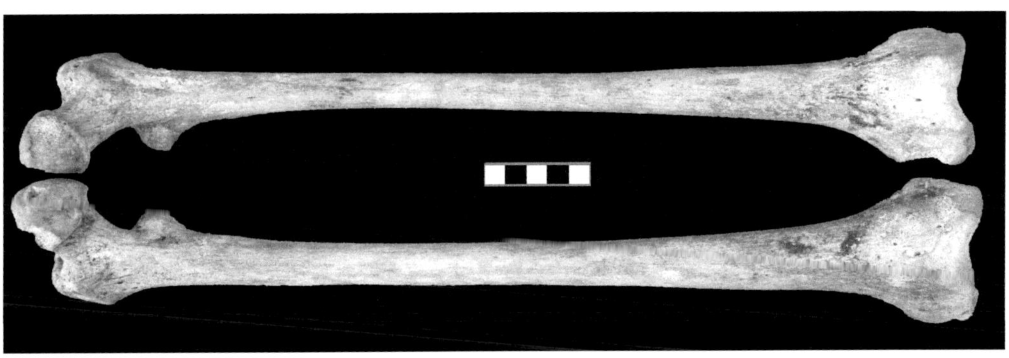

Figure 2.24 Developmental dysplasia of the hip of the most severe form, hip dislocation (see also Figures 2.25 and 2.26). Note the deformed femoral heads and the overall gracility of the bones. (Alkmaar-Grote Kerk, Medieval-Modern, 5099; photos by Efthymia Nikita, from the reference collection of the Cultural Heritage Agency of the Netherlands)

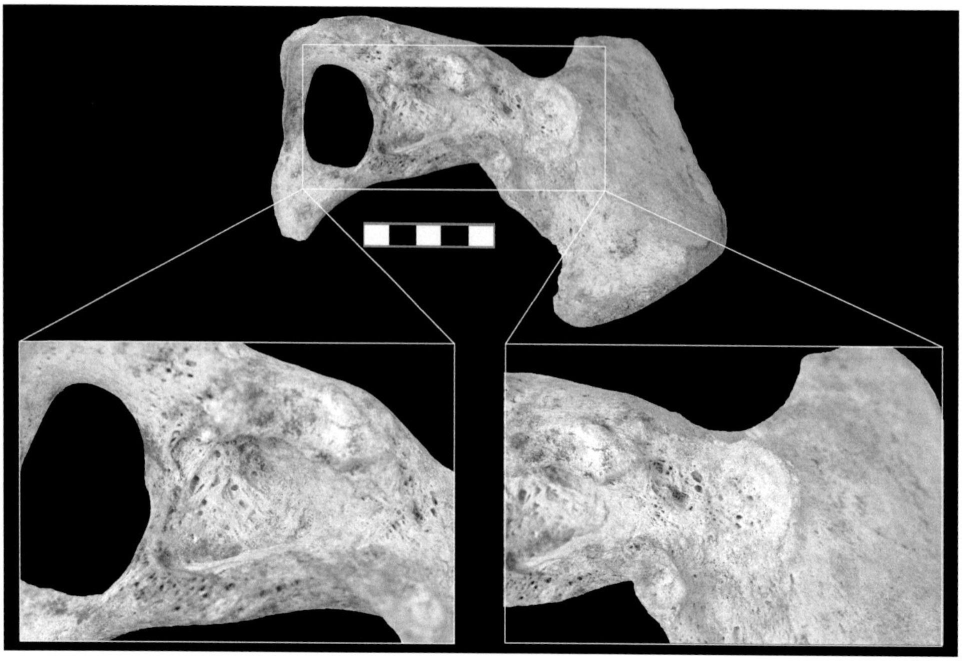

Figure 2.25 Developmental dysplasia of the hip seen in a right os coxa. Note the triangular/oval true acetabulum, and the false acetabulum superior to the true one. (Same individual as in Figure 2.24; photos by Efthymia Nikita, from the reference collection of the Cultural Heritage Agency of the Netherlands)

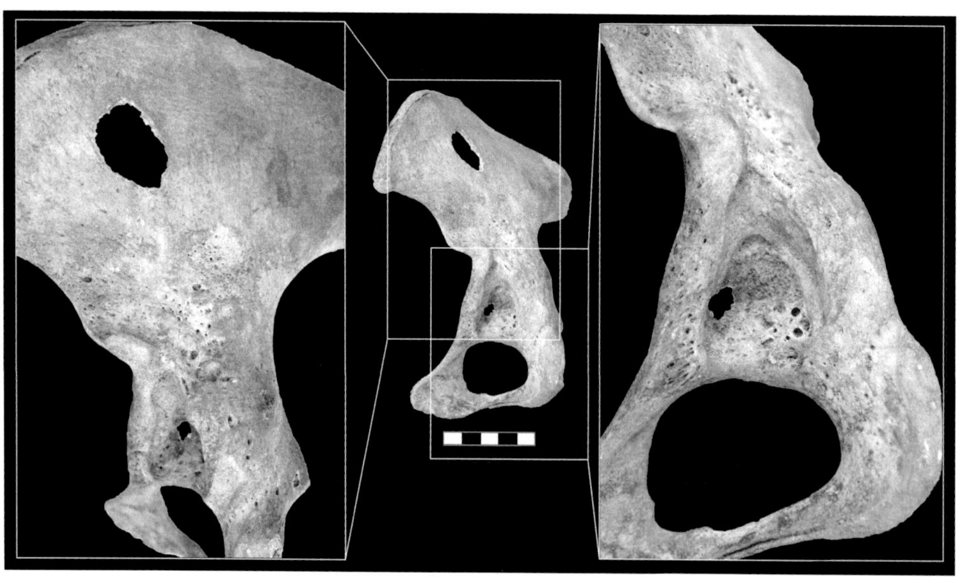

Figure 2.26 Developmental dysplasia of the hip seen in a left os coxa. Note the triangular true acetabulum with porous floor, and the false acetabulum superior to the true one. (Same individual as in Figures 2.24 and 2.25; photos by Efthymia Nikita, from the reference collection of the Cultural Heritage Agency of the Netherlands)

DDH is particularly high when foetal position in utero obstructs the abduction and external rotation of the femur, or when it applies mechanical pressure on the greater trochanter. Additionally, tight swaddling of the infant postnatally, as well as the use of cradleboards, have also been linked to DDH. Furthermore, hormonal influences may play a role in the appearance of DDH, as supported by the condition's higher prevalence in females.

Léri–Weill dyschondrosteosis

Léri–Weill dyschondrosteosis is a mesomelic dysplasia, predominantly linked to mutations in the *SHOX* gene or its enhancers. The condition is inherited as a pseudoautosomal trait, and its severity can vary greatly between individuals (Box 2.26).

Box 2.26 Skeletal manifestation of Léri–Weill dyschondrosteosis

- mesomelia → reduced stature
- Madelung's deformity (Box 2.27)
- forearm shortening more pronounced than lower leg shortening
- high arched palate
- scoliosis

(Data from Lewis 2017; Schiller et al. 2000)

Box 2.27 Madelung's deformity

Madelung's deformity is an abnormality of the wrist and forearm bones, characterised by a shortened and dorso-laterally bowed radius, dorsal dislocation of the shortened ulna at the wrist, an increase in the width of the interosseous space, and secondary deformations of the carpal bones (Figure 2.27). Its aetiology is unclear but genetics play a role. The disorder is not typically identifiable during infancy or early childhood; instead, bone deformities progressively develop and become distinct by late childhood or adolescence.

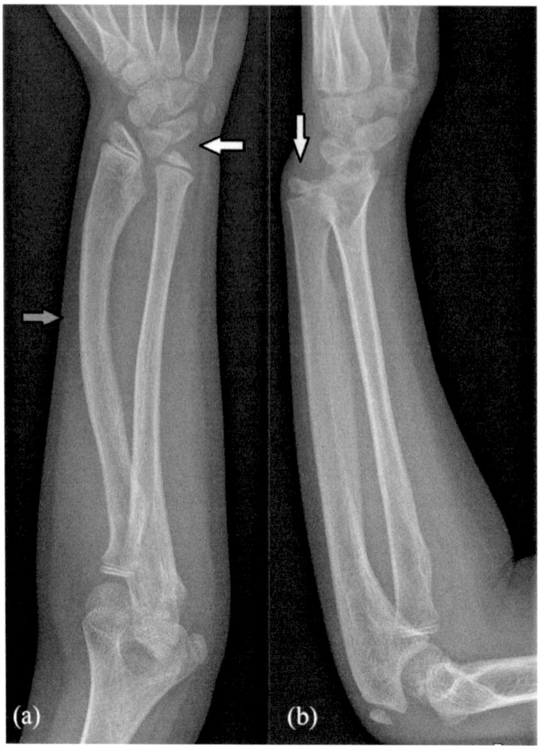

Figure 2.27 Radiographs of the left arm and wrist showing Madelung's deformity in an individual with Leri–Weill dyschondrosteosis. Note the short and bowed radius, dorsal dislocation of the ulna at the wrist, and pyramidalisation of the carpus. (Figure 1 from De Leucio et al. 2020; article licensed under a Creative Commons Attribution 4.0 International License)

Osteopetrosis

Osteopetrosis is a group of rare genetic disorders caused by a failure in osteoclast differentiation or function. This failure results in defective bone remodelling; thus, bones may appear denser and more compact, but have inferior mechanical properties. There are different variants of this condition; some follow an autosomal recessive inheritance pattern, while others are autosomal dominant, with the latter generally showing more benign symptoms compared to the former (Figures 2.28–2.31).

Achondroplasia

Achondroplasia is attributed to a mutation in the fibroblast growth factor receptor 3 (FGFR3) gene. While it can be inherited, most cases arise from a spontaneous mutation. This condition is a type of dwarfism whereby intramembranous ossification is normal, but endochondral ossification is impaired (Figures 2.32 and 2.33). Most individuals with achondroplasia have a normal or near-normal life span. However, individuals who inherit the homozygous genotype for achondroplasia die in utero or shortly after birth.

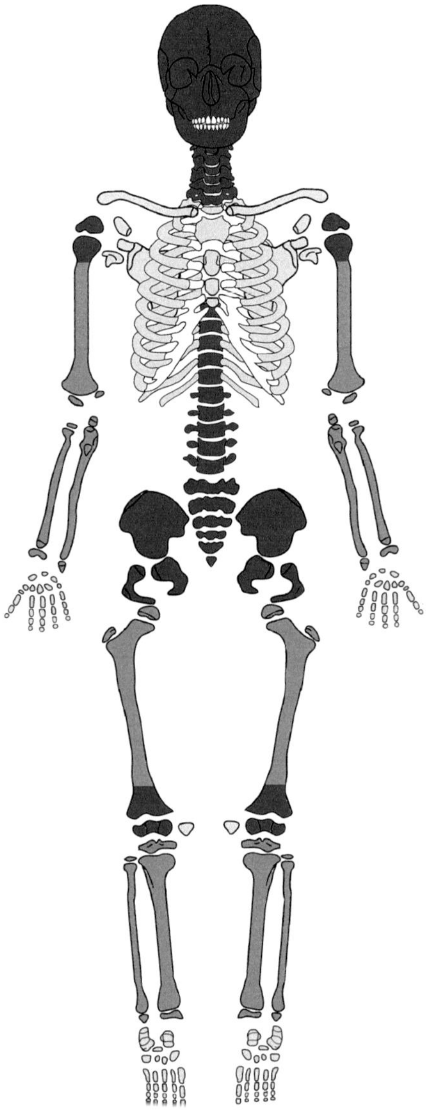

- equally common in males and females

General

- develops in late childhood/adolescence
- subnormal to normal life expectancy
- generalised osteosclerosis (increased cortical thickening and bone density)
- heavy bones
- pathological fractures

Skull

- rarely osteomyelitis (particularly mandibular)
- mild osteosclerosis of cranial base
- narrow foramina
- dense facial bones

Vertebrae

- endplate sclerosis
- scoliosis

Pelvic girdle

- osteosclerosis

Arm/leg

- reduced medullary cavity diameter
- flared metaphyses (particularly proximal humerus, distal femur)
- hip osteoarthritis

Figure 2.28 Skeletal manifestation of osteopetrosis – autosomal dominant type. (Data from Beighton and Cremin 1980; Bode and Peters 2002; Loría-Cortés et al. 1977; Waldron 2020)

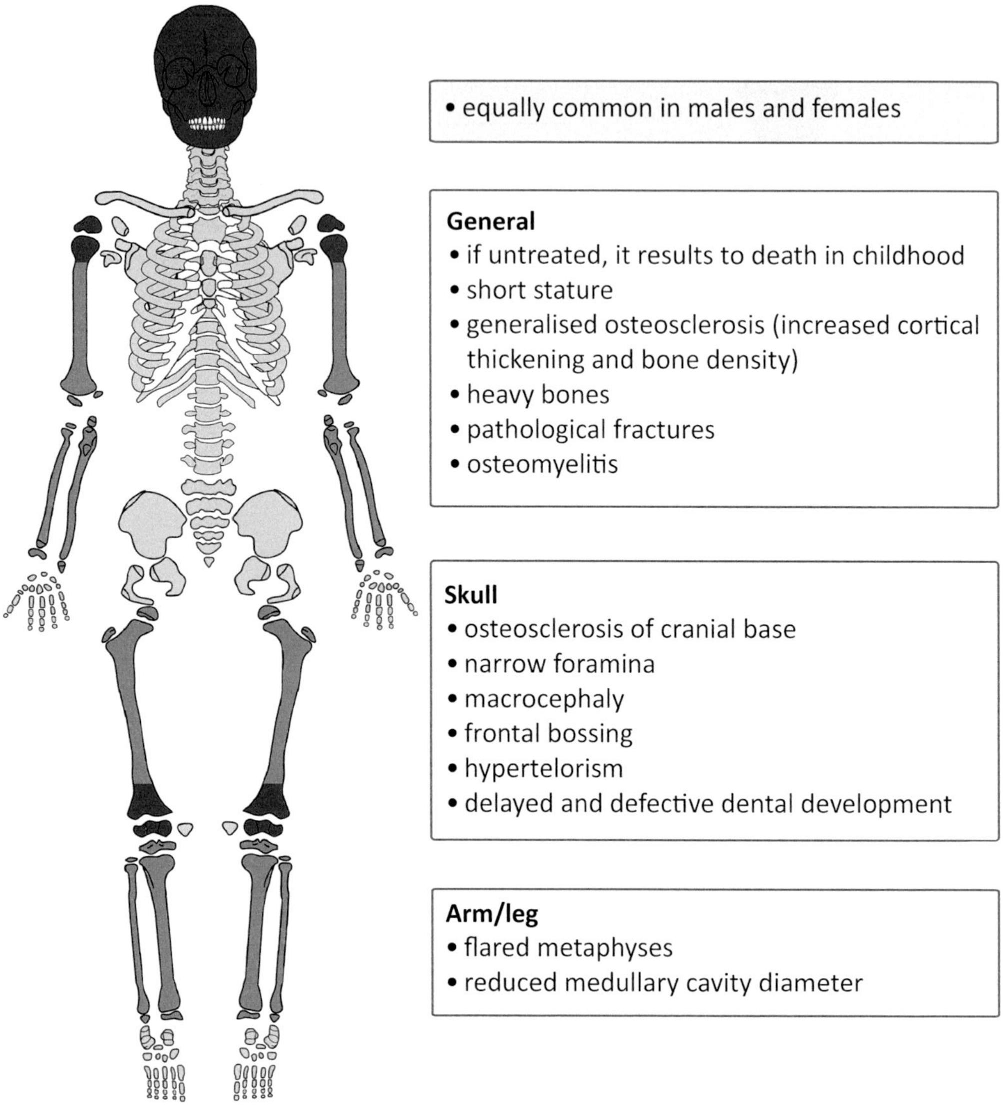

Figure 2.29 Skeletal manifestation of osteopetrosis – autosomal recessive type. (Data from Beighton and Cremin 1980; Bode and Peters 2002; Loría-Cortés et al. 1977; Waldron 2020)

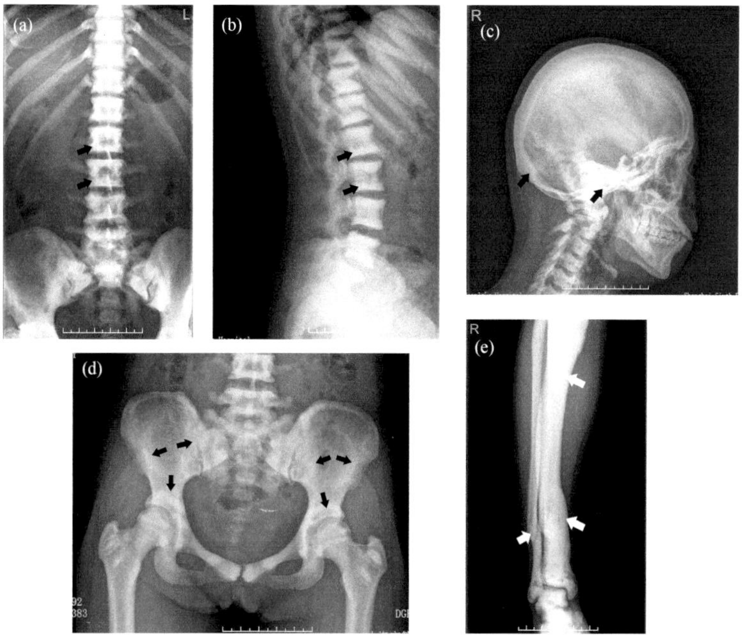

Figure 2.30 Radiographs of individuals affected by osteopetrosis (autosomal dominant type). Note the diffuse osteosclerosis in the vertebrae (a, b), skull base (c), and pelvis (d), as well as the tibial deformity due to multiple fractures (e). (Figure 1 in Wang et al. 2022; article licensed under a Creative Commons Attribution 4.0 International License)

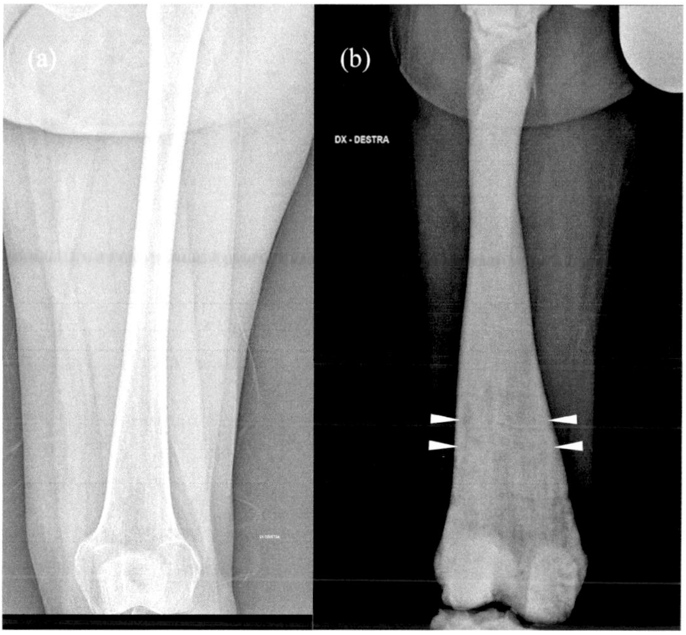

Figure 2.31 Radiograph of the femur of healthy individual (a) and individual affected by osteopetrosis (autosomal recessive type) (b). Note the metaphyseal enlargement of the distal femur, and increased bone radiolucency suggesting increased bone density. (Figure 2 in Spinnato et al. 2022; article licensed under a Creative Commons Attribution 4. 0 International License)

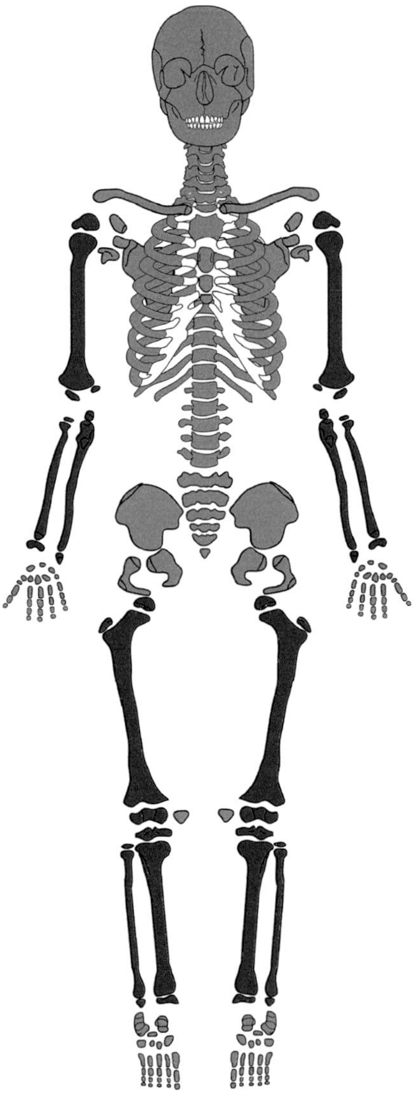

- equally common in males and females

General
- maximum height in adulthood up to 140 cm
- bones with fastest growth and fewer growth plates most severely shortened (disproportionate type of dwarfism)
- early onset osteoarthritis
- osteoporosis

Skull
- undersized base, unaffected vault → large, bulbous, brachycephalic skull
- frontal bossing
- depressed nasal bridge
- midfacial hypoplasia
- prognathism
- small foramen magnum
- hydrocephalus in 30% of cases

Thorax
- shortened and thickened ribs

Figure 2.32 Skeletal manifestation of achondroplasia. (Data from Arita et al. 2012; Aufderheide and Rodríguez-Martín 1998; Lewis 2017, 2019a; Richette et al. 2008; Waldron 2020)

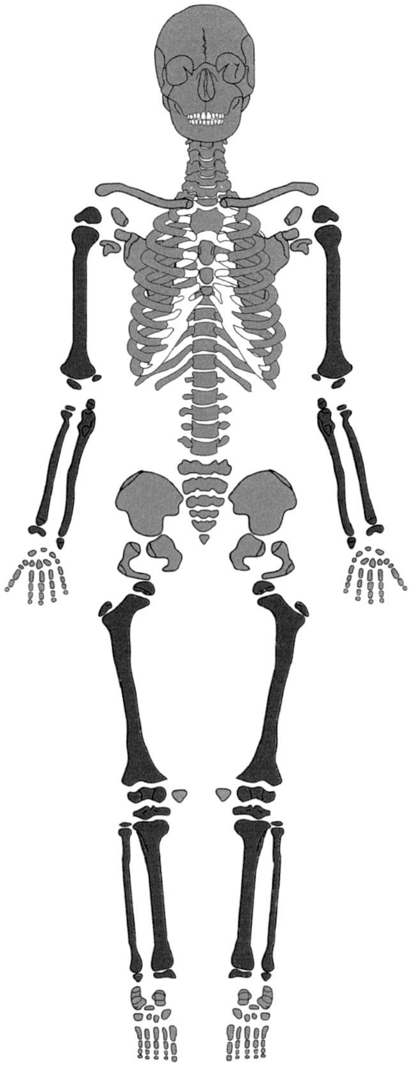

Vertebrae
- short vertebrae
- narrow spinal canal
- lumbar lordosis
- kyphosis

Pelvic girdle
- squared iliac bones
- wide and flaring iliac alae
- narrowed greater sciatic notch
- reduced antero-posterior diameter of pelvic inlet

Hand/foot
- "trident" hand

Arm/leg
- short limbs
- wide epiphyses and metaphyses
- pronounced muscle markings
- coxa vara
- bowing

Figure 2.32 (Continued)

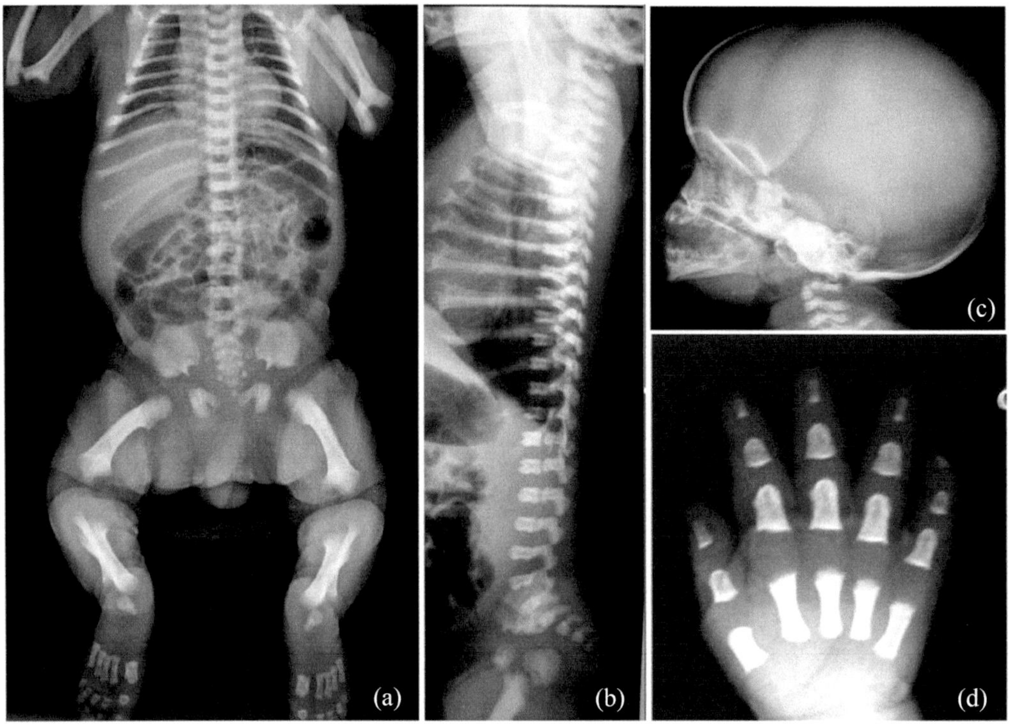

Figure 2.33 Radiographs of newborns with achondroplasia. Note the platyspondyly, squared pelvis, and metaphyseal irregularity of the long bones (a), lumbar lordosis (b), frontal bossing (c), and short hand bones (d). (Figure 1 in Llerena et al. 2022; article licensed under a Creative Commons Attribution 4.0 International License)

Hypochondroplasia

Hypochondroplasia is a type of short-limbed dwarfism associated with a mutation in the fibroblast growth factor receptor 3 (FGFR3) gene. This condition is similar to achondroplasia, but is generally milder. The diagnosis of hypochondroplasia can be challenging, as its phenotypic manifestation is variable (Figures 2.34–2.36).

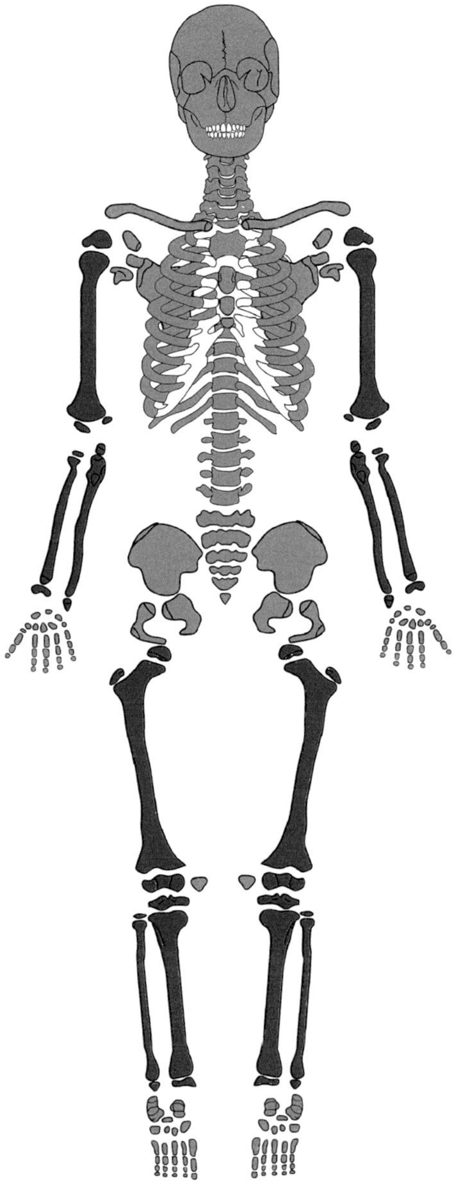

- equally common in males and females

General
- short stature
- stocky skeleton

Skull
- normal to large in size (macrocephaly)

Vertebrae
- platyspondyly
- lumbar lordosis
- short lumbar pedicles

Pelvic girdle
- short and square ilia

Hand/foot
- broad and short tubular bones

Arm/leg
- disproportionately short limbs
- thick diaphyses
- mild metaphyseal flaring
- lower limb long bone bowing
- short femoral neck with coxa vara
- pronounced muscle markings

Figure 2.34 Skeletal manifestation of hypochondroplasia. (Data from Oberklaid et al. 1979; Panda et al. 2014; Sargar et al. 2017; Traversari et al. 2020)

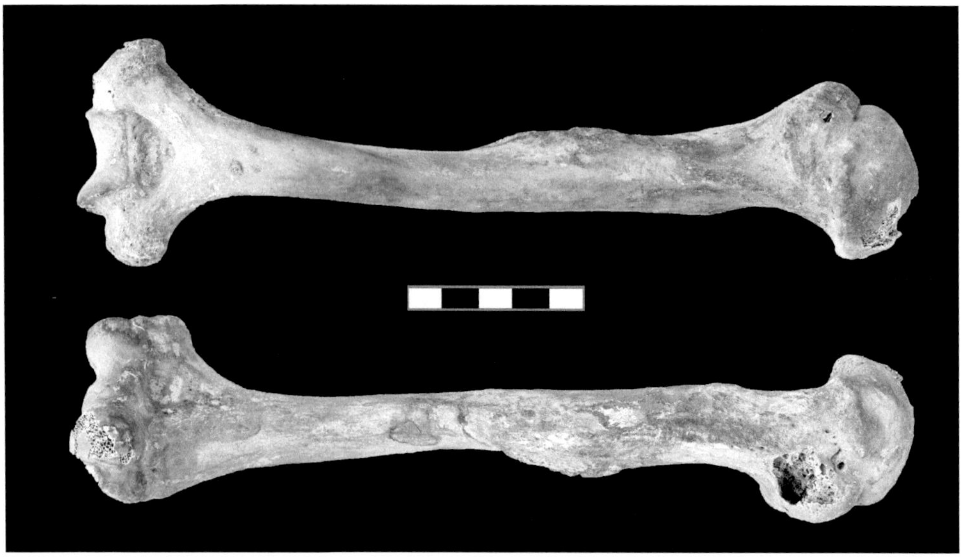

Figure 2.35 Possible hypochondroplasia. Note that the humerus is shorter than normal, with strongly developed deltoid tuberosity and greater tubercle. (5061; photos by Efthymia Nikita, from the reference collection of the Cultural Heritage Agency of the Netherlands)

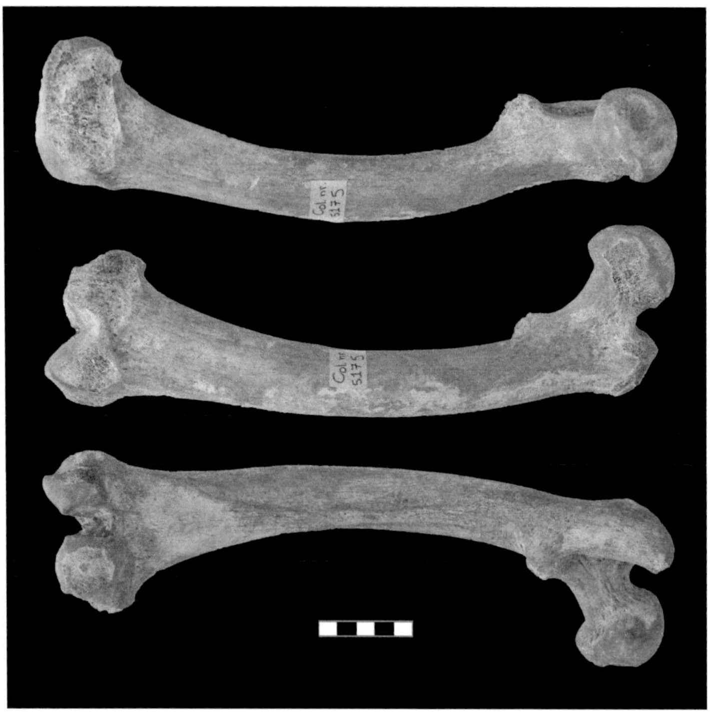

Figure 2.36 Possible hypochondroplasia. Note that the femur is shorter than normal, with pronounced mediolateral and anteroposterior bowing. (5175; photos by Efthymia Nikita, from the reference collection of the Cultural Heritage Agency of the Netherlands)

Turner's syndrome

Turner's syndrome (TS) is a disorder that affects females (Figures 2.37 and 2.38). It is characterised by the complete or partial lack of one of the X chromosomes. Its phenotypic manifestations are highly variable. As a result, the condition may be diagnosed at different ages: prenatally, shortly after birth, or in early childhood when the phenotypic manifestations are pronounced, but in adolescence or early adulthood when the symptoms are milder.

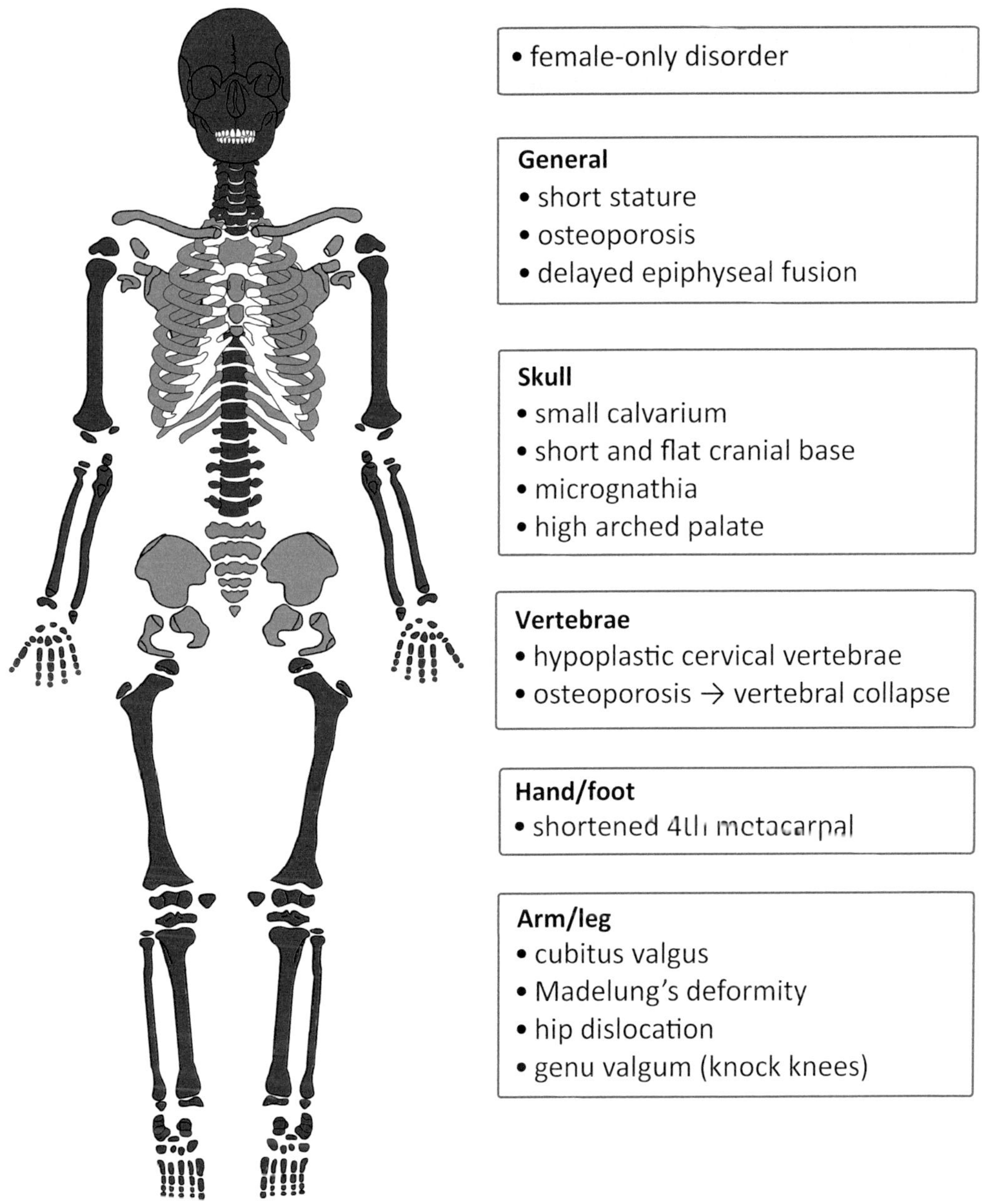

Figure 2.37 Skeletal manifestation of Turner's syndrome. (Data from Doswell et al. 2006; Goldberg et al. 1968; Jensen 1985; Sybert and McCauley 2004; Tauber et al. 2004; Trzcińska et al. 2011)

(a) (b)

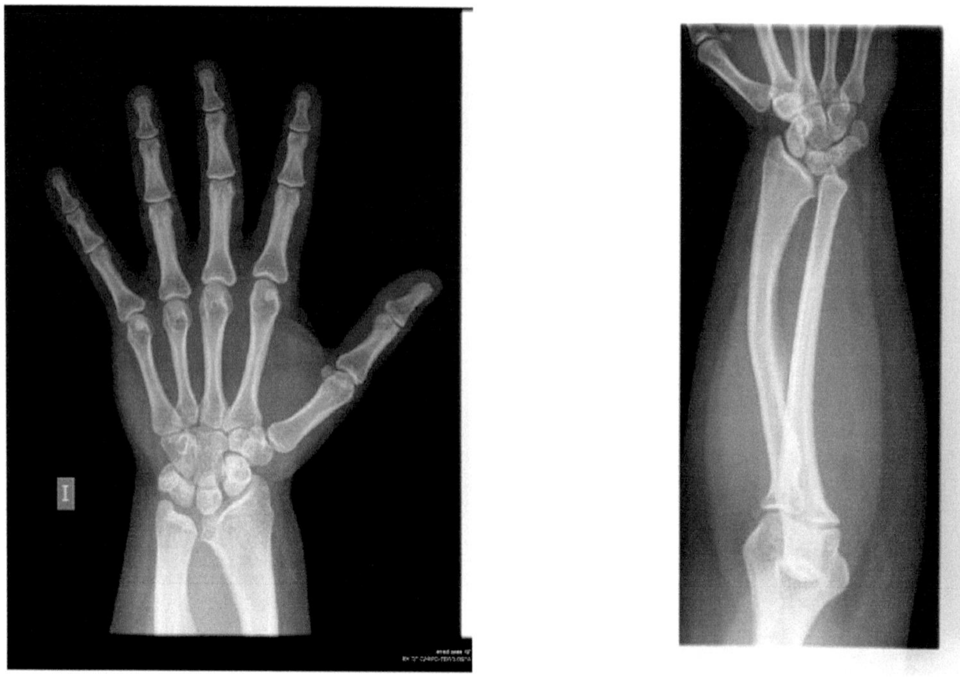

Figure 2.38 Radiograph of the hand and radius/ulna of individual with Turner's syndrome. Note the slight shortening of the IV metacarpal (a) and Madelung's deformity (b). (Figure 7 in Pereda et al. 2013; article licensed under a Creative Commons Attribution 2.0 International License)

Spondyloepiphyseal dysplasia

Spondyloepiphyseal dysplasia (SED) is a rare genetic disorder and has two forms: SED congenita and SED tarda (Figure 2.39). SED congenita is transmitted through an autosomal dominant inheritance pattern. It is associated with short stature, angular deformities of the limbs, and spinal deformities (e.g. scoliosis, lordosis, kyphosis). Additional skeletal manifestations may include genu valgum, coxa vara, clubfoot deformity, osteoarthritis, as well as craniofacial anomalies like cleft palate and hypertelorism. In contrast, SED tarda is mostly inherited in an X-linked recessive pattern and represents a milder form of the disorder. This variant is often unidentifiable at birth, and its manifestations start being obvious around the age of four years, though clinical onset can vary widely. In SED tarda, skeletal involvement is mostly limited to the spine and the larger joints.

Osteogenesis imperfecta

Osteogenesis imperfecta is a genetic disorder associated with defective type I collagen. It is characterised by fragile bones that fracture easily (Figure 2.40). Thus, it is often referred to as "brittle bone disease." There are several types of osteogenesis imperfecta, classified according to their mode of inheritance and clinical manifestations.

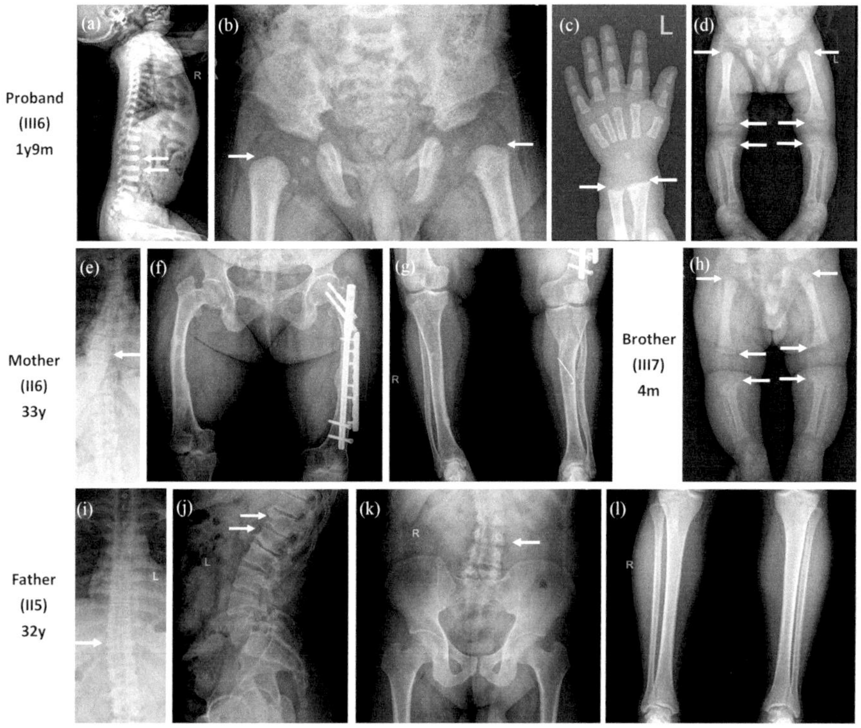

Figure 2.39 Radiographs of individuals with spondyloepiphyseal dysplasia in the same family. Note the flattened and transverse bottles-like vertebral bodies, small femoral heads, widened metaphyses, and scoliosis. (Figure 2 in Ma et al. 2023; article licensed under a Creative Commons Attribution 4.0 International License)

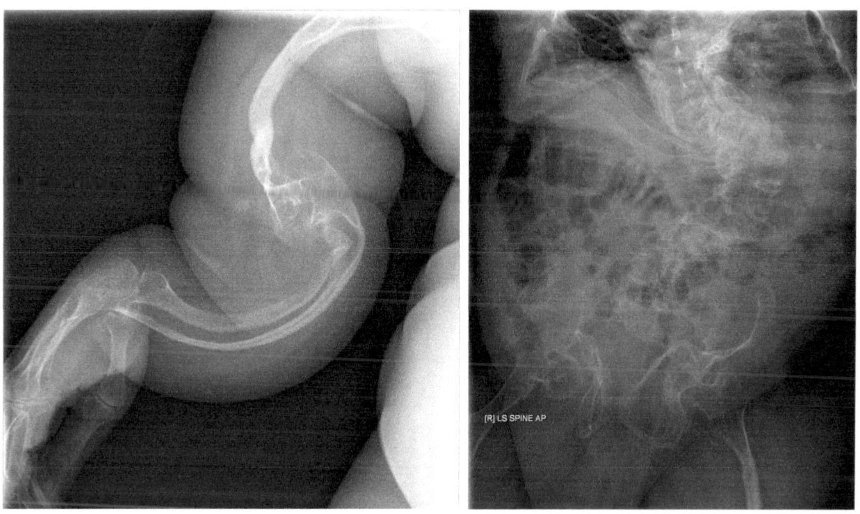

Figure 2.40 Radiographs of a 24-year-old male with osteogenesis imperfecta Type IVB. Note the severe scoliosis as well as extreme bending deformity of the upper limb long bones. (Images uploaded by the patient himself to Wikimedia Commons and attributed to the public domain: https://commons.wikimedia.org/wiki/File:Osteogenesis_imperfecta_X-ray_(clinically_type_IV)_of_spine,_chest,_and_pelvis.png, https://commons.wikimedia.org/wiki/File:Osteogenesis_imperfecta_X-ray_(clinically_type_IV)_of_right_arm.png)

Fibrous dysplasia

Fibrous dysplasia is a non-hereditary genetic disorder; it is caused by a gene mutation that affects the differentiation of osteoblasts. This mutation results in the substitution of normal bone with immature, poorly organised osseous and fibrous tissues. As a result, the bones have inferior mechanical properties and are susceptible to pathological fractures.

The condition may be monostotic or polyostotic (Figure 2.41). Monostotic fibrous dysplasia is more common (70% of documented cases). Polyostotic fibrous dysplasia may appear in isolation or in association with various syndromes. In addition, there is a third subtype called craniofacial fibrous dysplasia, which is characterised by the involvement of multiple bones of the craniofacial skeleton (Figures 2.42 and 2.43); however, it does not qualify as polyostotic fibrous dysplasia since bones beyond the craniofacial region are generally unaffected. Note that cherubism, a rare genetic disorder affecting the maxilla and mandible, is similar to fibrous dysplasia but is distinguished by its autosomal dominant mode of inheritance.

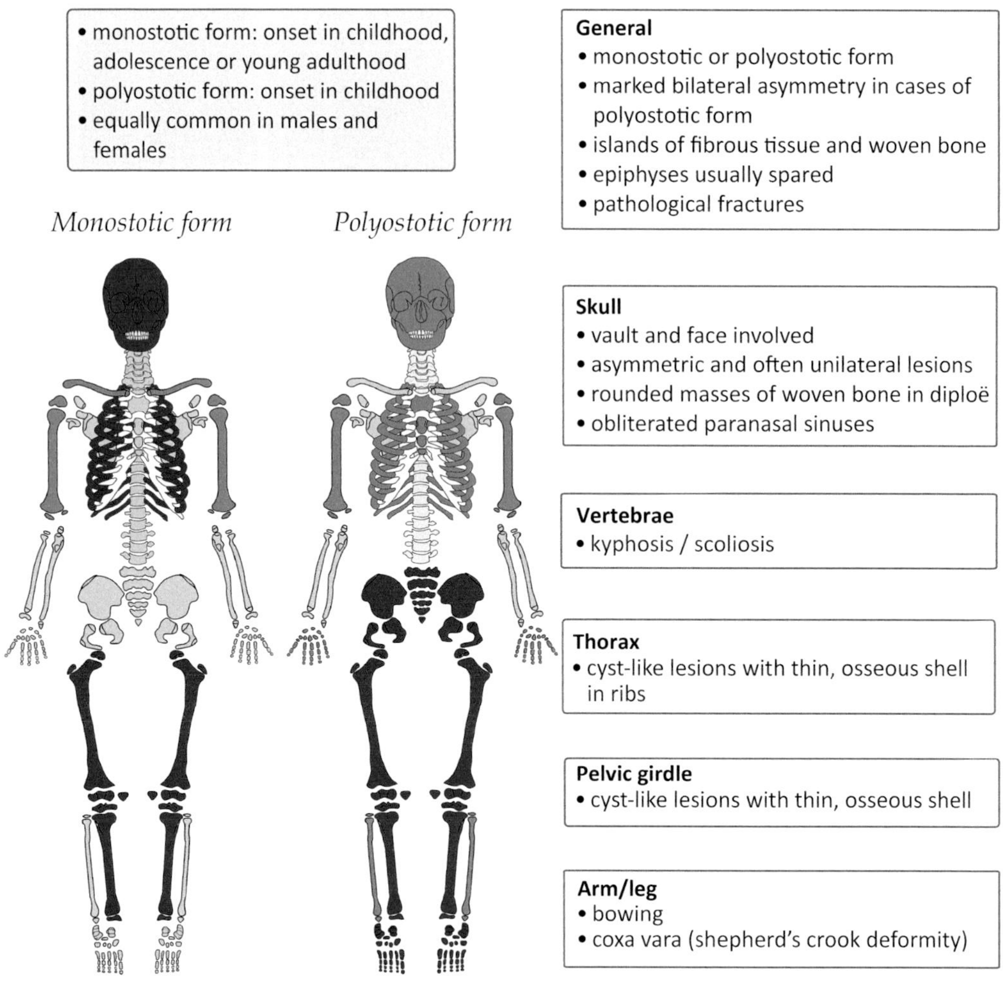

Figure 2.41 Skeletal manifestation of fibrous dysplasia. (Data from Chapurlat and Orcel 2008; DiCaprio and Enneking 2005; Eversole et al. 2008; Marques 2019; Waldron 2020)

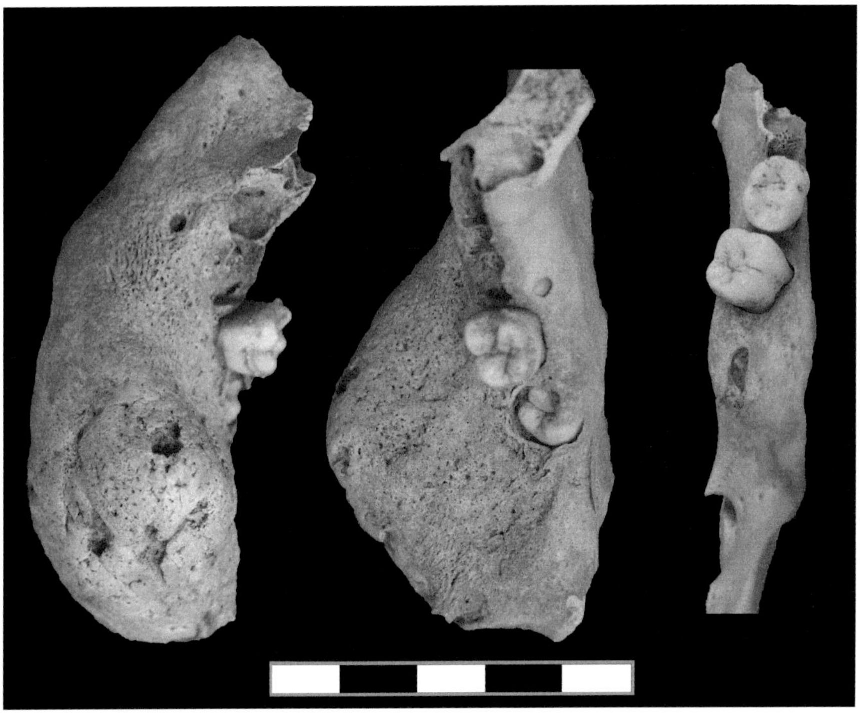

Figure 2.42 Craniofacial fibrous dysplasia. Note the gross and irregular bone expansion on the buccal aspect of the left part of the mandible compared to the normal right side of this element. This case has been published in detail in Craig and Craig (2013). (6–7 years old, Village Farm, Spofforth, North Yorkshire, 7th-9th c. CE, Spofforth 177; photos by Efthymia Nikita; copyright: Human Skeletal Collection, University of Sheffield)

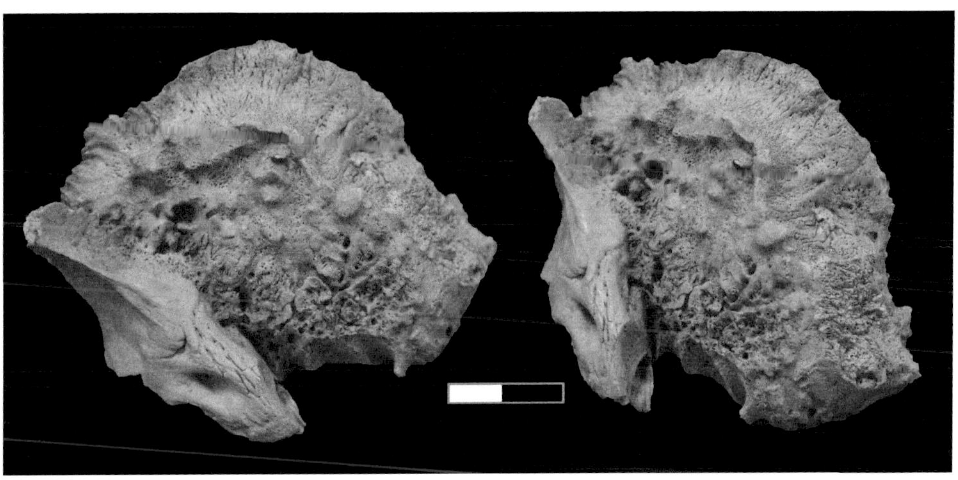

Figure 2.43 Craniofacial fibrous dysplasia. Note the gross bone expansion on the squamous part of the left temporal bone. The right temporal bone of the same individual was unaffected. (Same individual as in Figure 2.42; photos by Efthymia Nikita; copyright: Human Skeletal Collection, University of Sheffield)

Cleidocranial dysostosis

Cleidocranial dysostosis is a rare congenital disorder; it has an autosomal dominant inheritance pattern, and primarily affects intramembranous ossification (Figures 2.44 and 2.45).

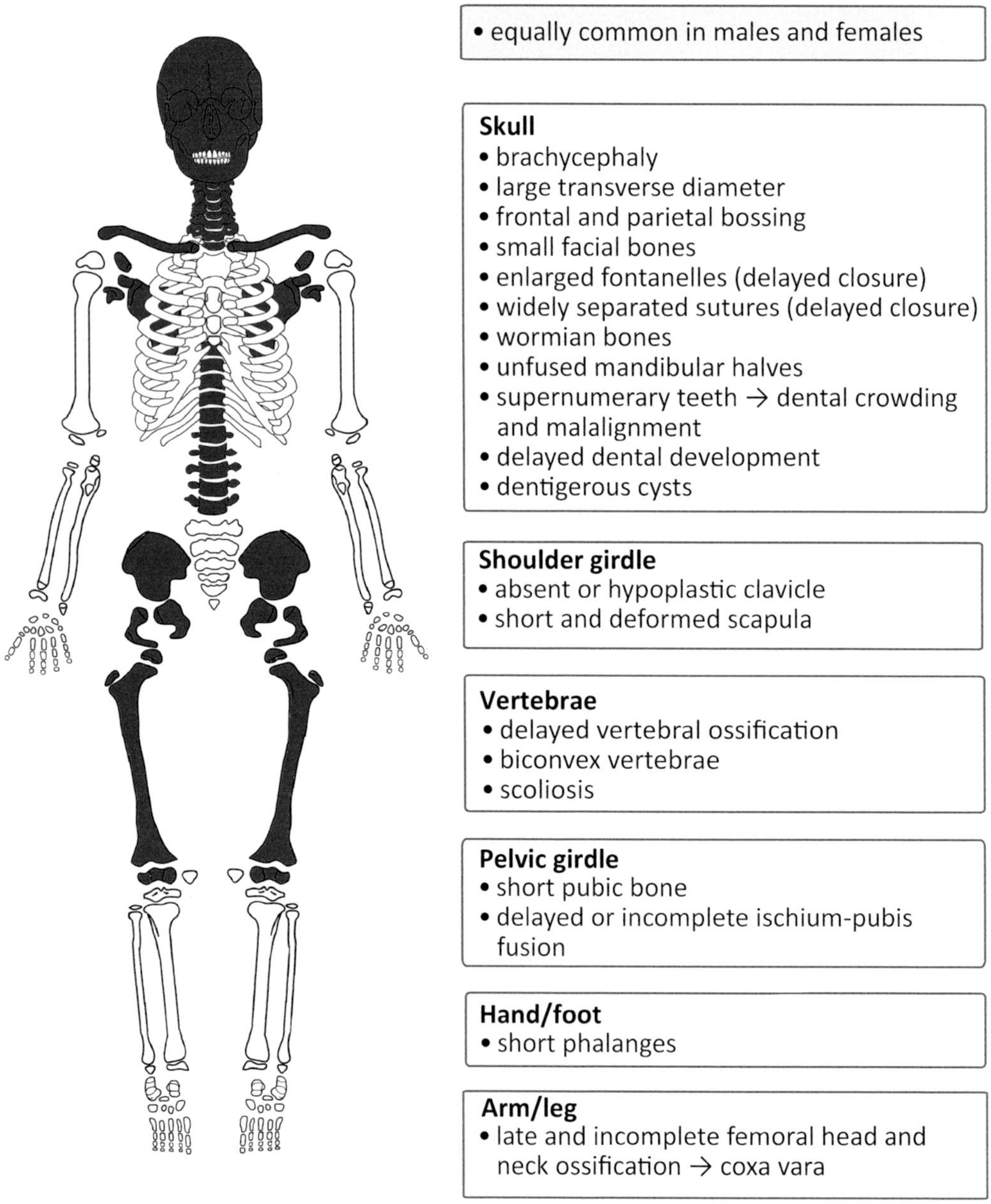

Figure 2.44 Skeletal manifestation of cleidocranial dysostosis. (Data from Lewis 2019a; Mehta and Verma 1992)

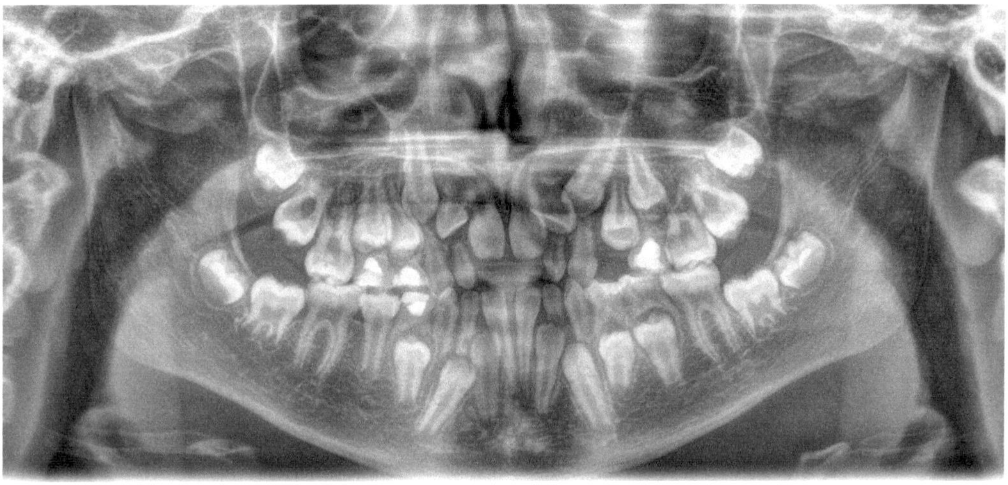

Figure 2.45 Multiple impacted permanent teeth in an 11.4-year-old girl with cleidocranial dysostosis. (Figure 3 in Papadopoulou et al. 2024; article licensed under a Creative Commons Attribution 4.0 International License)

Melorheostosis

Melorheostosis is a rare disorder. In many cases, it is associated with a gene mutation that affects a protein that controls bone cell growth. However, in many other cases, its aetiology is unknown. The condition affects both endochondral and intramembranous ossification, and involves the skeleton and surrounding soft tissues (Figures 2.46 and 2.47).

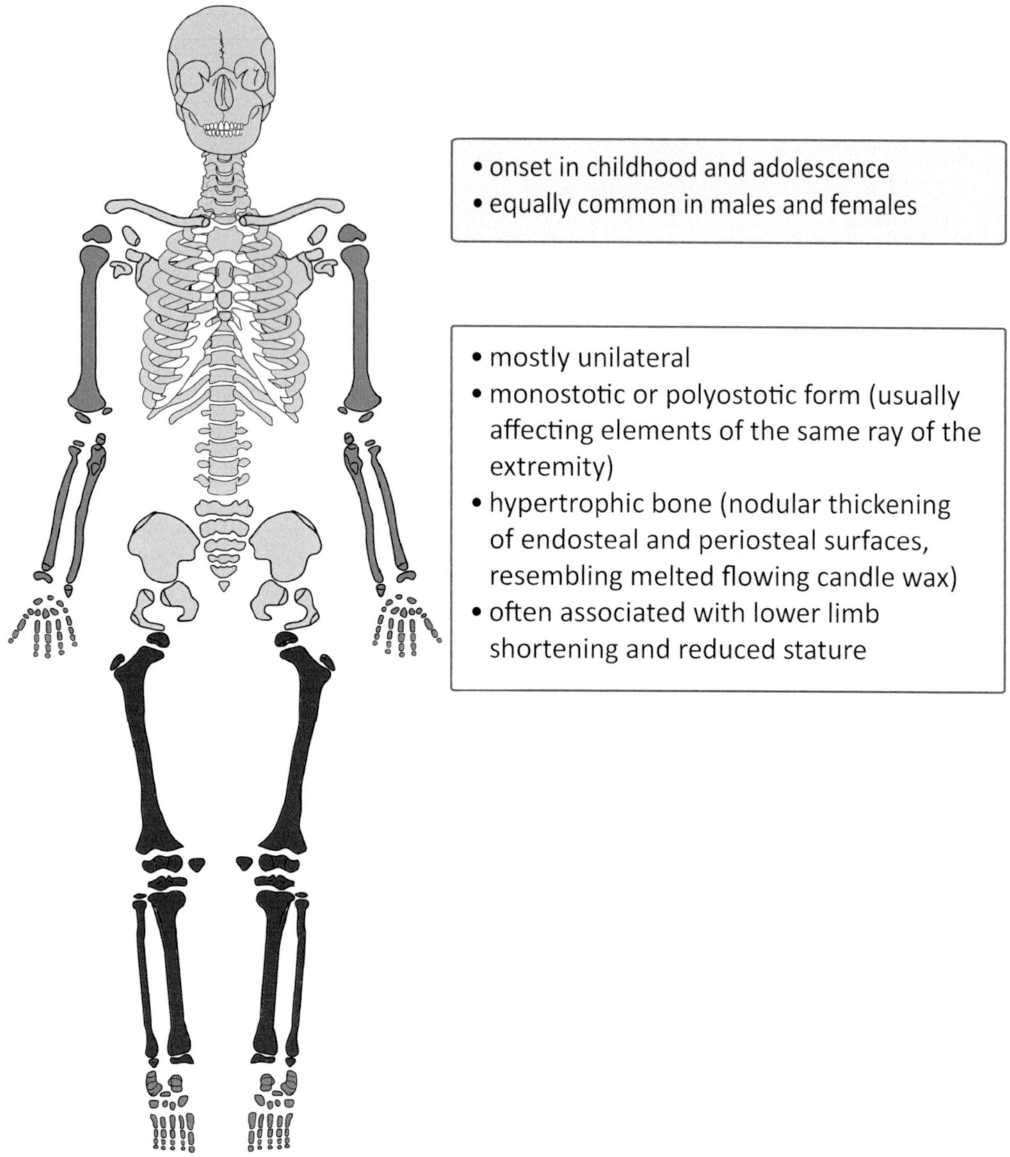

Figure 2.46 Skeletal manifestation of melorheostosis. (Data from Jurenka and Van Allen 1995; Kalbermatten et al. 2001; Lewis 2019b; Mariaud-Schmidt et al. 2002; Suresh et al. 2010; Werner and Scheimer 1987; Younge et al. 1979)

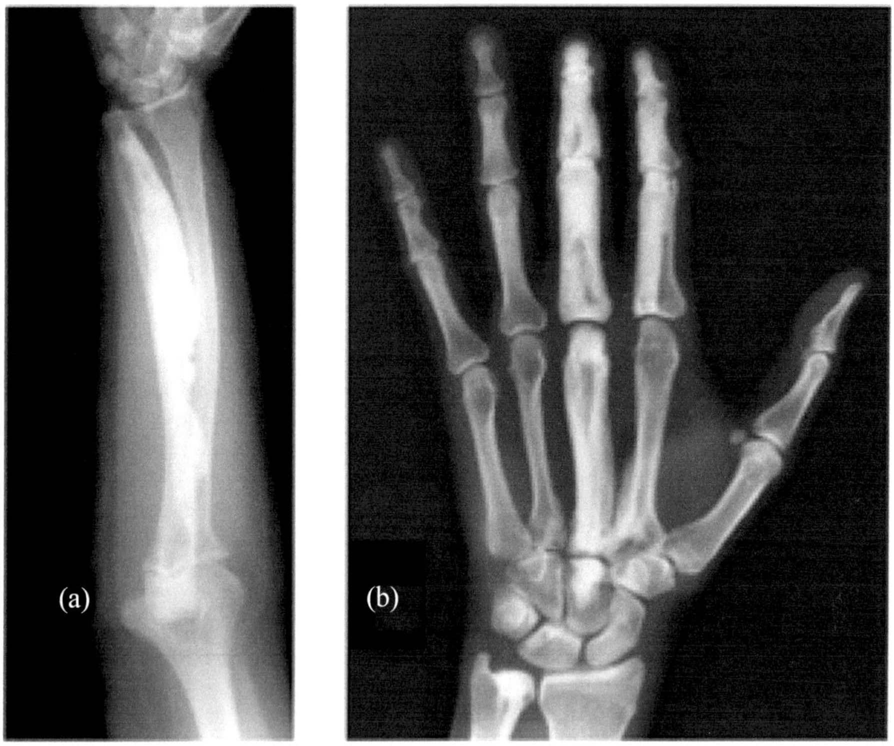

Figure 2.47 Radiographs of upper limbs with typical signs of melorheostosis. Note the "melting candle wax" in the ulna (a) and bone hypertrophy in some of the hand bones (b). (Figure 1 in Wordsworth and Chan 2019; article licensed under a Creative Commons Attribution 4.0 International License)

References and suggested readings

Alghamdi, M.A., Ziermann, J.M., Gregg, L., Diogo, R. (2017). A detailed musculoskeletal study of a fetus with anencephaly and spina bifida (craniorachischisis), and comparison with other cases of human congenital malformations. *Journal of Anatomy* 230:842–858. https://doi.org/10.1111/joa.12601

Al-Mutabagani, M.A., Surendra, M. (2006). Total occipitalization of the atlas. *Anatomical Science International* 81:173–180. https://doi.org/10.1111/j.1447-073X.2006.00129.x

Anderson, T. (1987). A Medieval biparte cuneiform I with attempted unilateral fusion. *Ossa* 13:39–48.

Antón, S.C., Polidoro, G.M. (2000). Prehistoric radio-ulnar synostosis: Implications for function. *International Journal of Osteoarchaeology* 10:189–197. https://doi.org/10.1002/1099-1212(200005/06)10:3%3C189::AID-OA521%3E3.0.CO;2-G

Arita, E.S., Pippa, M.G.B., Marcucci, M., Cardoso, R., Cortes, A.R.G., Watanabe, P.C.A., Oliveira, J.X. (2012). Assessment of osteoporotic alterations in achondroplastic patients: A case series. *Clinical Rheumatology* 32:399–402. https://doi.org/10.1007/s10067-012-2126-x

Aufderheide, A.C., Rodríguez-Martín, C. (1998). *The Cambridge Encyclopedia of Paleopathology*. Cambridge: Cambridge University Press.

Barnes, E. (1994). *Developmental Defects of the Axial Skeleton in Paleopathology*. Denver, CO: University Press of Colorado.

Barnes, E. (2008). Congenital anomalies. In *Advances in Human Paleopathology*, edited by Pinhasi, R., Mays, S., pp. 329–362. Hoboken, NJ: John Wiley & Sons.

Barnes, E. (2012a). *Atlas of Developmental Field Anomalies of the Human Skeleton: A Paleopathology Perspective*. Hoboken, NJ: John Wiley & Sons.

Barnes, E. (2012b). Developmental disorders in the skeleton. In *A Companion to Paleopathology*, edited by Grauer, A.L., pp. 380–400. Hoboken, NJ: Wiley-Blackwell.

Beighton, P., Cremin, B.J. (1980). Osteopetrosis. In *Sclerosing Bone Dysplasias*, edited by Beighton, P., Cremin, B.J., pp. 19–31. Berlin: Springer.

Blatt, S. (2015). To swaddle, or not to swaddle? Paleoepidemiology of developmental dysplasia of the hip and the swaddling dilemma among the indigenous populations of North America. *American Journal of Human Biology* 27:116–128. https://doi.org/10.1002/ajhb.22622

Bode, M., Peters, K.M. (2002). Osteopetrose. In *Knochenkrankheiten*, edited by Peters, K.M., pp. 6–8. Heidelberg: Steinkopff.

Brasili, P., Bonfiglioli, B., Ventrella, A.R. (2002). A case of 'butterfly' vertebra from Sardinia. *International Journal of Osteoarchaeology* 12:415–419. https://doi.org/10.1002/oa.643

Case, D., Burnett, S. (2012). Identification of tarsal coalition and frequency estimates from skeletal samples. *International Journal of Osteoarchaeology* 22:667–684. https://doi.org/10.1002/oa.1228

Chapurlat, R.D., Orcel, P. (2008). Fibrous dysplasia of bone and McCune-Albright syndrome. *Best Practice & Research Clinical Rheumatology* 22:55–69. https://doi.org/10.1016/j.berh.2007.11.004

Clements, W., Mezue, W., Mathew, B. (1995). Os odontoideum – congenital or acquired? That's not the question. *Injury* 26:640–642. https://doi.org/10.1016/0020-1383(95)00123-Q

Cohen, M. Jr. (2000). History, terminology, and classification of craniosynostosis. In *Craniosynostosis: Diagnosis, Evaluation, and Management*, edited by Cohen, M.M. Jr, MacLean, R.E., 2nd edition, pp. 103–111. New York: Oxford University Press.

Craig, E., Craig, G. (2013). The diagnosis and context of a facial deformity from an Anglo-Saxon cemetery at Spofforth, North Yorkshire. *International Journal of Osteoarchaeology* 23:631–639. https://doi.org/10.1002/oa.1288

De la Cruz, A., Linthicum, Jr. F.H., Luxford, W.M. (1985). Congenital atresia of the external auditory canal. *Laryngoscope* 95:421–427.

De Leucio, A., Castelein, S., Bellemans, M., Simoni, P. (2020). Radiotriquetral ligament in Madelung's deformity associated with Leri-Weill's dyschondrosteosis. *Cureus* 12:e7100. https://doi.org/10.7759/cureus.7100

Dewan, M.C., Rattani, A., Mekary, R., Glancz, L.J., Yunusa, I., Baticulon, R.E., Fieggen, G., Wellons III, J.C., Park, K.B., Warf, B.C. (2018). Global hydrocephalus epidemiology and incidence: Systematic review and meta-analysis. *Journal of Neurosurgery* 130:1065–1079. https://doi.org/10.3171/2017.10.JNS17439

DiCaprio, M.R., Enneking, W.F. (2005). Fibrous dysplasia: Pathophysiology, evaluation, and treatment. *The Journal of Bone & Joint Surgery* 87:1848–1864.

Dobbs, M.B., Gurnett, C.A. (2009). Update on clubfoot: Etiology and treatment. *Clinical Orthopaedics and Related Research* 467:1146–1153. https://doi.org/10.1007/s11999-009-0734-9

Doswell, B.H., Visootsak, J., Brady, A.N., Graham Jr, J.M. (2006). Turner syndrome: An update and review for the primary pediatrician. *Clinical Pediatrics* 45:301–313. https://doi.org/10.1177/000992280604500402

Drew, R., Kjellström, A. (2021). Sacralization in the Mary Rose and Kronan assemblages: An inconsistently recorded anomaly. *International Journal of Osteoarchaeology* 31:683–700. https://doi.org/10.1002/oa.2982

Dunn, P.M. (1976). The anatomy and pathology of congenital dislocation of the hip. *Clinical Orthopaedics and Related Research* 119:23–27.

Eversole, L.R., Su, L., El Mofty, S.K. (2008). Benign fibro-osseous lesions of the craniofacial complex: A review. *Head and Neck Pathology* 2:177–202. https://doi.org/10.1007/s12105-008-0057-2

Frantz, C.H., O'Rahilly, R. (1961). Congenital skeletal limb deficiencies. *The Journal of Bone & Joint Surgery* 43:1201–1224.

Gholve, P.A., Hosalkar, H.S., Ricchetti, E.T., Pollock, A.N., Dormans, J.P., Drummond, D.S. (2007). Occipitalization of the atlas in children. Morphologic classification, associations, and clinical relevance. *The Journal of Bone & Joint Surgery* 89:571–578. https://doi.org/10.2106/jbjs.f.00527

Glorieux, F.H., Rauch, F. (2006). Osteogenesis imperfecta. In *Dynamics of Bone and Cartilage Metabolism: Principles and Clinical Applications*, edited by Seibel, M.J., Robins, S.P., Bilezikian, J.P., 2nd edition, pp. 831–842. San Diego: Academic Press.

Goldberg, M.B., Scully, A.L., Solomon, I.L., Steinbach, H.L. (1968). Gonadal dysgenesis in phenotypic female subjects. A review of eighty-seven cases, with cytogenetic studies in fifty-three. *The American Journal of Medicine* 45:529–543. https://doi.org/10.1016/0002-9343(68)90169-1

Graham, H.K., Parsch, K. (2009). Neural tube defects, spina bifida, and spinal dysraphism. In *Children's Orthopaedics and Fractures*, edited by Benson, M., Fixsen, J., Macnicol, M., Parsch, K., 3rd edition, pp. 265–286. London: Springer.

Gresky, J., Dellú, E., Favia, M., Ferorelli, D., Radina, F., Scardapane, A., Petiti, E. (2021). A critical review of the anthropological and paleopathological literature on osteopetrosis as an ancient rare disease (ARD). *International Journal of Paleopathology* 33:280–288. https://doi.org/10.1016/j.ijpp.2021.05.006

Gunderson, C.H., Greenspan, R.H., Glaser, G.H., Lubs, H.A. (1967). The Klippel-Feil syndrome: Genetic and clinical reevaluation of cervical fusion. *Medicine* 46:491–512.

Haque, S., Alam, M.K. (2015). Common dental anomalies in cleft lip and palate patients. *The Malaysian Journal of Medical Sciences* 22:55–60.

Hassan, N.M.M., Dhillon, A., Huang, B. (2016). Cleidocranial dysplasia: Clinical overview and genetic considerations. *Pediatric Dental Journal* 26:45–50. https://doi.org/10.1016/j.pdj.2016.04.001

Irurita, J., Alemán, I., Viciano, J., López-Lázaro, S., Botella, M.C. (2015). Alterations of skull bones found in anencephalic skeletons from an identified osteological collection. Two case reports. *International Journal of Legal Medicine* 129:903–912. https://doi.org/10.1007/s00414-014-1123-9

Jensen, B.L. (1985). Craniofacial morphology in Turner syndrome. *Journal of Craniofacial Genetics and Developmental Biology* 5:327–340.

Jurenka, S.B., Van Allen, M.I. (1995). Mixed sclerosing bone dysplasia, small stature, seizure disorder, and mental retardation: A syndrome? *American Journal of Medical Genetics* 57:6–9. https://doi.org/10.1002/ajmg.1320570103

Kalbermatten, N.T., Vock, P., Rüfenacht, D., Anderson, S.E. (2001). Progressive melorheostosis in the peripheral and axial skeleton with associated vascular malformations: Imaging findings over three decades. *Skeletal Radiology* 30:48–52. https://doi.org/10.1007/s002560000283

Katz, J., Chaushu, G., Rotstein, I. (2001). Stafne's bone cavity in the anterior mandible: A possible diagnostic challenge. *Journal of Endodontics* 27:304–307. https://doi.org/10.1097/00004770-200104000-00020

Keenleyside, A. (2011). Congenital aural atresia in an adult female from Apollonia Pontica, Bulgaria. *International Journal of Paleopathology* 1:63–67. https://doi.org/10.1016/j.ijpp.2011.01.001

Kösling, S., Omenzetter, M., Bartel-Friedrich, S. (2009). Congenital malformations of the external and middle ear. *European Journal of Radiology* 69:269–279. https://doi.org/10.1016/j.ejrad.2007.10.019

Kosowski, T.R., Weathers, W.M., Wolfswinkel, E.M., Ridgway, E.B. (2012). Cleft palate. *Seminars in Plastic Surgery* 26:164–169. https://doi.org/10.1055/s-0033-1333883

Kumar, A., Tubbs, R.S. (2011). Spina bifida: A diagnostic dilemma in paleopathology. *Clinical Anatomy* 24:19–33. https://doi.org/10.1002/ca.21058

Latief, B.S., Lekkas, C., Kuijpers, M.A.R. (2010). Maxillary arch width in unoperated adult bilateral cleft lip and alveolus and complete bilateral cleft lip and palate. *Orthodontics & Craniofacial Research* 13:82–88. https://doi.org/10.1111/j.1601-6343.2009.01479.x

Lewis, M. (2017). *Paleopathology of Children: Identification of Pathological Conditions in the Human Skeletal Remains of Non-Adults*. San Diego: Academic Press.

Lewis, M. (2019a). Skeletal dysplasias and related conditions. In *Ortner's Identification of Pathological Conditions in Human Skeletal Remains*, edited by Buikstra, J., pp. 615–637. San Diego: Academic Press.

Lewis, M. (2019b). Congenital and neuromechanical abnormalities of the skeleton. In *Ortner's Identification of Pathological Conditions in Human Skeletal Remains*, edited by Buikstra, J., pp. 585–614. San Diego: Academic Press.

Llerena Jr, J., Kim, C.A., Fano, V., Rosselli, P., Collett-Solberg, P.F., de Medeiros, P.F.V., del Pino, M., Bertola, D., Lourenço, C.M., Cavalcanti, D.P., Félix, T.M., Rosa-Bellas, A., Rossi, N.T., Abreu, F., Cavalcanti, N., Hervias Ruz, M.C., Baratela, W. (2022). Achondroplasia in Latin America: Practical recommendations for the multidisciplinary care of pediatric patients. *BMC Pediatrics* 22:492. https://doi.org/10.1186/s12887-022-03505-w

Loría-Cortés, R., Quesada-Calvo, E., Cordero-Chaverri, E. (1977). Osteopetrosis in children: A report of 26 cases. *The Journal of Pediatrics* 91:43–47. https://doi.org/10.1016/s0022-3476(77)80441-1

Ma, J., Zhang, Y., Ding, X., Liang, Z., Yang, C., Deng, Z., He, H., Guan, Z., Zeng, C., Lin, Y., Luo, X. (2023). Co-occurrence of spondyloepiphyseal dysplasia and X-linked hypophosphatemia in a three-generation Chinese family. *Calcified Tissue International* 113:266–275. https://doi.org/10.1007/s00223-023-01104-0

Mann, R.W. (2001). *Stafne's Defects of the Human Mandible*. Doctoral Dissertation, University of Hawaii, Manoa.

Mann, R.W., Hunt, D.R. (2012). *Photographic Regional Atlas of Bone Disease: A Guide to Pathologic and Normal Variation in the Human Skeleton*, 3rd edition. Springfield, IL: Charles C. Thomas.

Mann, R.W., Tuamsuk, P., Hefner, J.T. (2013). Aplasia of the os odontoideum: Skeletal manifestation from Thailand. *International Journal of Paleopathology* 3:302–306. https://doi.org/10.1016/j.ijpp.2013.08.001

Mariaud-Schmidt, R.P., Bitar, W.E., Pérez-Lamero, F., Barros-Nuñez, P. (2002). Melorheostosis: Unusual presentation in a girl. *Clinical Imaging* 26:58–62. https://doi.org/10.1016/S0899-7071(01)00351-5

Marques, C. (2019). Tumors of bone. In *Ortner's Identification of Pathological Conditions in Human Skeletal Remains*, edited by Buikstra, J., pp. 639–717. San Diego: Academic Press.

McIntyre, J.D., Benson, M.K. (2002). An aetiological classification for developmental synostoses at the elbow. *Journal of Pediatric Orthopaedics* 11:313–319.

Mehta, L., Verma, I.C. (1992). Cleidocranial dysplasia: Underdiagnosed and misdiagnosed?. *The Indian Journal of Pediatrics* 59:633–636. https://doi.org/10.1007/bf02833006

Meltzer, R.M. (1987). Polydactyly. *Clinics in Podiatric Medicine and Surgery* 4:57–62.

Menezes, R., Vieira, A.R. (2008). Dental anomalies as part of the cleft spectrum. *Cleft Palate-Craniofacial Journal* 45:414–419. https://doi.org/10.1597/07-064.1

Mitchell, P.D., Redfern, R.C. (2008). Diagnostic criteria for developmental dislocation of the hip in human skeletal remains. *International Journal of Osteoarchaeology* 18:61–71. https://doi.org/10.1002/oa.919

Mitchell, P.D., Redfern, R.C. (2011). Brief communication: Developmental dysplasia of the hip in medieval London. *American Journal of Physical Anthropology* 144:479–484. https://doi.org/10.1002/ajpa.21448

Morris, J.K., Rankin, J., Garne, E., Loane, M., Greenlees, R., Addor, M.C., Arriola, L., Barisic, I., Bergman, J.E.H., Csaky-Szunyogh, M., Dias, C., Draper, E.S., Gatt, M., Khoshnood, B., Klungsoyr, K., Kurinczuk, J.J., Lynch, C., McDonnell, R., Nelen, V., Neville, A.J., O'Mahony, M.T., Pierini, A., Randrianaivo, H., Rissmann, A., Tucker, D., Verellen-Dumoulin, C., de Walle, H.E.K., Wellesley, D., Wiesel, A., Dolk, H. (2016). Prevalence of microcephaly in Europe: Population based study. *BMJ* 354:i4721. https://doi.org/10.1136/bmj.i4721

Müller, F., O'Rahilly, R., Benson, D.R. (1986). The early origin of vertebral anomalies, as illustrated by a "butterfly vertebra." *Journal of Anatomy* 149:157–169.

O'Rahilly, R. (1953). A survey of carpal and tarsal anomalies. *The Journal of Bone & Joint Surgery* 35:626–642.

Oberklaid, F., Danks, D.M., Jensen, F., Stace, L., Rosshandler, S. (1979). Achondroplasia and hypochondroplasia. Comments on frequency, mutation rate, and radiological features in skull and spine. *Journal of Medical Genetics* 16:140–146. https://doi.org/10.1136/jmg.16.2.140

Panda, A., Gamanagatti, S., Jana, M., Gupta, A.K. (2014). Skeletal dysplasias: A radiographic approach and review of common non-lethal skeletal dysplasias. *World Journal of Radiology* 6:808–825. https://doi.org/10.4329/wjr.v6.i10.808

Papadopoulou, C.I., Sifakakis, I., Tournis, S. (2024). Metabolic bone diseases affecting tooth eruption: A narrative review. *Children* 11:748. https://doi.org/10.3390/children11060748

Pereda, A., Garin, I., Garcia-Barcina, M., Gener, B., Beristain, E., Ibañez, A.M., Perez de Nanclares, G. (2013). Brachydactyly E: Isolated or as a feature of a syndrome. *Orphanet Journal of Rare Diseases* 8:141. https://doi.org/10.1186/1750-1172-8-141

Philipsen, H., Takata, T., Reichart, P., Sato, S., Suei, Y. (2002). Lingual and buccal mandibular bone depressions: A review based on 583 cases from a worldwide literature survey, including 69 new cases from Japan. *Dentomaxillofacial Radiology* 31:281–290. https://doi.org/10.1038/sj.dmfr.4600718

Resnick, D.J. (2002). *Diagnosis of Bone and Joint Disorders*, 4th edition. Philadelphia: Saunders.

Richards, G.D., Anton, S.C. (1991). Craniofacial configuration and postcranial development of a hydrocephalic child (ca. 2500 B.C.–500 A.D.): With a review of cases and comment on diagnostic criteria. *American Journal of Physical Anthropology* 85:185–200. https://doi.org/10.1002/ajpa.1330850207

Richette, P., Bardin, T., Stheneur, C. (2008). Achondroplasia: From genotype to phenotype. *Joint, Bone, Spine* 75:125–130. https://doi.org/10.1016/j.jbspin.2007.06.007

Samartzis, D., Herman, J., Lubicky, J.P. (2006). Classification of congenitally fused cervical patterns in Klippel-Feil patients: Epidemiology and role in the development of cervical spine-related symptoms. *Spine* 31:798–804. https://doi.org/10.1097/01.brs.0000239222.36505.46

Sargar, K.M., Singh, A.K., Kao, S.C. (2017). Imaging of skeletal disorders caused by fibroblast growth factor receptor gene mutations. *RadioGraphics* 37:1813–1830. https://doi.org/10.1148/rg.2017170017

Schiller, S., Spranger, S., Schechinger, B., Fukami, M., Merker, S., Drop, S.L., Tröger, J., Knoblauch, H., Kunze, J., Seidel, J., Rappold, G.A. (2000). Phenotypic variation and genetic heterogeneity in Léri-Weill syndrome. *European Journal of Human Genetics* 8:54–62. https://doi.org/10.1038/sj.ejhg.5200402

Silva, A.M. (2011). Foot anomalies in the Late Neolithic/Chalcolithic population exhumed from the rock cut cave of São Paulo 2 (Almada, Portugal). *International Journal of Osteoarchaeology* 21:420–427. https://doi.org/10.1002/oa.1148

Solomon, L.B., Rühli, F.J., Taylor, J., Ferris, L., Pope, R., Henneberg, M. (2003). A dissection and computer tomograph study of tarsal coalitions in 100 cadaver feet. *Journal of Orthopaedic Research* 21:352–358. https://doi.org/10.1016/s0736-0266(02)00131-6

Spinnato, P., Pedrini, E., Petrera, M.R., Zarantonello, P., Trisolino, G., Sangiorgi, L., Carpenzano, M., Crombé, A., Tetta, C. (2022). Spectrum of skeletal imaging features in osteopetrosis: Inheritance pattern and radiological associations. *Genes* 13:1965. https://doi.org/10.3390/genes13111965

Stafne, E.C. (1942). Bone cavities situated near the angle of the mandible. *Journal of the American Dental Association* 23:553–556. https://doi.org/10.14219/jada.archive.1942.0315

Suresh, S., Muthukumar, T., Saifuddin, A. (2010). Classical and unusual imaging appearances of melorheostosis. *Clinical Radiology* 8:593–600. https://doi.org/10.1016/j.crad.2010.02.004

Sybert, V.P., McCauley, E. (2004). Turner's syndrome. *The New England Journal of Medicine* 351:1227–1238. https://doi.org/10.1056/nejmra030360

Taneja, T., Shetty, V., Ramachandran, M. (2021). Congenital radioulnar synostosis. In *Congenital Anomalies of the Upper Extremity*, edited by Laub, Jr. D.R., 2nd edition, pp. 163–170. Berlin: Springer.

Tauber, M., Lounis, N., Coulet, J., Baunin, C., Cahuzac, J.P., Rochiccioli, P. (2004). Wrist anomalies in Turner syndrome compared with Leri-Weill dyschondrosteosis: A new feature in Turner syndrome. *European Journal of Pediatrics* 163:475–481. https://doi.org/10.1007/s00431-004-1471-4

Tini, P.G., Wieser, C., Zinn, W.M. (1977). The transitional vertebra of the lumbosacral spine: Its radiological classification, incidence, and clinical significance. *Rheumatology and Rehabilitation* 16:180–185. https://doi.org/10.1093/rheumatology/16.3.180

Titelbaum, A.R., Burnett, S.E., Case, D.T. (2023). Developmental conditions in paleopathology. In *The Routledge Handbook of Paleopathology*, edited by Grauer, A.L., pp. 250–270. London: Routledge.

Traversari, M., Da Via, S., Petrella, E., Feeney, R.N., Benazzi, S. (2020). A case of dwarfism in 6th century Italy: Bioarchaeological assessment of a hereditary disorder. *International Journal of Paleopathology* 30:110–117. https://doi.org/10.1016/j.ijpp.2020.03.003

Trzcińska, D., Olszewska, E., Wiśniewski, A., Mildc, K., Madej, M. (2011). The knee alignment and the foot arch in patients with Turner syndrome. *Pediatric Endocrinology, Diabetes and Metabolism* 17:138–144.

Venning, P. (1956). Radiological studies of variations in the segmentation and ossification of the digits of the human foot. I. Variation in the number of phalanges and centers of ossification of the toes. *American Journal of Physical Anthropology* 14:1–34. https://doi.org/10.1002/ajpa.1330140117

Waldron, T. (2020). *Palaeopathology*, 2nd edition. Cambridge: Cambridge University Press.

Wang, Z., Li, X., Wang, Y., Fu, W., Liu, Y., Zhang, Z., Wang, C. (2022). Natural history of type II autosomal dominant osteopetrosis: A single center retrospective study. *Frontiers in Endocrinology* 13:819641. https://doi.org/10.3389/fendo.2022.819641

Werner, M.S., Scheimer, R.A. (1987). Melorheostosis: A review of the literature and case report. *Journal of the American Podiatric Medical Association* 77:95–98. https://doi.org/10.7547/87507315-77-2-96

Whyte, M.P., Gottesman, G.S., Eddy, M.C., McAlister, W.H. (1999). X-linked recessive spondyloepiphyseal dysplasia tarda. Clinical and radiographic evolution in a 6-generation kindred and review of the literature. *Medicine* 78:9–25. https://doi.org/10.1097/00005792-199901000-00002

Wordsworth, P., Chan, M. (2019). Melorheostosis and osteopoikilosis: A review of clinical features and pathogenesis. *Calcified Tissue International* 104:530–543. https://doi.org/10.1007/s00223-019-00543-y

Wynne-Davies, R., Hall, C. (1982). Two clinical variants of spondylo-epiphysial dysplasia congenita. *The Journal of Bone & Joint Surgery* 64:435–441. https://doi.org/10.1302/0301-620x.64b4.6807992

Younge, D., Drummond, D., Herring, J., Cruess, R. (1979). Melorheostosis in children: Clinical features and natural history. *The Journal of Bone & Joint Surgery* 61:415–418. https://doi.org/10.1302/0301-620x.61b4.500749

Chapter 3

Circulatory disorders

Circulatory disorders are associated with a reduced blood flow to various tissues of the body, and they may have different aetiologies. The circulatory system is essential for a healthy skeleton as it supplies the bones with oxygen, nutrients, and hormones, and facilitates the removal of carbon dioxide and other waste products. Therefore, circulatory disorders can have a severe effect on bone growth and maintenance. The decrease in blood flow may appear gradually, in which case the affected skeletal elements usually atrophy, or suddenly, which can cause bone necrosis (Box 3.1). This chapter covers osteochondroses, osteochondritis dissecans, slipped femoral capital epiphysis, and hypertrophic osteoarthropathy.[1]

Osteochondroses

Osteochondroses are circulatory disorders that share key characteristics: (1) they affect young individuals, particularly children and adolescents; (2) they are more common among males; (3) they target the epiphyseal or apophyseal centers; and (4) they are often followed by reossification.

Scheuermann's disease

Scheuermann's disease affects the vertebrae and causes kyphosis (Figures 3.1 and 3.2). Its aetiology is unclear, but it has been associated with mechanical stress, trauma, weakened vertebral endplates due to defective collagen fibril formation, elevated growth hormone levels,

Box 3.1 Osteonecrosis

Osteonecrosis is the death of bone cells as a result of reduced or eliminated blood supply, which ultimately leads to bone destruction. Depending on which parts of a bone are affected by osteonecrosis, different terms are used to describe this process: *avascular necrosis* refers to osteonecrosis in the epiphyses and subchondral bone, whereas *bone infarct* covers osteonecrosis in the metaphyses or diaphyses. Osteonecrosis may be caused by trauma, developmental and haematopoietic disorders, infections, metabolic, and other conditions. Irrespective of its aetiology, osteonecrosis is characterised by cellular death and repair, which manifest as bone resorption and formation.

DOI: 10.4324/9781003475026-3

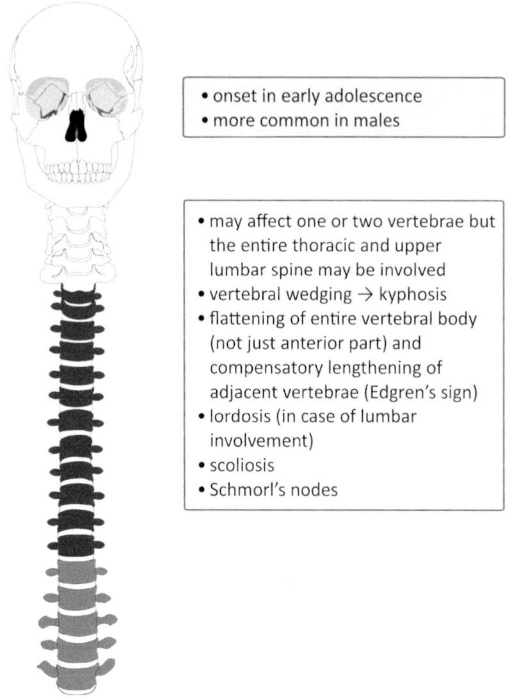

Figure 3.1 Skeletal manifestation of Scheuermann's disease. (Data from Grauer 2019; Lowe and Line 2007; Palazzo et al. 2014; Üstündağ and Deveci 2011)

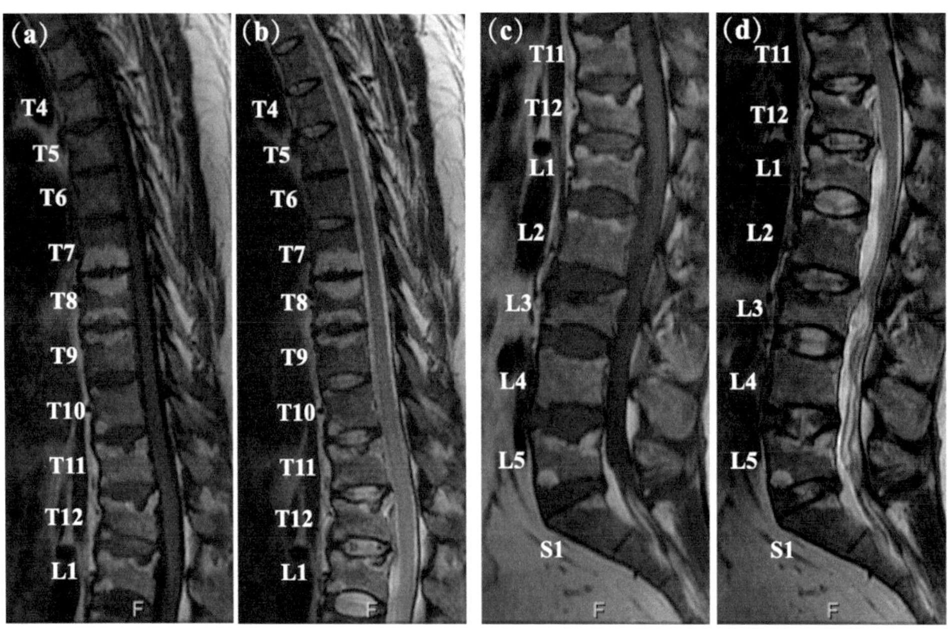

Figure 3.2 Magnetic resonance imaging of the vertebrae of an individual with Scheuermann's disease. Note the compression fracture in L3, as well as vertebral endplate alterations and Schmorl's nodes in multiple vertebrae. (Figure 1 from Wang et al. 2021; article licensed under a Creative Commons Attribution 4.0 International License)

juvenile osteoporosis, vitamin A deficiency, poliomyelitis, epiphysitis, and genetic factors since the condition is often shared among family members.

Osgood–Schlatter disease

Osgood–Schlatter disease is characterised by an avulsion of the tibial tuberosity and the separation of part of the tuberosity from the rest of the tibia (Figures 3.3 and 3.4). During growth, the tibial tuberosity has not fused yet with the proximal tibial metaphysis. Therefore, avulsion of part of the tuberosity is possible when repetitive strain is applied to the insertion of the

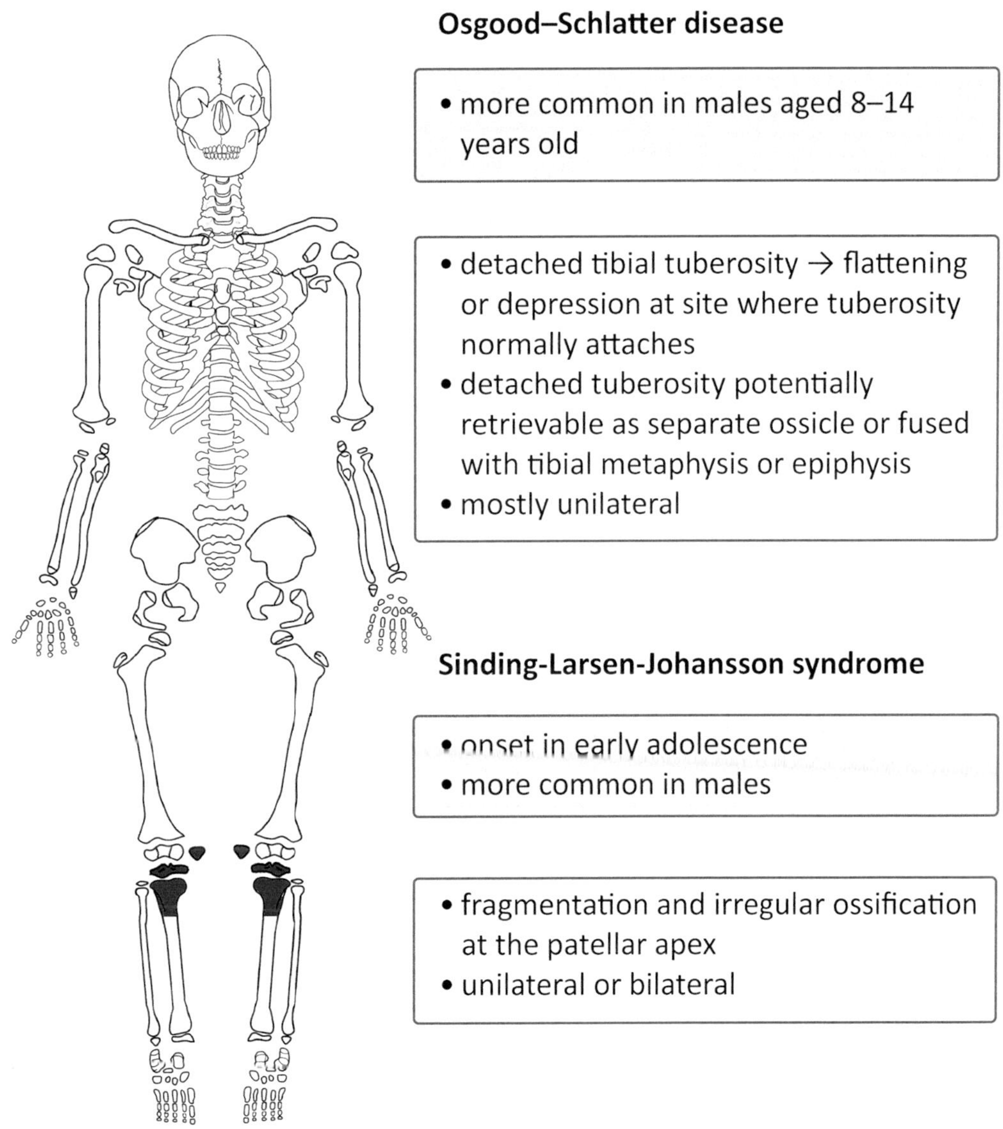

Figure 3.3 Skeletal manifestation of Osgood–Schlatter disease and Sinding–Larsen–Johansson syndrome. (Data from Aufderheide and Rodríguez-Martín 1998; Gholve et al. 2007; Grauer 2019; Hirano et al. 2002)

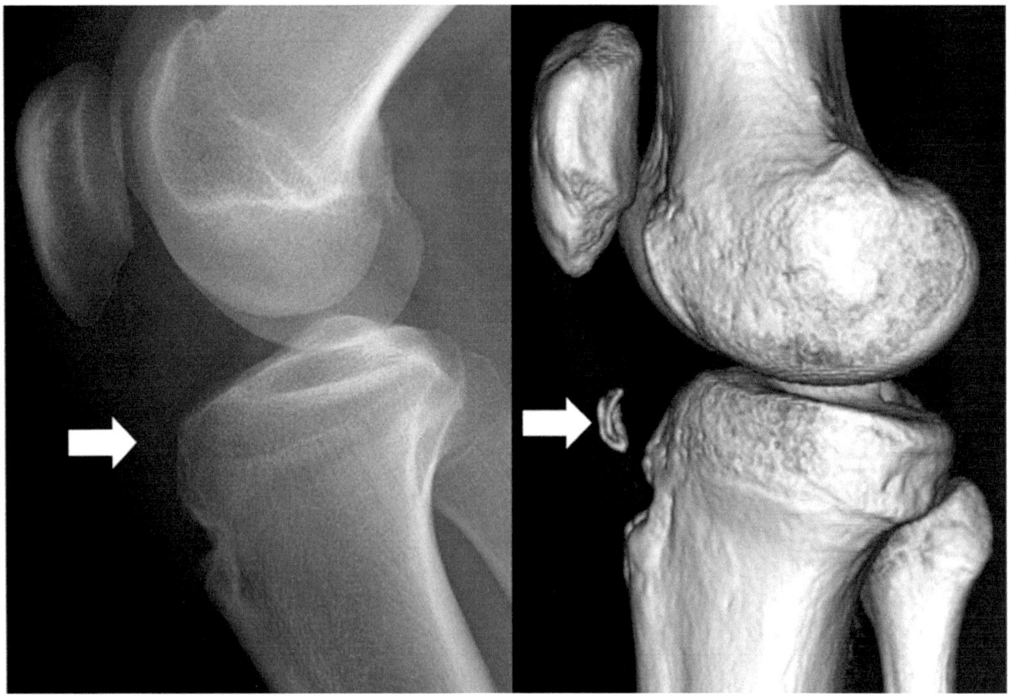

Figure 3.4 Radiograph (left) and 3D CT scan (right) showing ossicle detached from the tibial tuberosity; the ossicle (arrow) is minimally visible in the radiograph, highlighting the importance of using proper imaging means. (Figure 11 in Fujita et al. 2022; article licensed under a Creative Commons Attribution 4.0 International License)

patellar tendon. The resulting bone fragment may later fuse with the metaphysis or epiphysis of the tibia, or it may form a separate ossicle. Osgood–Schlatter disease is unlikely to occur after the age of 14–18 years, when the tibial tuberosity fuses with the proximal metaphysis.

Sinding–Larsen–Johansson syndrome

Sinding–Larsen–Johansson syndrome is a traction apophysitis at the attachment of the patellar tendon to the inferior pole of the patella, caused by excessive repetitive strain (Figure 3.3).

Freiberg's disease

Freiberg's disease is the necrosis of the metatarsal heads, particularly the second metatarsal (Figures 3.5 and 3.6). Trauma is often associated with this condition, but developmental anomalies may also contribute to its aetiology.

Köhler's disease

Köhler's disease is the necrosis of the navicular bone (Figures 3.5 and 3.7). Its aetiology is unclear, but it has been associated with trauma. It often heals without complications, even without treatment.

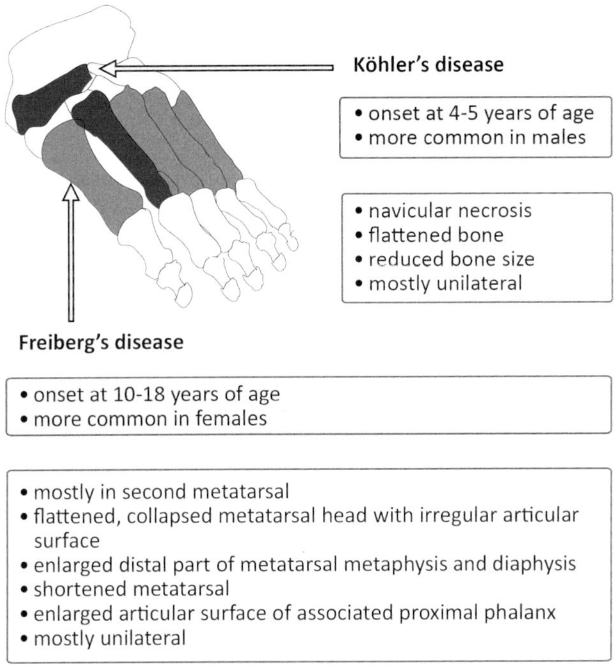

Figure 3.5 Skeletal manifestation of Freiberg's disease and Köhler's disease. (Data from Aufderheide and Rodríguez-Martín 1998; Grauer 2019; Khoury et al. 2007)

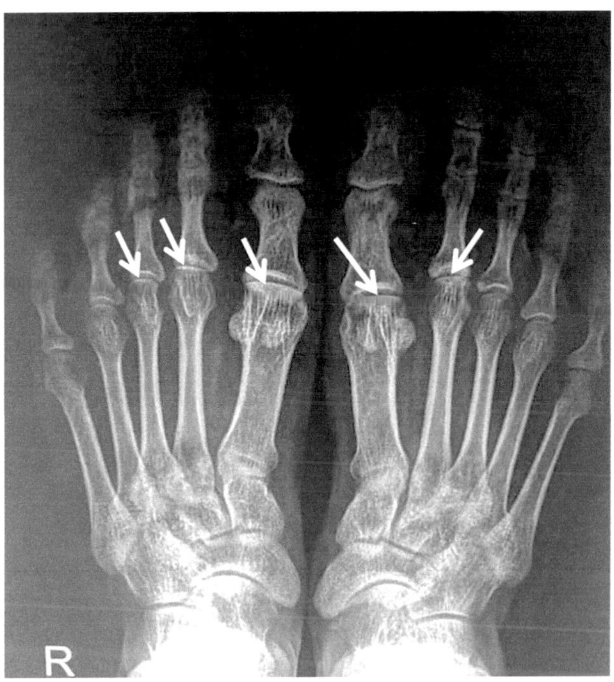

Figure 3.6 Radiograph of the feet of an individual with Freiberg's disease. Note the flattening and sclerosis of the metatarsal heads. (Figure 1 in El-Amin et al. 2023; article licensed under a Creative Commons Attribution 4.0 International License)

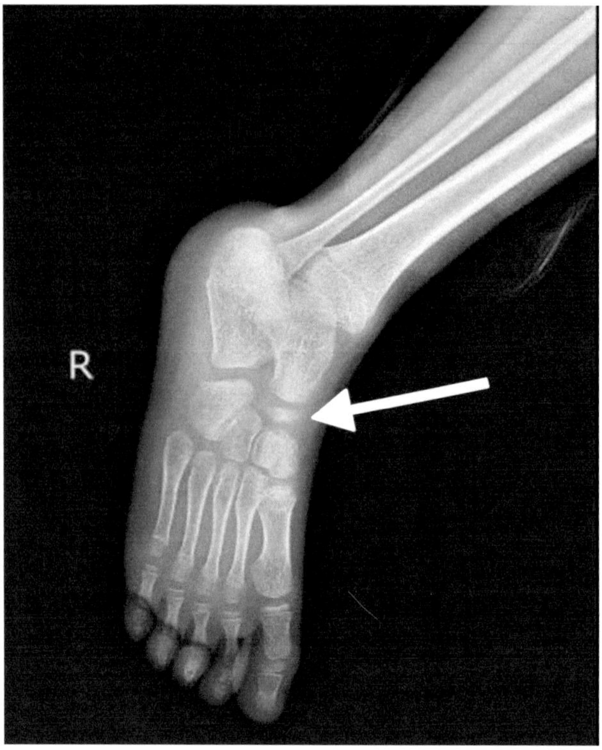

Figure 3.7 Radiograph of the foot and ankle of an individual with Köhler's disease. Note the irregular shape, sclerosis, and increased density of the navicular bone. (Figure 2 in Deshpande et al. 2023; article licensed under a Creative Commons Attribution 4.0 International License)

Legg–Calvé–Perthes disease

Legg–Calvé–Perthes disease (LCPD) is the osteonecrosis of the femoral head due to a prolonged interruption of blood supply during childhood, which is then restored (Figures 3.8–3.11). Many factors can restrict the blood supply of the femoral head, resulting in LCPD, such as mechanical stress, trauma, genetic predisposition, endocrine and haematopoietic disorders.

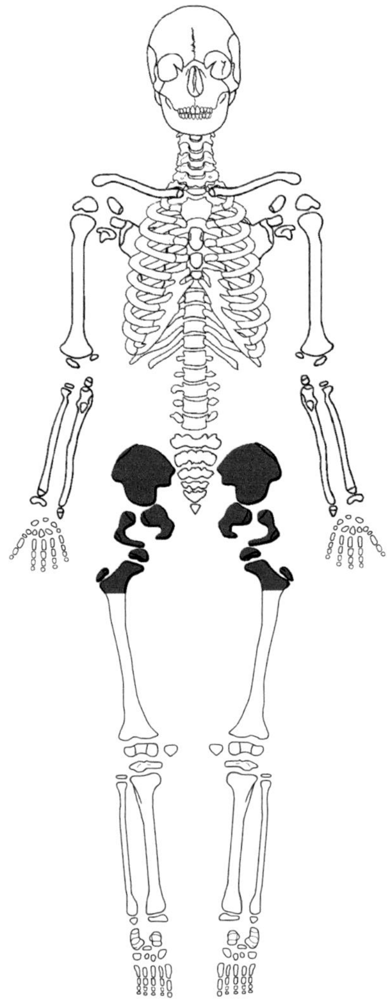

Slipped femoral capital epiphysis

- more common in male adolescents

- inferior-posterior displacement of femoral proximal epiphysis and fusion with neck
- mild to severe slippage
- head deformity
- neck and head osteoporosis
- neck shortening, broadening and buttressing (reactive new bone formation)
- necrosis
- limb shortening and gracility → lordosis and/or scoliosis
- early-onset hip osteoarthritis
- mostly unilateral

Legg–Calvé–Perthes disease

- onset at 4-8 years of age
- more common in males

- femoral head necrosis (head flattened and mushroom-shaped)
- enlarged head and neck (coxa magna)
- lower head position compared to greater trochanter
- no significant dislocation of head center relative to neck axis
- neck thickening and shortening with varus deformity
- enlarged, flattened acetabulum
- secondary osteoarthritis
- shortened limb on affected side → additional deformities in lower limbs due to abnormal gait (e.g. periostitis, pathological fractures, enlarged tibia and foot bones contralateral to affected hip)
- mostly unilateral

Figure 3.8 Skeletal manifestation of Legg–Calvé–Perthes disease and slipped femoral capital epiphysis. (Data from Georgiadis et al. 2015; Grauer 2019; Huhnstock et al. 2014; Jingushi and Suenaga 2004; Kim et al. 2006; Knüsel et al. 1992; Lewis 2017; Peck et al. 2017; Smrčka et al. 2009; Waldron 2020)

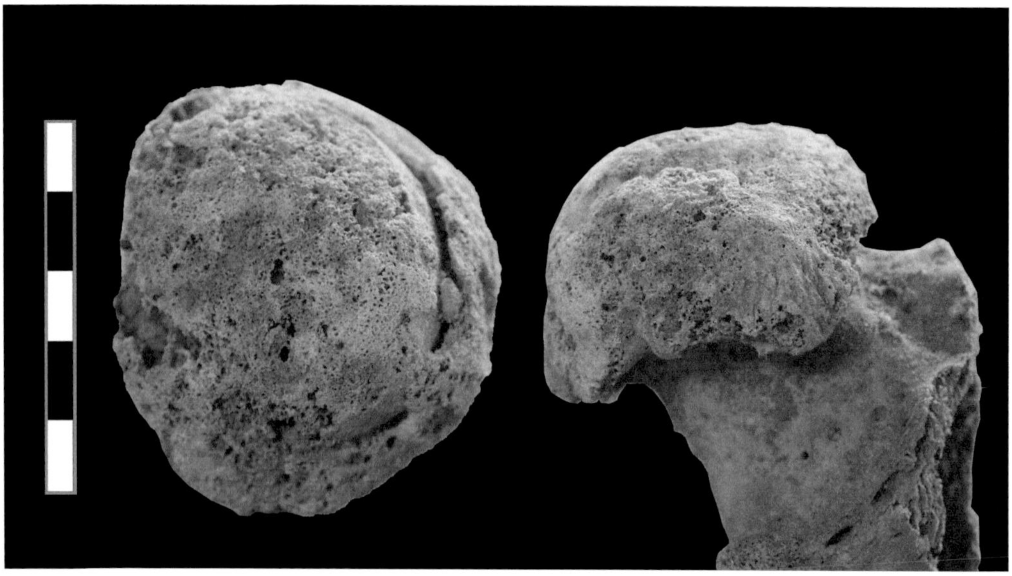

Figure 3.9 Legg–Calvé–Perthes disease in a right femur. Note the flattened and mushroom-shaped head and secondary osteoarthritic changes. (Terschelling-Midsland, Collection NAD Nuis inv. Nr. F 2009-II-40; photos by Efthymia Nikita, with permission from the Noordelijk Archeologisch Depot)

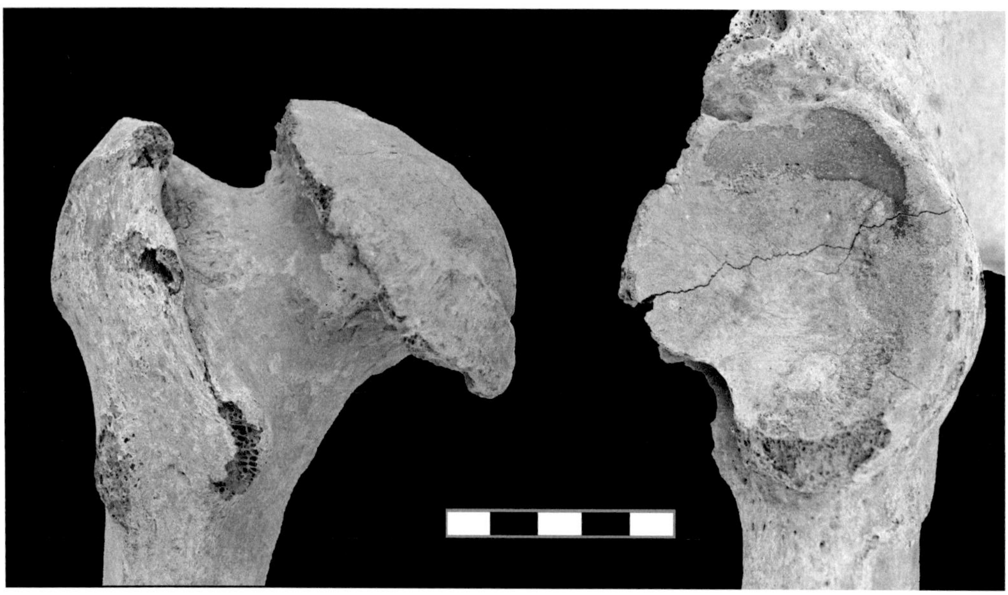

Figure 3.10 Legg–Calvé–Perthes disease in a left femur. Note the flattened and mushroom-shaped head, with marginal lipping, and eburnation on the acetabulum due to secondary osteoarthritis. (Probable male, Adult, Dokkum-Kerkplein, Medieval-Modern, 5100; photos by Efthymia Nikita, from the reference collection of the Cultural Heritage Agency of the Netherlands)

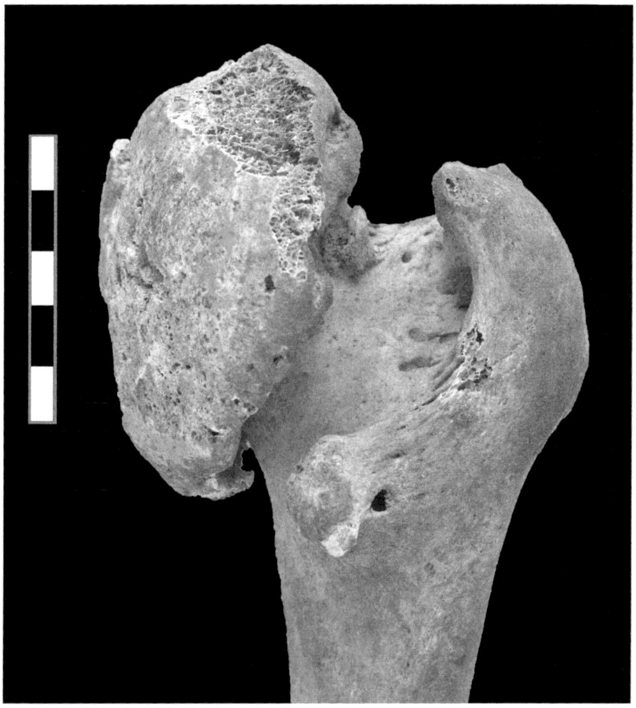

Figure 3.11 Legg–Calvé–Perthes disease in a right femur. Note the flattened, deformed head, with marginal lipping. (Adult, 5194; photo by Efthymia Nikita, from the reference collection of the Cultural Heritage Agency of the Netherlands)

Slipped femoral capital epiphysis

Slipped femoral capital epiphysis is the slippage of the proximal femoral epiphysis relative to the femoral neck, when the integrity of the growth plate has been compromised (Figures 3.8, 3.12, and 3.13). This condition has been associated with endocrine disorders, mechanical stress, genetic predisposition, and other factors.

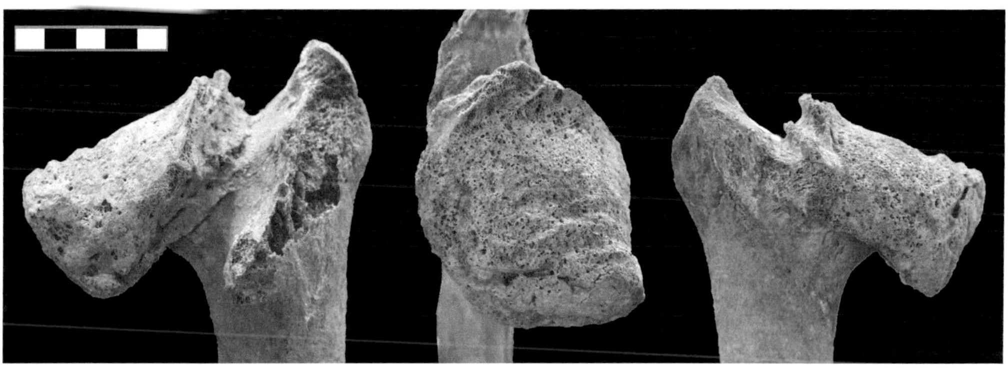

Figure 3.12 Slipped femoral capital epiphysis in a right femur. Note the severe head deformity, neck shortening, and the fact that the greater trochanter is now the most superior part of the bone. (Male, Middle adult, Emmen-Marktplein, Collection NAD Nuis inv. Nr. D 2017-V.43; photos by Efthymia Nikita, with permission from the Noordelijk Archeologisch Depot)

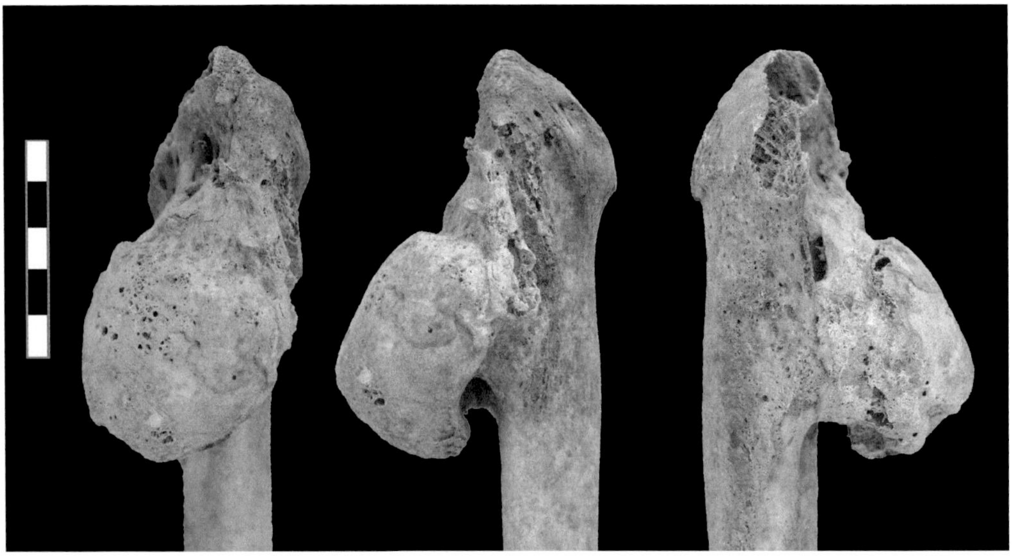

Figure 3.13 Slipped femoral capital epiphysis in a left femur. Note the severe inferior displacement of the capital epiphysis and resultant head deformity. (Amersfoort, 5192; photos by Efthymia Nikita, from the reference collection of the Cultural Heritage Agency of the Netherlands)

Osteochondritis dissecans

In osteochondritis dissecans, part of the articular cartilage and subchondral bone in a synovial joint detach from the underlying bone (Figures 3.14–3.17). The resulting fragment may reattach to the articular surface (possibly slightly displaced), or it may free-float in the joint capsule. Over time, the defect on the articular surface may become partially covered by a layer of new bone; however, a depression will persist. Contemporary cases are often found in young athletes, suggesting a link to physical activity that results in acute macrotrauma or repeated microtrauma, while genetic susceptibility may also play a role in the development of the condition.

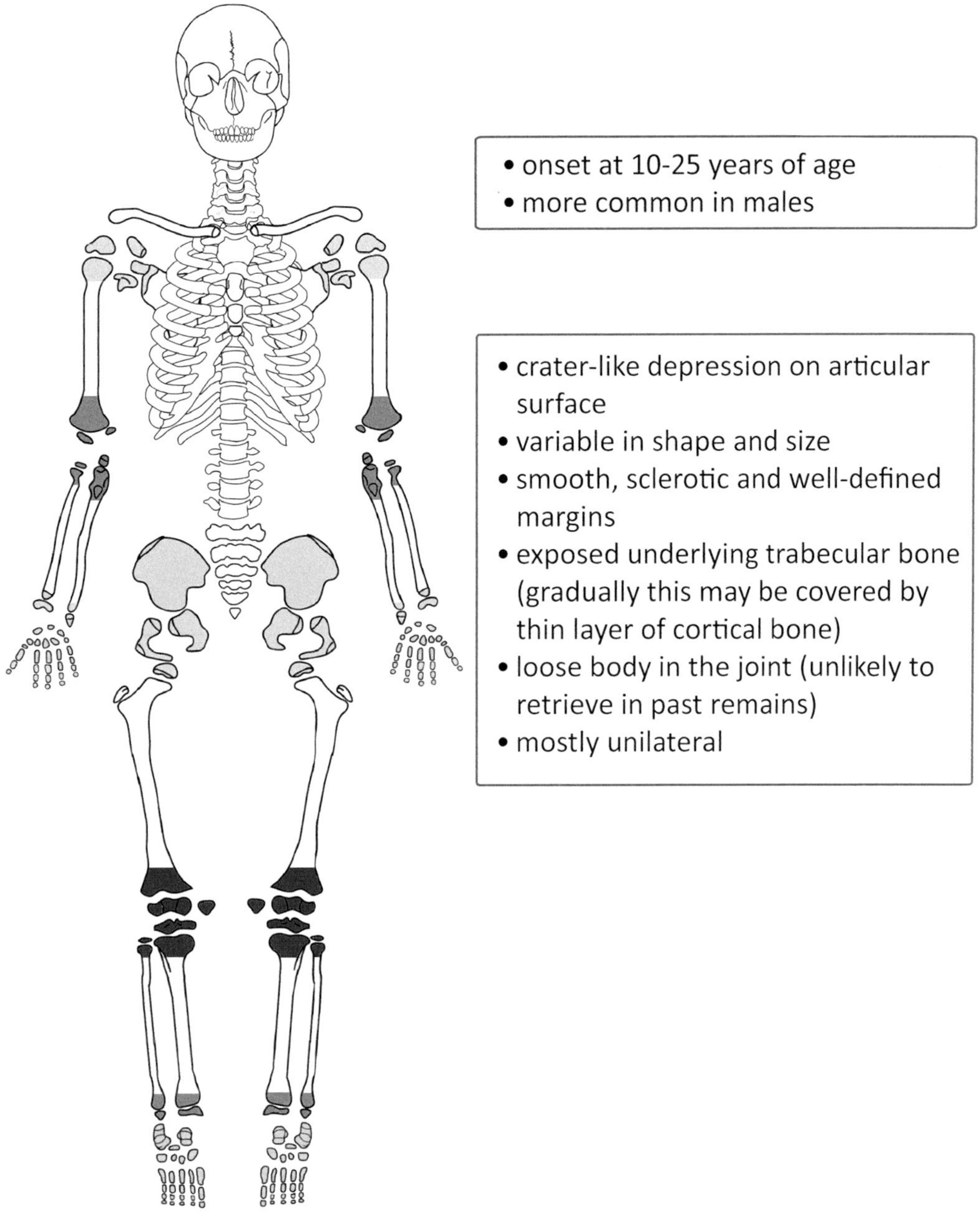

Figure 3.14 Skeletal manifestation of osteochondritis dissecans. (Data from Aufderheide and Rodríguez-Martín 1998; Backes et al. 2014; Kessler et al. 2014; Schindler 2007; Waldron 2020)

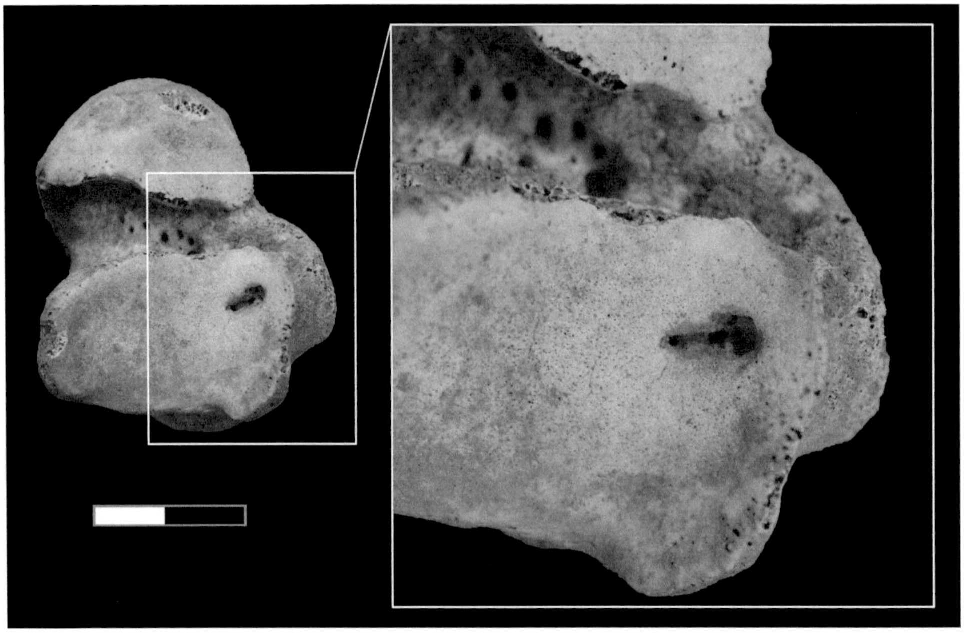

Figure 3.15 Osteochondritis dissecans in the posterior subtalar facet of a right talus. (Female, 45–60 years old, All Saints Church, Fishergate, York, Medieval, Y-2357; photos by Efthymia Nikita; copyright: Human Skeletal Collection, University of Sheffield)

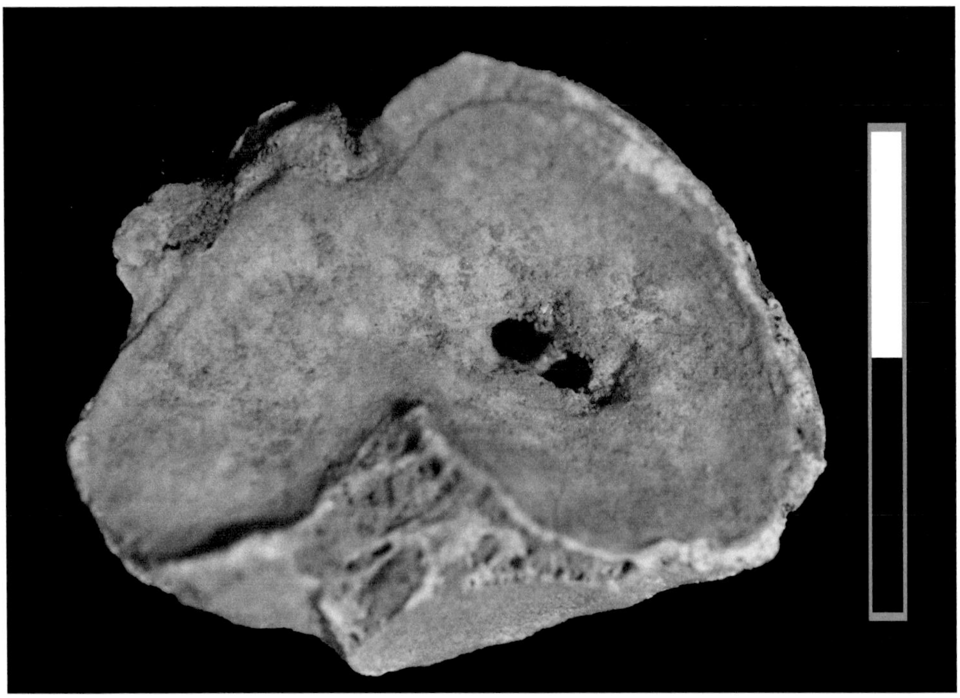

Figure 3.16 Osteochondritis dissecans in the proximal articular facet of a first metatarsal. (Medieval Nonsuch Palace, Burial 80; photo by Efthymia Nikita; copyright: Duckworth Laboratory, University of Cambridge)

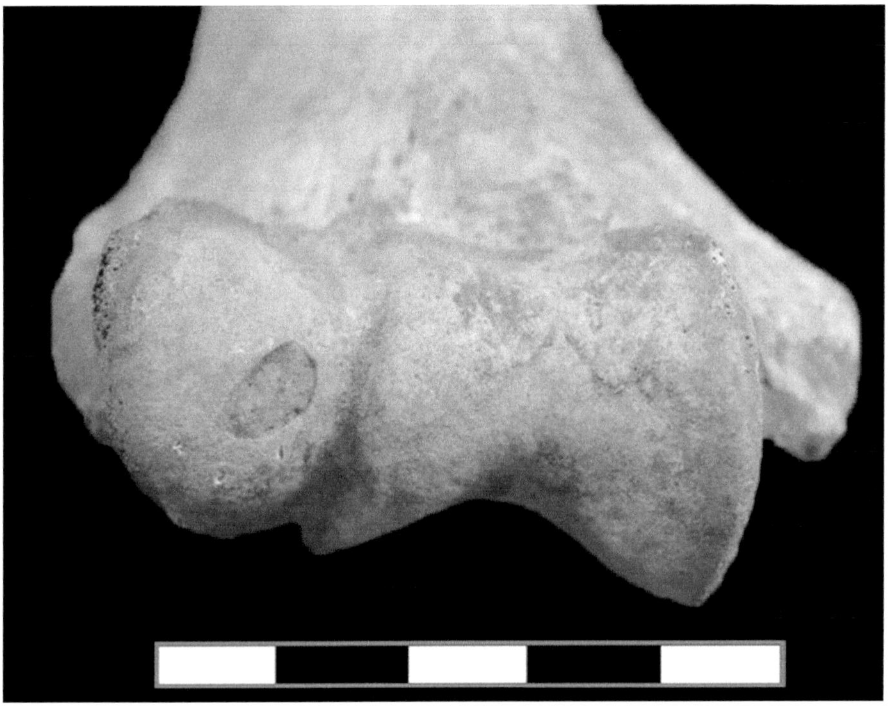

Figure 3.17 Osteochondritis dissecans in the capitulum of a right humerus. (Male, 23–39 years old, All Saints Church, Fishergate, York, Medieval, Y-3861; photo by Efthymia Nikita; copyright: Human Skeletal Collection, University of Sheffield)

Hypertrophic osteoarthropathy

Hypertrophic osteoarthropathy appears as periosteal bone formation and may be primary or secondary (Figures 3.18 and 3.19). The primary or idiopathic type is a rare genetic disorder that mostly affects males during the first year of life and puberty. Many individuals with this type of condition become asymptomatic in adulthood. The secondary type (hypertrophic pulmonary osteoarthropathy) is more common and typically occurs in adults. It is often associated with lung carcinoma, pulmonary tuberculosis, and other chronic lung diseases, as well as gastrointestinal, cardiovascular, hepatobiliary, infectious, and endocrine disorders.

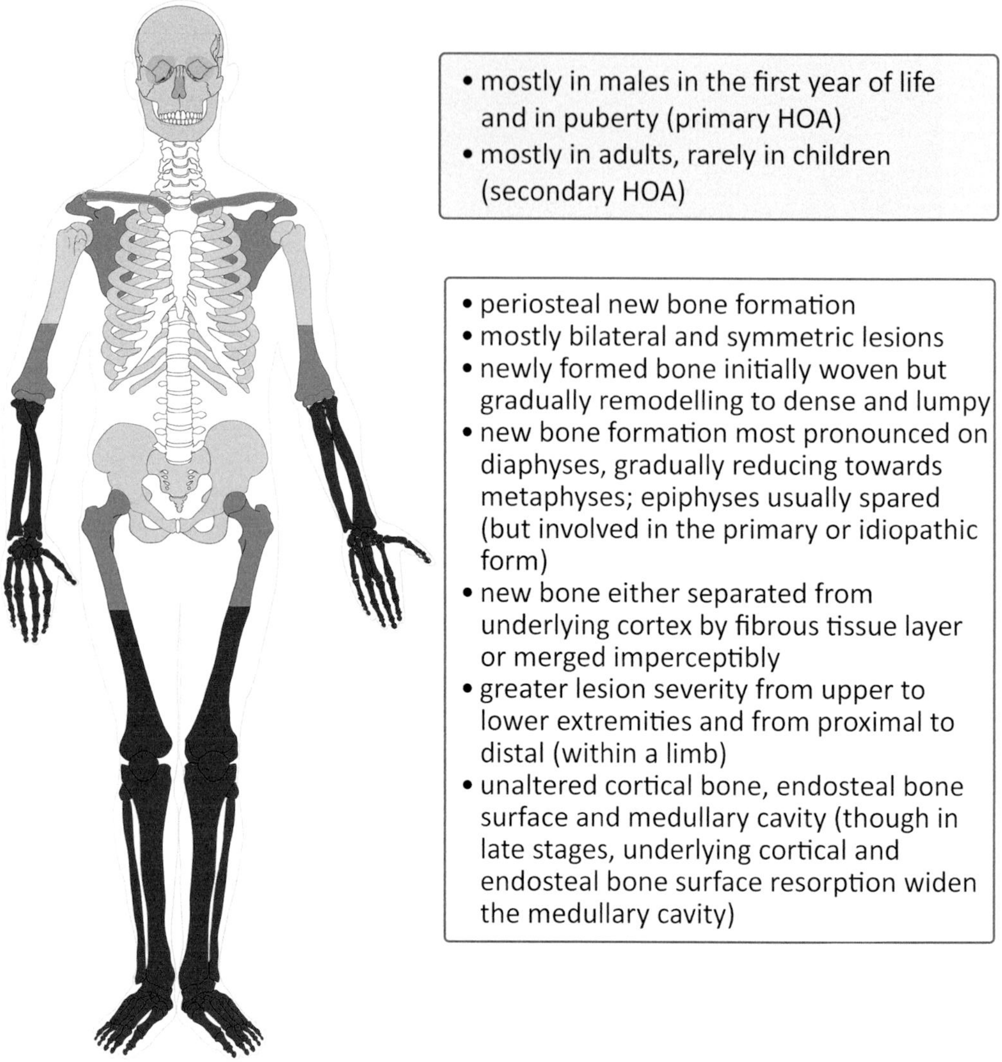

Figure 3.18 Skeletal manifestation of hypertrophic osteoarthropathy. (Data from Ali et al. 1980; Assis et al. 2011; Aufderheide and Rodríguez-Martín 1998; Gall et al. 1951; Grauer 2019; Rothschild and Rothschild 1998)

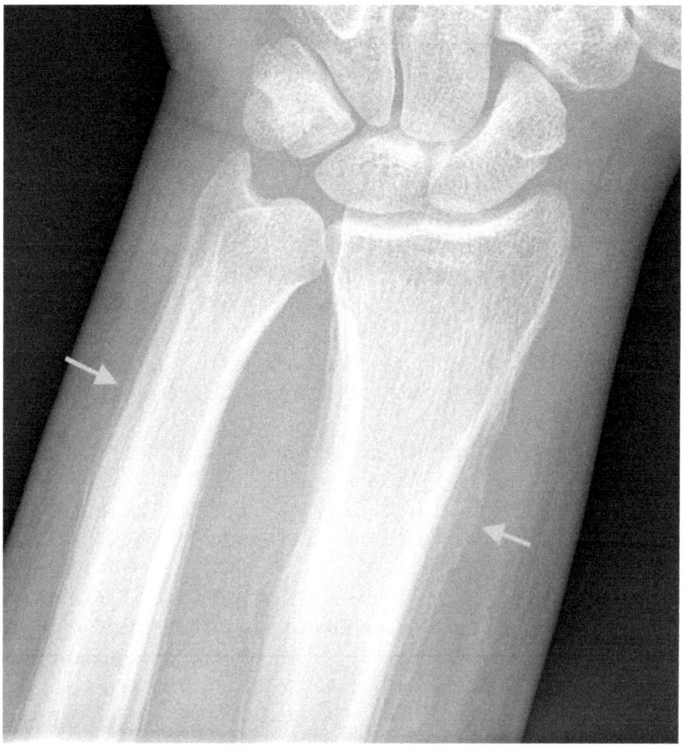

Figure 3.19 Left wrist radiograph of an individual with hypertrophic pulmonary osteoarthropathy. Note the periosteal new bone formation in the distal radius and ulna. (Figure 3 in Tekiteki et al. 2020; article licensed under a Creative Commons Attribution 4.0 International License)

Note

1 Evidence for cardiovascular disease has also been identified in skeletal remains through atherosclerotic calcifications appearing as yellow-brown plaques. However, these are not covered in this chapter, as they are not pathological lesions directly affecting the skeleton.

References and suggested readings

Ali, A., Tetalman, M.R., Fordham, E.W., Turner, D.A., Chiles, J.T., Patel, S.L., Schmidt, K.D. (1980). Distribution of hypertrophic pulmonary osteoarthropathy. *American Journal of Roentgenology* 134:771–780. https://doi.org/10.2214/ajr.134.4.771

Assis, S., Santos, A.L., Roberts, C.A. (2011). Evidence of hyperotrophic osteoarthropathy in individuals from the Coimbra Skeletal Identified Collection (Portugal). *International Journal of Paleopathology* 1:155–163. https://doi.org/10.1016/j.ijpp.2012.02.009

Aufderheide, A.C., Rodríguez-Martín, C. (1998). *The Cambridge Encyclopedia of Human Paleopathology*. Cambridge: Cambridge University Press.

Backes, J.R., Durbin, T.C., Bentley, J.C., Klingele, K.E. (2014). Multifocal juvenile osteochondritis dissecans of the knee: A case series. *Journal of Pediatric Orthopaedics* 34:453–458. https://doi.org/10.1097/bpo.0000000000000121

Biehler-Gomez, L., Maderna, E., Brescia, G., Caruso, V., Rizzi, A., Cattaneo, C. (2019). Distinguishing atherosclerotic calcifications in dry bone: Implications for forensic identification. *Journal of Forensic Sciences* 64:839–844. https://doi.org/10.1111/1556-4029.13948

Deshpande, S.V., Channawar, R.A., Wamborikar, H., Patil, B., Pundkar, A. (2023). Bilateral Kohler's disease: A case report. *Cureus* 15:e44929. https://doi.org/10.7759/cureus.44929

Edmonds, E., Polousky, J. (2013). A review of knowledge in osteochondritis dissecans: 123 years of minimal evolution from König to the ROCK study group. *Clinical Orthopaedics and Related Research* 471:1118–1126. https://doi.org/10.1007/s11999-012-2290-y

El-Amin, H., Ali, A.M.A., Elmansour, O.K.O., Abbas, R., Mohamed, E., Biraima, W.H., Ahmed, O.K., Mohamedali, A.O., Arja, A., Babikir, A.O.A. (2023). Freiberg's disease involving first metatarsal bone bilaterally in an African male patient: A case report. *Cureus* 15: e49093. https://doi.org/10.7759/cureus.49093

Fujita, K., Nakase, J., Yoshimizu, R., Kimura, M., Kanayama, T., Tsuchiya, H. (2022). Bursoscopic ultrasound-guided ossicle resection for Osgood-Schlatter disease. *Arthroscopy Techniques* 11:e841–e846. https://doi.org/10.1016/j.eats.2021.12.043

Gall, E.A., Bennett, G.A., Bauer, W. (1951). Generalized hypertrophic osteoarthropathy: A pathologic study of seven cases. *American Journal of Patholology* 27:349–381.

Georgiadis, A.G., Seeley, M.A., Yellin, J.L., Sankar, W.N. (2015). The presentation of Legg-Calvé-Perthes disease in females. *Journal of Children's Orthopaedics* 9:243–247. https://doi.org/10.1007/s11832-015-0671-y

Gholve, P.A., Scher, D.M., Khakharia, S., Widmann, R.F., Green, D.W. (2007). Osgood Schlatter syndrome. *Current Opinion in Pediatrics* 19:44–50. https://doi.org/10.1097/MOP.0b013e328013dbea

Grauer, A.L. (2019). Circulatory, reticuloendothelial, and hematopoietic disorders. In *Ortner's Identification of Pathological Conditions in Human Skeletal Remains*, edited by Buikstra, J., pp. 491–530. San Diego: Academic Press.

Hirano, A., Fukubayashi, T., Ishii, T., Ochiai, N. (2002). Magnetic resonance imaging of Osgood-Schlatter disease: The course of the disease. *Skeletal Radiology* 31:334–342. https://doi.org/10.1007/s00256-002-0486-z

Huhnstock, S., Svenningsen, S., Pripp, A.H., Terjesen, T., Wiig, O. (2014). The acetabulum in Perthes' disease: A prospective study of 123 children. *Journal of Children's Orthopaedics* 8:457–465.

Jaffe, H.L. (1972). *Metabolic, Degenerative and Inflammatory Diseases of Bone and Joints*. Philadelphia: Lea and Febiger.

Jingushi, S., Suenaga, E. (2004). Slipped capital femoral epiphysis: Etiology and treatment. *Journal of Orthopedic Science* 9:214–219. https://doi.org/10.1007/s00776-003-0755-2

Kessler, J.I., Nikizad, H., Shea, K.G., Jacobs Jr, J.C., Bebchuk, J.D., Weiss, J.M. (2014). The demographics and epidemiology of osteochondritis dissecans of the knee in children and adolescents. *The American Journal of Sports Medicine* 42:320–326. https://doi.org/10.1177/0363546513510390

Khoury, J., Jerushalmi, J., Loberant, N., Shtarker, H., Militianu, D., Zohar, K. (2007). Kohler disease: Diagnoses and assessment by bone scintigraphy. *Clinical Nuclear Medicine* 32:179–181. https://doi.org/10.1097/01.rlu.0000255026.52044.85

Kim, W.-C., Hiroshima, K., Imaeda, T. (2006). Multicenter study for Legg-Calvé-Perthes disease in Japan. *Journal of Orthopedic Science* 11:333–341. https://doi.org/10.1007/s00776-006-1021-1

Knüsel, C.J., Chundun, Z.C., Cardwell, P. (1992). Slipped proximal femoral epiphysis in a priest from the medieval period. *International Journal of Osteoarchaeology* 2:109–119. https://doi.org/10.1002/oa.1390020203

Lewis, M. (2017). *Paleopathology of Children: Identification of Pathological Conditions in the Human Skeletal Remains of Non-Adults*. San Diego: Academic Press.

Lowe, T.G., Line, B.G. (2007). Evidence based medicine: Analysis of Scheuermann kyphosis. *Spine* 32:115–119. https://doi.org/10.1097/BRS.0b013e3181354501

Martínez-Lavín, M. (2020). Hypertrophic osteoarthropathy. *Best Practice & Research Clinical Rheumatology* 34:101507. https://doi.org/10.1016/j.berh.2020.101507

Palazzo, C., Sailhan, F., Revel, M. (2014). Scheuermann's disease: An update. *Joint Bone Spine* 81:209–214. https://doi.org/10.1016/j.jbspin.2013.11.012

Pavone, V., Chisari, E., Vescio, A., Lizzio, C., Sessa, G., Testa, G. (2019). Aetiology of Legg-Calvé-Perthes disease: A systematic review. *World Journal of Orthopedics* 10:145–165. https://doi.org/10.5312/wjo.v10.i3.145

Peck, D., Voss, L.M., Voss, T.T. (2017). Slipped capital femoral epiphysis: Diagnosis and management. *American Family Physician* 95:779–784.

Resnick, D.J. (2002). *Diagnosis of Bone and Joint Disorders*, 4th edition. Philadelphia: Saunders.

Resnick, M., Jacobson, J.A., Chung, C.B., Kransdorf, M.J., Pathria, M.N. (2024). *Resnick's Bone and Joint Imaging*, 4th edition. Philadelphia: Saunders.

Rothschild, B.M., Rothschild, C. (1998). Recognition of hypertrophic osteoarthropathy in skeletal remains. *The Journal of Rheumatology* 21:2221–2227.

Schindler, O.S. (2007). Osteochondritis dissecans of the knee. *Current Orthopaedics* 21:47–58. https://doi.org/10.1016/j.cuor.2006.11.006

Shah, K.N., Racine, J., Jones, L.C., Aaron, R.K. (2015). Pathophysiology and risk factors for osteonecrosis. *Current Reviews in Musculoskeletal Medicine* 8:201–209. https://doi.org/10.1007/s12178-015-9277-8

Smrčka, V., Marik, I., Svenssonova, M., Likovsky, J. (2009). Legg-Calvé-Perthes disease in Czech archaeological material. *Clinical Orthopaedics and Related Research* 467:293–297. https://doi.org/10.1007/s11999-008-0527-6

Sorenson, K.H. (1964). *Scheuermann's Juvenile Kyphosis*. Copenhagen: Munksgaard.

Tekiteki, A., Good, W.R., Diggins, B., Anderson, G., Wong, C.A. (2020). Recurrent hypertrophic pulmonary osteoarthropathy in an adult with bronchiectasis. *Respirology Case Reports* 8:e00602. https://doi.org/10.1002/rcr2.602

Üstündağ, H., Deveci, A. (2011). A possible case of Scheuermann's disease from Akarçay Höyük, Birecik (Şanlıurfa, Turkey). *International Journal of Osteoarchaeology* 21:187–196. https://doi.org/10.1002/oa.1120

Waldron, T. (2020). *Palaeopathology*, 2nd edition. Cambridge: Cambridge University Press.

Wang, S., Wang, X., Teng, X., Li, S., Zhang, H., Shan, Z., Li, Y. (2021). Lumbar Scheuermann's disease found in a patient with osteogenesis imperfecta (OI) caused by a heterozygous mutation in *COL1A2* (c. 4048G> A): A case report. *BMC Musculoskeletal Disorders* 22:525. https://doi.org/10.1186/s12891-021-04401-7

Yap, F.Y., Skalski, M.R., Patel, D.B., Schein, A.J., White, E.A., Tomasian, A., Masih, S., Matcuk Jr, G.R. (2017). Hypertrophic osteoarthropathy: Clinical and imaging features. *RadioGraphics* 37:157–195. https://doi.org/10.1148/rg.2017160052

Chapter 4

Haematopoietic disorders

Haematopoietic disorders affect the haematopoietic system, that is, the system responsible for blood cell synthesis. These disorders may be caused by genetic or environmental factors. This chapter examines haematopoietic disorders with varied underlying aetiologies, including anaemias (both iron deficiency anaemia and genetic anaemias) and blood cancers (leukaemia and multiple myeloma).

Anaemias

Anaemias are characterised by a deficiency in red blood cells (also called erythrocytes), or a reduction in the haemoglobin content in these cells, or the presence of haemoglobin with abnormal morphology. Anaemias may be acquired or inherited. Acquired anaemias can arise from excessive red blood cell destruction or from significant loss of red blood cells due to other infections, trauma, menstruation, childbirth, and other factors. In addition, acquired anaemias may result from inadequate haemoglobin in the red blood cells because of insufficient dietary intake or absorption of iron. Therefore, while iron deficiency is a major cause for anaemia, many other factors contribute to the development of this disorder, and these factors often coexist in the same individual (e.g. malnutrition and infection). In addition, red blood cell production may be considered inadequate relative to the body's requirements under certain conditions, such as during childhood with its associated accelerated growth or during pregnancy when there are increased nutritional demands.

As mentioned above, anaemias are characterised by a deficiency in red blood cells, or reduced or abnormal haemoglobin. Haemoglobin is a protein with four polypeptide chains (two alpha and two beta). Each chain has haem (heme in American English), an iron-containing molecule important for the transportation of oxygen throughout the body. Individuals with anaemia have abnormally low haemoglobin levels, and their body suffers from oxygen deficiency. The lack of oxygen promotes the secretion of erythropoietin, a hormone that stimulates red blood cell production.

Red blood cells are synthesised in the red bone marrow. At birth, all bone marrow is red. Therefore, if there is a need for additional red blood cell production at this stage, additional marrow would need to be formed, occupying all available space within the bones. By the age of 25, a significant part of red bone marrow has transformed to fatty, yellow marrow, and the remaining red marrow is mostly found in the axial skeleton as well as the proximal femora and humeri. When there is increased demand for red blood cells after marrow conversion has started, existing areas of red marrow may expand, but there is also the possibility of

DOI: 10.4324/9781003475026-4

re-conversion of yellow marrow to red marrow. Age affects the efficiency of marrow re-conversion; individuals younger than 40 are better able to perform such a re-conversion.

As a consequence of the above processes, increased synthesis of red blood cells produces a limited hyperplastic response in the skeleton of adults, while the bone marrow is more reactive in juveniles, resulting in more pronounced skeletal changes. Furthermore, children have less mineralised and more highly vascularised bones compared to adolescents and adults; thus, their bones are affected more by marrow expansion. This explains why cribra orbitalia (CO) and porotic hyperostosis (PH), two cranial porotic lesions often associated with anaemias, typically develop during childhood, though healed CO and PH lesions often remain visible into adulthood (Box 4.1).

Several studies have examined the association between porous skeletal lesions, particularly CO and PH, but also cribra femoralis and cribra humeralis, with specific types of anaemia. The nature of these lesions has been so contested in paleopathology that a two-day meeting, the International Meeting on Porous Skeletal Lesions, was organised in 2023 at the Department of Life Sciences of the University of Coimbra. Traditionally, PH and CO have been linked to

Box 4.1 Porotic hyperostosis and cribra orbitalia

Porotic hyperostosis is the presence of porosity on the external surface of the cranial vault (Figures 4.1 and 4.2); it results from an expansion of the diploë and resultant resorption of the outer table. The lesion may appear as scattered, isolated, fine foramina or as large, potentially coalescent apertures, or even as protruding trabeculae. Porotic hyperostosis is mostly found in the parietal bones, though it may also occur in the frontal and occipital bones. Typically, the lesions are symmetric and do not affect the inner table. It is important to use the term porotic hyperostosis only for cranial bones that demonstrate both porosity and thickening due to the expansion of the diploë.

CO manifest as porosity on the orbital roofs and are usually found bilaterally (Figures 4.3 and 4.4). Similar to PH, these lesions are due to the expansion of the diploë.

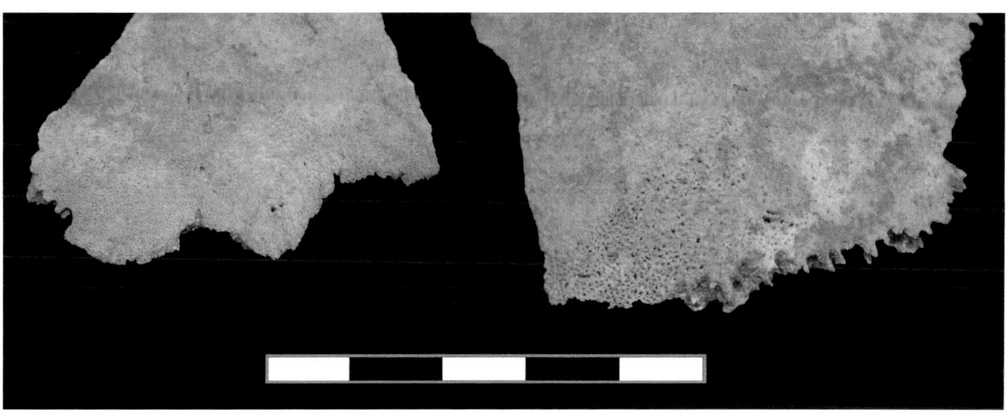

Figure 4.1 Mild porosity on parietal bones, though it is unclear whether this is associated with marrow hyperplasia. (Right: Infant, Ayia Napa Monastery, Cyprus, B3; left: Child, Ayia Napa Monastery, Cyprus, GBP34; photos by Anna Karligkioti; permission to use this image has been granted by the Director of the Department of Antiquities, Cyprus)

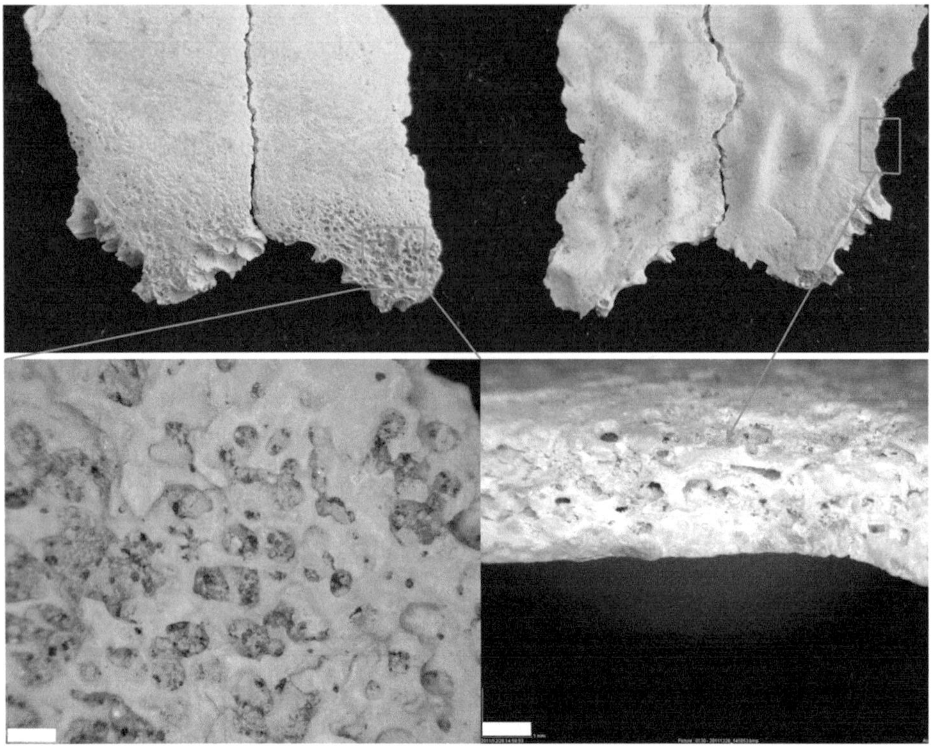

Figure 4.2 Porotic hyperostosis on the parietal bone of a Pleistocene hominin. (Figure 3 in Domínguez-Rodrigo et al. 2012; article licensed under a Creative Commons Attribution 4.0 International License)

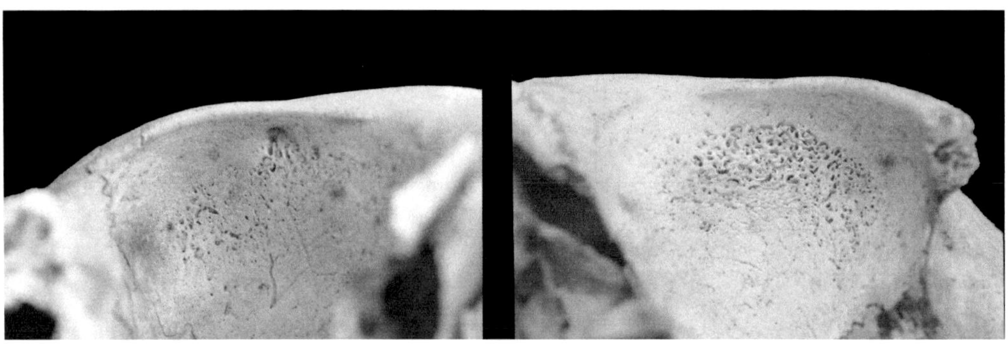

Figure 4.3 Cribra orbitalia; scattered fine porosity on the right orbit (left) and larger, often coalescent apertures on the left orbit (right). (Sbide, Roman/Byzantine; photos by Efthymia Nikita, with the kind permission of Dr. Ahmet Ihsan Aytek, Burdur Mehmet Akif Ersoy University)

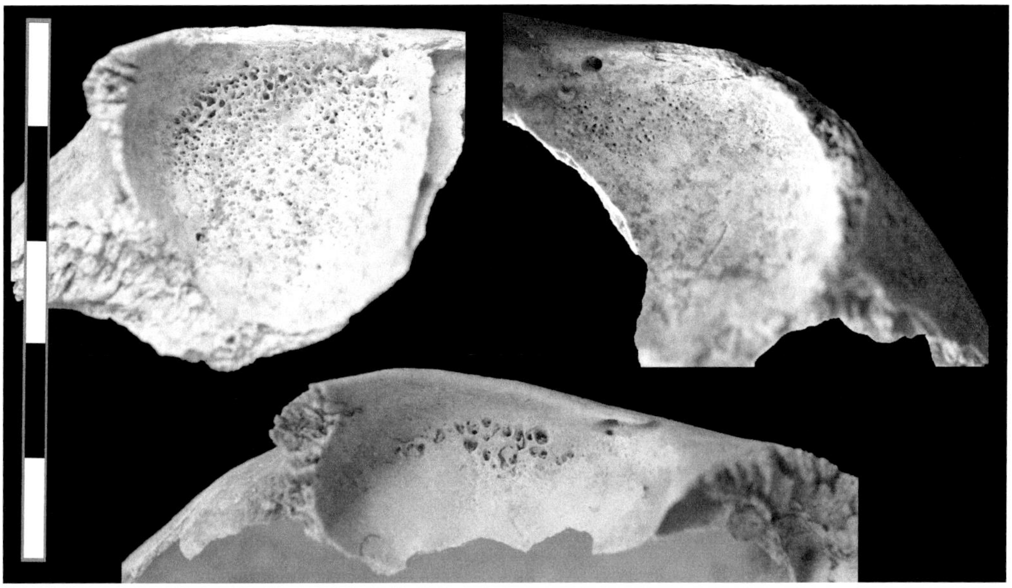

Figure 4.4 Cribra orbitalia; combination of large apertures and fine porosity that cover the orbital roof in the right orbit (upper left), fine porosity restricted to the anterior medial part of the left orbital roof (upper right), and large apertures in the anterior part of the right orbital roof (bottom). (Top: Kibyra, Roman Imperial; bottom: Philadelphia, Roman/Byzantine; photos by Efthymia Nikita, with the kind permission of Dr. Ahmet Ihsan Aytek, Burdur Mehmet Akif Ersoy University)

iron deficiency anaemia (IDA), which is the most common type of anaemia. However, more recently, it has been supported that iron deficiency may inhibit the proliferation of bone marrow and the formation of new erythrocytes, thereby raising doubts about whether iron deficiency alone is sufficient to cause CO and PH. These lesions have also been associated with haemolytic anaemias, including thalassaemia and sickle cell anaemia, as well as with megaloblastic anaemias resulting from deficiencies in vitamins B12 and B9. Beyond anaemia, the presence of porosities in the cranial vault and orbital roofs has been associated with rickets, scurvy, respiratory infections, subperiosteal inflammation, neoplastic conditions, osteoporosis, trauma, and other conditions. Importantly, PH and CO may not have the same aetiology. Given the several conditions associated with these lesions, PH and CO are often used in bioarchaeological studies as indicators of physiological stress occurring during childhood, mostly associated with infectious disease and malnutrition. Cribra humeralis and cribra femoralis have not been as extensively studied as CO and PH, and the correlation between these porous postcranial and cranial lesions in different skeletal assemblages has produced mixed results. Nonetheless, the aetiology of cribra humeralis and cribra femoralis has also been linked to physiological stress, namely infectious diseases resulting in anaemia, particularly when these occur during periods of accelerated growth. The complex aetiology of porous cranial and postcranial lesions, and its potential association with anaemias, but also with age, has been further supported by recent research focused on bone elemental concentrations in juveniles (Gomes et al. 2025). This research found an association between CO and cribra femoralis with lower Fe and higher S; the development of cribra femoralis was also linked to higher P, Ca, and Sr levels, while age was an important factor in the appearance of CO, cribra femoralis, and cribra humeralis.

Iron deficiency anaemia

IDA is the result of an iron deficit in the body (Figure 4.5). Iron is important for haemoglobin synthesis; thus, it is important in oxygen transport, as briefly noted above. Iron is also important for various physiological processes, including the transmission of nerve impulses, immune system functions, collagen synthesis, and the conversion of nutrients into energy. When red blood cells are deficient in iron, they become smaller than normal (microcytic) and have a pale colour (hypochromic) due to their reduced haemoglobin. These cells also have a shorter lifespan and are less capable of transporting oxygen.

IDA can have several aetiologies, including insufficient dietary intake of iron, increased physiological demands associated with growth or pregnancy, gastrointestinal malabsorption of iron, loss of blood (e.g. due to trauma, infections, or neoplastic conditions), genetics (e.g. genetic iron-refractory IDA), or a combination of these factors. In contemporary contexts, it is uncommon to develop IDA exclusively due to dietary deficiencies. Nonetheless, the increased nutritional requirements associated with growth in children and the reproductive needs of women may lead to diet-related forms of acquired anaemia, which are rarely seen in other parts of the population. Red meat, organ meats (e.g. liver), shellfish, certain fish (e.g. tuna, sardines, mackerel), poultry, as well as spinach, broccoli, legumes (e.g. peas, beans, lentils), and eggs are rich in iron. Haem iron, present in meat, poultry, and seafood, is more efficiently absorbed by the body than non-haem iron from plant-based sources. Calcium can inhibit the absorption of iron in the gastrointestinal tract when both are consumed together; however, the effect of this inhibition is unlikely to be clinically significant in the long term. Conversely, vitamin A tends to enhance iron absorption, and vitamin C promotes the absorption of non-haem iron. Individuals may be unable to absorb sufficient amounts of iron from dietary sources if they suffer from diarrhoea and/or vomiting due to infections. Indeed, anaemia in archaeological assemblages is often interpreted as the outcome of an interplay between diet and disease.

Iron deficiency during the first six months of life is rare because neonates rely on iron stores that have accumulated during gestation. Nevertheless, by the end of the fifth or sixth month, these iron reserves are depleted, thus iron deficiency is common among infants and children. Iron deficiency is common during weaning as children start consuming carbohydrate staples that are often low in iron, and they are also more exposed to gastrointestinal infections. This can have important implications since IDA has been associated with severe effects on child development, including growth delays and hindered cognitive development.

Thalassaemia

Thalassaemia is a hereditary type of anaemia where there is reduced or no synthesis of the alpha or beta globin chains of the haemoglobin molecule. As a result, the newly formed erythrocytes have inadequate haemoglobin content; thus, they are hypochromic and microcytic, with reduced capacity to transport oxygen throughout the body. Moreover, these red blood cells have a reduced lifespan. Thus, thalassaemia is characterised as a haemolytic anaemia.

Thalassaemia offers some resistance to malaria, and as a result of the selective pressures associated with malaria resistance, it shows a high prevalence in regions where malaria has been endemic. Nonetheless, the migration of individuals from endemic regions has led to the introduction of thalassaemia into previously unaffected parts of the world.

The classification of thalassaemias derives from the haemoglobin polypeptide chain affected by the disease. Most α-thalassaemias arise from deletions, while most β-thalassaemias

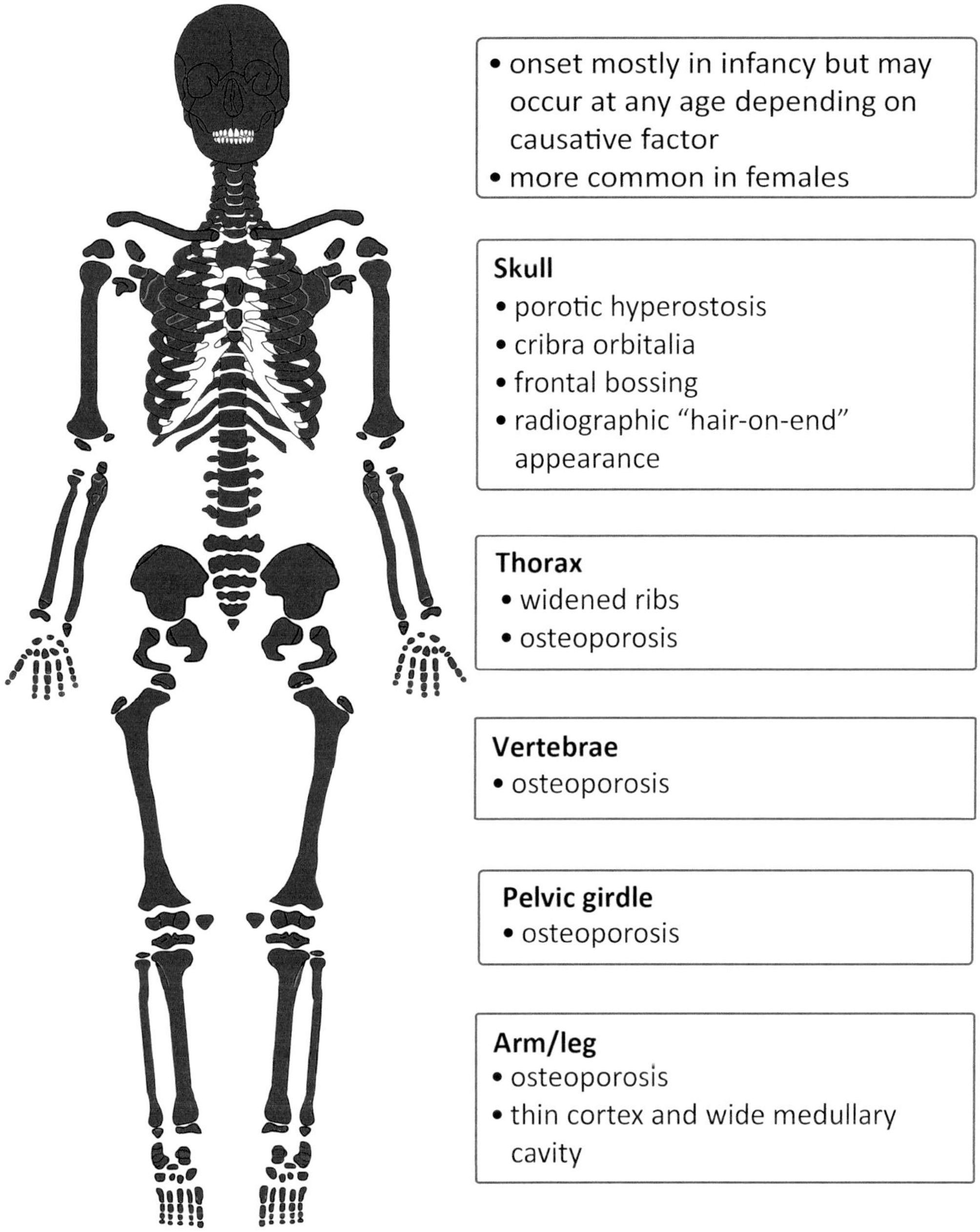

Figure 4.5 Skeletal manifestation of iron deficiency anaemia. Note that in children the entire skeleton may be affected, while in adults bone changes occur in areas of permanent haematopoietic activity (skull, spine, ribs, sternum, pelvis, proximal humerus and femur). (Data from Hershkovitz et al. 1997; Lanzkowsky 1977; Lewis 2017)

are linked to point mutations. The clinical manifestations of α-thalassaemia depend on the number of affected alpha globin genes, and range from asymptomatic to death in utero. The most common type of thalassaemia is β-thalassaemia; similarly, to α-thalassaemia this shows considerable variability in phenotypic expression, which is categorised into major, minor, and intermedia forms.

β-thalassaemia minor (T-minor) is typically asymptomatic and does not usually result in skeletal changes.

β-thalassaemia major (T-major) is the most severe form of this disorder. Affected individuals require regular blood transfusions for their survival; in the absence of treatment, there is a high risk of skeletal complications (e.g. thinning and brittleness of bones), as well as growth delay, and pronounced enlargement of the liver and spleen. In the past, most children diagnosed with T-major died in early childhood in the absence of regular blood transfusions.

β-thalassaemia intermedia is more severe than T-minor but less severe than T-major. Its symptoms usually appear at the age of two to four years and include pallor, fatigue, growth delay, enlarged liver and spleen, and skeletal deformities. Patients with β-thalassaemia intermedia often survive into adulthood without requiring blood transfusions, but they show significant bone marrow hyperplasia and associated skeletal changes. This particular form of thalassaemia is likely to be found more frequently in archaeological contexts and shows variable phenotypic expressions (Boxes 4.2 and 4.3, Figures 4.6–4.8).

Box 4.2 Diagnosing thalassaemia

The abnormal and premature fusion of the growth plates, especially in the proximal humerus, which is accompanied by limb shortening, varus deformity of the head, and lytic cortical defects in the shaft, is considered pathognomonic for thalassaemia by Hershkovitz et al. (1991). In contrast, Lagia et al. (2007) proposed that the odontofacial changes associated with thalassaemia are diagnostic of this condition. Vlok et al. (2021) argued that both the odontofacial features and the characteristic "rib-within-a-rib" radiographic appearance are strongly diagnostic of thalassaemia, while lack or poor pneumatisation of the sinuses, enlargement of the tubular hand and foot bones caused by marrow hyperplasia, premature fusion of the proximal humeral and distal femoral epiphyses, and widening of the ribs were deemed diagnostic of the condition.

Box 4.3 Eva-BeTa

Scianò et al. (2021) created a diagnostic tool for β-thalassaemia, called Eva-BeTa. This tool records various skeletal markers associated with this condition as present or absent; however, for cribra orbitalia and porotic hyperostosis, additional values are used depending on the results of microscopic and radiological analyses. Each marker is assigned a weight that reflects its diagnostic value: *non-specific indicators* include porotic hyperostosis, cribra orbitalia, growth arrest lines, long bone porosity, and premature fusion of the humeral epiphyses; *indicative/non-diagnostic indicators* include vertebral body deformity; *indicative/diagnostic indicators* include maxillary and mid-facial bone hypertrophy, hair-on-end, rib-within-a-rib, and enlarged foramina of the manual phalanges.

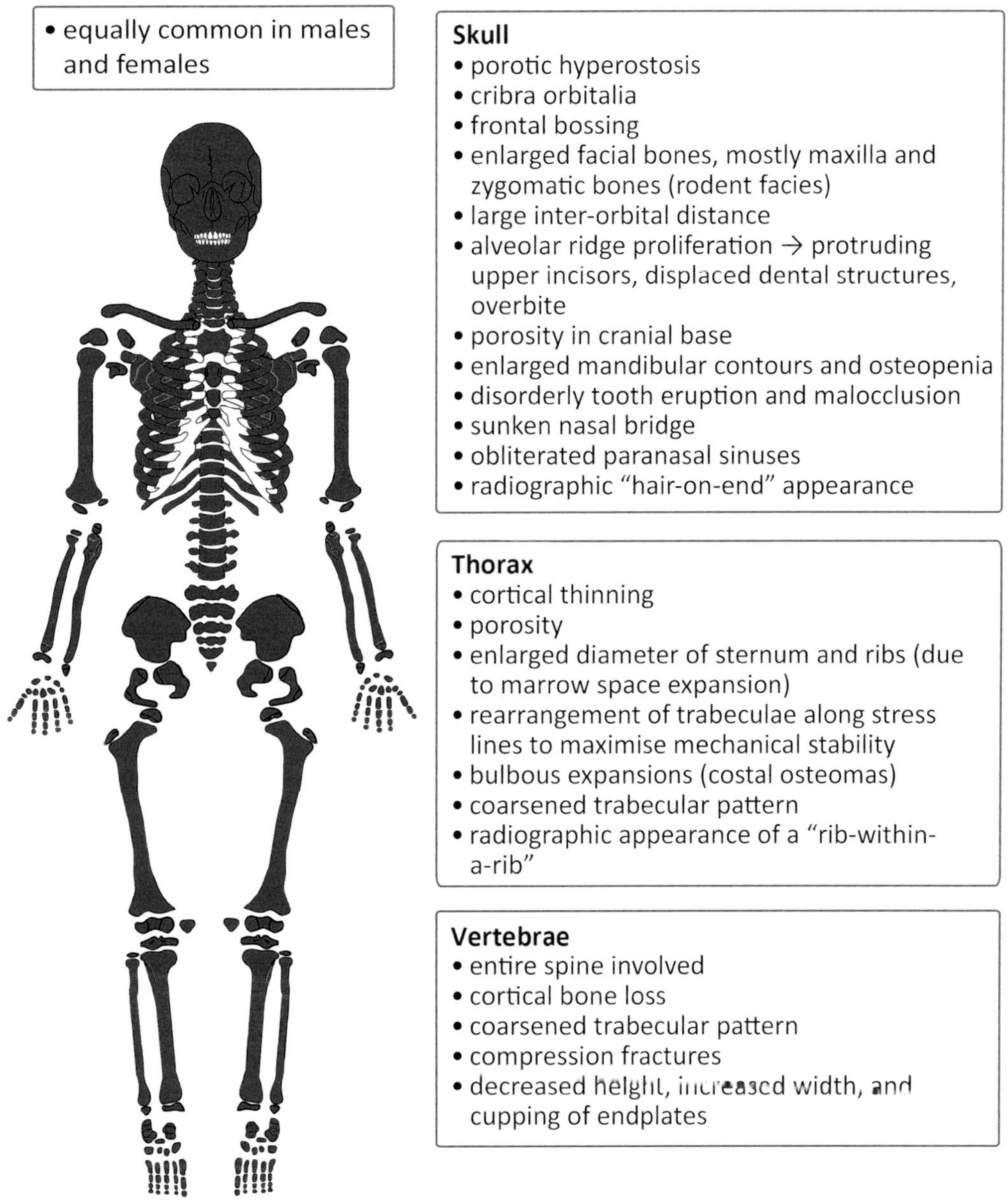

Figure 4.6 Skeletal manifestation of thalassaemia. Note that in children the entire skeleton may be affected, while in adults bone changes occur in areas of permanent haematopoietic activity. (Data from Caffey 1957; Grauer 2019; Hershkovitz et al. 1991; Lagia et al. 2007; Lawson et al. 1981; Scianò et al. 2021; Techataweewan et al. 2021)

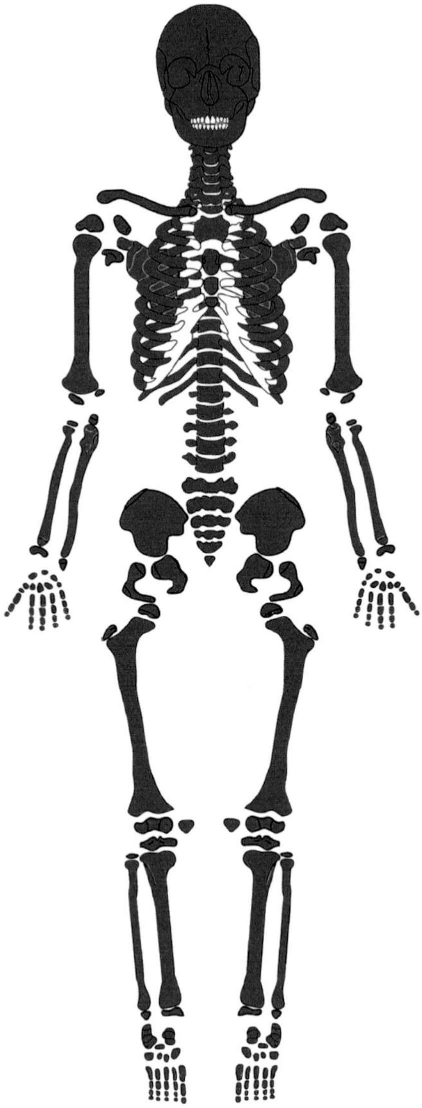

Shoulder girdle
- cortical thinning and porosity on clavicles and scapulae
- rearrangement of trabeculae along stress lines to maximise mechanical stability

Pelvic girdle
- thin and porous cortices
- protrusio acetabuli
- coarsened trabecular pattern
- rearrangement of trabeculae along stress lines to maximise mechanical stability

Hand/foot
- enlarged phalanges, metacarpals and metatarsals
- enlarged nutrient foramina
- thin and porous cortices
- widened medullary cavity
- rearrangement of trabeculae along stress lines to maximise mechanical stability
- pathological fractures

Arm/leg
- expanded medullary cavities
- thin and porous cortical bone
- enlarged nutrient foramina
- early and irregular proximal humeral or distal femoral, tibial or fibular epiphyseal union (unilateral or bilateral) → deformed shoulder (humerus varus) or other joints
- widened metaphyses and epiphyses
- pathological fractures
- coarsened trabecular pattern

Figure 4.6 (Continued)

Sickle cell anaemia

Sickle cell anaemia is another hereditary type of anaemia; it is due to a mutation that causes the substitution of valine for glutamic acid as the sixth amino acid in the beta globin chain. As a result of this substitution, the newly formed red blood cells have an elongated, sickle-like morphology. These cells have a short lifespan and are less efficient at oxygen transport. Furthermore, the sickle-shaped erythrocytes cannot effectively traverse capillaries and may aggregate, causing an obstruction in blood flow. Therefore, in sickle cell anaemia, bone changes result from two mechanisms: marrow hyperplasia due to an increased demand for erythropoiesis, and the formation of blood clots, mostly within the long bones. These clots inhibit the delivery of essential

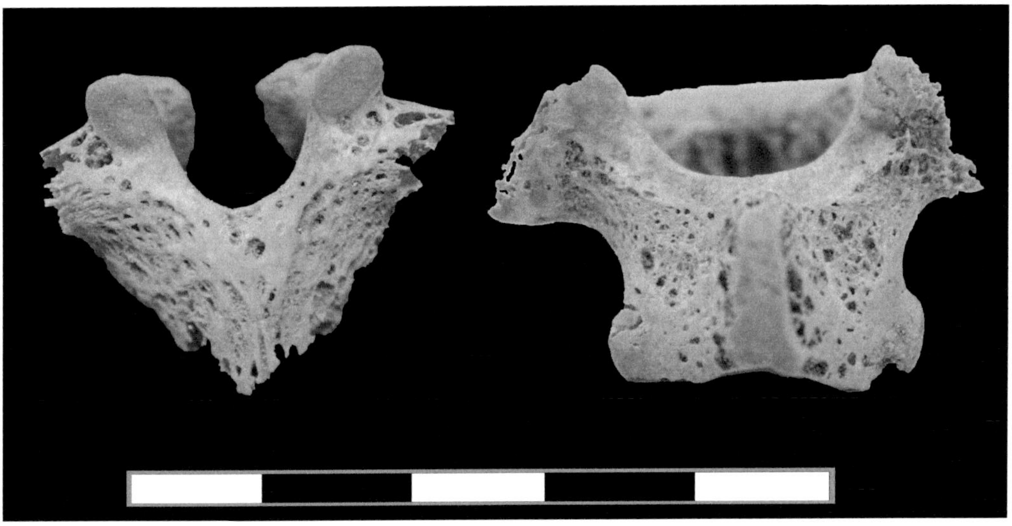

Figure 4.7 Thoracic and lumbar vertebrae with diffuse porosity, probably associated with marrow expansion due to thalassaemia, also taking into account the high prevalence of thalassaemia in Cyprus, where these elements were excavated. (Child, Ayia Napa Monastery, Cyprus, B1-GBP3; photos by Anna Karligkioti; permission to use this image has been granted by the Director of the Department of Antiquities, Cyprus)

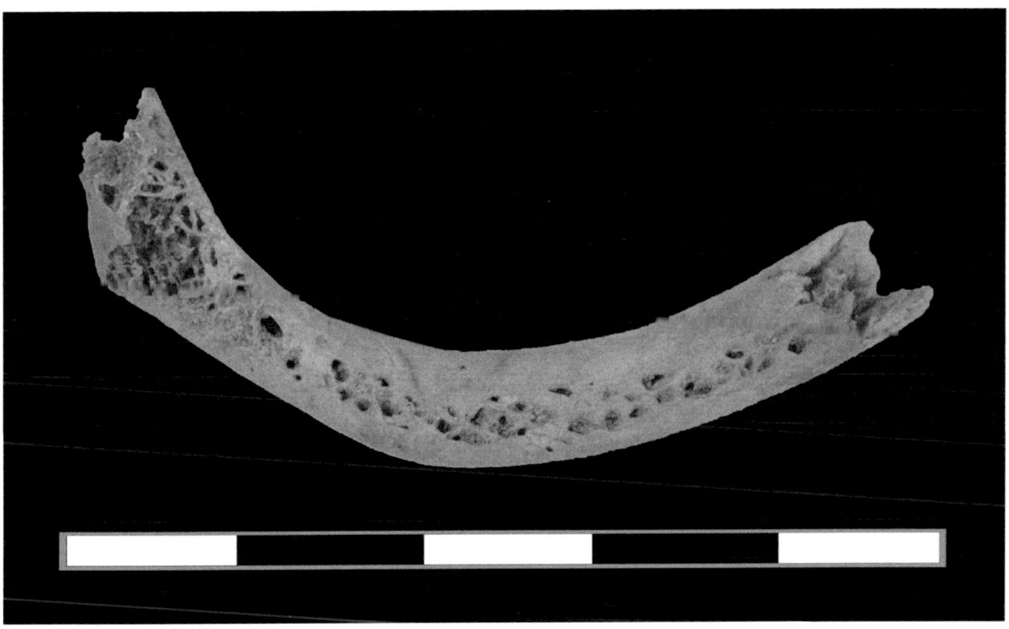

Figure 4.8 Rib with diffuse porosity, probably associated with marrow expansion due to thalassaemia. (Child, Ayia Napa Monastery, Cyprus, B1-GBP3; photo by Anna Karligkioti; permission to use this image has been granted by the Director of the Department of Antiquities, Cyprus)

nutrients to the bones and surrounding tissues, leading to necrosis and secondary infections (Figures 4.9 and 4.10). Similarly to thalassaemia, carriers of the sickle cell trait show some resistance to malaria, which may influence the geographic distribution of this disease.

Sickle cell anaemia manifests in homozygous individuals, while carriers of the sickle cell trait may remain asymptomatic. Infants with sickle cell anaemia will develop symptoms after six months of age. In the absence of treatment, especially in past contexts, most affected individuals died by the age of ten years, often much sooner. Therefore, skeletal manifestations of sickle cell anaemia are rarely identified in adolescents or adults in bioarchaeological assemblages.

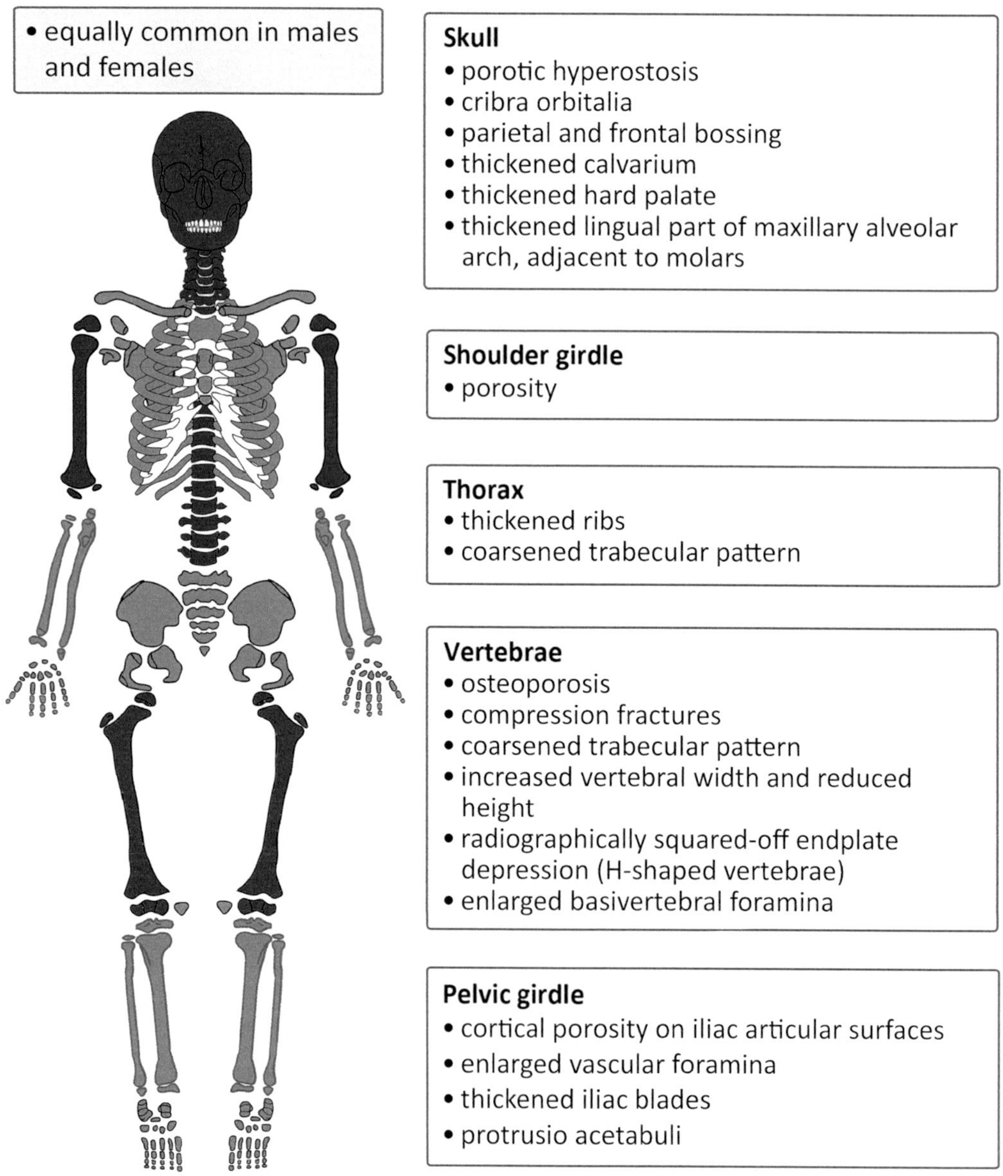

Figure 4.9 Skeletal manifestation of sickle cell anaemia. (Data from Aguilar et al. 2005; Almeida and Roberts 2005; Ganguly et al. 2011; Grauer 2019; Hershkovitz et al. 1997; Lewis 2017)

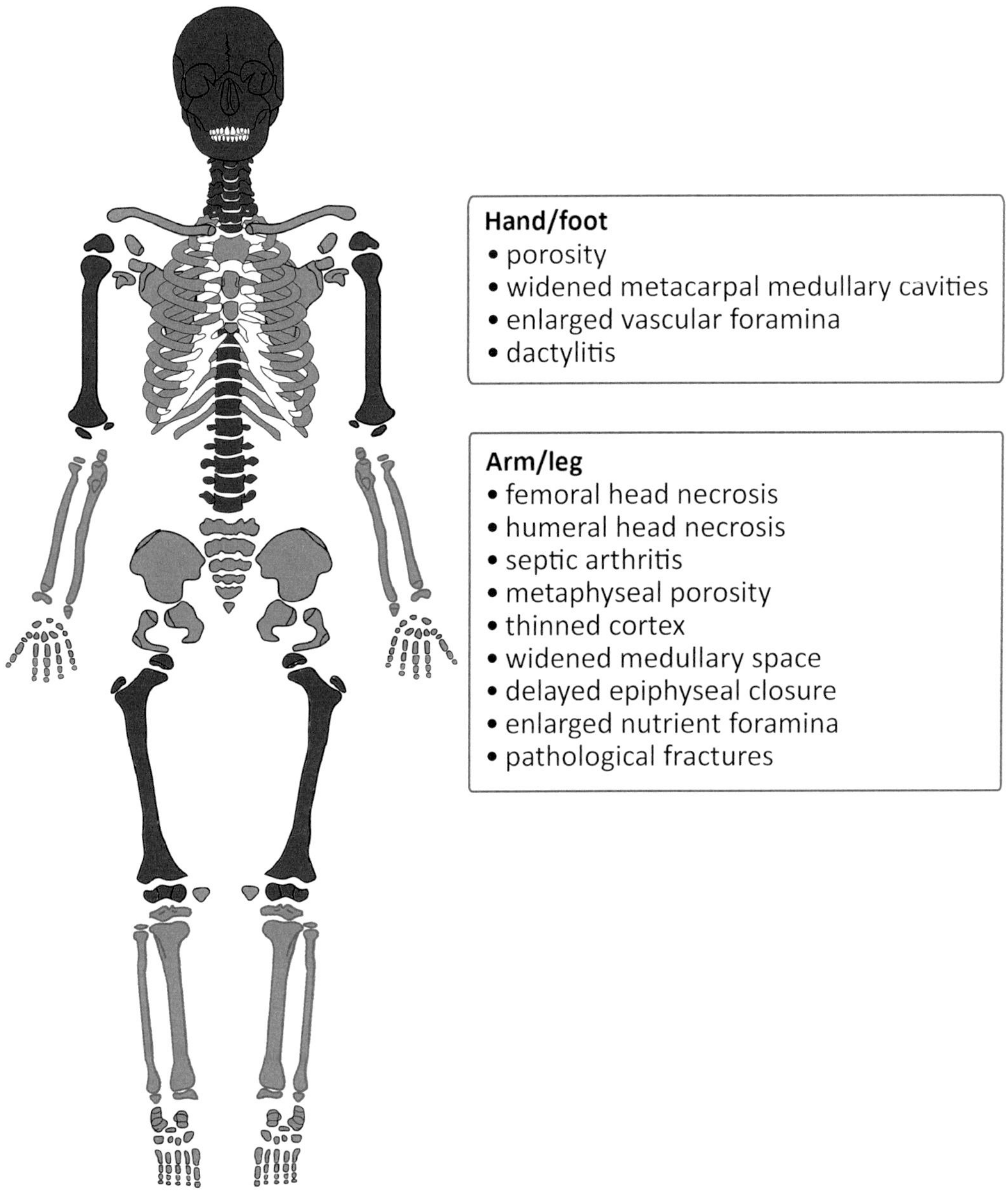

Figure 4.9 (Continued)

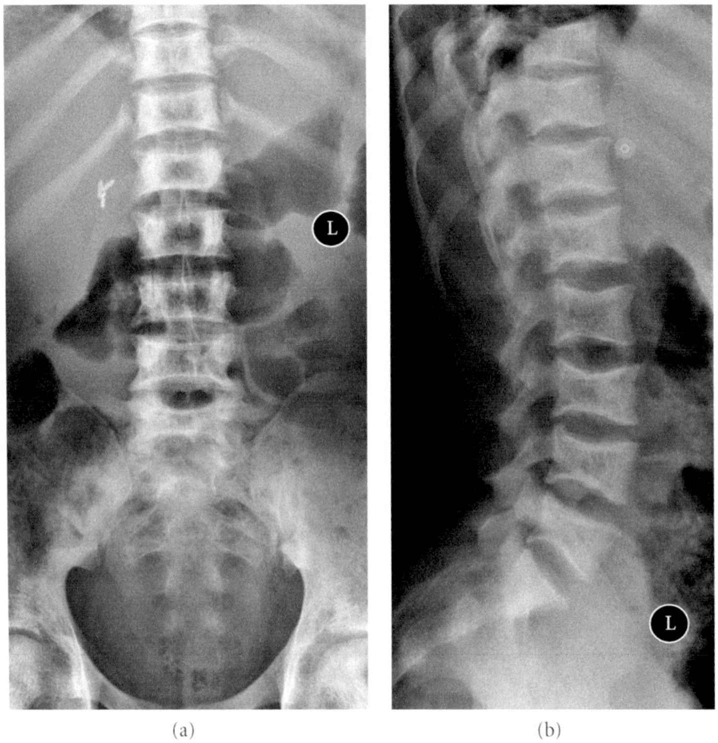

Figure 4.10 Radiographs of the lumbar spine of an individual with sickle cell anaemia. Note the H-shaped vertebrae due to endplate depressions. (Figure 11 in Ganguly et al. 2011; article licensed under a Creative Commons Attribution 3.0 Unported License)

Leukaemia

Leukaemia is a type of cancer associated with the uncontrolled proliferation of abnormal blood cells (Figures 4.11–4.13). These aberrant cells are called leukaemia cells, and they occupy an increasing part of the space within the bone marrow, inhibiting the development of healthy mature blood cells. Leukaemia mostly affects the white blood cells, but it may involve other blood cells as well. According to its progression, leukaemia may be acute or chronic. Acute leukaemia progresses aggressively and rapidly; the abnormal cells are immature, and the condition hinders their maturation and functionality. In contrast, chronic leukaemia is less aggressive and involves mature or partially mature cells that proliferate at a slower rate. While acute leukaemia affects both children and adults, chronic leukaemia is primarily seen in adults.

- mostly affecting children (peak prevalence between 2-5 years), though it may occur at any age
- more common in males

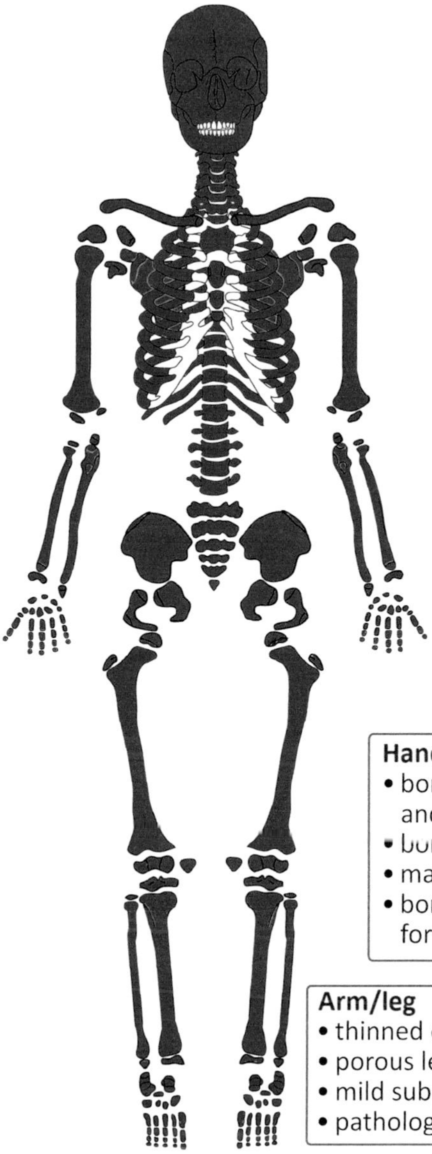

General
- diffuse osteopenia
- lytic lesions of variable size (multiple lytic lesions and large single lesions)
- enlarged vascular foramina
- mild subperiosteal new bone formation
- lesions observed on a few elements or throughout the skeleton
- pathological fractures

Skull
- ectocranial pitting (mostly in parietal, occipital, temporal and frontal bones)
- endocranial pitting
- sutural diastasis

Shoulder girdle
- pitting on clavicle and scapula

Thorax
- bone resorption in sternum and ribs
- subperiosteal new bone formation on ribs

Vertebrae
- porosity (mostly in the bodies) without marginal reactions
- compression fractures

Pelvic girdle
- pitting

Hand/foot
- bone resorption in metacarpal/metatarsal diaphyses and metaphyses
- bone resorption in phalangeal diaphyses
- marginal joint erosions
- bone resorption and subperiosteal new bone formation on tarsals

Arm/leg
- thinned cortices
- porous lesions on metaphyses without marginal reactions
- mild subperiosteal new bone formation
- pathological fractures in lower limbs (usually bilateral)

Figure 4.11 Skeletal manifestation of leukaemia in juveniles. (Data from Angsubhakorn and Suvannasankha 2018; Grauer 2019; Isidro et al. 2019; Klaus 2016; Pear 1974; Riccio et al. 2013; Rothschild et al. 1997)

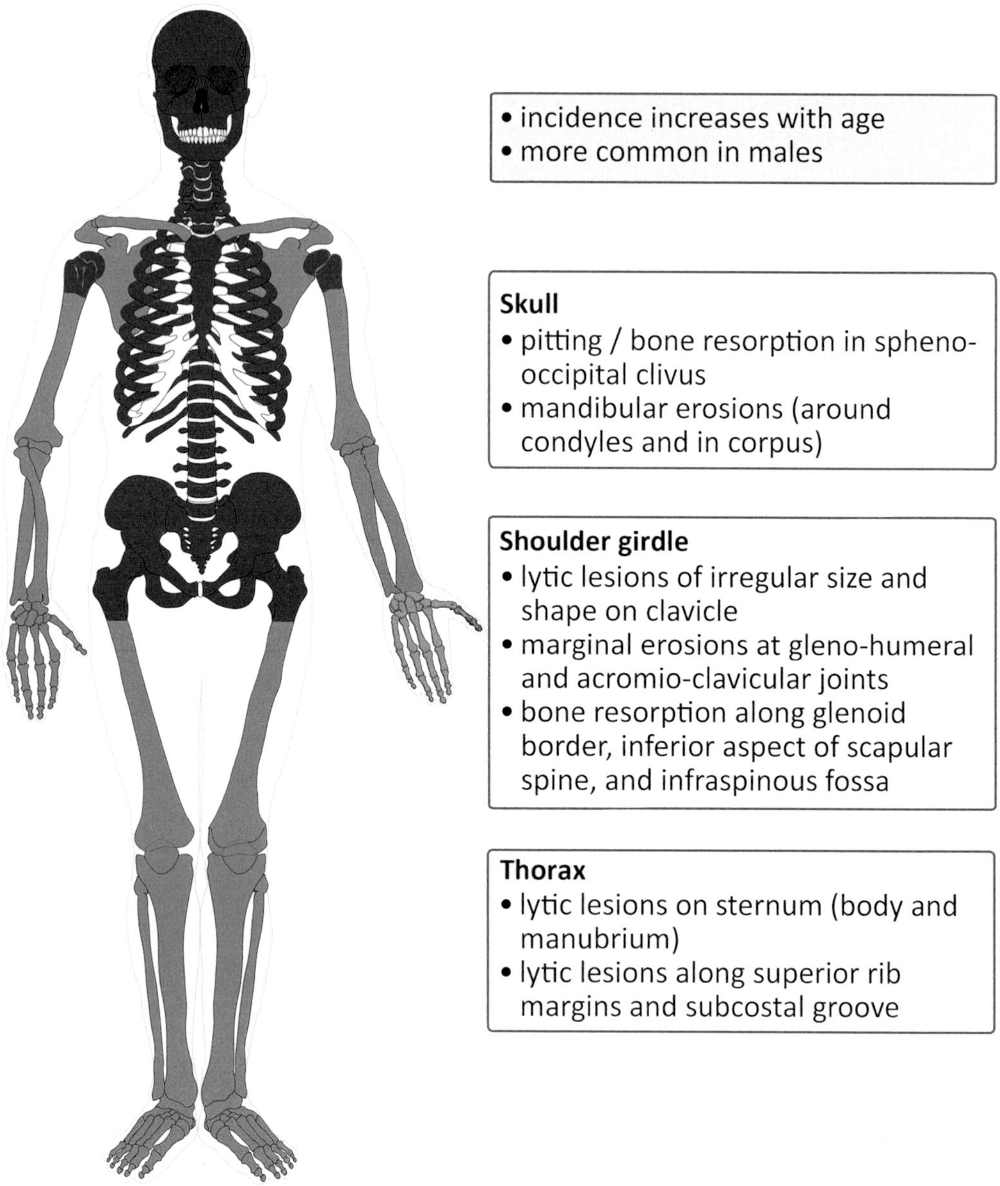

Figure 4.12 Skeletal manifestation of leukaemia in adults. (Data from Angsubhakorn and Suvannasankha 2018; Isidro et al. 2019; Rothschild et al. 1997)

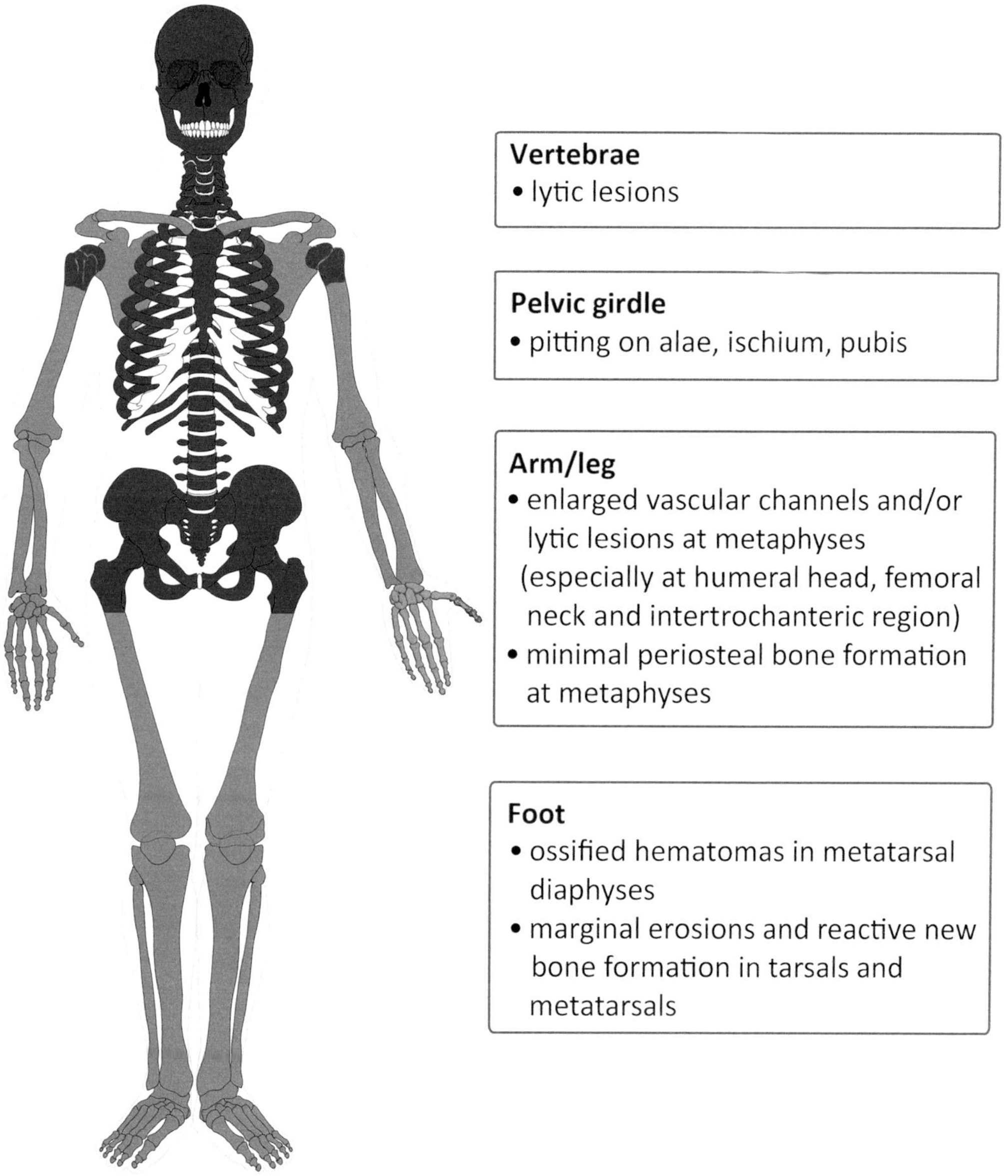

Figure 4.12 (Continued)

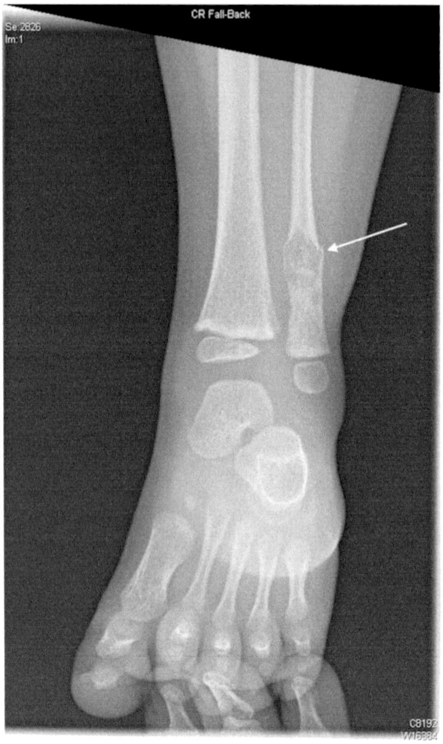

Figure 4.13 Radiograph of the ankle of an individual with leukaemia. Note the lytic lesion on the distal fibular metaphysis. (Figure 2 in Iyer et al. 2022; article licensed under a Creative Commons Attribution-ShareAlike 4.0 International license)

Multiple myeloma

Multiple myeloma is a cancer that involves abnormal plasma cells, which are a type of white blood cell (Figures 4.14–4.17). Plasma cells are important in immune response as they synthesise antibodies that fight infections. However, in cases of multiple myeloma, neoplastic plasma cells (myeloma cells) accumulate within the bone marrow. This accumulation leads to the displacement of normal haematopoietic cells in the bone marrow and causes bone tissue damage.

Multiple myeloma arises from an interplay of genetic and environmental factors. Clinical studies indicate that advancing age, male sex, ancestry (individuals of African descent are much more frequently affected than individuals of European descent), and family history are significant risk factors. Additionally, environmental factors, such as contact with certain chemicals used in metalworking, agriculture, and other industries, as well as exposure to ionising radiation, have been associated with the development of multiple myeloma. Finally, obesity and autoimmunity may contribute to increased risk for developing multiple myeloma.

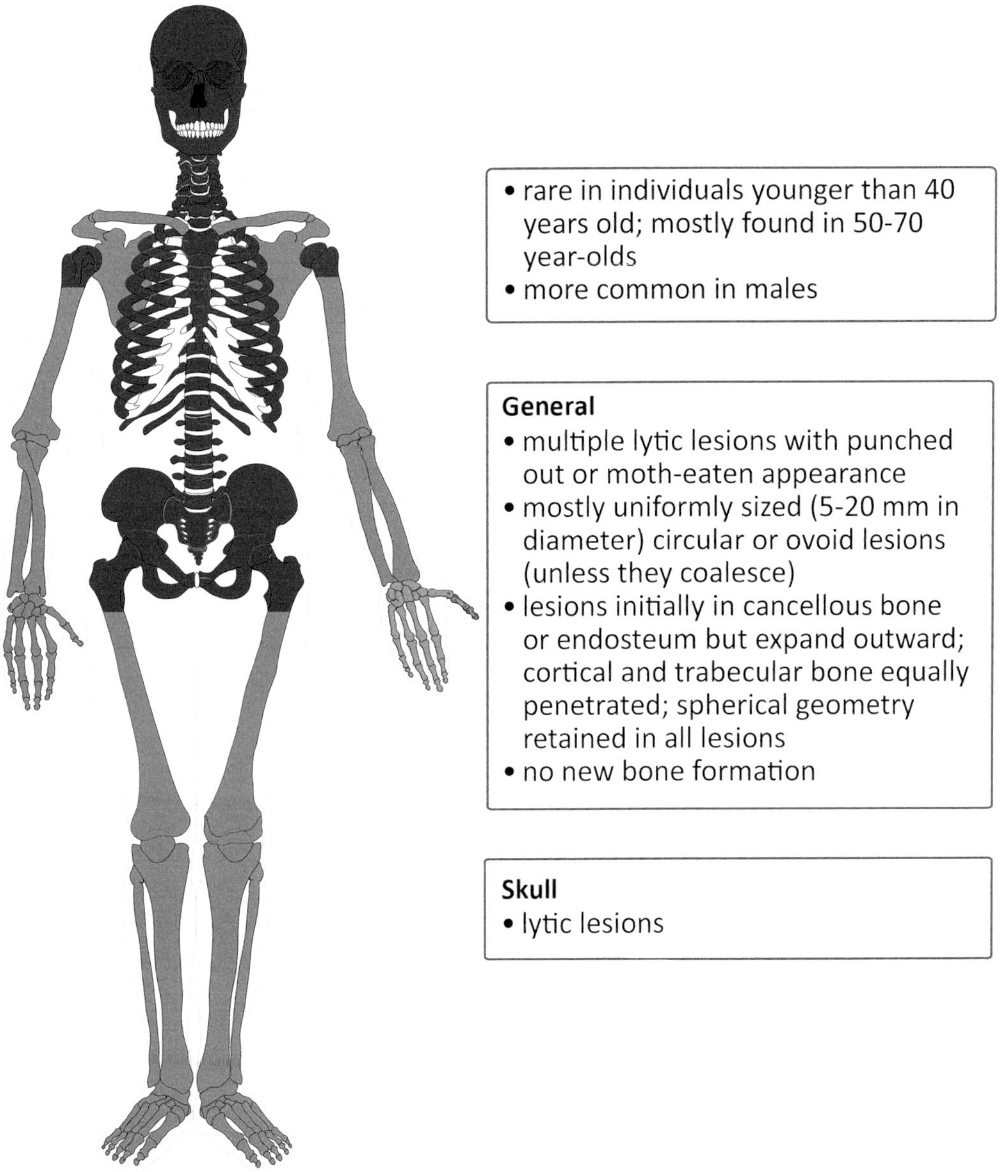

Figure 4.14 Skeletal manifestation of multiple myeloma. (Data from Borggrefe et al. 2015; Grauer 2019; Hameed et al. 2014; Kuehl and Bergsagel 2002; Rothschild et al. 1998; Strouhal 1991)

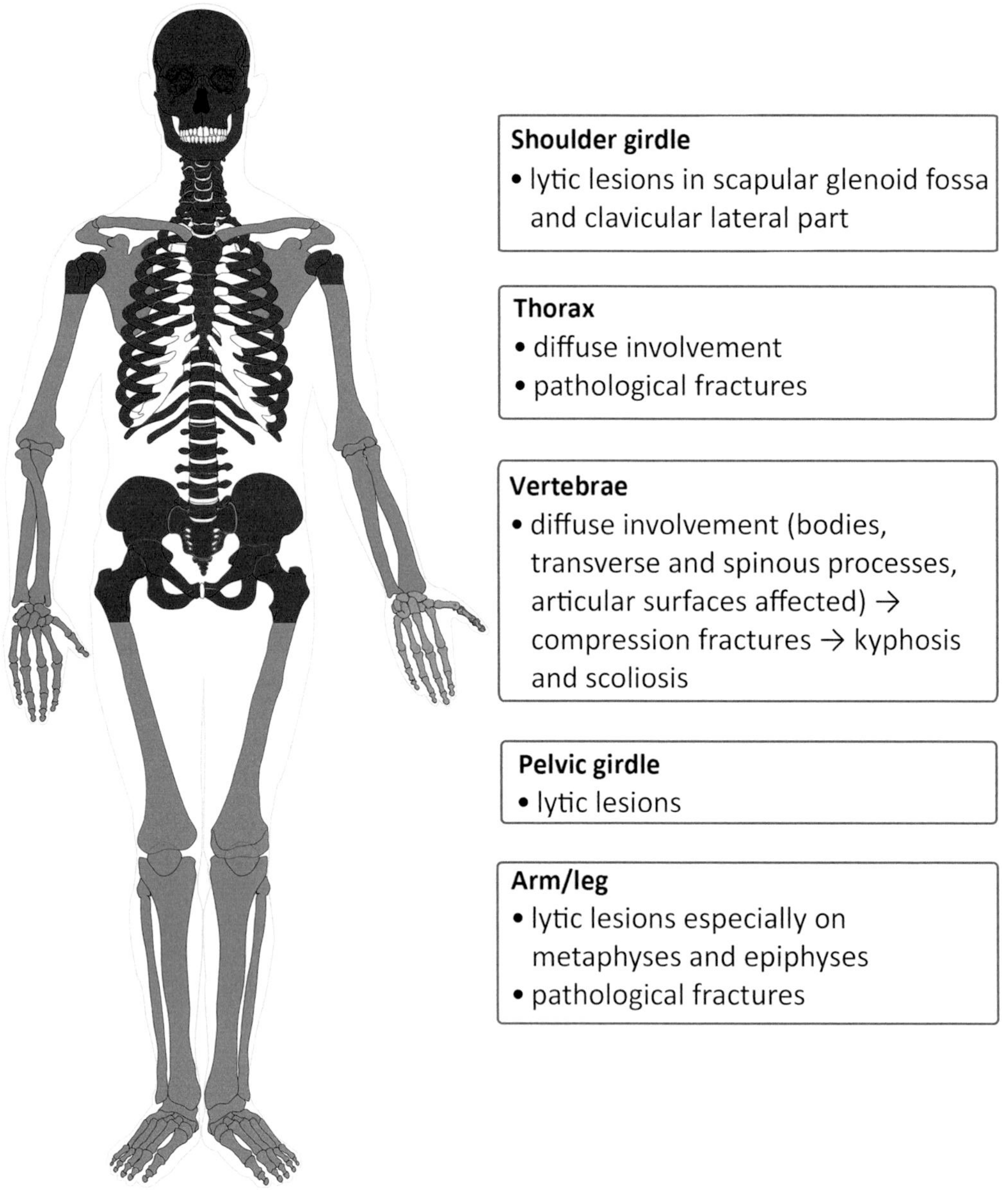

Figure 4.14 (Continued)

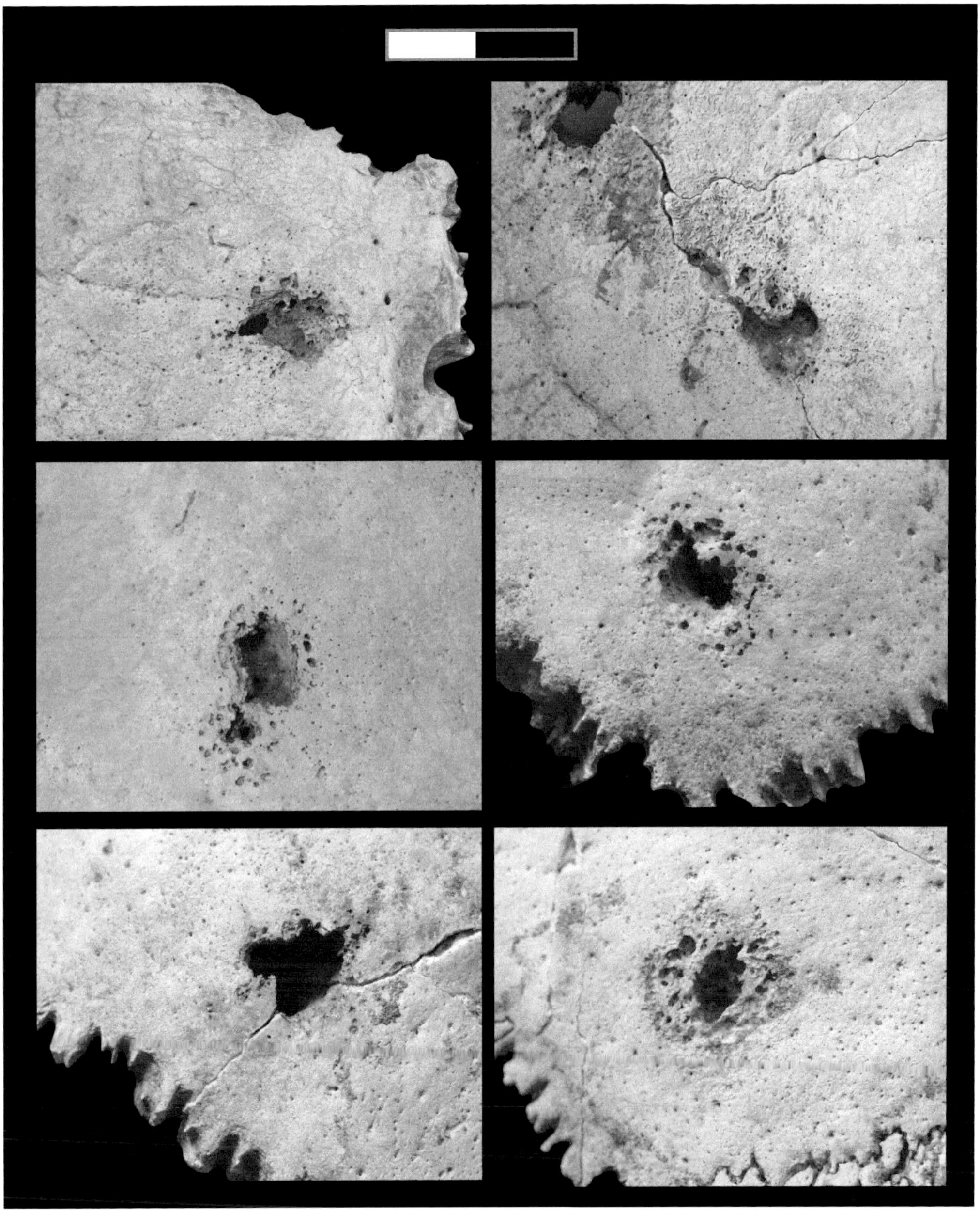

Figure 4.15 Probable multiple myeloma. Note the multiple, small, and uniformly sized circular/ovoid lytic lesions on the cranial vault, coupled with a lack of new bone formation in all cases except for the lesion in the upper right panel where minimal new bone formation is visible. (Male, Old adult, All Saints Church, Fishergate, York, Medieval, Y-2635; photos by Efthymia Nikita; copyright: Human Skeletal Collection, University of Sheffield)

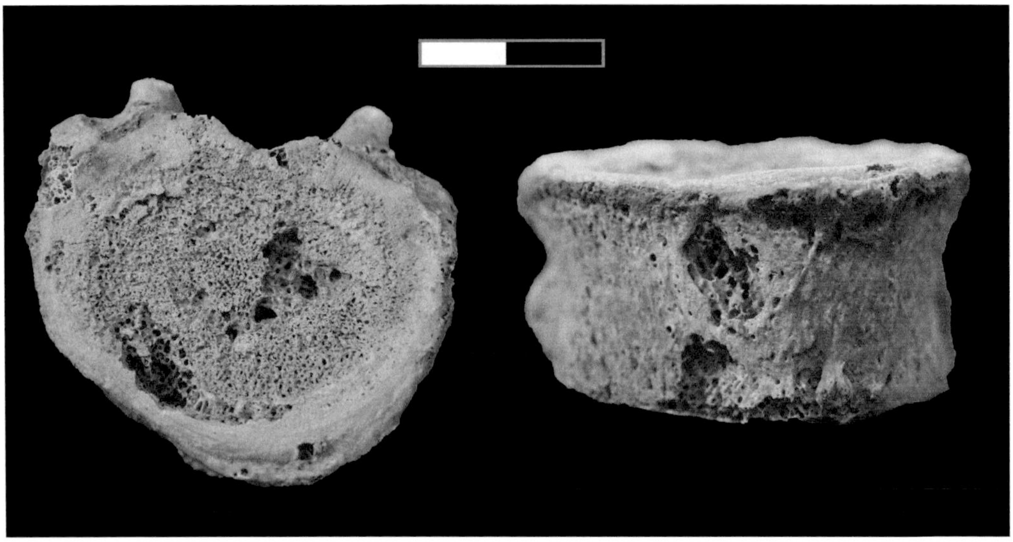

Figure 4.16 Probable multiple myeloma. Note the multiple, small, and uniformly sized lytic lesions on different parts of the vertebral body. (Same individual as in Figure 4.15; photos by Efthymia Nikita; copyright: Human Skeletal Collection, University of Sheffield)

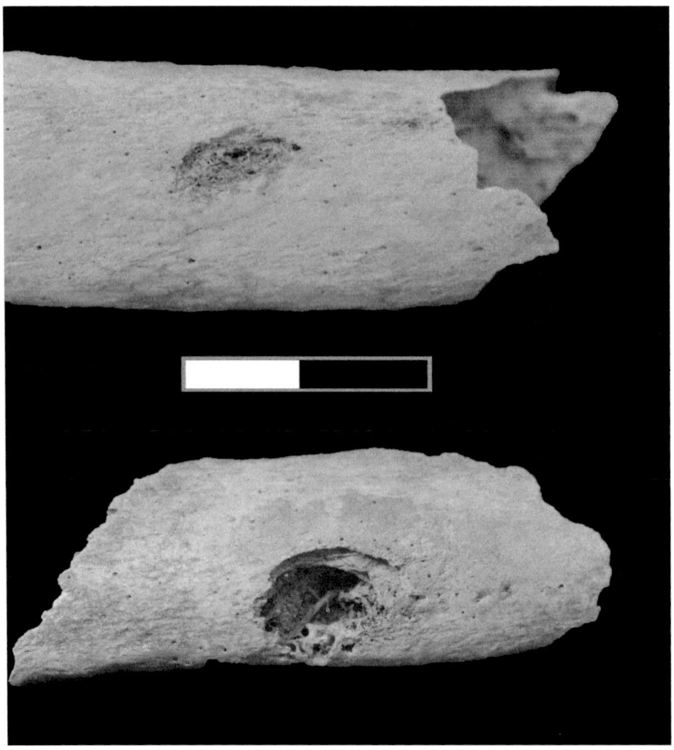

Figure 4.17 Probable multiple myeloma. Note the small and uniformly sized lytic lesions on different rib shafts; no new bone formation is seen in the upper image but minimal in the lower one. (Same individual as in Figures 4.15 and 4.16; photos by Efthymia Nikita; copyright: Human Skeletal Collection, University of Sheffield)

References and suggested readings

Aguilar, C., Vichinsky, E., Neumayr, L. (2005). Bone and joint disease in sickle cell disease. *Hematology/Oncology Clinics* 19:929–941.

Almeida, A., Roberts, I. (2005). Bone involvement in sickle cell disease. *British Journal of Haematology* 129:482–490. https://doi.org/10.1111/j.1365-2141.2005.05476.x

Angsubhakorn, N., Suvannasankha, A. (2018). Acute lymphoblastic leukaemia with osteolytic bone lesions: Diagnostic dilemma. *BMJ Case Reports 2018*: bcr-2018-225008. https://doi.org/10.1136/bcr-2018-225008

Biehler-Gomez, L., Giordano, G., Cattaneo, C. (2019). Multiple myeloma bone lesions in skeletal remains: Report of two known cases from the 20th century CAL Milano Cemetery Skeletal Collection. *International Journal of Osteoarchaeology* 29:101–107. https://doi.org/10.1002/oa.2721

Borggrefe, J., Giravent, S., Campbell, G., Thomsen, F., Chang, D., Franke, M., Günther, A., Heller, M., Wulff, A. (2015). Association of osteolytic lesions, bone mineral loss and trabecular sclerosis with prevalent vertebral fractures in patients with multiple myeloma. *European Journal of Radiology* 84:2269–2274. https://doi.org/10.1016/j.ejrad.2015.07.024

Brickley, M.B. (2018). *Cribra orbitalia* and porotic hyperostosis: A biological approach to diagnosis. *American Journal of Physical Anthropology* 167:896–902. https://doi.org/10.1002/ajpa.23701

Brickley, M.B. (2024). Perspectives on anemia: Factors confounding understanding of past occurrence. *International Journal of Paleopathology* 44:90–104. https://doi.org/10.1016/j.ijpp.2023.12.001

Caffey, J. (1957). Cooley's anaemia: A review of the roentgenographic findings in the skeleton. *The American Journal of Roentgenology* 78:381–391.

Cole, G., Waldron, T. (2019). Cribra orbitalia: Dissecting an ill-defined phenomenon. *International Journal of Osteoarchaeology* 29:613–621. https://doi.org/10.1002/oa.2757

De Sanctis, V., Soliman, A.T., Elsefdy, H., Soliman, N., Bedair, E., Fiscina, B., Kattamis, C. (2018). Bone disease in β thalassemia patients: Past, present and future perspectives. *Metabolism* 80:66–79. https://doi.org/10.1016/j.metabol.2017.09.012

Djuric, M., Milovanovic, P., Janovic, A., Draskovic, M., Djukic, K., Milenkovic, P. (2008). Porotic lesions in immature skeletons from Stara Torina, late medieval Serbia. *International Journal of Osteoarchaeology* 18:458–475. https://doi.org/10.1002/oa.955

Domínguez-Rodrigo, M., Pickering, T.R., Diez-Martín, F., Mabulla, A., Musiba, C., Trancho, G., Baquedano, E., Bunn, H.T., Barboni, D., Santonja, M., Uribelarrea, D., Ashley, G.M., Martínez-Ávila, M.S., Barba, R., Gidna, A., Yravedra, J., Arriaza, C. (2012). Earliest porotic hyperostosis on a 1.5-million-year-old hominin, Olduvai Gorge, Tanzania. *PLoS ONE* 7: e46414. https://doi.org/10.1371/journal.pone.0046414

Faerman, M., Nebel, A., Filon, D., Thomas, M.G., Bradman, N., Ragsdale, B.D., Schultz, M., Oppenheim, A. (2000). From a dry bone to a genetic portrait: A case study of sickle cell anemia. *American Journal of Physical Anthropology* 111:153–163. https://doi.org/10.1002/(SICI)1096-8644(200002)111:2%3C153::AID-AJPA2%3E3.0.CO;2-O

Ganguly, A., Boswell, W., Aniq, H. (2011). Musculoskeletal manifestations of sickle cell anaemia: A pictorial review. *Anemia* 2011:794283. https://doi.org/10.1155/2011/794283

Gomes, R.A.M.P., Petit, J., Dutour, O., Santos, A.L. (2022). Frequency and co-occurrence of porous skeletal lesions in identified non-adults from Portugal (19th to 20th centuries) and its association with respiratory infections as cause of death. *International Journal of Osteoarchaeology* 32:1061–1072. https://doi.org/10.1002/oa.3132

Gomes, R.A.M.P., Catarino, L., Santos, A.L. (2025). The role of Fe, S, P, Ca, and Sr in porous skeletal lesions: A study on non-adult individuals using pXRF. *Biological Trace Element Research* 203:591–607. https://doi.org/10.1007/s12011-024-04187-4

Grauer, A.L. (2019). Circulatory, reticuloendothelial, and hematopoietic disorders. In *Ortner's Identification of Pathological Conditions in Human Skeletal Remains*, edited by Buikstra, J., pp. 491–530. San Diego: Academic Press.

Hameed, A., Brady, J.J., Dowling, P., Clynes, M., O'Gorman, P. (2014). Bone disease in multiple myeloma: Pathophysiology and management. *Cancer Growth Metastasis* 7:33–42. https://doi.org/10.4137/CGM.S16817

Hershkovitz, I., Ring, B., Speirs, M., Galili, E., Kislev, M., Edelson, G., Hershkovitz, A. (1991). Possible congenital hemolytic anemia in prehistoric coastal inhabitants of Israel. *American Journal of Physical Anthropology* 85:7–13. https://doi.org/10.1002/ajpa.1330850103

Hershkovitz, I., Rothschild, B.M., Latimer, B., Dutour, O., Léonetti, G., Greenwald, C.M., Rothschild, C., Jellema, L.M. (1997). Recognition of sickle cell anemia in skeletal remains of children. *American Journal of Physical Anthropology* 104:213–226. https://doi.org/10.1002/(SICI)1096-8644(199710)104:2%3C213::AID-AJPA8%3E3.0.CO;2-Z

Isidro, A., Seiler, R., Seco, M. (2019). Leukemia in ancient Egypt: Earliest case and state-of-the-art techniques for diagnosing generalized osteolytic lesions. *International Journal of Osteoarchaeology* 29:273–280. https://doi.org/10.1002/oa.2736

Iyer, A., Mangal, R., Stead, T., Barbera, A. (2022). Acute lymphoblastic leukemia presenting as a pathologic fibular fracture. *Orthopedic Reviews* 14. https://doi.org/10.52965/001c.37419

Johnson, E.E., Wessling-Resnick, M. (2012). Iron metabolism and the innate immune response to infection. *Microbes and Infection* 14:207–216. https://doi.org/10.1016/j.micinf.2011.10.001

Klaus, H.D. (2016). A probable case of acute childhood leukemia: Skeletal involvement, differential diagnosis, and the bioarchaeology of cancer in South America: Acute childhood leukemia in Lambayeque, Peru. *International Journal of Osteoarchaeology* 26:348–358. https://doi.org/10.1002/oa.2411

Kuehl, W.M., Bergsagel, P.L. (2002). Multiple myeloma: Evolving genetic events and host interactions. *Nature Reviews Cancer* 2:175–187. https://doi.org/10.1038/nrc746

Lagia, A., Eliopoulos, C., Manolis, S. (2007). Thalassemia: Macroscopic and radiological study of a case. *International Journal of Osteoarchaeology* 17:269–285. https://doi.org/10.1002/oa.881

Lanzkowsky, P. (1977). Osseous changes in iron deficiency anemia – implications for paleopathology. In *Porotic Hyperostosis: An Enquiry*, edited by Cockburn, E., pp. 23–34. Detroit: Paleopathology Association.

Lawson, J., Ablow, R., Pearson, H. (1981). The ribs in thalassemia I: The relationship to therapy. *Pediatric Radiology* 140:663–672. https://doi.org/10.1148/radiology.140.3.7280233

Lewis, M.E. (2012). Thalassaemia: Its diagnosis and interpretation in past skeletal populations. *International Journal of Osteoarchaeology* 22:685–693. https://doi.org/10.1002/oa.1229

Lewis, M. (2017). *Paleopathology of Children: Identification of Pathological Conditions in the Human Skeletal Remains of Non-Adults*. San Diego: Academic Press.

McIlvaine, B.K. (2015). Implications of reappraising the iron-deficiency anemia hypothesis. *International Journal of Osteoarchaeology* 25:997–1000. https://doi.org/10.1002/oa.2383

O'Donnell, L., Hill, E.C., Anderson, A.S., Edgar, H.J.H. (2020). Cribra orbitalia and porotic hyperostosis are associated with respiratory infections in a contemporary mortality sample from New Mexico. *American Journal of Physical Anthropology* 173:721–733. https://doi.org/10.1002/ajpa.24131

O'Donnell, L., Buikstra, J.E., Hill, E.C., Anderson, A.S., O'Donnell Jr, M.J. (2023). Skeletal manifestations of disease experience: Length of illness and porous cranial lesion formation in a contemporary juvenile mortality sample. *American Journal of Human Biology* 35:e23896. https://doi.org/10.1002/ajhb.23896

Oxenham, M.F., Cavill, I. (2010). Porotic hyperostosis and cribra orbitalia: The erythropoietic response to iron-deficiency anaemia. *Anthropological Science* 118:199–200. https://doi.org/10.1537/ase.100302

Pear, B.L. (1974). Skeletal manifestations of the lymphomas and leukemias. *Seminars in Roentgenology* 9:229–240. https://doi.org/10.1016/0037-198X(74)90020-0

Perisano, C., Marzetti, E., Spinelli, M.S., Callà, C.A., Graci, C., Maccauro, G. (2012). Physiopathology of bone modifications in β-thalassemia. *Anemia* 2012:320737. https://doi.org/10.1155/2012/320737

Riccio, I., Marcarelli, M., Del Regno, N., Fusco, C., Di Martino, M., Savarese, R., Gualdiero, G., Oreste, M., Indolfi, C., Porpora, G., Esposito, M. (2013). Musculoskeletal problems in pediatric acute leukemia. *Journal of Pediatric Orthopaedics B* 22:264–269. https://doi.org/10.1097/bpb.0b013e32835d731c

Riccomi, G., Fornaciari, G., Giuffra, V. (2019). Multiple myeloma in paleopathology: A critical review. *International Journal of Paleopathology* 24:201–212. https://doi.org/10.1016/j.ijpp.2018.12.001

Rivera, F., Mirazón Lahr, M. (2017). New evidence suggesting a dissociated etiology for *cribra orbitalia* and porotic hyperostosis. *American Journal of Physical Anthropology* 164:76–96. https://doi.org/10.1002/ajpa.23258

Rothschild, B.M., Hershkovitz, I., Dutour, O., Latimer, B., Rothschild, C., Jellema, L.M. (1997). Recognition of leukemia in skeletal remains: Report and comparison of two cases. *American Journal of Physical Anthropology* 10:481–496. https://doi.org/10.1002/(SICI)1096-8644(199704)102:4%3C481::AID-AJPA5%3E3.0.CO;2-V

Rothschild, B.M., Hershkovitz, I., Dutour, O. (1998). Clues potentially distinguishing lytic lesions of multiple myeloma from those of metastatic carcinoma. *American Journal of Physical Anthropology* 105:241–250. https://doi.org/10.1002/(SICI)1096-8644(199802)105:2%3C241::AID-AJPA10%3E3.0.CO;2-0

Schats, R. (2021). Cribriotic lesions in archaeological human skeletal remains. Prevalence, co-occurrence, and association in medieval and early modern Netherlands. *International Journal of Paleopathology* 35:81–89. https://doi.org/10.1016/j.ijpp.2021.10.003

Scianò, F., Bramanti, B., Gualdi-Russo, E. (2021). A new investigative strategy to diagnose β-thalassemia syndrome in past human populations. *Archaeological and Anthropological Sciences* 13:26. https://doi.org/10.1007/s12520-020-01261-5

Strouhal, E. (1991). Myeloma multiplex versus osteolytic metastatic carcinoma: Differential diagnosis in dry bones. *International Journal of Osteoarchaeology* 1:219–224. https://doi.org/10.1002/oa.1390010314

Stuart-Macadam, P. (1992). Porotic hyperostosis: A new perspective. *American Journal of Physical Anthropology* 87:39–47. https://doi.org/10.1002/ajpa.1330870105

Stuart-Macadam, P. (2006). Integrative anthropology: A focus on iron-deficiency anemia. *Archeological Papers of the American Anthropological Association* 16:129–137. https://doi.org/10.1525/ap3a.2006.16.1.129

Techataweewan, N., Mann, R.W., Vlok, M., Ruengdit, S., Panthongviriyakul, C., Buckley, H.R. (2021). Thalassemia major in a 49-year-old Thai female: Gross and x-ray examination of dry bone. *International Journal of Osteoarchaeology* 31:866–880. https://doi.org/10.1002/oa.3003

Vlok, M., Buckley, H.B., Miszkiewicz, J.J., Walker, M.M., Domett, K., Willis, A., Trinh, H.H., Minh, T.A., Nguyen, M.H.T., Nguyen, L.C., Matsumura, H., Wang, T., Nghia, H.T., Oxenham, M.F. (2021). Forager and farmer evolutionary adaptations to malaria evidenced by 7000 years of thalassemia in Southeast Asia. *Scientific Reports* 11:5677. https://doi.org/10.1038/s41598-021-83978-4

Walker, P.L., Bathurst, R.R., Richman, R., Gjerdrum, T., Andrushko, V.A. (2009). The causes of porotic hyperostosis and cribra orbitalia: A reappraisal of the iron-deficiency-anemia hypothesis. *American Journal of Physical Anthropology* 139:109–125. https://doi.org/10.1002/ajpa.21031

Wander, K., Shell Duncan, B., McDade, T. (2009). Evaluation of iron deficiency as a nutritional adaptation to infectious disease: An evolutionary medicine perspective. *American Journal of Human Biology* 21:172–179. https://doi.org/10.1002/ajhb.20839

Wapler, U., Crubezy, E., Schultz, M. (2004). Is cribra orbitalia synonymous with anemia? Analysis and interpretation of cranial pathology in Sudan. *American Journal of Physical Anthropology* 123:333–339. https://doi.org/10.1002/ajpa.10321

Chapter 5

Metabolic disorders

Metabolic disorders disrupt the body's normal metabolic processes and can cause skeletal changes by affecting bone formation, resorption, and/or mineralisation. This chapter covers a range of such disorders that have been identified in palaeopathological contexts, including osteoporosis, vitamin C deficiency, vitamin D deficiency, Paget's disease of bone, fluorosis, and hyperostosis frontalis interna.

Osteoporosis

Osteoporosis is characterised by an increased rate of bone resorption relative to bone formation, which results in decreased bone mass per unit volume. This imbalance in bone formation and resorption affects both cortical and trabecular bone and leads to lower bone quantity and quality (Figure 5.1). As a result, individuals with osteoporosis are susceptible to fractures, which may occur even after minimal trauma.

Osteoporosis is classified as primary and secondary to reflect its causative factors. Primary osteoporosis mostly affects older individuals, especially post-menopausal women, although idiopathic osteoporosis can be found in juveniles and young adults. Primary osteoporosis is further grouped into type I and type II, as described below. In contrast, secondary osteoporosis may affect individuals of any age and is associated with lifestyle factors, medical procedures, and other pathological conditions.

Type I osteoporosis is linked to menopause. As oestrogen levels decrease, bone is resorbed at a faster rate, while bone formation is slowed down. As a result, within 20 years of the cessation of oestrogen secretion, up to 50% of trabecular and 30% of cortical bone may be lost. As bone loss in type I osteoporosis impacts mostly trabecular bone, it often leads to vertebral fractures and kyphosis (Figure 5.2). In addition, fractures at the distal radius are often found in cases of type I osteoporosis, as this anatomical area is also rich in trabecular bone (Figure 5.3). Nonetheless, not all women experience bone loss severe enough to lead to osteoporosis or fractures; factors such as inadequate nutrition or a genetic predisposition can increase fracture risk.

Type II osteoporosis affects older males and females. In this type of osteoporosis, bone loss is equally notable in trabecular and cortical bone. Ageing contributes to bone loss through various mechanisms, including reducing the number of existing osteoprogenitor cells and restricting their ability to differentiate into new bone cells. Furthermore, dietary calcium intake is reduced with advancing age, as is the efficiency of its intestinal absorption, while vitamin D levels also decrease as individuals age. A reduction in calcium levels and/or a deficiency in vitamin D may trigger secondary hyperparathyroidism, elevated bone turnover, loss

DOI: 10.4324/9781003475026-5

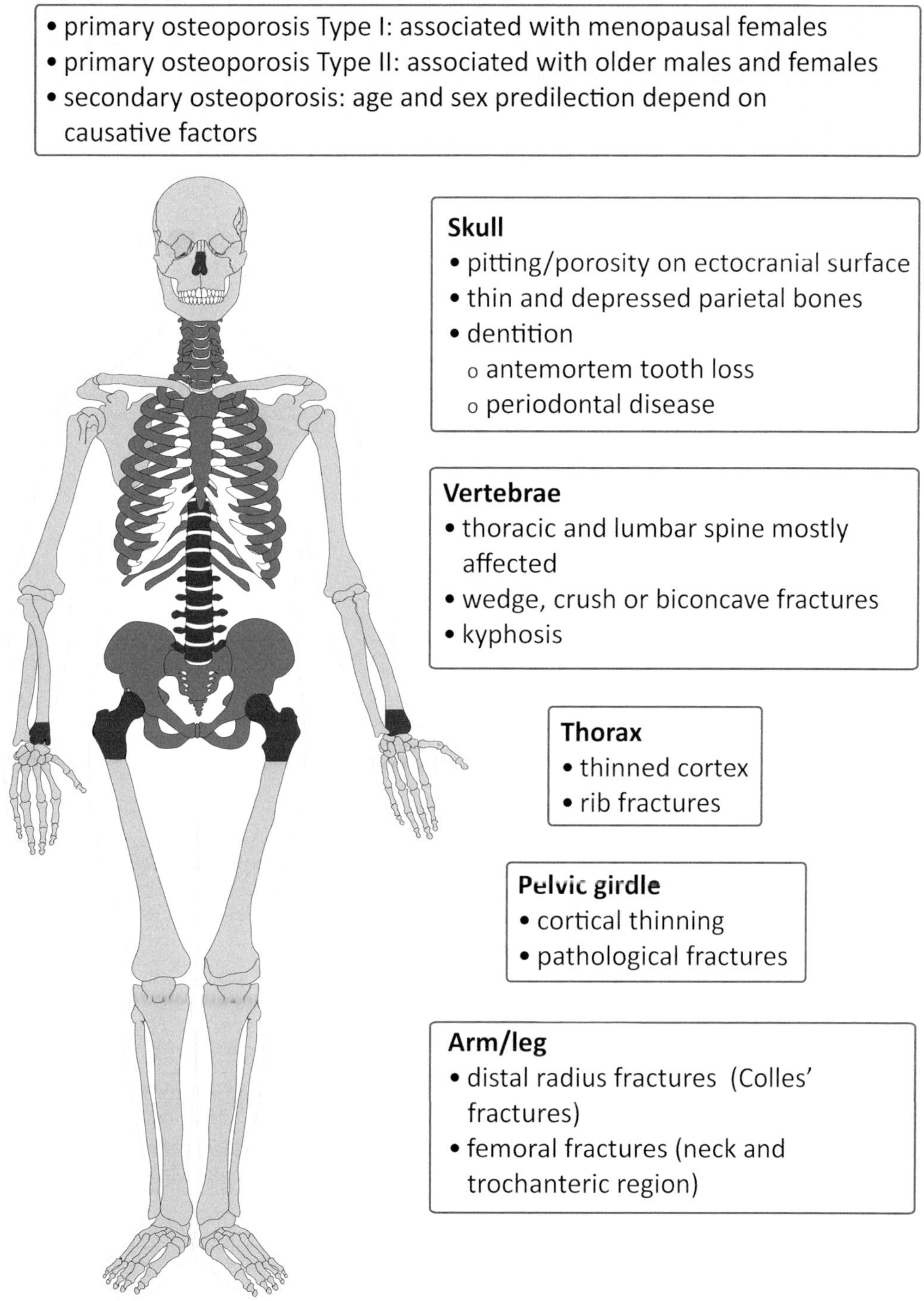

Figure 5.1 Skeletal manifestation of osteoporosis. (Data from Brickley 2002; Brickley and Agarwal 2003; Brickley et al. 2020; Curate 2014; Curate et al. 2016; Hegeman et al. 2004; Ives et al. 2017; Mays 2006)

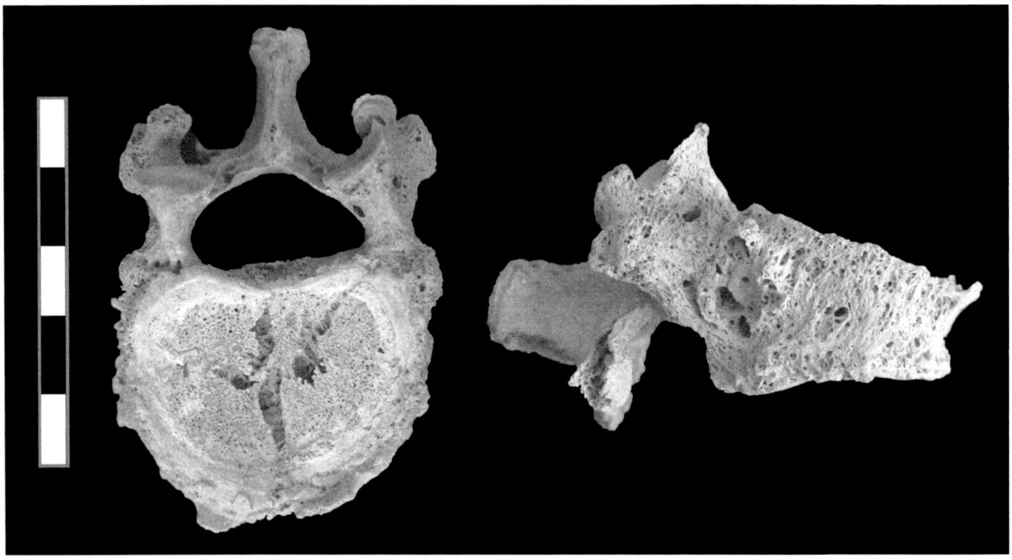

Figure 5.2 Compression fracture of the body of a lower thoracic vertebra. (Sbide, Roman/Byzantine; photos by Efthymia Nikita, with the kind permission of Dr. Ahmet Ihsan Aytek, Burdur Mehmet Akif Ersoy University)

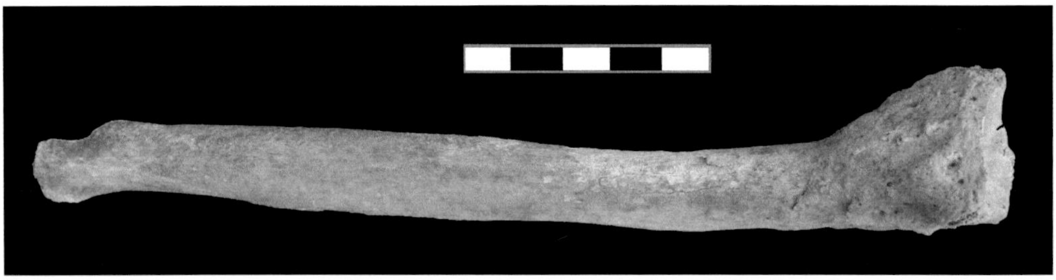

Figure 5.3 Colles' fracture of a left radius. Note the dorsal displacement of the distal part of the bone. (Sbide, Byzantine; photo by Efthymia Nikita, with the kind permission of Dr. Ahmet Ihsan Aytek, Burdur Mehmet Akif Ersoy University)

of bone mass, defects in mineralisation, and an increased risk of fractures. The role of other nutrients can also be important; for example, dietary protein or phosphorus could affect calcium absorption, though this has not been a consistent finding in relevant research. Type II osteoporosis is mostly associated with hip fractures (Figures 5.4 and 5.5). While it affects both males and females, bone loss and its clinical manifestations generally appear earlier in females. This pattern can be partly attributed to the lower peak bone mass attained by females compared to males (Box 5.1).

Secondary osteoporosis may arise from multiple factors, including underlying pathological conditions, medical procedures, and lifestyle choices. In what concerns pathologies, several conditions may contribute to the development of secondary osteoporosis. An increased risk of osteoporosis has been identified in patients with persistent infections, such as tuberculosis, poliomyelitis, and Hansen's disease. In addition, type 1 diabetes can also result in lower bone

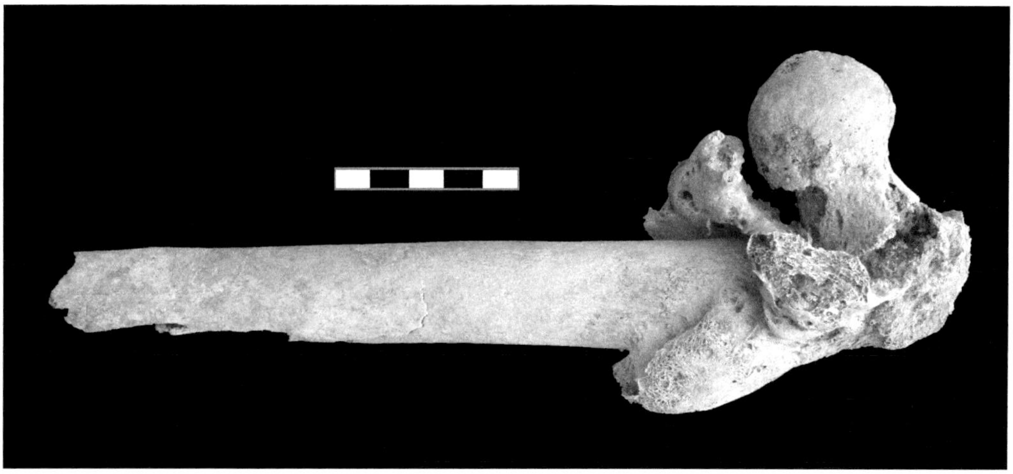

Figure 5.4 Healed femoral fracture with extensive new bone formation. (Tefenni, Byzantine; photo by Efthymia Nikita, with the kind permission of Dr. Ahmet Ihsan Aytek, Burdur Mehmet Akif Ersoy University)

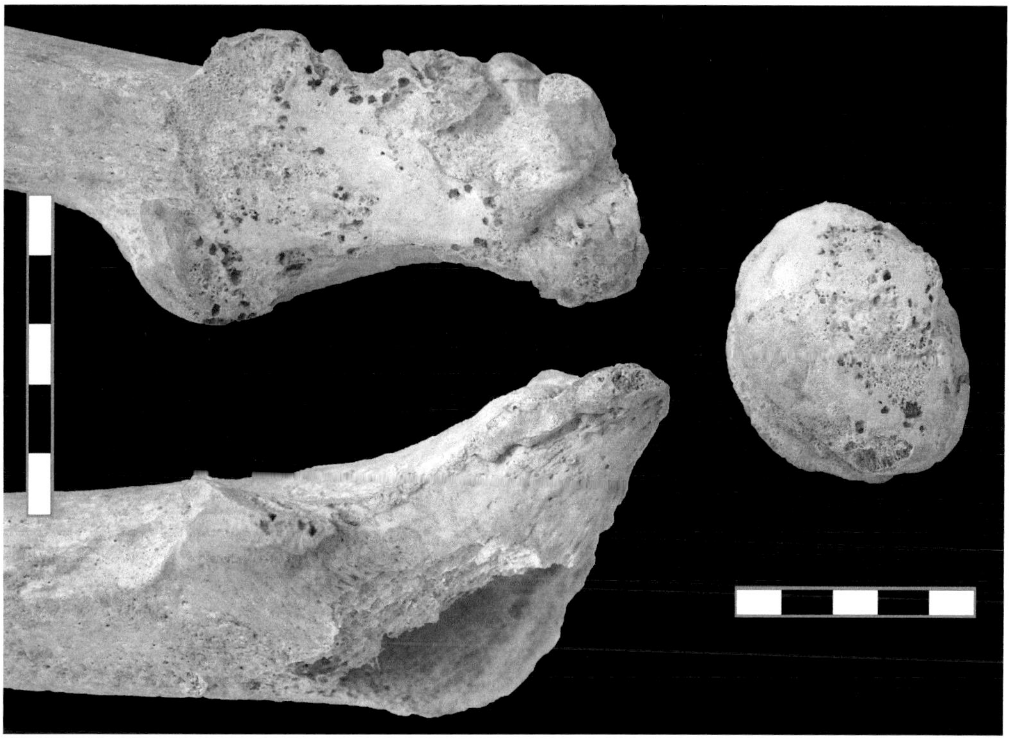

Figure 5.5 Fractured right femur. Note that although the head has completely detached from the rest of the bone, the fracture has healed, resulting in marginal osteophytes, porosity, and eburnation both on the head and the area where the neck used to be. (Oosterblokker, 5158; photos by Efthymia Nikita, from the reference collection of the Cultural Heritage Agency of the Netherlands)

Box 5.1 Peak bone mass

Peak bone mass is the greatest amount of bone tissue attained at the end of skeletal maturity. While peak bone mass is largely determined genetically, it is also affected by an individual's health during childhood, the quality of diet, levels of physical activity, reproductive history, smoking, and drinking alcohol. Inadequate attainment of peak bone mass results in increased susceptibility to fractures at an earlier age later in life.

mineral density. Rheumatoid arthritis can also cause osteoporosis, both due to chronic inflammation associated with the disease, as well as the effects of the medication used to treat it. Anorexia nervosa and other conditions that cause undernutrition can impair collagen synthesis. Many other conditions can compromise bone health, such as hyperthyroidism, hyperparathyroidism, kidney diseases, and neoplastic conditions, especially metastatic bone disease. An example of medical procedure that may result in osteoporosis is the surgical removal of the ovaries, which can disrupt the individual's endocrine status and accelerate bone loss, unless oestrogen replacement therapy is applied. With regard to lifestyle factors, smoking and alcohol consumption increase the risk of bone fractures. Another critical lifestyle factor is physical activity. Engaging in exercise, particularly when ten to 18 years old, stimulates bone formation, maximising peak bone mass. In adulthood, a lack of physical activity, restricted mobility, and conditions such as weightlessness (e.g. during space travel) contribute to bone loss. In contrast, engaging in multi-component exercise that includes strength training, aerobic activities, high-impact exercises, and/or weight-bearing workouts can mitigate bone loss. Nevertheless, excessive exercise can lead to amenorrhea in women, which has a negative effect on bone health. For women, reproductive history is also important for bone health; childlessness, the number of childbirths, and the onset of menstruation have a complex relationship to bone mineral density.

In bioarchaeological studies, osteoporosis may be identified macroscopically (see Figure 5.1); however, macroscopic assessments will certainly underestimate its prevalence, while pathological fractures associated with this condition may be caused by other factors. Therefore, the diagnosis of osteoporosis in bioarchaeological contexts relies on methods that allow measuring bone mineral density (e.g. dual-energy X-ray absorptiometry), or cortical bone loss (e.g. radiogrammetry). Skeletal histomorphometry, radiography, light microscopy, and scanning electron microscopy have also occasionally been used to assess the extent of bone remodelling and loss.

Scurvy

Scurvy results from a prolonged deficiency of vitamin C (ascorbic acid). Most vertebrate species can synthesise vitamin C; however, humans and other primates obtain this nutrient from dietary sources. Many vegetables and fruits are rich sources of vitamin C, with high concentrations found in citrus fruits, strawberries, tomatoes, Brussels sprouts, guava, potatoes, cabbage, broccoli, spinach, and peppers. Organ meats and fish roe are also important sources of vitamin C. However, the concentration of vitamin C in foods may decrease in cases of prolonged storage and when using various processing methods, such as cooking, drying, pickling, and salting. In bioarchaeological research, the identification of scurvy can provide information regarding past dietary practices, subsistence strategies, and environmental conditions. Furthermore, the presence of scurvy can reflect underlying issues such as parasitic infections, which may inhibit the absorption of vitamin C, even when an individual's diet is sufficiently rich in fresh fruits and vegetables.

In adults, symptoms of scurvy typically appear two to three months after the onset of vitamin C deficiency, because the body can store ascorbic acid for this duration of time. In contrast, juveniles show clinical symptoms after a deficiency period of six to ten months, although initial signs may be observed as early as two to four months. While the condition mostly affects individuals aged between five months and two years, scurvy can impact children of any age, as well as adults. It is rare in neonates because fetuses acquire adequate levels of ascorbic acid through the placenta during gestation, building inborn stores of vitamin C. Furthermore, under normal conditions, the maternal breast milk contains sufficient vitamin C; thus, scurvy among breastfed infants is also rare. As a result, it is uncommon for infants under the age of five months to develop scurvy. Scurvy heals quickly once vitamin C is reintroduced to the diet, with most symptoms typically disappearing within two weeks.

Vitamin C has several critical roles, including the regulation of collagen synthesis. It serves as a cofactor in the hydroxylation of proline and lysine amino acid residues, a process that is essential for the formation of mature collagen. Therefore, a deficiency in vitamin C can negatively affect both the quality and quantity of collagen formation. Inadequate collagen synthesis produces blood vessels that are prone to rupture, and periosteal membranes that tear easily. In addition, vitamin C is crucial for iron metabolism and immune defence; thus, vitamin C-deficient individuals are more susceptible to anaemia and infections.

Scurvy can be caused by insufficient intake or malabsorption of vitamin C, as well as by elevated physiological demands for this nutrient, or a genetic predisposition to reduced levels of vitamin C. Insufficient intake is often associated with low socioeconomic status, eating disorders, mental disabilities, parental neglect, and other factors. Individuals suffering from diabetes, anaemia, infections, and other conditions typically have increased vitamin C requirements; thus, they are more susceptible to scurvy. This is also the case for pregnant women and individuals who have experienced significant trauma or burns. Vitamin C malabsorption is commonly seen in patients with gastrointestinal disorders, while a genetic predisposition to low vitamin C levels has been proposed, since some studies have found a potential link between the Hp 2–2 phenotype and reduced vitamin C availability.

The symptoms of scurvy include fatigue and irritability, musculoskeletal pain, and general weakness. Swollen and bleeding gums are also commonly seen in scorbutic individuals. Moreover, as the blood vessels are fragile, bleeding under the skin (purpura or petechiae) is often seen. Skeletal lesions associated with scurvy result from the primary effects of vitamin C deficiency on the skeleton (e.g. changes in collagen structure, increased bone loss, defective osteoid accumulation) but also from trauma to weakened bone and blood vessels. Concerning the latter, compromised collagen synthesis results in vascular fragility and predisposes individuals to haemorrhages following even minimal trauma. Subperiosteal haemorrhages may appear in various parts of the skeleton, particularly where blood vessels lie near the skin surface or are subjected to mechanical stress from muscle activity. Haemorrhaging may trigger a periosteal response, resulting in new bone formation and porosity at affected sites.[1] Once vitamin C is reintroduced into the diet, new bone formation is stimulated. Even minimal amounts of vitamin C can promote an osteoblastic response; therefore, proliferative lesions can be found both during the healing and the active phase of the disease.

Juvenile scurvy

Skeletal lesions due to scurvy are more prominent in juveniles, as their skeleton is still growing (Boxes 5.2 and 5.4, Figures 5.6–5.14). Moreover, in developing skeletons, the periosteum is less firmly attached to the underlying bone; thus, it is more susceptible to form bone in response to haemorrhage. Nonetheless, the distribution and severity of skeletal lesions can vary considerably.

Box 5.2 Skeletal manifestation of scurvy in juveniles

Skull

- calvarium
  - porosity and/or SNB with or without vascular impressions on ectocranial surface
  - porosity and/or SNB with or without vascular impressions on endocranial surface
- frontal bone
  - porosity and/or SNB on orbital roofs
- occipital bone
  - porosity and/or SNB on inferior surface of pars basilaris*
- maxillae
  - porosity and/or SNB on anterior surface and/or around infraorbital foramina
  - porosity and/or SNB on posterior surface, superior to alveolar margins
  - porosity and/or SNB on hard palate and alveolar process
  - palatine torus
- zygomatic bones
  - porosity and/or SNB on lateral part of external surface
  - porosity on internal surface
  - porosity and/or SNB on lateral orbit
- temporal bones
  - porosity and/or SNB on external surfaces of temporal squama
- sphenoid bone
  - porosity and/or SNB on greater wings
  - porosity and/or SNB around foramen rotundum
  - porosity and/or SNB on lesser wings
  - porosity and/or SNB on pterygoid fossae
- mandible
  - porosity and/or SNB on medial surface of ramus/coronoid process
  - SNB along mylohyoid line
  - porosity and/or SNB on alveolar processes and sockets

- dentition
    - antemortem tooth loss
    - enamel hypoplasia

Shoulder girdle

- porosity and/or SNB (especially in supraspinous and infraspinous fossae)

Thorax

- rib fractures adjacent to costochondral junction
- rib flaring adjacent to costochondral junction (scorbutic rosary)
- SNB on anterior/lateral rib shaft

Pelvic girdle

- porosity and/or SNB on iliac surface

Arm/leg

- bones experiencing rapid growth (e.g. distal femur) most severely affected
- transverse fractures through epiphyseal growth plate; microfracture repair may manifest as bony spurs at metaphyseal margins (Pelkan's spurs)
- porosity and/or SNB on diaphysis and metaphyses (extending more than a centimetre from metaphyseal plate)
- SNB on femoral linea aspera
- ossified hematomas resulting from repeated haemorrhage and healing

Key: SNB = subperiosteal new bone
*Microporosity on the inferior pars basilaris should not be included in the assessment of scurvy in individuals younger than 3.5 years, based on the findings by Eggington et al. (2024)

(Data from Aufderheide and Rodríguez-Martín 1998; Brickley and Ives 2006; Brickley and Morgan 2023a; Brickley et al. 2020; Brown and Ortner 2011; Eggington et al. 2024; Fain 2005; Geber and Murphy 2012; Klaus 2017; Moore and Koon 2017; Murphy et al. 2024; Ortner and Ericksen 1997; Ortner et al. 1999, 2001; Snoddy et al. 2018; Stark 2014)

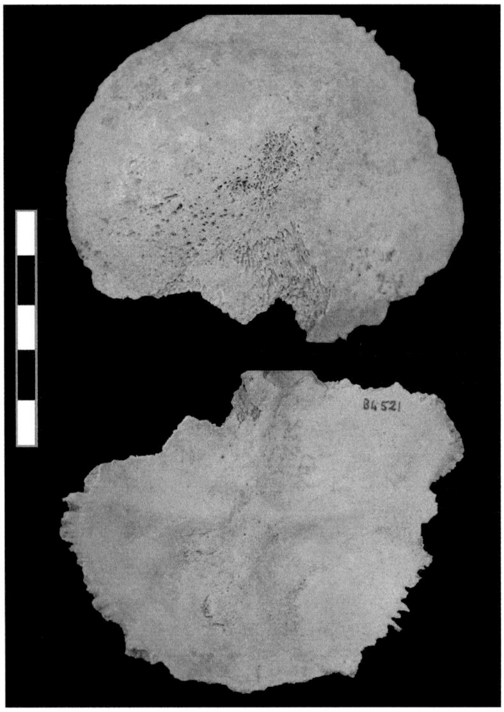

Figure 5.6 Scurvy. Porosity and SNB on the ectocranial (top) and endocranial (bottom) surface of the occipital bone. (1–2 years old, Black Gate cemetery, Newcastle-Upon-Tyne, 8th–12th c. CE, BG-521; photos by Efthymia Nikita; copyright: Human Skeletal Collection, University of Sheffield)

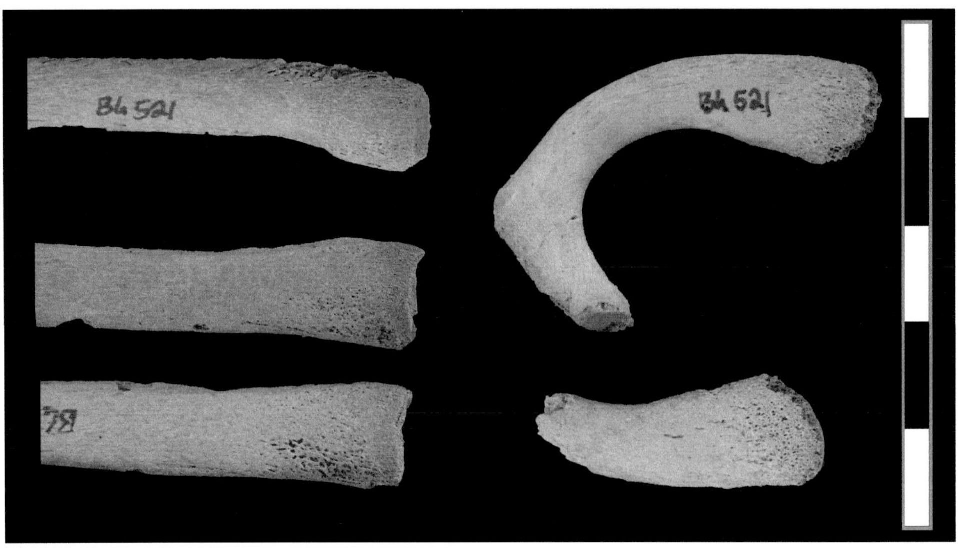

Figure 5.7 Scurvy. Porosity and flaring adjacent to the costochondral junction of multiple ribs. (Same individual as in Figure 5.6; photos by Efthymia Nikita; copyright: Human Skeletal Collection, University of Sheffield)

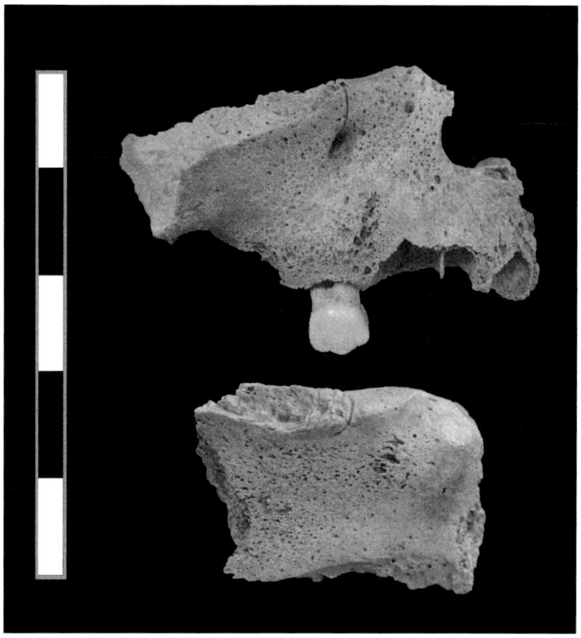

Figure 5.8 Scurvy. Porosity and SNB on the anterior maxilla, around the infraorbital foramen and superior to the alveolar margins (top); porosity on the greater wing of the sphenoid bone (bottom). (Same individual as in Figures 5.6 and 5.7; photos by Efthymia Nikita; copyright: Human Skeletal Collection, University of Sheffield)

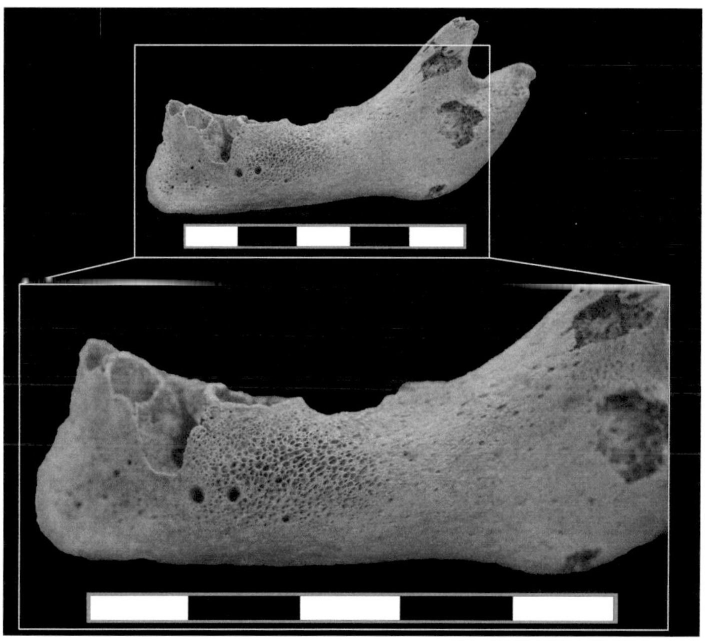

Figure 5.9 Scurvy. Porosity on the mandibular corpus as well as on the ramus. (Same individual as in Figures 5.6–5.8; photos by Efthymia Nikita; copyright: Human Skeletal Collection, University of Sheffield)

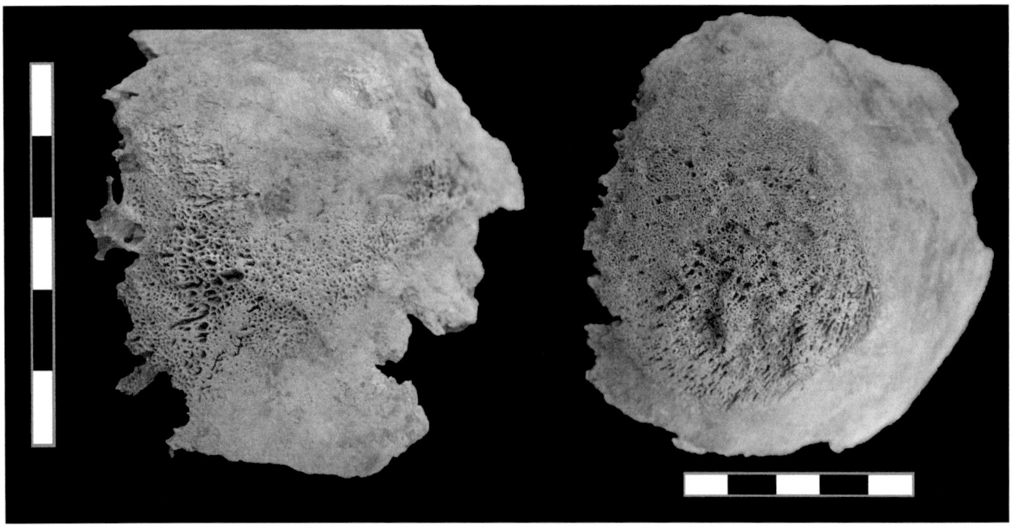

Figure 5.10 Scurvy. Severe porotic alterations on the ectocranial surface. (1–1.5 years old, Black Gate cemetery, Newcastle-Upon-Tyne, 8th–12th c. CE, BG-281; photos by Efthymia Nikita; copyright: Human Skeletal Collection, University of Sheffield)

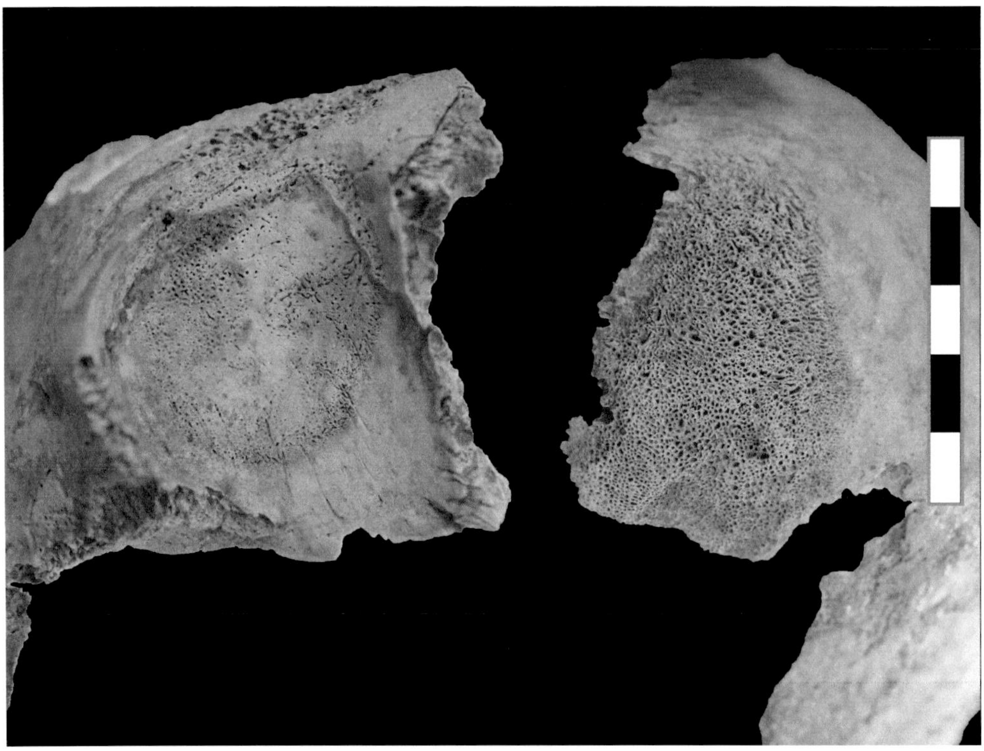

Figure 5.11 Scurvy. Porosity on the orbital roof (left) and severe porotic alterations on the ectocranial surface (right). Note that the scale corresponds only to the ectocranial lesion. (Same individual as in Figure 5.10; photos by Efthymia Nikita; copyright: Human Skeletal Collection, University of Sheffield)

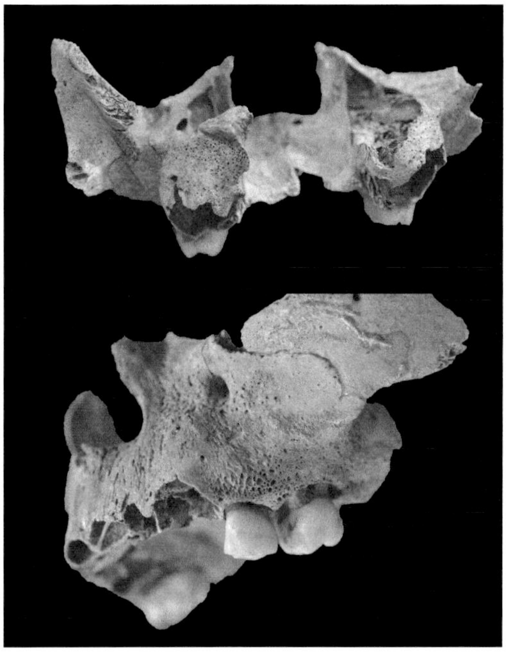

Figure 5.12 Scurvy. Porosity on the posterior surface of the maxilla (top); porosity and SNB on the anterior surface of the maxilla, superior to the alveolar margins and around the infraorbital foramen (bottom). (Same individual as in Figures 5.10 and 5.11; photos by Efthymia Nikita; copyright: Human Skeletal Collection, University of Sheffield)

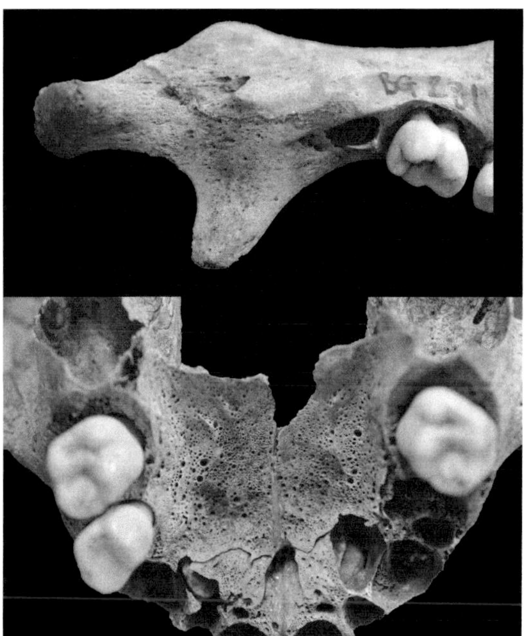

Figure 5.13 Scurvy. Porosity and SNB on the coronoid process (top), and porosity on the hard palate (bottom). (Same individual as in Figures 5.10–5.12; photos by Efthymia Nikita; copyright: Human Skeletal Collection, University of Sheffield)

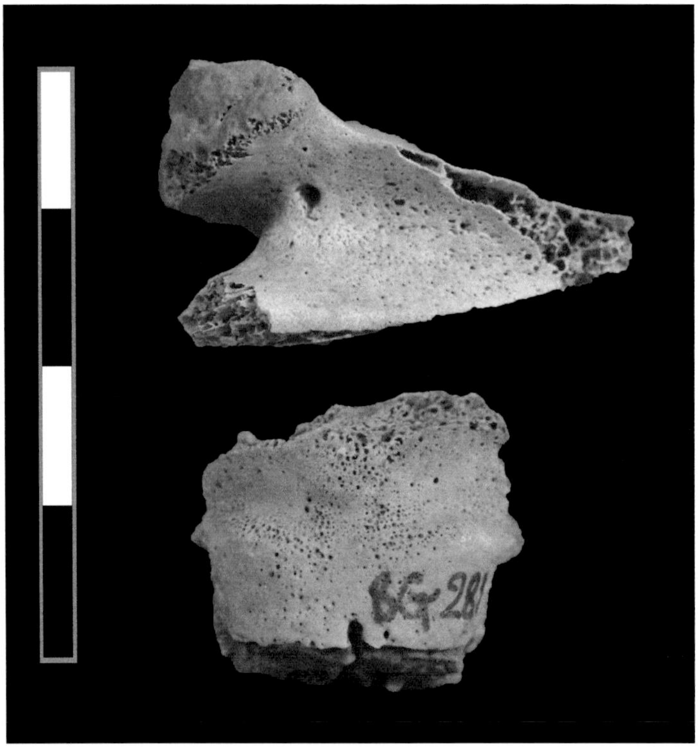

Figure 5.14 Scurvy. Porosity in the supraspinous fossa (top) and pars basilaris (bottom). (Same individual as in Figures 5.10–5.13; photos by Efthymia Nikita; copyright: Human Skeletal Collection, University of Sheffield)

Adult scurvy

Many of the skeletal lesions described above for juveniles may also be used to diagnose scurvy in adults, although differences in skeletal maturity mean the presentation in adults is generally less pronounced and often non-specific (Boxes 5.3 and 5.4, Figures 5.15–5.18).

Box 5.3 Skeletal manifestation of scurvy in adults

Skull

- porosity and/or SNB on ectocranial surface of parietal and/or squamous part of temporal bones
- porosity and/or SNB with vascular impressions on endocranial surface
- porosity and/or SNB on orbital roofs/lateral orbit
- porosity and/or SNB on anterior maxillary surface and/or in infraorbital foramina region

- porosity and/or SNB on posterior maxillary surface, superior to alveolar margins
- porosity and/or SNB on maxillary palate, outside alveolar margins
- porosity and/or SNB on maxillary alveolar process
- porosity and/or SNB on lateral part of anterior zygomatic bone surface
- porosity on internal/posterior zygomatic bone surface
- porosity and/or SNB on greater wing of sphenoid bone
- porosity and/or SNB at foramen rotundum of sphenoid bone
- porosity and/or SNB on lesser wings of sphenoid bone
- porosity and/or SNB on pterygoid fossae of sphenoid bone
- porosity and/or SNB on interior surface of mandibular rami/coronoid process
- SNB along mandibular mylohyoid line
- dentition
    - antemortem tooth loss
    - periodontal disease

Shoulder girdle

- porosity and/or SNB in supra and/or infraspinous scapular fossae

Thorax

- transverse fractures at osteocartilaginous rib junction
- SNB on anterior/lateral rib shaft surfaces

Vertebrae

- osteopenia
- biconcave bodies
- vertebral collapse

Arm/leg

- ossified haematomas
- porosity and/or SNB on diaphyses/metaphyses

Pelvic girdle

- porosity and/or SNB, particularly on visceral iliac surface

(Data compiled from Brickley et al. 2020; Geber and Murphy 2012; Holck 1984; Reikersdorfer et al. 2024; Snoddy et al. 2018)

Box 5.4 Pathognomonic or not?

While there is broad agreement regarding the skeletal changes linked to scurvy, there is no consensus on the diagnostic strength of these changes. For example, the presence of macroscopic lesions on the external surface of the greater wing of the sphenoid bone has been regarded as virtually pathognomonic for scurvy, provided that other potential disorders have been adequately ruled out (Ortner and Ericksen 1997). However, Melikian and Waldron (2003) observed that clinical cases of scurvy showed more pronounced and different manifestations in the cranial bones than those identified in archaeological contexts, which raised questions regarding the diagnosis of scurvy using previously established criteria. Brickley and Morgan (2023b) suggest that in juvenile skeletons, macroscopic lesions *diagnostic of* scurvy include the bilateral presence of unambiguous porosity on the greater wing of the sphenoid bone, along with additional lesions that have few alternative aetiologies. Lists of traits with different diagnostic confidence have also been proposed by Snoddy et al. (2018), Geber and Murphy (2012), and others.

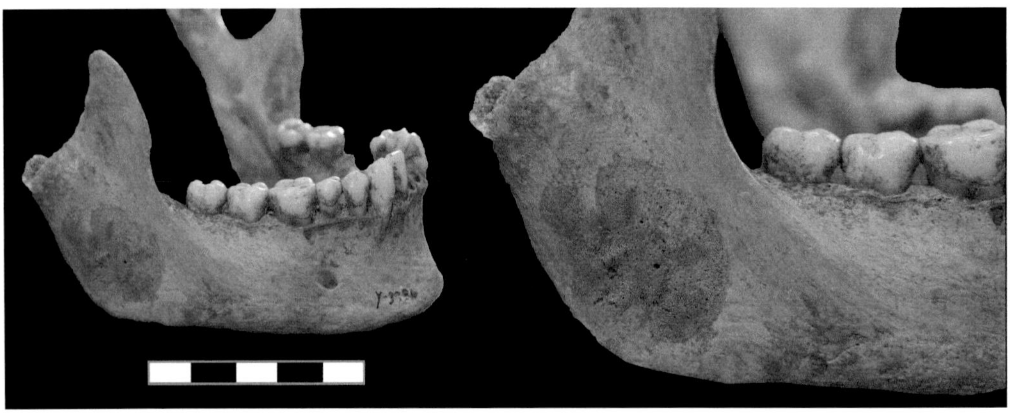

Figure 5.15 Adult scurvy. SNB on the mandibular ramus. (18–24 years old, All Saints Church, Fishergate, York, Medieval, Y-3936; photos by Efthymia Nikita; copyright: Human Skeletal Collection, University of Sheffield)

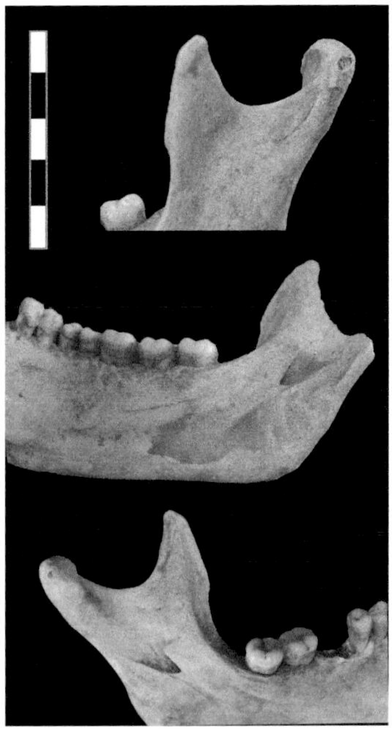

Figure 5.16 Adult scurvy. SNB below the condylar process (top), along the mylohyoid line (middle) and on the interior surface of the coronoid process (bottom). (Same individual as in Figure 5.15; photos by Efthymia Nikita; copyright: Human Skeletal Collection, University of Sheffield)

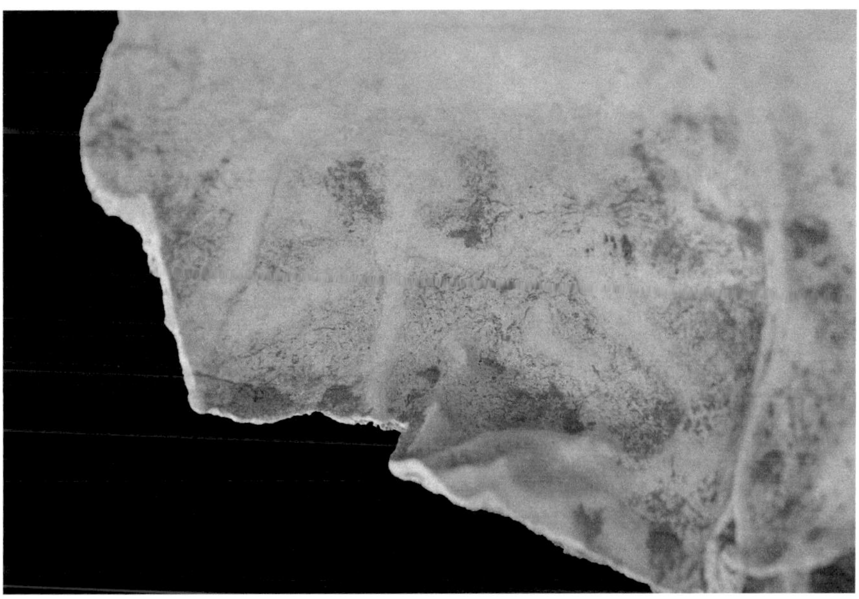

Figure 5.17 Adult scurvy. SNB with vascular impressions on the endocranial surface of the frontal bone. (Same individual as in Figures 5.15 and 5.16; photo by Efthymia Nikita; copyright: Human Skeletal Collection, University of Sheffield)

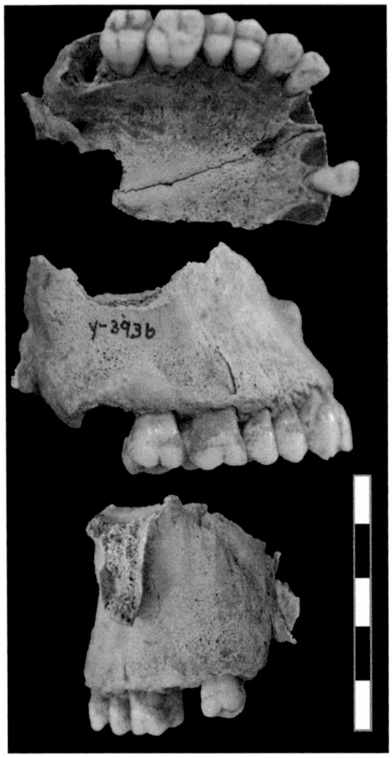

Figure 5.18 Adult scurvy. Porosity on the hard palate (top), maxillary alveolar process (middle), and posterior maxillary surface, superior to the alveolar margins (bottom). (Same individual as in Figures 5.15–5.17; photos by Efthymia Nikita; copyright: Human Skeletal Collection, University of Sheffield)

Rickets/osteomalacia

Rickets in juveniles and osteomalacia in adults result from a deficiency of vitamin D (see Box 5.5 regarding terminology). Vitamin D can be obtained through the consumption of oily fish, egg yolks, mushrooms, and liver. However, it is mostly synthesised within the skin when exposed to sunlight. Vitamin D deficiency is largely affected by geographical latitude, cloud cover, and altitude. Skin pigmentation is also important; individuals with darker skin require longer exposure to UVB radiation to synthesise vitamin D. Furthermore, diseases that impair the absorption of vitamin D or calcium (e.g. cystic fibrosis and coeliac disease), but also chronic kidney disease and liver failure, can contribute to this deficiency. Vitamin D deficiency has further been linked to genetic factors (e.g. hypophosphatemic rickets). Cultural factors are also important in the development of rickets. These factors include diets low in phosphorus and calcium, as well as the consumption of foods that decrease vitamin D bioaccessibility, such as cereal grains and legumes that are rich in phytates. In infants, a deficiency in vitamin D reflects maternal vitamin D deficiency, which impacts the infant both in utero and during the postpartum period through breastfeeding. In addition, the dietary choices made during weaning are critical because nutritional rickets can arise from deficiencies in vitamin D, calcium, or both. The use of heavy clothing (including cases of swaddling infants), the application of sunscreens that inhibit ultraviolet light absorption by the skin,

Box 5.5 Clinical and palaeopathological terminology

In clinical contexts, the term "rickets" denotes deficient mineralisation at the growth plates; thus, it applies exclusively to juveniles, whose growth plates have not closed yet. In paleopathology, "rickets" is also used to describe vitamin D deficiency in juveniles. In contrast, whereas in paleopathology the term "osteomalacia" refers to skeletal changes caused by vitamin D deficiency occurring in adulthood, in clinical contexts, "osteomalacia" refers to areas of inadequately mineralised osteoid that develop within remodelling areas of pre-existing bone. Thus, in clinical contexts, juveniles may have simultaneously rickets and osteomalacia. Finally, the term "residual rickets" describes bone lesions observed in adults but associated with an episode of rickets that occurred earlier in life, before the growth plates closed.

spending too much time indoors, and living in densely populated urban environments with tall buildings, narrow streets, and industrial pollutants also restrict skin exposure to sunlight and may result in vitamin D deficiency. Finally, advanced age is a risk factor for vitamin D deficiency. Older individuals generally show lower concentrations of vitamin D compared to younger ones, irrespective of diet and sunlight exposure. This pattern has been associated with a reduction in skin thickness and in the levels of 7-dehydrocholesterol in the skin of older adults, coupled with a decline in kidney function, which restricts the synthesis of active vitamin D.

Vitamin D contributes to the intestinal absorption of calcium and phosphate and facilitates the reabsorption of these minerals in the kidneys. This process elevates the levels of calcium and phosphate in the bloodstream, which is essential for cartilage and bone mineralisation. Thus, in individuals with vitamin D deficiency, mineralisation is disrupted, and unmineralised matrix (osteoid) accumulates. The growth plate cartilage and osteoid keep expanding, and this becomes visible as widening of the bone metaphyses. In addition, the underlying trabecular bone shows inadequate mineralisation and irregular vascularisation. The skeleton overall becomes weaker and more susceptible to fractures or deformity. Since vitamin D is important for the immune system, its deficiency can also affect the skeleton indirectly as it renders individuals more vulnerable to infections.

Rickets can cause muscle weakness and cramps, bone pain, skeletal fragility and associated deformities, impaired growth and development, as well as twitching and tingling in the extremities, and potentially seizures due to low levels of calcium in the blood. In adults, osteomalacia can cause similar symptoms, including bone pain, muscle weakness, increased susceptibility to fractures, muscle cramps, and tingling in the hands and feet.

Rickets

Rickets results from a deficiency of vitamin D during childhood. It is most common among children aged between three and 18 months, particularly affecting juveniles who cannot yet engage independently in outdoor activities that allow sun exposure, as well as those whose dietary intake of vitamin D is insufficient. Adolescents may also develop rickets because of their accelerated growth and associated increased demands for vitamin D, while neonates may develop rickets if their mothers are vitamin D deficient during pregnancy.

The skeletal changes caused by rickets depend on the severity of malnutrition, the age of onset of the disease, and the individual's growth rate and levels of mobility (Boxes 5.6 and 5.7, Figures 5.19–5.20). These changes fall into two groups. The first group includes lesions that arise from defective mineralisation of bone during periods of growth. These lesions mostly occur in parts of the skeleton characterised by active growth; an example of such lesions is the fraying and flaring of the growth plates. The second group includes changes that result from biomechanical deformation, such as bowing or twisting, in bones that are structurally weak. These deformities are particularly pronounced in weight-bearing skeletal elements. In children who do not walk yet, there may be bowing in the upper limb long bones, while in children who are old enough to walk, similar deformities may appear in the lower limb long bones. Tightly swaddled infants may also display bowing and angular deformities, as well as metaphyseal fractures in the long bones and ribs. Cranial bone deformities can be pronounced in

Box 5.6 Skeletal manifestation of rickets

Skull

- cranial vault porosity
- orbital roof porosity
- cranial vault thickening
- new porous bone on ectocranium (e.g. on glabella)
- areas of demineralisation manifesting as parietal and occipital bone thinning and flattening (craniotabes)
- frontal and parietal bossing
- widening of sutures and delayed fontanelle closure
- mandibular ramus deformation/medial angulation
- dentition
    - delayed or disordered tooth eruption
    - enamel hypoplasia
    - dental caries

Thorax

- rib bending deformity
- costochondral junction cupping and beading (rachitic rosary)
- porous cortex at costochondral ends
- anterior sternal protrusion (pectus carinatum)
- posterior sternal curvature (pectus excavatum)
- fractures

Shoulder girdle

- abnormal curvature
- blunting, flattening, squaring, cupping of inferior scapular angle (scapula sign)
- porous, coarse, or striated bone at the inferior scapular angle

Vertebrae

- kyphosis or scoliosis

Pelvic girdle

- iliac curvature
- protrusio acetabuli
- abnormal sacral angulation

Arm/leg

- growth stunting
- thickening
- cortical porosity (especially at metaphyses)
- flared metaphyses
- porosity/roughening of bone underlying growth plates
- cupping deformities in growth plate
- abnormal curvature/bending (as a result of weight-bearing stresses experienced by the forearms during crawling and by the legs during walking)
- porosity on concave side of deformed bones
- coxa vara
- superior flattening of femoral metaphysis
- genu valgum (knock knees)

(Data from Brickley and Morgan 2023b; Brickley et al. 2018, 2020; Ives and Humphrey 2018; Ives et al. 2023; Lewis 2017; Mankin 1974; Mays et al. 2006; Ortner and Mays 1998; Prentice 2013)

Box 5.7 Diagnosing rickets

According to Brickley and Morgan (2023a), macroscopic lesions *diagnostic of* active rickets include distinct lesions of the bone underlying the growth plate and, when pertinent, the metaphysis; macroscopic lesions *diagnostic of* healed rickets include biomechanical deformities in the bones and/or bone thickening. Lesions *highly consistent/ typical of* active rickets include low-grade porosity and roughening of the bone surfaces underlying the growth plate, and/or other lesions with few alternative causes, while for healed rickets, there should be evidence of biomechanical deformities indicative of defective bone mineralisation and/or other lesions with few alternative causes. Finally, *consistent with* rickets are porotic lesions and/or biomechanical deformities that are consistent with this condition, but have alternative causes.

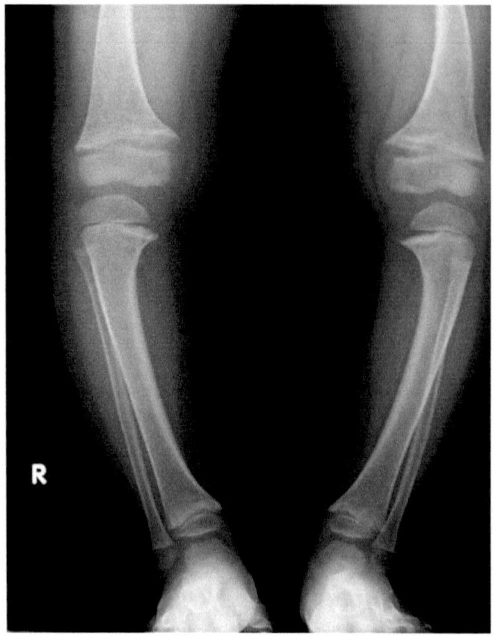

Figure 5.19 Radiograph of the lower limbs of a 5-year-old girl with hypophosphatemic rickets. Note the bowing deformity of the femora and tibiae. (Figure 2 in Michałus et al. 2022; article licensed under a Creative Commons Attribution 4.0 International License)

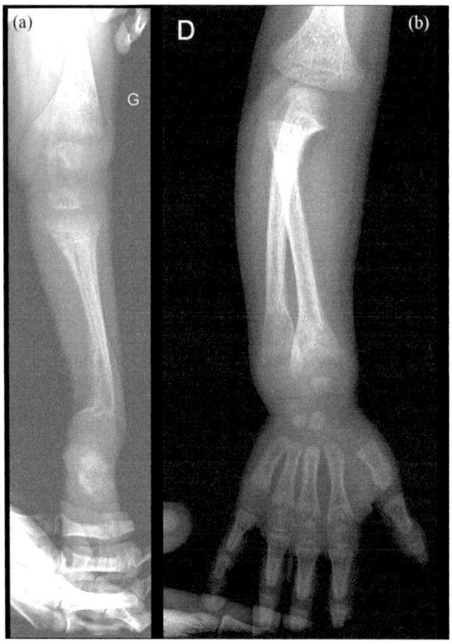

Figure 5.20 Rachitic changes in a 30-month-old female. Note the flared and frayed metaphyses, as well as the metaphyseal cupping and bowing deformities. (Figure 1 in Nicolescu et al. 2018; article licensed under a Creative Commons Attribution 4.0 International License)

young children who spend long periods in a prone position. Finally, whereas in malnourished children the skeleton shows generalised atrophy, and has thin cortices, sparse trabeculae, and enlarged marrow spaces, well-nourished children show thickened but porous bone cortices, as well as more pronounced bowing, cupping, and flaring deformities, as they are more likely to remain mobile.

When examining rickets, it is important to consider its potential co-occurrence with scurvy or other conditions with different aetiologies (see Boxes 5.8 and 5.9).

Residual rickets

Residual rickets is found in adults who experienced rickets during infancy, childhood, or adolescence, but the condition has healed since then. The skeletal changes associated with residual rickets are often subtle, as the lesions caused by juvenile rickets tend to resolve over time. However, the resultant deformities may become permanent (Box 5.10, Figures 5.21–5.27).

Box 5.8 Scurvy-rickets co-occurrence

Scurvy can affect the expression of rickets by inhibiting the activity of osteoblasts, thus impeding the accumulation of unmineralised osteoid. Conversely, rickets can affect the expression of scurvy by impairing bone mineralisation, thus hindering the accumulation of calcified matrix and new bone formation. The manifestation of these co-occurring diseases depends on several factors, such as the sequence of disease onset, the severity of each condition, the duration, and possible recurrent appearance of illness. Frequently, one disease will dominate and obscure many features of the secondary condition. In infants and children, scurvy tends to be the predominant disease in cases of co-occurrence with rickets.

Box 5.9 Rickets-neoplastic disease co-occurrence

Experimental research in rodents has found that vitamin D slows or impedes cancer development by promoting cellular differentiation, reducing the proliferation rate of cancer cells, stimulating apoptosis, decreasing tumour angiogenesis, and mitigating tumour progression and metastasis. Vitamin D can also enhance immune responses to cancer. Observational studies have found an association between elevated levels of vitamin D and a decreased risk of colorectal and bladder cancers; however, no significant relationship has been identified between vitamin D and the risk of breast, lung, or other cancers. In contrast, higher concentrations of vitamin D in the blood may be linked to an increased risk of prostate cancer and potentially pancreatic cancer.

Box 5.10 Skeletal manifestation of residual rickets

Shoulder girdle

- scapular curvature

Thorax

- rib curvature
- sternal curvature
- pseudofractures

Vertebrae

- compression fractures → kyphosis or scoliosis

Pelvic girdle

- angled sacrum
- pseudofractures

Arm/leg

- residual bending, mostly in lower limbs (most frequently anterior curvature of proximal femur below lesser trochanter)
- osseous ridge on anterior aspect of proximal femur
- genu valgum (knock knees)

(Data from Brickley et al. 2010, 2018, 2020, Tschinkel and Gowland 2020)

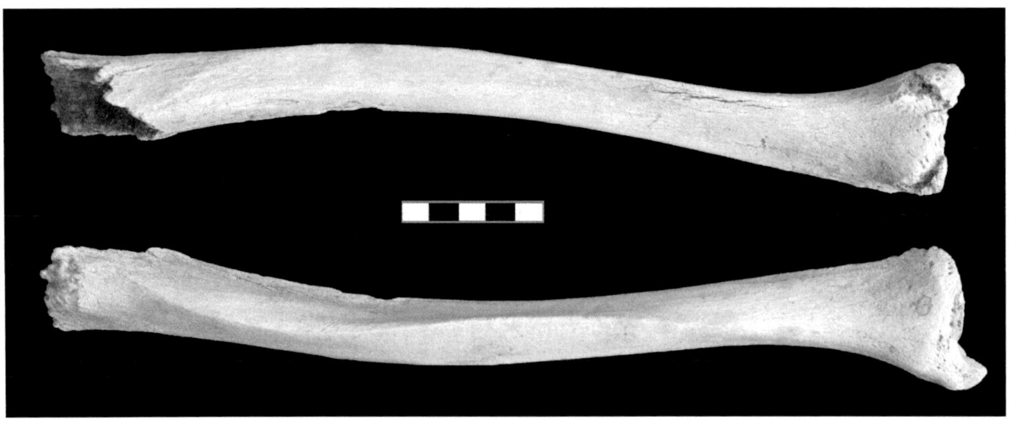

Figure 5.21 Bending deformity of the left tibia. (Sbide, Roman/Byzantine; photos by Efthymia Nikita, with the kind permission of Dr. Ahmet Ihsan Aytek, Burdur Mehmet Akif Ersoy University)

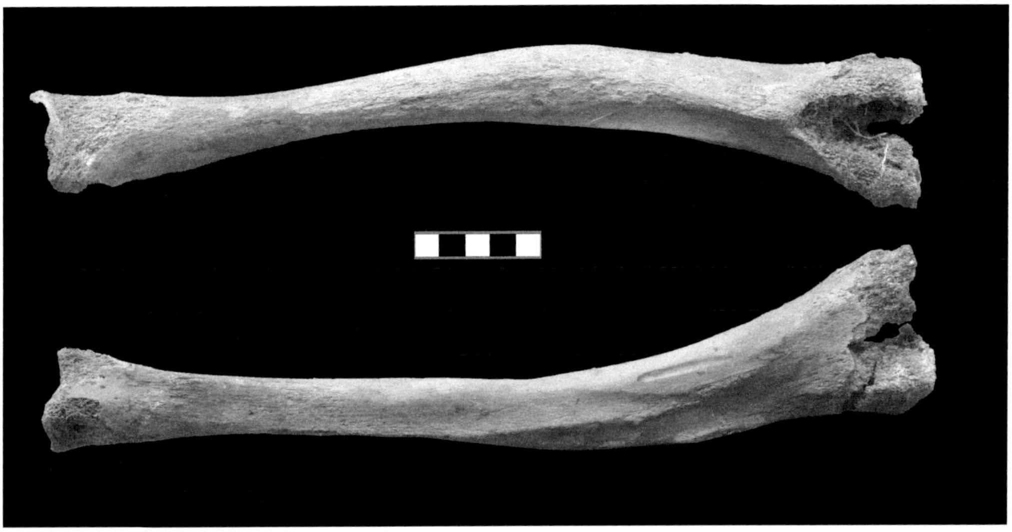

Figure 5.22 Bending deformity of the left tibia. (Female, 40–80 years old, Emmen-Marktplein, Collection NAD Nuis inv. Nr. D 2017-V.104; photos by Efthymia Nikita, with permission from the Noordelijk Archeologisch Depot)

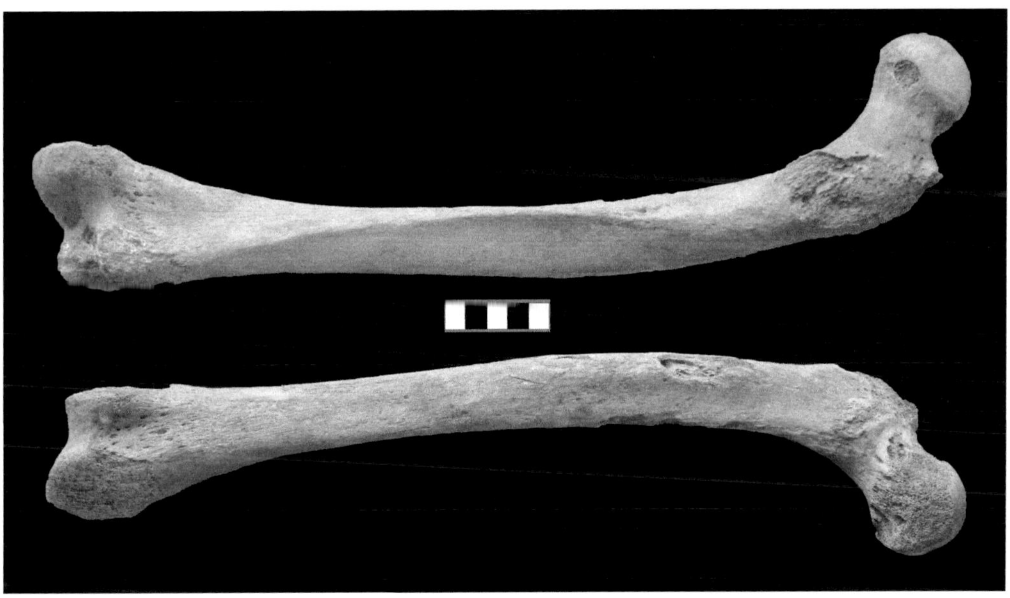

Figure 5.23 Bending deformity of the right femur. (Same individual as in Figure 5.22; photos by Efthymia Nikita, with permission from the Noordelijk Archeologisch Depot)

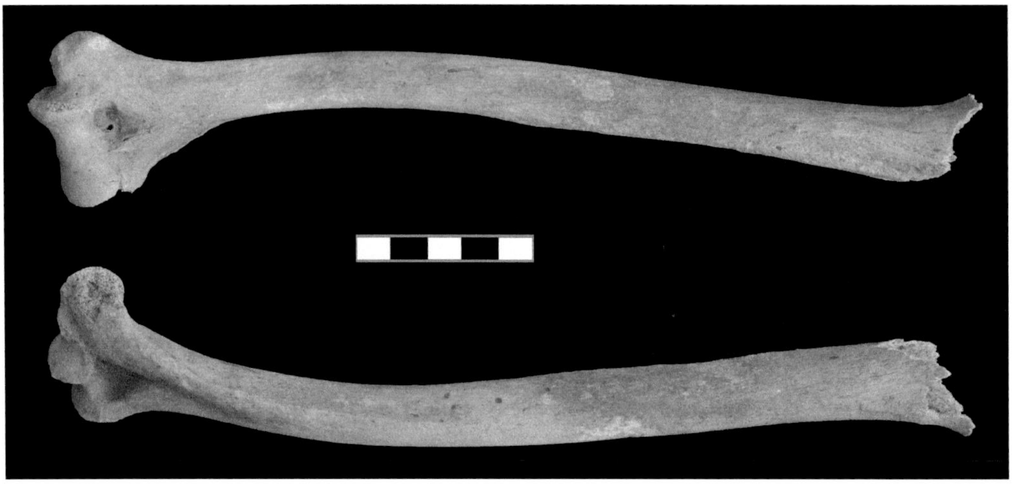

Figure 5.24 Bending deformity of the left humerus. (Sbide, Roman/Byzantine; photos by Efthymia Nikita, with the kind permission of Dr. Ahmet Ihsan Aytek, Burdur Mehmet Akif Ersoy University)

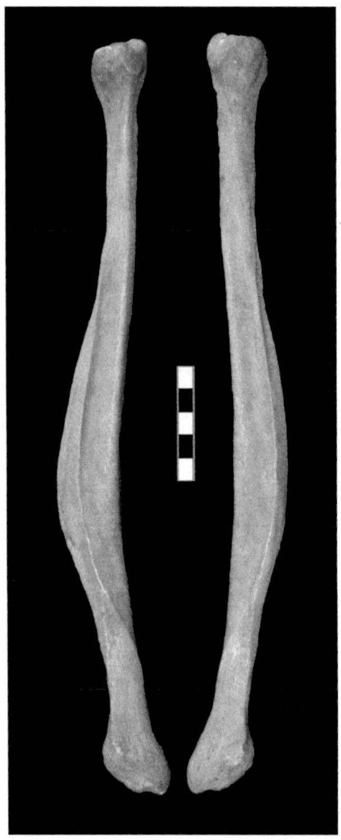

Figure 5.25 Bending deformity of the fibulae. (Photos by Efthymia Nikita; copyright: Duckworth Laboratory, University of Cambridge)

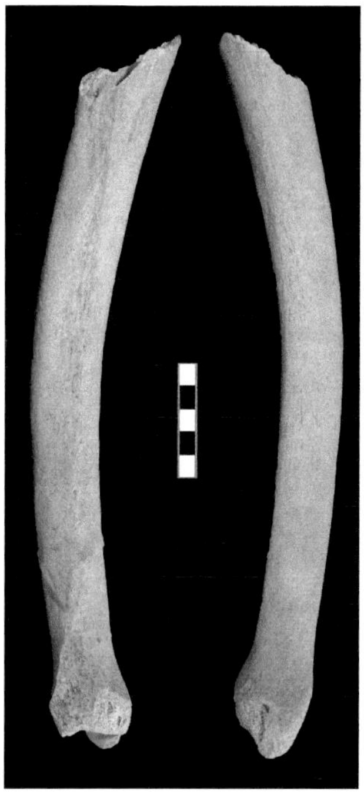

Figure 5.26 Bending deformity of the left tibia. (Photos by Efthymia Nikita; copyright: Duckworth Laboratory, University of Cambridge)

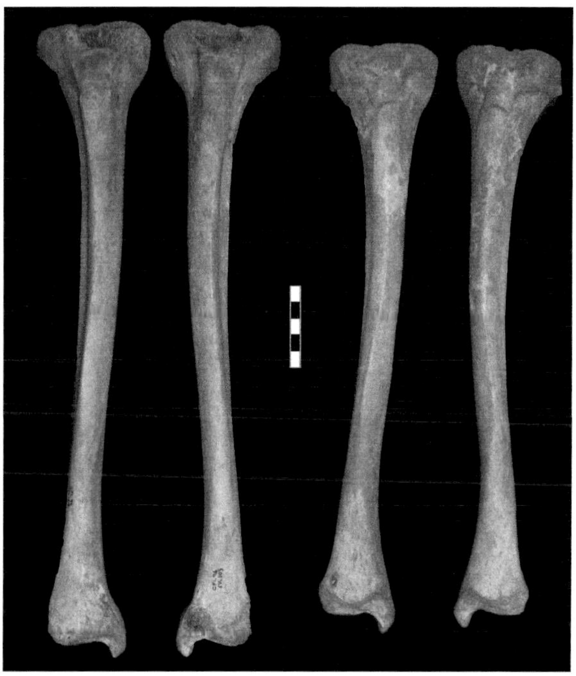

Figure 5.27 Bending deformity of two pairs of tibiae. (Left: Male, 26–35 years old, Centre For Life, Newcastle Infirmary at The Forth, 18th–19th c. CE, CFL-105; right: Female, Young adult, Centre For Life, Newcastle Infirmary at The Forth, 18th–19th c. CE, CFL-210; photos by Efthymia Nikita; copyright: Human Skeletal Collection, University of Sheffield)

Osteomalacia

Osteomalacia arises from a deficiency of vitamin D during adulthood, when impaired mineralisation disrupts the process of bone remodelling (see above for a discussion on the terminological differences between the clinical and palaeopathological literature). As a result of the accumulation of unmineralised osteoid, the skeleton is softened and weakened, leading to bone deformities and pseudofractures, which may progress to true fractures (Boxes 5.11 and 5.12, Figures 5.28–5.31).

Box 5.11 Skeletal manifestation of osteomalacia

Skull

- fine pitting/diffuse porosity
- basilar invagination
- antemortem tooth loss

Shoulder girdle

- clavicular fractures/pseudofractures*
- posterior curvature of scapular blade
- buckling/collapse of superior scapular border
- pseudofractures* on scapular lateral border, inferior lateral spine margin, and inferior angle

Thorax

- flattening/straightening of lateral rib shaft border
- rib neck angulation
- thinned cortex
- rib fractures/pseudofractures*
- anterior sternal protrusion (pectus carinatum)
- posterior sternal curvature (pectus excavatum)

Hand/foot

- metacarpal/metatarsal pseudofractures*

Vertebrae

- buckling/folding of vertebral bodies
- wedging/biconcave compression → kyphosis or scoliosis
- pseudofractures on transverse processes

Pelvic girdle

- iliac crest folding over or collapsing into iliac body
- cortical thinning in central ilium

- pseudofractures* on superior/inferior pubic rami
- anteriorly protruding pubic rami (anterior projection of pubic symphyseal faces)
- protrusio acetabuli
- sacral angulation → obstructed pelvic inlet

Arm/leg

- pseudofractures* (especially in femoral neck and subtrochanteric region)
- antero-lateral bending of proximal femur
- coxa vara
- antero-posteriorly flattened proximal femur (subtrochanteric platymeria)
- genu valgum (knock knees)
- upper limb long bone bending
- poorly mineralised bone at muscle attachment sites
- cortical thinning

*typically bilateral and symmetric; minimal fractures where unmineralised osteoid accumulates; may evolve to true fractures; bony spicule formation facilitates recognition

(Data from Brickley et al. 2005, 2007, 2018, 2020; Ives and Brickley 2014; Mankin 1974)

Box 5.12 Diagnosing osteomalacia

According to Van der Merwe et al. (2018), lesions *highly suggestive* for osteomalacia include a) unilateral or bilateral pseudofractures at the scapular spine inferior lateral margin, b) healing rib (pseudo)fractures, and/or c) pelvic (pseudo)fractures. *Possible* osteomalacia lesions include a) lesions on the scapular spine when no other strongly diagnostic or diagnostic lesions are present, b) no scapular lesions, but possible rib, pelvic, and/or femoral pseudofractures coupled with some of the general features.

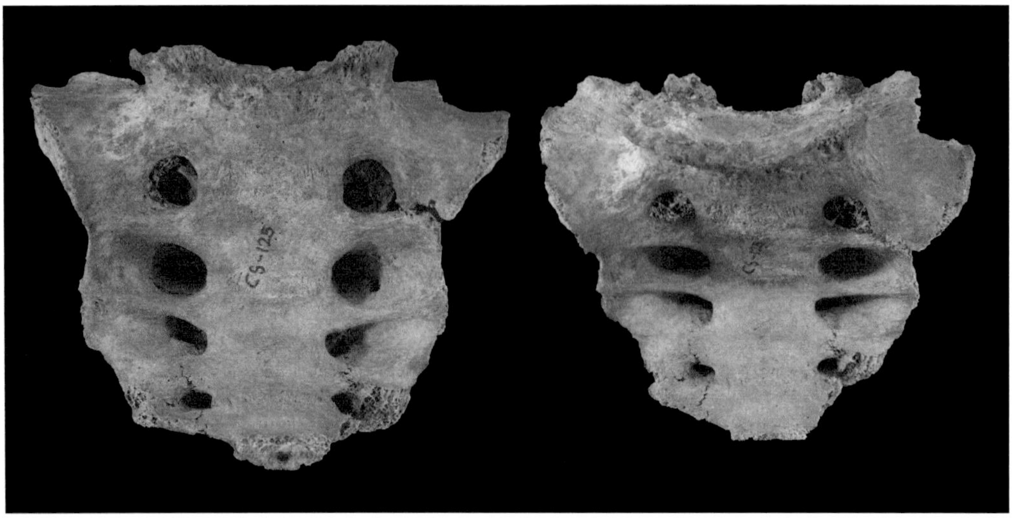

Figure 5.28 Angulated sacrum. (Male, 50–80 years old, St Hilda's Church, Coronation Street, South Shields, Newcastle, 19th c., CS06-125; photos by Efthymia Nikita; copyright: Human Skeletal Collection, University of Sheffield)

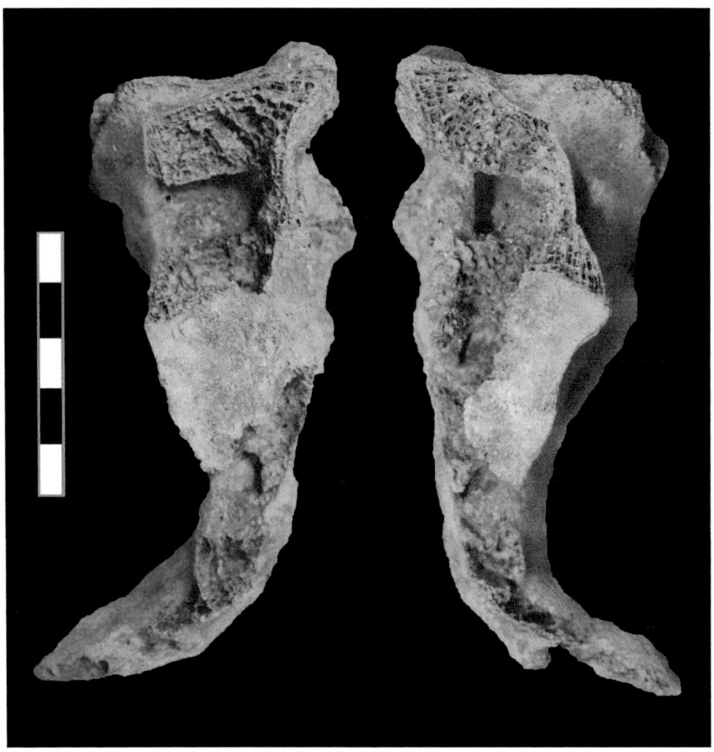

Figure 5.29 Abnormal angulation of the inferior part of the sacrum. (Male, Old adult, Centre For Life, Newcastle Infirmary at The Forth, 18th-19th c. CE, CFL 138; photos by Efthymia Nikita; copyright: Human Skeletal Collection, University of Sheffield)

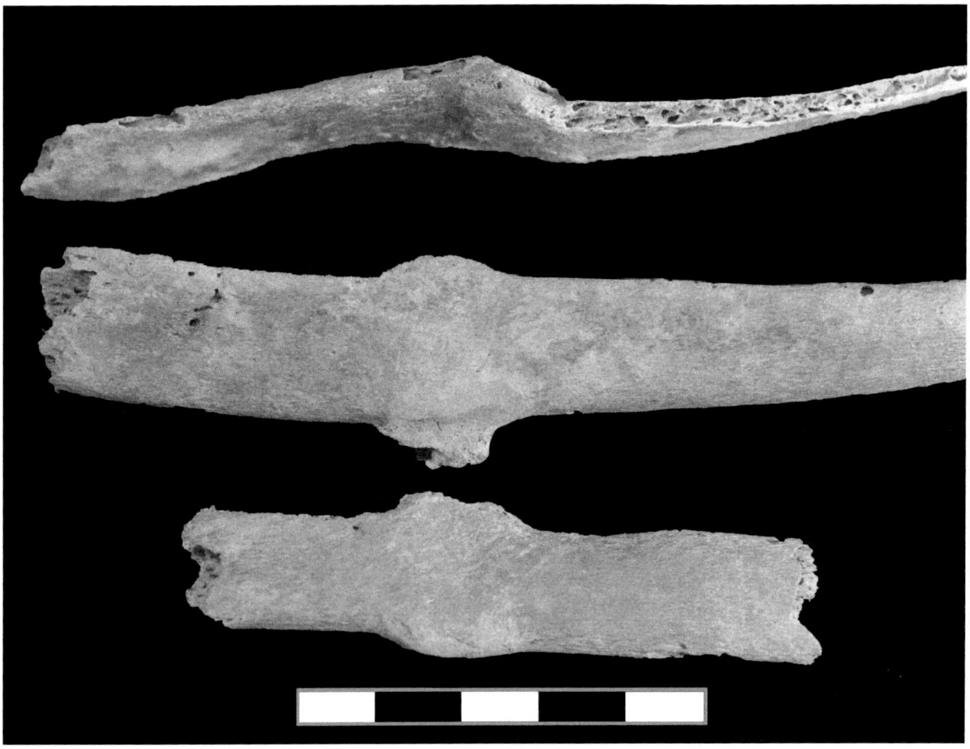

Figure 5.30 Healed rib fractures; note callus formation. (Same individual as in Figure 5.29; photos by Efthymia Nikita; copyright: Human Skeletal Collection, University of Sheffield)

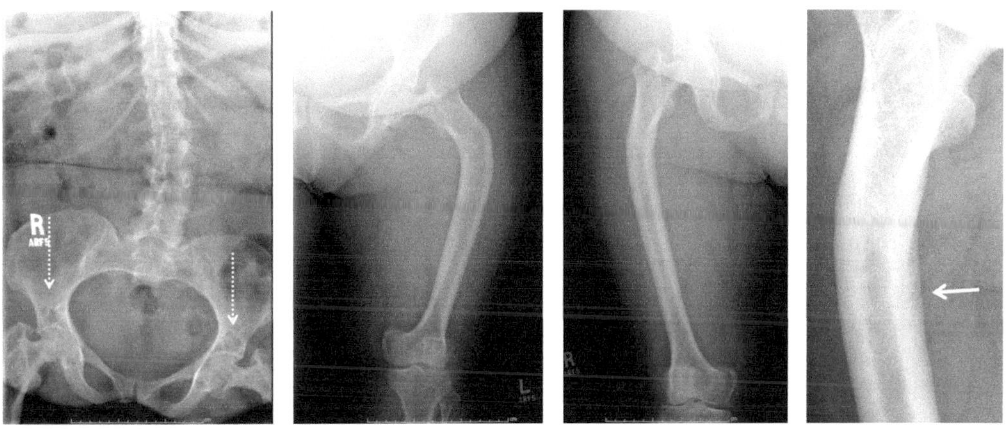

(a) (b) (c) (d)

Figure 5.31 Osteomalacia in a 51-year-old female. Note the heterogeneous bone density (dotted arrows) and bowing deformities of the femora. (Figure 5 in Patel et al. 2015; article licensed under a Creative Commons Attribution 3.0 Unported License)

Box 5.13 Osteomalacia-osteoporosis co-occurrence

Many risk factors are shared between osteoporosis and osteomalacia, both of which commonly affect elderly individuals, as described above. The co-occurrence of these conditions can exacerbate their individual effects. Specifically, vitamin D deficiency causes muscle weakness, increasing fall risk, which, when coupled with osteoporosis, implies a greater risk of fractures. Similarly, osteoporosis is characterised by increased rates of bone resorption; when vitamin D deficiency, which increases the accumulation of poorly mineralised osteoid, co-occurs with osteoporosis, the fracture risk is further increased.

Box 5.14 Metabolic and infectious disease co-occurrence

Infections and dietary deficiencies have a synergistic relationship, particularly in poor socio-economic contexts. Vitamin D controls important immune functions; thus, its deficiency can increase the susceptibility to infectious diseases and impair the immune system's capacity to respond effectively to infections. On the other hand, infections can affect normal vitamin D physiology. Similarly, individuals deficient in vitamin C are more vulnerable to infectious diseases, given the vital role that vitamin C plays in immune defence.

The issue of disease co-occurrence was briefly mentioned above, for scurvy. Osteomalacia may also co-occur with other conditions, especially osteoporosis (Box 5.13), while vitamin C and D deficiencies also have a complex relationship with infectious diseases (Box 5.14).

Paget's disease of bone

Paget's disease of bone (PDB) is characterised by abnormal bone remodelling, resulting in significant enlargement and deformity of the affected bones (Figures 5.32–5.38). Osteoclastic activity predominates during the initial phase of the disease, called the "lytic phase." The disease then progresses to the "mixed phase," where osteolytic and osteoblastic activities co-occur, with the latter being dominant. Collagen fibres in the newly formed bone are deposited in a disorganised manner; thus, the bone is of inferior mechanical quality. In the final phase of PDB ("sclerotic phase"), osteogenic activity is predominant; however, the newly formed bone again has a disorganised microarchitecture and reduced mechanical strength. Eventually,

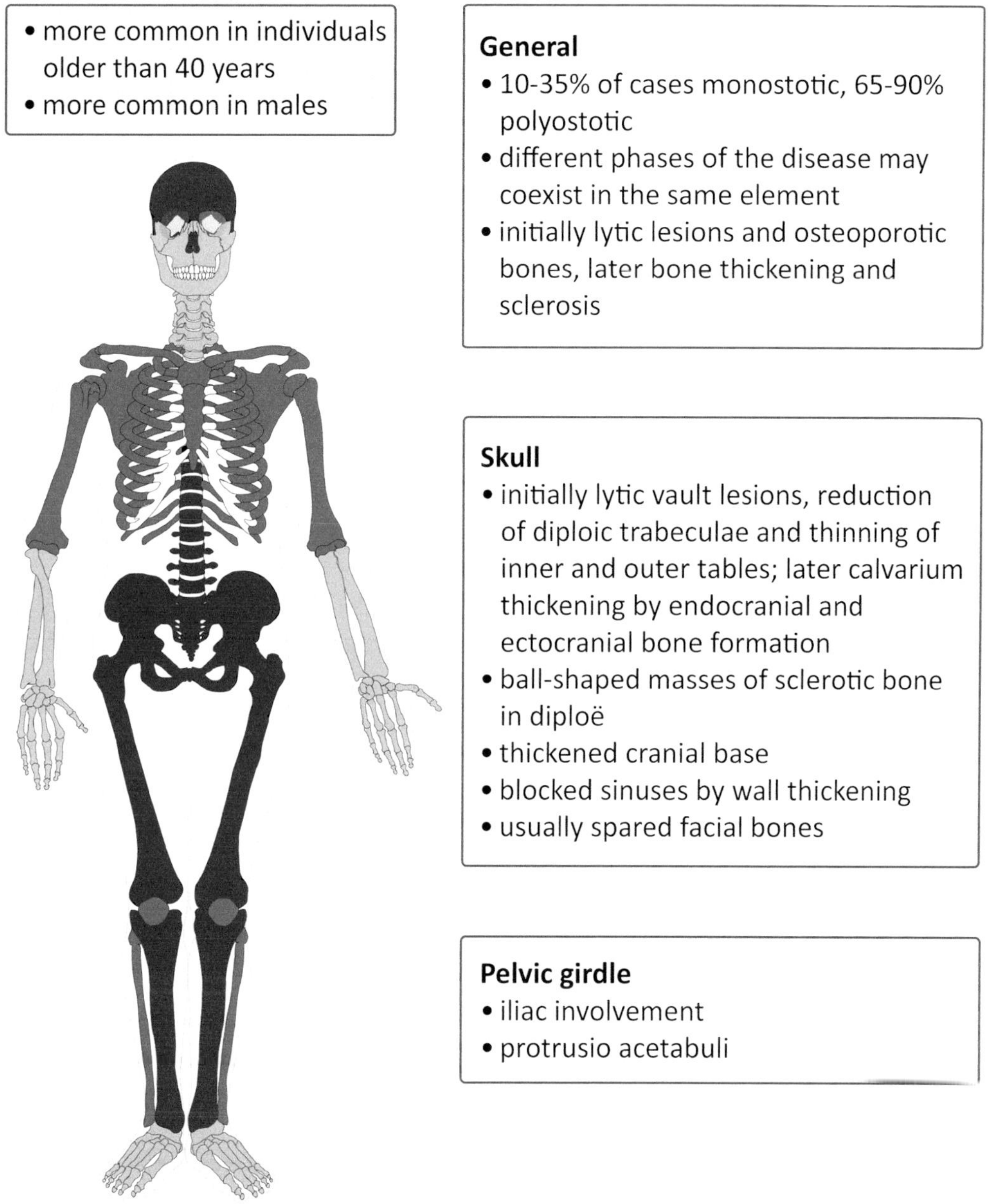

Figure 5.32 Skeletal manifestation of Paget's disease of bone. (Data from Brickley et al. 2020; Burrell et al. 2019; Cooper et al. 1999; Davie et al. 1999; Garnett and Lewis 2022; Grauer and Roberts 2019; Mays 2008; Nepal et al. 2021; Schneider et al. 2002; Shaker 2009; Tuck et al. 2017; Valenzuluela and Pietschmann 2017; Vallet and Ralston 2016; Whitehouse and Davies 2006)

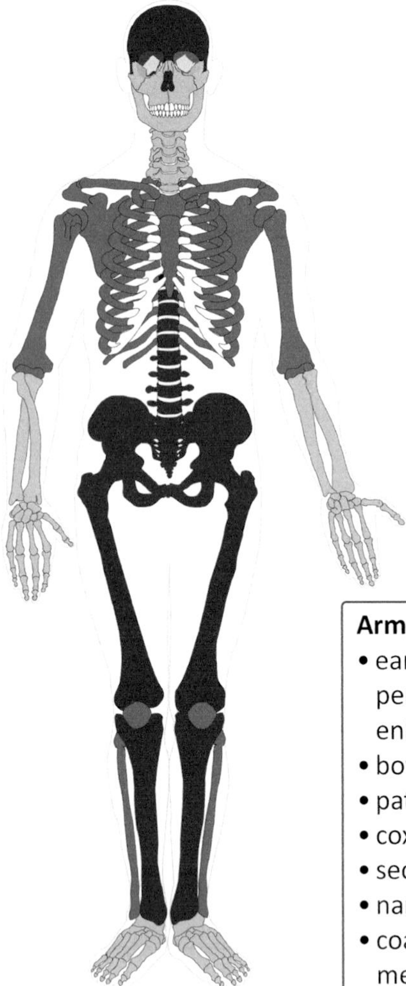

Figure 5.32 (Continued)

the disease enters a quiescent phase where both bone resorption and formation are diminished. PDB may affect a single bone (monostotic form), but it is more commonly observed in multiple bones (polyostotic form). Macroscopically, bones affected by PDB are enlarged, heavier, and show increased porosity compared to normal bone. However, macroscopic analysis alone has been found to lead to overdiagnosis; thus, it is important to complement it with radiographic and histological analysis (Garnett and Lewis 2022).

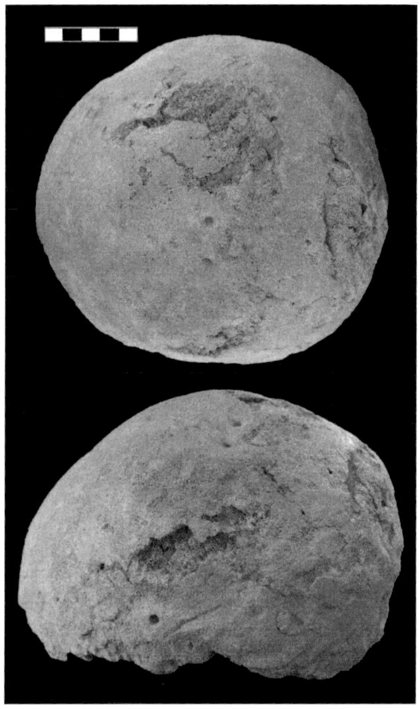

Figure 5.33 Paget's disease of bone. Note the extreme thickening of the cranial vault. (Female, Young adult, Black Gate cemetery, Newcastle-Upon-Tyne, 8th-12th c. CE, BG 90/92; photos by Efthymia Nikita; copyright: Human Skeletal Collection, University of Sheffield)

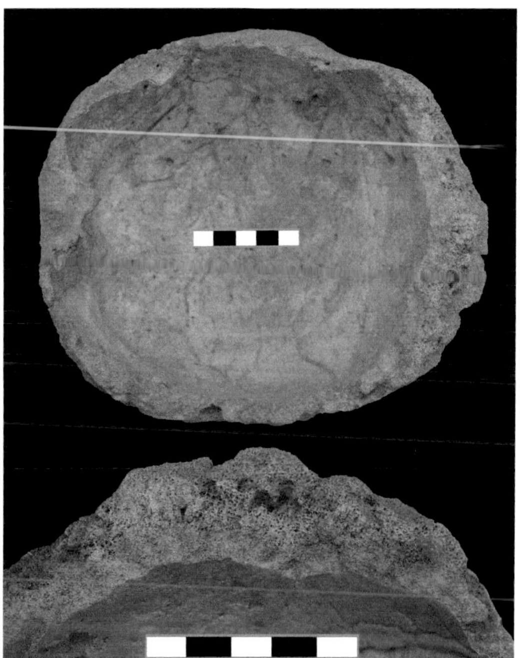

Figure 5.34 Paget's disease of bone. Note the extreme thickening of the cranial vault, particularly of the frontal bone. (Same individual as in Figure 5.33; photos by Efthymia Nikita; copyright: Human Skeletal Collection, University of Sheffield)

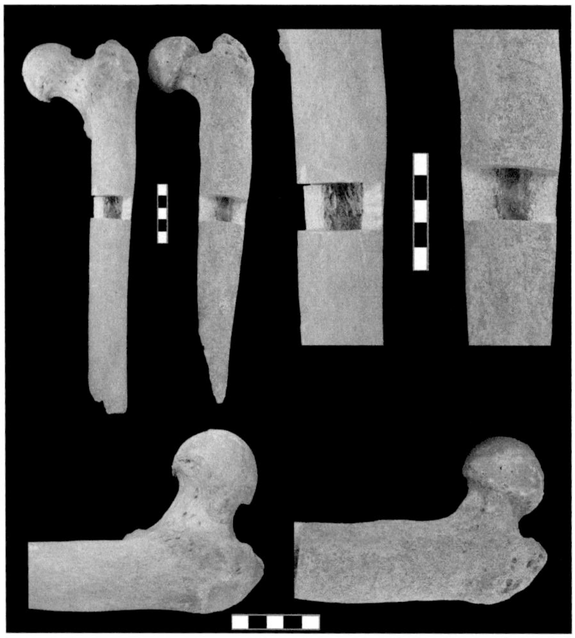

Figure 5.35 Paget's disease of bone. Note the thickening of the left femur (right) compared to a normal bone (left); also note the cut section showing cortical thickening and narrowing of the medullary canal. (Same individual as in Figures 5.33–5.34; photos by Efthymia Nikita; copyright: Human Skeletal Collection, University of Sheffield)

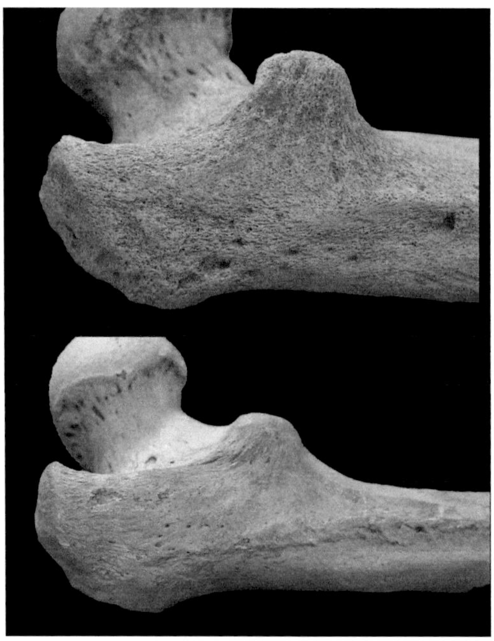

Figure 5.36 Paget's disease of bone. Note the thickening of the proximal left femur (top) compared to a normal bone (bottom); also note the porous, pumice-like bone surface of the affected element. (Same individual as in Figures 5.33–5.35; photos by Efthymia Nikita; copyright: Human Skeletal Collection, University of Sheffield)

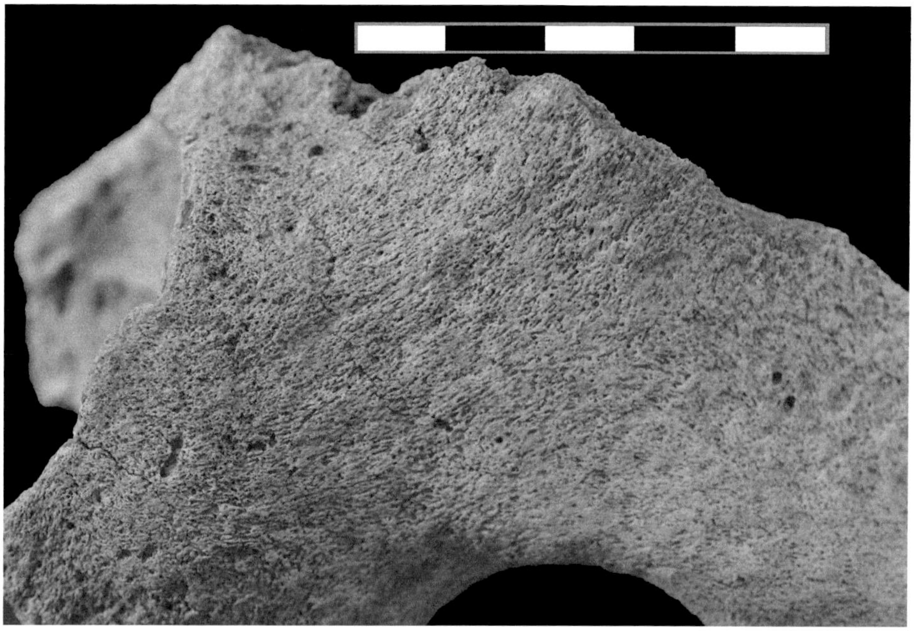

Figure 5.37 Paget's disease of bone. Note the porous, pumice-like surface of the left os coxa. (Same individual as in Figures 5.33–5.36; photo by Efthymia Nikita; copyright: Human Skeletal Collection, University of Sheffield)

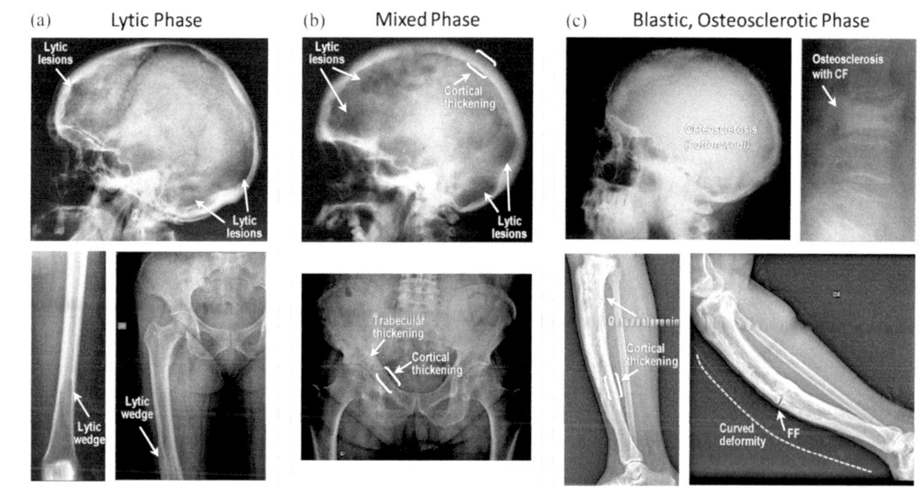

Figure 5.38 Radiographs of different skeletal elements affected by Paget's disease of bone during different stages of this condition. Lytic phase: lytic lesions in the frontal and occipital bones (top) and the distal femur (bottom). Mixed phase: lytic lesions, coupled with thickened diploë (top); cortical and trabecular thickening and lytic lesions in the right os coxa (bottom). Blastic, osteosclerotic phase: thickening of the cranial vault, and areas of focal sclerosis ("cotton wool" appearance) (top left); sclerotic vertebra with compression fracture (CF) (top right); bowed tibiae with loss of distinction between cortex and medullary cavity (bottom). (Figure 2 in Rendina et al. 2024; article licensed under a Creative Commons Attribution 4.0 International License)

The aetiology of PDB remains unknown; however, it has been associated with viral infections (especially those caused by paramyxoviruses), genetic predisposition, and exposure to toxins. Most patients remain asymptomatic; however, others may experience bone pain, secondary osteoarthritis, pathological fractures, skeletal deformities, and neurological problems resulting from bone overgrowth that causes nerve impingement. In rare cases, pagetic bone will undergo malignant transformation to a sarcoma.

Fluorosis

Fluorosis arises from prolonged consumption of excessive fluoride. Around 80% of ingested fluoride is absorbed in the gastrointestinal tract. About 50% of this in adults and 80% in young children is retained in the body, almost exclusively in the bones and teeth, and the rest is excreted. Within the skeleton, fluoride ions substitute for the hydroxyl groups in hydroxyapatite, resulting in the formation of fluorapatite.

In normal concentrations, fluoride contributes to skeletal health; however, prolonged excessive consumption of fluoride can have negative effects. These include gastrointestinal disturbances (e.g. nausea, constipation, bloating, diarrhoea), muscle wasting, joint pain, and skin rashes. As fluorosis progresses, the skeleton is involved (Box 5.15, Figures 5.39 and 5.40) and individuals may show bone deformities, fractures, osteosclerosis, radiculopathy (due to a pinched nerve in the spine), or myelopathy (due to compression of the spinal cord).

Box 5.15 Skeletal manifestation of fluorosis

Skull

- thickening
- obliterated diploë
- ossification of attachment sites for ligaments and tendons
- irregular margins of foramen magnum (due to ossified ligaments)
- dentition
    - discoloration/mottling
    - enamel pitting

Thorax

- rib enlargement (sclerotic new bone formation)
- rough rib surfaces (due to ligament ossification)
- intercostal muscle ossification
- ligamentous ossification resulting in fusion of ribs with vertebrae and sternum
- rib fractures
- trabecular bone thickening and sclerosis

Vertebrae

- cervical and lumbar vertebrae mostly affected
- trabecular bone thickening and sclerosis

- ossification of ligamentum flavum and other spinal ligaments
- fused vertebrae by thick osteophytes
- degenerative joint disease
- enlarged vertebral bodies
- kyphosis

Pelvic girdle

- ossified ligament attachment sites
- trabecular bone thickening and sclerosis

Arm/leg

- periosteal bone formation → bones heavy and irregular
- enthesophytes at muscle and tendon insertions
- genu varum
- genu valgum (knock knees)
- fractures
- thickened trabecular bone

(Data from Jolly et al. 1969; Littleton 1999; Petrone et al. 2019; Walser III et al. 2020)

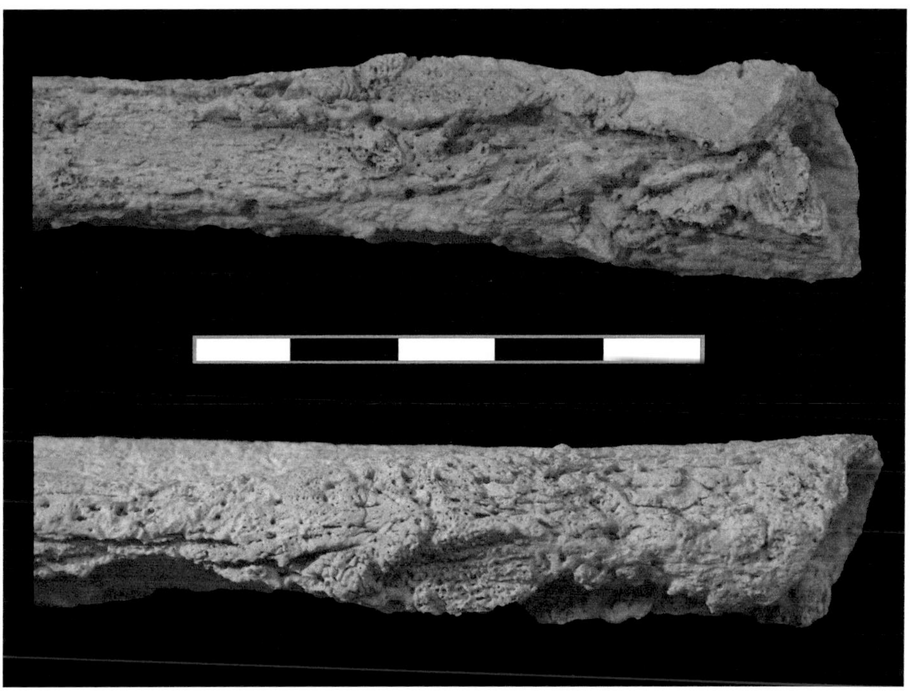

Figure 5.39 Possible fluorosis. Note the extensive periosteal new bone formation on the fibular shaft, resulting in a highly irregular bone surface. (Photos by Efthymia Nikita; copyright: Duckworth Laboratory, University of Cambridge)

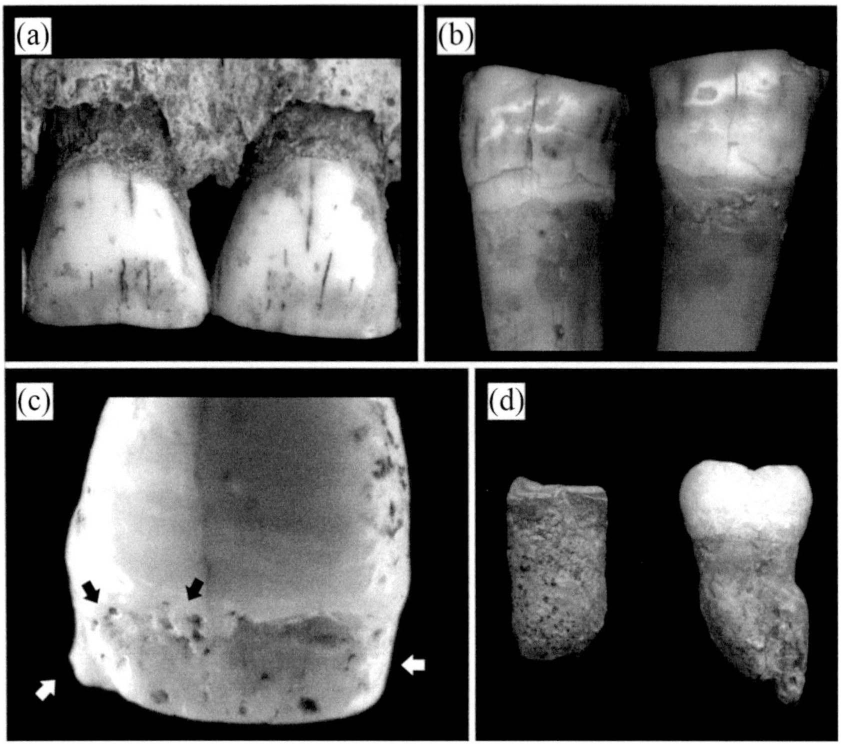

Figure 5.40 Dental pathological features of fluorosis. Note mottling and staining (a, b), pitting and enamel hypomineralisation (c), and root hypercementosis (d). (Figure 5 in Petrone et al. 2011; article licensed under a Creative Commons Attribution 4.0 International License)

Fluorosis is usually chronic, resulting from the prolonged consumption of excessive fluoride, especially through well and spring water where the surrounding geological formations have high fluoride concentrations. Various biological factors (e.g. genetics, sex, and age), cultural parameters (e.g. food additives and smoking), and environmental conditions (e.g. elevated temperatures and volcanic emissions) also play a significant role in the onset and severity of fluorosis.

Hyperostosis frontalis interna

Hyperostosis frontalis interna (HFI) appears as abnormal bone formation on the endocranial surface of the frontal bone, which may also be present in other cranial bones. It has diverse skeletal manifestations, ranging from isolated nodules to extensive areas of osseous overgrowth (Figures 5.41 and 5.42).

HFI is mostly found in postmenopausal females, while in males it is rather rare and often linked to hypogonadism. Although its aetiology is unclear, it has been associated with obesity, genetic factors, and various metabolic and endocrine disorders. The fact that HFI is rather common in contemporary populations, but rarely documented in human remains prior to the 18th century, has led to the proposal that it may be associated with the advent of

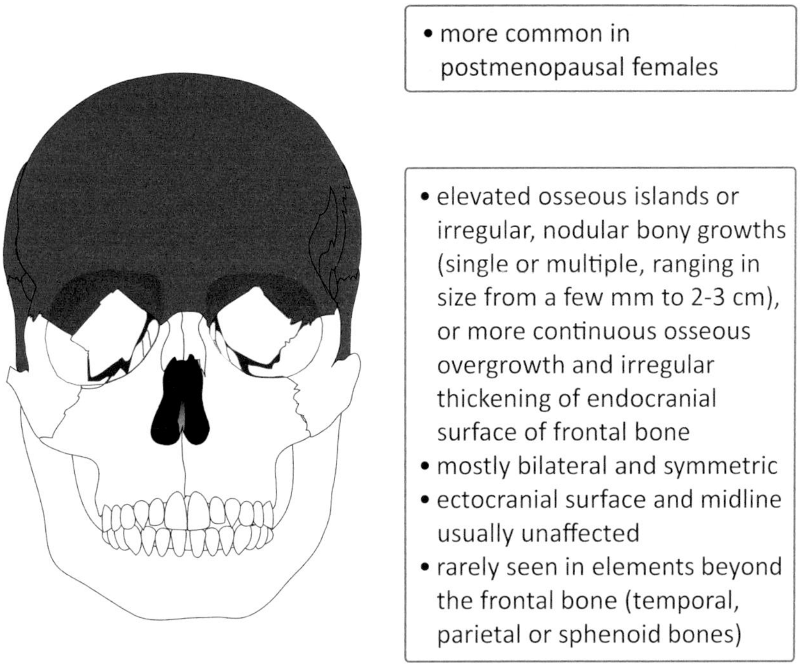

Figure 5.41 Skeletal manifestation of hyperostosis frontalis interna. (Data from Brickley and Mays 2019; Devriendt et al. 2005; Hershkovitz et al. 1999; Mulhern et al. 2006; Rühli and Henneberg 2002; Western and Bekvalac 2017)

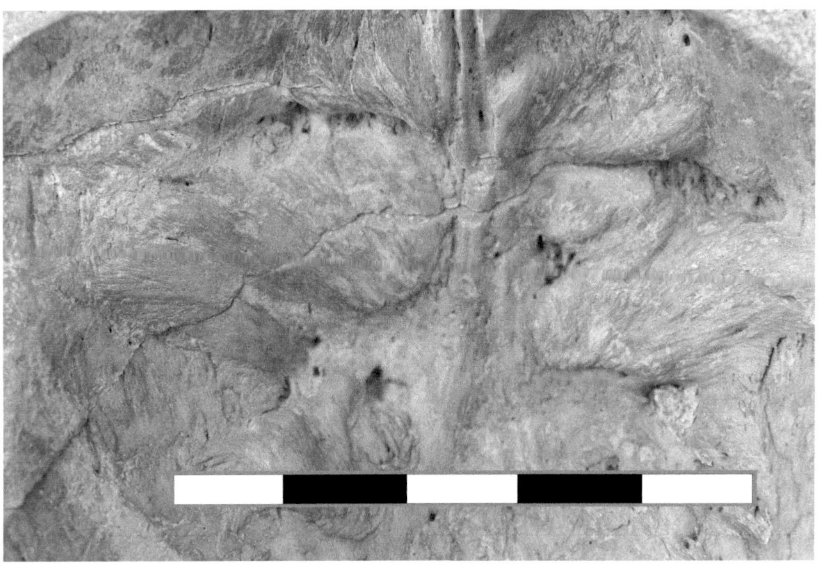

Figure 5.42 Hyperostosis frontalis interna. Note the bilateral extensive nodular bony overgrowth on the endocranial surface of the frontal bone. (Female, over 40 years old, Kampen Agnes klooster, 5164; photo by Efthymia Nikita, from the reference collection of the Cultural Heritage Agency of the Netherlands)

industrialisation and accompanying socioeconomic and lifestyle changes. Alternatively, this temporal pattern may be linked to an increase in longevity, which has led to changes in the human life cycle and associated fluctuations in hormone levels, or it may simply be an artefact of underreporting since HFI can be missed in well-preserved crania.

Individuals with HFI usually show no symptoms; however, compression due to thickened cranial bones may lead to cerebral atrophy, with subsequent cognitive deficits, neuropsychiatric symptoms, headaches, visual disturbances, and seizures. HFI is a hallmark feature of Morgagni–Stewart–Morel syndrome, which also includes virilism or hirsutism and obesity, but it can also develop as part of other syndromes, or as an independent entity.

Note

1 In cases of scurvy, bone porosity appears as localised penetrations in the cortical bone surface, specifically, as fine openings measuring less than 1 millimetre in diameter.

References and suggested readings

Agarwal, S.C. (2018). Understanding bone aging, loss and osteoporosis in the past. In *Biological Anthropology of the Human Skeleton*, edited by Katzenberg, M.A., Grauer, A.L., 3rd edition, pp. 385–414. Hoboken, NJ: John Wiley & Sons.

Agarwal, S.C., Stout, S.D. (2003). *Bone Loss and Osteoporosis: An Anthropological Perspective*. New York: Kluwer Academic/Plenum Publishers.

Aghajanian, P., Hall, S., Wongworawat, M.D., Mohan, S. (2015). The roles and mechanisms of actions of vitamin C in bone: New developments. *Journal of Bone and Mineral Research* 30:1945–1955. https://doi.org/10.1002/jbmr.2709

Aufderheide, A., Rodríguez-Martín, C. (1998). *The Cambridge Encyclopedia of Human Paleopathology*. Cambridge: Cambridge University Press.

Brickley, M. (2002). An investigation of historical and archaeological evidence for age-related bone loss and osteoporosis. *International Journal of Osteoarchaeology* 12:364–371. https://doi.org/10.1002/oa.635

Brickley, M.B. (2022). Commentary: Pathological fractures in osteomalacia, an underrecognized phenomenon. *International Journal of Osteoarchaeology* 32:536–540. https://doi.org/10.1002/oa.3024

Brickley, M., Agarwal, S.C. (2003). Techniques for the investigation of age-related bone loss and osteoporosis in archaeological bone. In *Bone Loss and Osteoporosis: An Anthropological Perspective*, edited by Agarwal, S.C., Stout, S.D., pp. 157–172. New York: Kluwer Academic/Plenum Publishers.

Brickley, M., Ives, R. (2006). Skeletal manifestations of infantile scurvy. *American Journal of Physical Anthropology* 129:163–172. https://doi.org/10.1002/ajpa.20265

Brickley, M., Mays, S. (2019). Metabolic disease. In *Ortner's Identification of Pathological Conditions in Human Skeletal Remains*, edited by Buikstra, J., pp. 531–566. San Diego: Academic Press.

Brickley, M.B., Morgan, B. (2023a). Assessing diagnostic certainty for scurvy and rickets in human skeletal remains. *American Journal of Biological Anthropology* 181:637–645. https://doi.org/10.1002/ajpa.24799

Brickley, M.B., Morgan, B. (2023b). Metabolic and endocrine diseases. In *The Routledge Handbook of Paleopathology*, edited by Grauer, A.L., pp. 338–359. London: Routledge.

Brickley, M., Mays, S., Ives, R. (2005). Skeletal manifestations of vitamin D deficiency osteomalacia in documented historical collections. *International Journal of Osteoarchaeology* 15:389–403. https://doi.org/10.1002/oa.794

Brickley, M., Mays, S., Ives, R. (2007). An investigation of skeletal indicators of vitamin D deficiency in adults: Effective markers for interpreting past living conditions and pollution levels in 18th and 19th century Birmingham, England. *American Journal of Physical Anthropology* 132:67–79. https://doi.org/10.1002/ajpa.20491

Brickley, M., Mays, S., Ives, R. (2010). Evaluation and interpretation of residual rickets deformities in adults. *International Journal of Osteoarchaeology* 20:54–66. https://doi.org/10.1002/oa.1007

Brickley, M.B., Mays, S., George, M., Prowse, T.L. (2018). Analysis of patterning in the occurrence of skeletal lesions used as indicators of vitamin D deficiency in subadult and adult skeletal remains. *International Journal of Paleopathology* 23:43–53. https://doi.org/10.1016/j.ijpp.2018.01.001

Brickley, M.B., Ives, R., Mays, S. (2020). *The Bioarchaeology of Metabolic Bone Disease*, 2nd edition. San Diego: Academic Press.

Brown, M., Ortner, D.J. (2011). Childhood scurvy in a medieval burial from Mačvanska Mitrovica, Serbia. *International Journal of Osteoarchaeology* 21:197–207. https://doi.org/10.1002/oa.1124

Burrell, C.L., Emery, M.M., Gonzalez, S. (2019). Paget's disease of bone in two medieval skeletons from Poulton Chapel, Cheshire, UK. *International Journal of Osteoarchaeology* 29:922–933. https://doi.org/10.1002/oa.2807

Cooper, C., Schafheutle, K., Dennison, E., Kellingray, S., Guyer, P., Barker, D. (1999). The epidemiology of Paget's disease in Britain: Is the prevalence decreasing? *Journal of Bone and Mineral Research* 14:192–197. https://doi.org/10.1359/jbmr.1999.14.2.192

Crandall, J.J., Klaus, H.D. (2014). Advancements, challenges, and prospects in the paleopathology of scurvy: Current perspectives on vitamin C deficiency in human skeletal remains. *International Journal of Paleopathology* 5:1–8. https://doi.org/10.1016/j.ijpp.2014.04.005

Curate, F. (2014). Osteoporosis and paleopathology: A review. *Journal of Anthropological Sciences* 92:119–146. https://doi.org/10.4436/JASS.92003

Curate, F., Silva, T.F., Cunha, E. (2016). Vertebral compression fractures: Towards a standard scoring methodology in paleopathology. *International Journal of Osteoarchaeology* 26:366–372. https://doi.org/10.1002/oa.2418

Davie, M., Davies, M., Francis, R., Fraser, W., Hosking, D., Tansley, R. (1999). Paget's disease of bone: A review of 889 patients. *Bone* 24:S11–S12. https://doi.org/10.1016/S8756-3282(99)00027-7

Devriendt, W., Piercecchi-Marti, M.D., Adalian, P., Sanvoisin, A., Dutour, O., Leonetti, G. (2005). Hyperostosis frontalis interna: Forensic issues. *Journal of Forensic Sciences* 50:143–146.

Eggington, J., Pitt, R., Hodson, C. (2024). A macroscopic assessment of porosity and new bone formation on the inferior pars basilaris: Normal growth or an indicator of scurvy?. *International Journal of Paleopathology* 45:62–72. https://doi.org/10.1016/j.ijpp.2024.05.001

Fain, O. (2005). Musculoskeletal manifestations of scurvy. *Joint Bone Spine* 72:124–128. https://doi.org/10.1016/j.jbspin.2004.01.007

Garnett, E.M., Lewis, M.E. (2022). The potential for over diagnosis of Paget's disease of bone using macroscopic analysis. *International Journal of Paleopathology* 38:55–63. https://doi.org/10.1016/j.ijpp.2022.07.001

Geber, J., Murphy, E. (2012). Scurvy in the Great Irish Famine: Evidence of vitamin C deficiency from a mid-19th century skeletal population. *American Journal of Physical Anthropology* 148:512–524. https://doi.org/10.1002/ajpa.22066

Gennari, L., Rendina, D., Falchetti, A., Merlotti, D. (2019). Paget's disease of bone. *Calcified Tissue International* 104:483–500. https://doi.org/10.1007/s00223-019-00522-3

Grauer, A.L., Roberts, C.A. (2019). Fungal, viral, multicelled parasitic, and protozoan infections. In *Ortner's Identification of Pathological Conditions in Human Skeletal Remains*, edited by Buikstra, J., pp. 441–478. San Diego: Academic Press.

Harvey, N., Dennison, E., Cooper, C. (2014). Osteoporosis: A lifecourse approach. *Journal of Bone and Mineral Research* 29:1917–1925. https://doi.org/10.1002/jbmr.2286

Hegeman, J., Oskam, J., Van der Palen, J., Ten Duis, H., Vierhout, P. (2004). The distal radial fracture in elderly women and the bone mineral density of the lumbar spine and hip. *Journal of Hand Surgery* 29:473–476. https://doi.org/10.1016/J.JHSB.2004.05.002

Hershkovitz, I., Greenwald, C., Rothschild, B.M., Latimer, B., Dutour, O., Jellema, L.M., Wish-Baratz, S. (1999). Hyperostosis frontalis interna: An anthropological perspective. *American Journal of Physical Anthropology* 109:303–325. https://doi.org/10.1002/(SICI)1096-8644(199907)109:3<303::AID-AJPA3>3.0.CO;2-I

Holck, P. (1984). Scurvy – a paleopathological problem. In *Proceedings of the Paleopathology Association 5th European Meeting*, edited by Cockburn, E., pp. 163–171, Siena.

Holick, M.F. (2007). Vitamin D deficiency. *The New England Journal of Medicine* 357:266–281. https://doi.org/10.1056/NEJMra070553

Ives, R., Brickley, M. (2014). New findings in the identification of adult vitamin D deficiency osteomalaica: Results from a large-scale study. *International Journal of Paleopathology* 7:45–56. https://doi.org/10.1016/j.ijpp.2014.06.004

Ives, R., Humphrey, L. (2018). Endochondral growth disruption during vitamin D deficiency rickets in a mid-19th century series from Bethnal Green, London, UK. *American Journal of Physical Anthropology* 167:585–601. https://doi.org/10.1002/ajpa.23687

Ives, R., Mant, M., De La Cova, C., Brickley, M. (2017). A large-scale palaeopathological study of hip fractures from post-medieval urban England. *International Journal of Osteoarchaeology* 27:261–275. https://doi.org/10.1002/oa.2536

Ives, R., Swan, K., Humphrey, L. (2023). Investigating the "scapula sign" as an indicator of rickets. *International Journal of Paleopathology* 41:59–68. https://doi.org/10.1016/j.ijpp.2023.02.004

Jablonski, N.G., Chaplin, G. (2018). The roles of vitamin D and cutaneous vitamin D production in human evolution and health. *International Journal of Paleopathology* 23:54–59. https://doi.org/10.1016/j.ijpp.2018.01.005

Jaffe, H. (1972). *Metabolic, Degenerative, and Inflammatory Diseases of Bones and Joints*. Philadelphia: Lea and Febiger.

Jolly, S., Singh, B., Mathur, O. (1969). Endemic fluorosis in Punjab (India). *The American Journal of Medicine* 47:553–563. https://doi.org/10.1016/0002-9343(69)90186-7

Kanis, J. (1998). *Pathophysiology and Treatment of Paget's Disease of Bone*, 2nd edition. London: Martin Dunitz.

Khosla, S., Riggs, B.L. (2005). Pathophysiology of age-related bone loss and osteoporosis. *Endocrinology & Metabolism Clinics* 34:1015–1030. https://doi.org/10.1016/j.ecl.2005.07.009

Klaus, H.D. (2017). Paleopathological rigor and differential diagnosis: Case studies involving terminology, description, and diagnostic frameworks for scurvy in skeletal remains. *International Journal of Paleopathology* 19:96–110. https://doi.org/10.1016/j.ijpp.2015.10.002

Kozłowski, T., Witas, H.W. (2012). Metabolic and endocrine diseases. In *A Companion to Paleopathology*, edited by Grauer, A.L., pp. 401–419. Hoboken, NJ: Wiley-Blackwell.

Krenz-Niedbała, M. (2016). Did children in medieval and post-medieval Poland suffer from scurvy? Examination of the skeletal evidence. *International Journal of Osteoarchaeology* 26:633–647. https://doi.org/10.1002/oa.2454

Lewis, M. (2017). *Paleopathology of Children: Identification of Pathological Conditions in the Human Skeletal Remains of Non-Adults*. San Diego: Academic Press.

Lips, P. (2001). Vitamin D deficiency and secondary hyperparathyroidism in the elderly: Consequences for bone loss and fractures and therapeutic implications. *Endocrine Reviews* 22:477–501. https://doi.org/10.1210/edrv.22.4.0437

Littleton, J. (1999). Paleopathology of skeletal fluorosis. *American Journal of Physical Anthropology* 109:465–483. https://doi.org/10.1002/(SICI)1096-8644(199908)109:4<465::AID-AJPA4>3.0.CO;2-T

Lockau, L., Atkinson, S.A. (2018). Vitamin D's role in health and disease: How does the present inform our understanding of the past? *International Journal of Paleopathology* 23:6–14. https://doi.org/10.1016/j.ijpp.2017.11.005

Lupsa, B.C., Insogna, K. (2015). Bone health and osteoporosis. *Endocrinology and Metabolism Clinics* 44:517–530. https://doi.org/10.1016/j.ecl.2015.05.002

Mankin, H. (1974). Rickets, osteomalacia and renal osteodystrophy. Part I. *The Journal of Bone & Joint Surgery* 56:101–128.

Mays, S. (2006). A palaeopathological study of Colles' fractures. *International Journal of Osteoarchaeology* 16:415–428. https://doi.org/10.1002/oa.845

Mays, S. (2008). Metabolic bone disease. In *Advances in Human Paleopathology*, edited by Pinhasi, R., Mays, S., pp. 215–252. Hoboken, NJ: John Wiley & Sons.

Mays, S., Brickley, M.B. (2018). Vitamin D deficiency in bioarchaeology and beyond: The study of rickets and osteomalacia in the past. *International Journal of Paleopathology* 23:1–5. https://doi.org/10.1016/j.ijpp.2018.05.004

Mays, S., Brickley, M.B. (2022). Is dietary deficiency of calcium a factor in rickets? Use of current evidence for our understanding of the disease in the past. *International Journal of Paleopathology* 36:36–44. https://doi.org/10.1016/j.ijpp.2021.11.001

Mays, S., Brickley, M.B., Ives, R. (2006). Skeletal manifestations of rickets in infants and young children in an historic population from England. *American Journal of Physical Anthropology* 129:362–374. https://doi.org/10.1002/ajpa.20292

Melikian, M., Waldron, T. (2003). An examination of skulls from two British sites for possible evidence of scurvy. *International Journal of Osteoarchaeology* 13:207–212. https://doi.org/10.1002/oa.674

Michałus, I., Łupińska, A., Woch, I., Wieczorek-Szukała, K., Chlebna-Sokół, D., Lewiński, A. (2022). Bone turnover markers and bone mineral density in children with hypophosphatemic rickets. *Journal of Clinical Medicine* 11:4622. https://doi.org/10.3390/jcm11154622

Moore, J., Koon, H.E. (2017). Basilar portion porosity: A pathological lesion possibly associated with infantile scurvy. *International Journal of Paleopathology* 18:92–97. https://doi.org/10.1016/j.ijpp.2017.05.010

Mulhern, D.M., Wilczak, C.A., Dudar, J.Ch. (2006). Brief communication: Unusual finding at Pueblo Bonito: Multiple cases of hyperostosis frontalis interna. *American Journal of Physical Anthropology* 130:480–484. https://doi.org/10.1002/ajpa.20396

Murphy, K., Weisman, Q., Makeneni, S., Faerber, J., Bonafide, C.P., Kenyon, C.C. (2024). Characteristics of pediatric scurvy hospitalizations: 2006–2021. *Pediatrics* 154:e2024065782. https://doi.org/10.1542/peds.2024-065782

Nepal, S., Jarusriwanna, A., Unnanuntana, A. (2021). Stress fracture of the femoral shaft in Paget's disease of bone: A case report. *Journal of Bone Metabolism* 28:171–178. https://doi.org/10.11005/jbm.2021.28.2.171

Nicolescu, R.C., Lombet, J., Cavalier, E. (2018). Vitamin D-resistant rickets and cinacalcet—one more favorable experience. *Frontiers in Pediatrics* 6:376. https://doi.org/10.3389/fped.2018.00376

Ortner, D.J., Ericksen, M.F. (1997). Bone changes in the human skull probably resulting from scurvy in infancy and childhood. *International Journal of Osteoarchaeology* 7:212–220. https://doi.org/10.1002/(SICI)1099-1212(199705)7:3<212::AID-OA346>3.0.CO;2-5

Ortner, D.J., Mays, S. (1998). Dry-bone manifestations of rickets in infancy and early childhood. *International Journal of Osteoarchaeology* 8:45–55. https://doi.org/10.1002/(SICI)1099-1212(199801/02)8:1<45::AID-OA405>3.0.CO;2-D

Ortner, D.J., Kimmerle, E.H., Diez, M. (1999). Probable evidence of scurvy in subadults from archeological sites in Peru. *American Journal of Physical Anthropology* 108:321–331. https://doi.org/10.1002/(SICI)1096-8644(199903)108;3<321::AID-AJPA7>3.0.CO;2-7

Ortner, D.J., Butler, W., Cafarella, J., Miligan, L. (2001). Evidence of probable scurvy in subadults from archaeological sites in North America. *American Journal of Physical Anthropology* 114:343–351. https://doi.org/10.1002/ajpa.1046

Patel, A.A., Ramanathan, R., Kuban, J., Willis, M.H. (2015). Imaging findings and evaluation of metabolic bone disease. *Advances in Radiology* 2015:812794. https://doi.org/10.1155/2015/812794

Petrone, P., Giordano, M., Giustino, S., Guarino, F.M. (2011). Enduring fluoride health hazard for the Vesuvius area population: The case of AD 79 Herculaneum. *PLoS ONE* 6:e21085. https://doi.org/10.1371/journal.pone.0021085

Petrone, P., Graziano, V., Sastri, C., Sauvage, T., Mezzasalma, M., Paternoster, M., Guarino, F.M. (2019). Dental fluorosis in the Vesuvius towns in AD 79: A multidisciplinary approach. *Annals of Human Biology* 46:388–392. https://doi.org/10.1080/03014460.2019.1640791

Pettifor, J.M. (2014). Calcium and vitamin D metabolism in children in developing countries. *Annals of Nutrition and Metabolism* 64:15–22. https://doi.org/10.1159/000365124

Prentice, A. (2013). Nutritional rickets around the world. *The Journal of Steroid Biochemistry and Molecular Biology* 136:201–206. https://doi.org/10.1016/j.jsbmb.2012.11.018

Ray, D., Goswami, R., Gupta, N., Tomar, N., Singh, N., Sreenivas, V. (2009). Predisposition to vitamin D deficiency osteomalacia and rickets in females is linked to their 25 (OH) D and calcium intake rather than vitamin D receptor gene polymorphism. *Clinical Endocrinology* 71:334–340. https://doi.org/10.1111/j.1365-2265.2008.03500.x

Reikersdorfer, K.N., Singh, A., Young, J.D., Batty, M.B., Steele, A.E., Yuen, L.C., Momtaz, D.A., Weissert, J.N., Liu, D.S., Hogue, G.D. (2024). The troubling rise of scurvy: A review and national analysis of incidence, associated risk factors, and clinical manifestations. *Journal of the American Academy of Orthopaedic Surgeons, Globall Research & Reviews* 8:e24. https://doi.org/10.5435/JAAOSGlobal-D-24-00162

Rendina, D., Falchetti, A., Diacinti, D., Bertoldo, F., Merlotti, D., Giannini, S., Cianferotti, L., Girasole, G., Di Monaco, M., Gonnelli, S., Malavolta, N., Minisola, S., Vescini, F., Rossini, M., Frediani, B., Chiodini, I., Asciutti, F., Gennari, L. (2024). Diagnosis and treatment of Paget's disease of bone: Position paper from the Italian Society of Osteoporosis, Mineral Metabolism and Skeletal Diseases (SIOMMMS). *Journal of Endocrinological Investigation* 47:1335–1360. https://doi.org/10.1007/s40618-024-02318-1

Rühli, F.J., Henneberg, M. (2002). Are hyperostosis frontalis interna and leptin linked? A hypothetical approach about hormonal influence on human microevolution. *Medical Hypotheses* 58:378–381. https://doi.org/10.1054/mehy.2001.1481

Schattmann, A., Bertrand, B., Vatteoni, S., Brickley, M. (2016). Approaches to co-occurrence: Scurvy and rickets in infants and young children of 16–18th century Douai, France. *International Journal of Paleopathology* 12:63–75. https://doi.org/10.1016/j.ijpp.2015.12.002

Schneider, D., Hofmann, M.T., Peterson, J.A. (2002). Diagnosis and treatment of Paget's disease of bone. *American Family Physician* 65:2069–2072.

Shaker, J.L. (2009). Paget's disease of bone: A review of epidemiology, pathophysiology and management. *Therapeutic Advances in Musculoskeletal Disease* 1:107–125. https://doi.org/10.1177/1759720X09351779

Snoddy, A.M.E., Buckley, H.R., Halcrow, S.E. (2016). More than metabolic: Considering the broader paleoepidemiological impact of vitamin D deficiency in bioarchaeology. *American Journal of Physical Anthropology* 160:183–196. https://doi.org/10.1002/ajpa.22968

Snoddy, A.M.E., Buckley, H.R., Elliott, G.E., Standen, V.G., Arriaza, B.T., Halcrow, S.E. (2018). Macroscopic features of scurvy in human skeletal remains: A literature synthesis and diagnostic guide. *American Journal of Physical Anthropology* 167:876–895. https://doi.org/10.1002/ajpa.23699

Song, S.Y., Kim, Y., Park, H., Kim, Y.J., Kang, W., Kim, E.Y. (2017). Effect of parity on bone mineral density: A systematic review and meta-analysis. *Bone* 101:70–76. https://doi.org/10.1016/j.bone.2017.04.013

Stark, R.J. (2014). A proposed framework for the study of paleopathological cases of subadult scurvy. *International Journal of Paleopathology* 5:18–26. https://doi.org/10.1016/j.ijpp.2014.01.005

Tschinkel, K., Gowland, R. (2020). Knock-knees: Identifying genu valgum and understanding its relationship to vitamin D deficiency in 18th to 19th century northern England. *International Journal of Osteoarchaeology* 30:891–902. https://doi.org/10.1002/oa.2919

Tuck, S., Layfield, R., Walker, J., Mekkayil, B., Francis, R. (2017). Adult Paget's disease of bone: A review. *Rheumatology* 56:2050–2059. https://doi.org/10.1093/rheumatology/kew430

Valenzuluela, E.N., Pietschmann, P. (2017). Epidemiology and pathology of Paget's disease of bone—A review. *Wiener Medizinische Wochenschrift* 167:2–8. https://doi.org/10.1007/s10354-016-0496-4

Vallet, M., Ralston, S.H. (2016). Biology and treatment of Paget's disease of bone. *Journal of Cellular Biochemistry* 117:289–299. https://doi.org/10.1002/jcb.25291

Van der Merwe, A.E., Veselka, B., Van Veen, H.A., Van Rijn, R.R., Colman, K.L., De Boer, H.H. (2018). Four possible cases of osteomalacia: The value of a multidisciplinary diagnostic approach. *International Journal of Paleopathology* 23:15–25. https://doi.org/10.1016/j.ijpp.2018.03.004

Vlok, M., Snoddy, A.M.E., Ramesh, N., Wheeler, B.J., Standen, V.G., Arriaza, B.T. (2023). The role of dietary calcium in the etiology of childhood rickets in the past and the present. *American Journal of Human Biology* 35:e23819. https://doi.org/10.1002/ajhb.23819

Waldron, T. (2020). *Palaeopathology*, 2nd edition. Cambridge: Cambridge University Press.
Walser III, J.W., Gowland, R.L., Desnica, N., Kristjánsdóttir, S. (2020). Hidden dangers? Investigating the impact of volcanic eruptions and skeletal fluorosis in medieval Iceland. *Archaeological and Anthropological Sciences* 12:77. https://doi.org/10.1007/s12520-020-01026-0
Western, A.G., Bekvalac, J.J. (2017). Hyperostosis frontalis interna in female historic skeletal populations: Age, sex hormones and the impact of industrialization. *American Journal of Physical Anthropology* 162:501–515. https://doi.org/10.1002/ajpa.23133
Whitehouse, R.W., Davies, M.A. (2006). Paget's disease of bone. In *Imaging of the Hip and Bony Pelvis: Techniques and Applications*, edited by Davies, M.A., Johnson, K.J., Whitehouse, R.W., pp. 381–392. Berlin: Springer.

Chapter 6

Endocrine disorders

The endocrine system consists of glands that synthesise and secrete hormones, which play an important role in regulating metabolism, reproduction, growth, and other vital functions. The hypersecretion or hyposecretion of hormones can affect bone size, shape, and density, especially if it occurs during the years of active growth and development. This chapter will focus on disorders associated with the pituitary, parathyroid, thyroid, and adrenal glands, as well as the gonads. Note that endocrine disorders are frequently examined in conjunction with metabolic bone diseases because the metabolism is regulated by the endocrine system. For organisational purposes, endocrine and metabolic disorders have been kept separate in this book, with metabolic diseases discussed in Chapter 5.

Pituitary disturbances

The pituitary gland is a small gland found at the base of the brain within a cavity of the sphenoid bone (sella turcica). This gland has several important functions, including playing a key role in regulating the functions of other endocrine glands. Specifically, the pituitary gland synthesises the growth hormone, as well as hormones that stimulate testosterone and sperm production in males and oestrogen production in females (gonadotrophins), and promote lactation in females (prolactin). It also stores and releases anti-diuretic hormone that is synthesised in the hypothalamus. Moreover, the pituitary gland secretes the thyroid-stimulating hormone, which stimulates the thyroid gland to secrete hormones essential for the regulation of metabolism and other vital functions. Similarly, it secretes adrenocorticotropic hormone that stimulates the adrenal glands to produce cortisol, which regulates the body's response to stress, maintains constant blood pressure and blood sugar levels, and suppresses inflammation. In addition, the pituitary stores oxytocin, a hormone that is synthesised in the hypothalamus, which promotes uterine contractions during childbirth and stimulates milk ejection during breastfeeding. Disorders affecting the pituitary gland typically manifest as either a hypofunction or hyperfunction of the organs it regulates.

Hyperpituitarism

Hyperpituitarism is characterised by the overproduction of hormones synthesised by the pituitary gland, due to the hyperfunction of this gland. This condition is often linked to the presence of a pituitary adenoma, a benign neoplasm; however, it may also arise from intrinsic abnormalities such as hyperplasia of the gland, or even from factors that affect the function of the hypothalamus and, thus, indirectly impact the pituitary gland.

DOI: 10.4324/9781003475026-6

Pituitary gigantism

Pituitary gigantism is a rare condition caused by the hypersecretion of growth hormone. It appears when this hypersecretion takes place while the epiphyseal plates are still open. This hypersecretion promotes an abnormal proliferation and differentiation of chondrocytes at the growth plates, causing accelerated linear growth but maintaining normal body proportions. Affected individuals have a much greater height than normal (Figure 6.1).

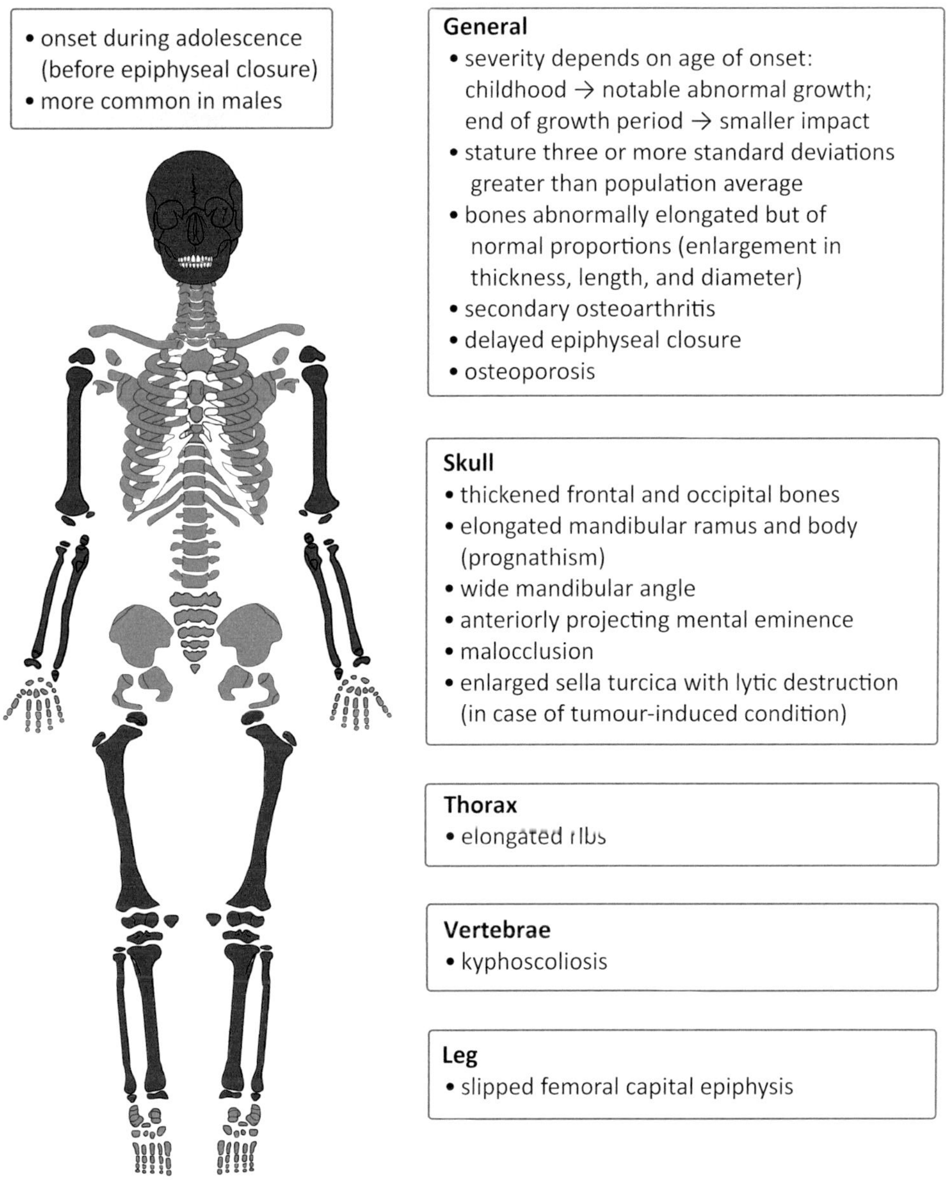

Figure 6.1 Skeletal manifestation of pituitary gigantism. (Data from Aufderheide and Rodríguez-Martín 1998; Lewis 2019; Reeves et al. 1978)

Acromegaly

Acromegaly is more common than gigantism and develops when excessive amounts of growth hormone are secreted after the closure of the growth plates. In acromegaly, the excessive production of growth hormone promotes bone growth; however, because the epiphyses have closed, linear growth is no longer possible. Consequently, this process results in periosteal new bone formation (Figures 6.2–6.4). Acromegaly may coexist with gigantism in cases where the hormonal imbalance starts during childhood and persists after epiphyseal closure.

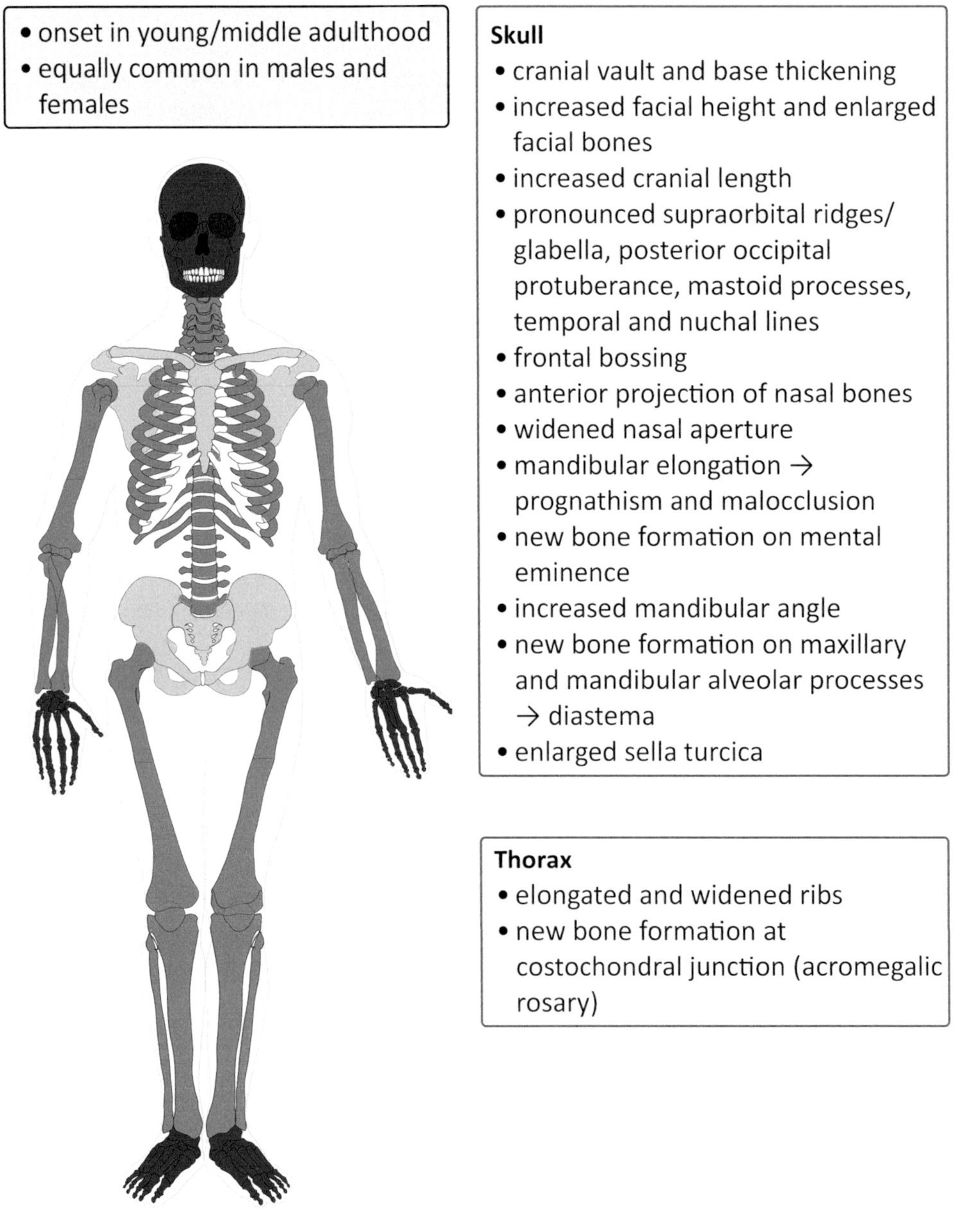

Figure 6.2 Skeletal manifestation of acromegaly. (Data from Aufderheide and Rodríguez-Martín 1998; Claessen et al. 2016; Cordero and Barkan 2008; Lewis 2019; van der Lely et al. 2005)

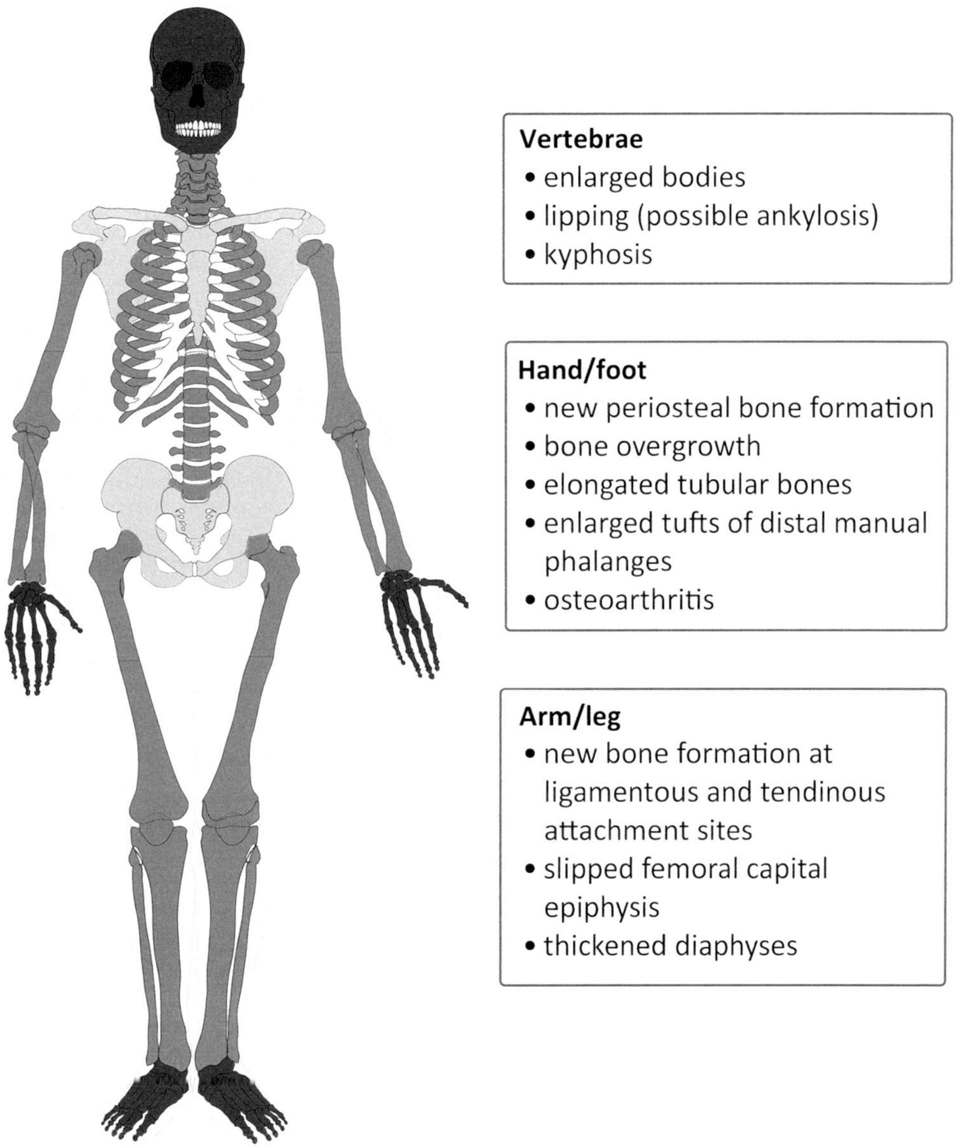

Figure 6.2 (Continued)

Hypopituitarism

Hypopituitarism is a disorder characterised by insufficient production of hormones by the pituitary gland. This condition may be caused by an impairment of the pituitary gland itself, for example, in cases of pituitary tumours, infections, traumatic injuries, or genetic disorders. Alternatively, these factors may affect the function of the hypothalamus and exert an indirect influence on the pituitary gland.

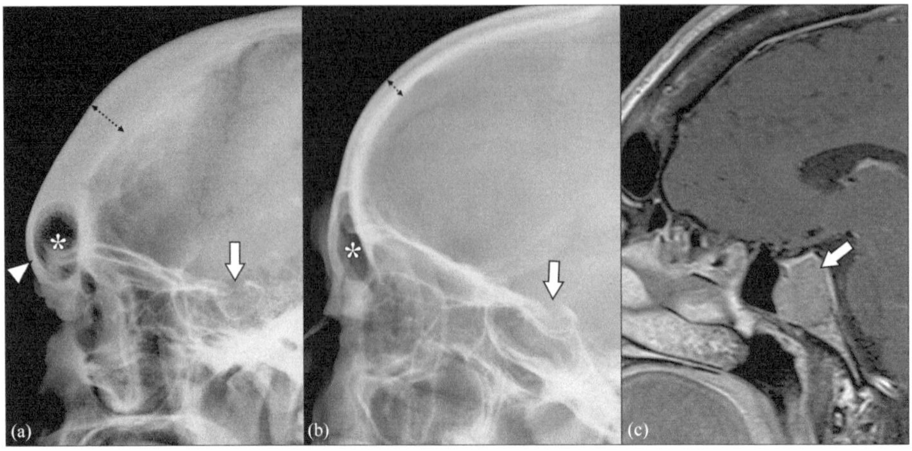

Figure 6.3 Radiograph of the skull of an individual with acromegaly (a). Note the thickness of the frontal bone, pronounced glabella, enlarged frontal sinus and sella turcica. Radiograph of the skull of healthy individual for comparison (b). MRI scan of the individual in (a), showing pituitary macroadenoma that has enlarged the sella turcica (c). (Figure 3 in Baptista et al. 2023; article licensed under a Creative Commons Attribution 4.0 International License)

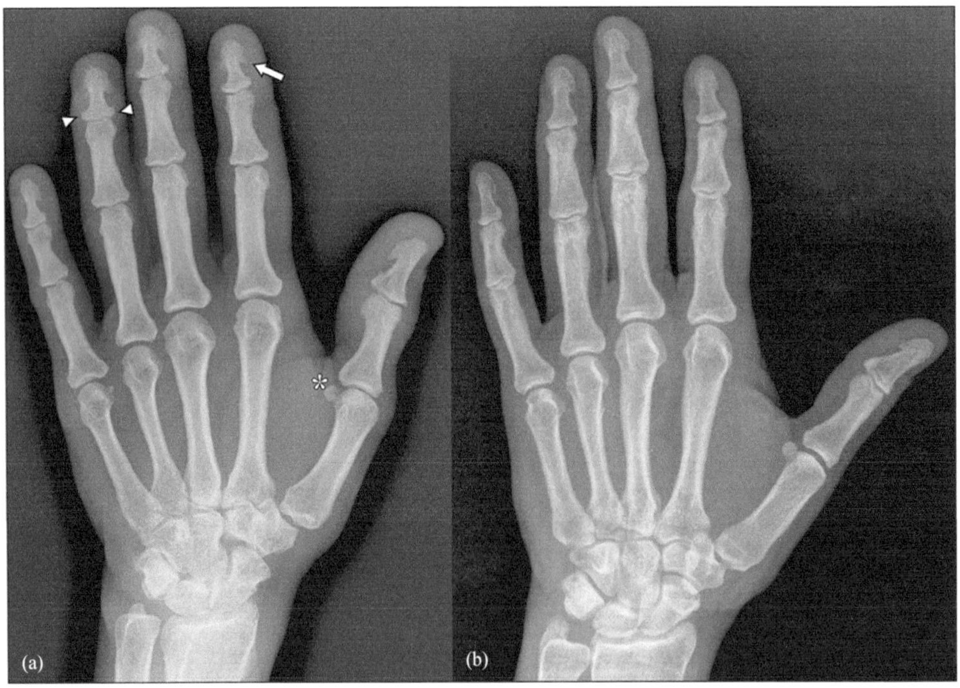

Figure 6.4 Radiograph of the hand of an individual with acromegaly (a). Note the hypertrophy of the distal phalangeal tufts, enlargement of the phalangeal bases as well as enlarged sesamoid bone. Radiograph of the hand of healthy individual for comparison (b). (Figure 4 in Baptista et al. 2023; article licensed under a Creative Commons Attribution 4.0 International License)

Pituitary dwarfism

Pituitary dwarfism is associated with inadequate amounts of growth hormone. In individuals with pituitary dwarfism, both intramembranous and endochondral ossification are impaired, resulting in short stature but maintaining normal body proportions (Figure 6.5). It is important to note that if hypopituitarism appears during adulthood, it does not typically result in skeletal deformities but may contribute to osteoporosis.

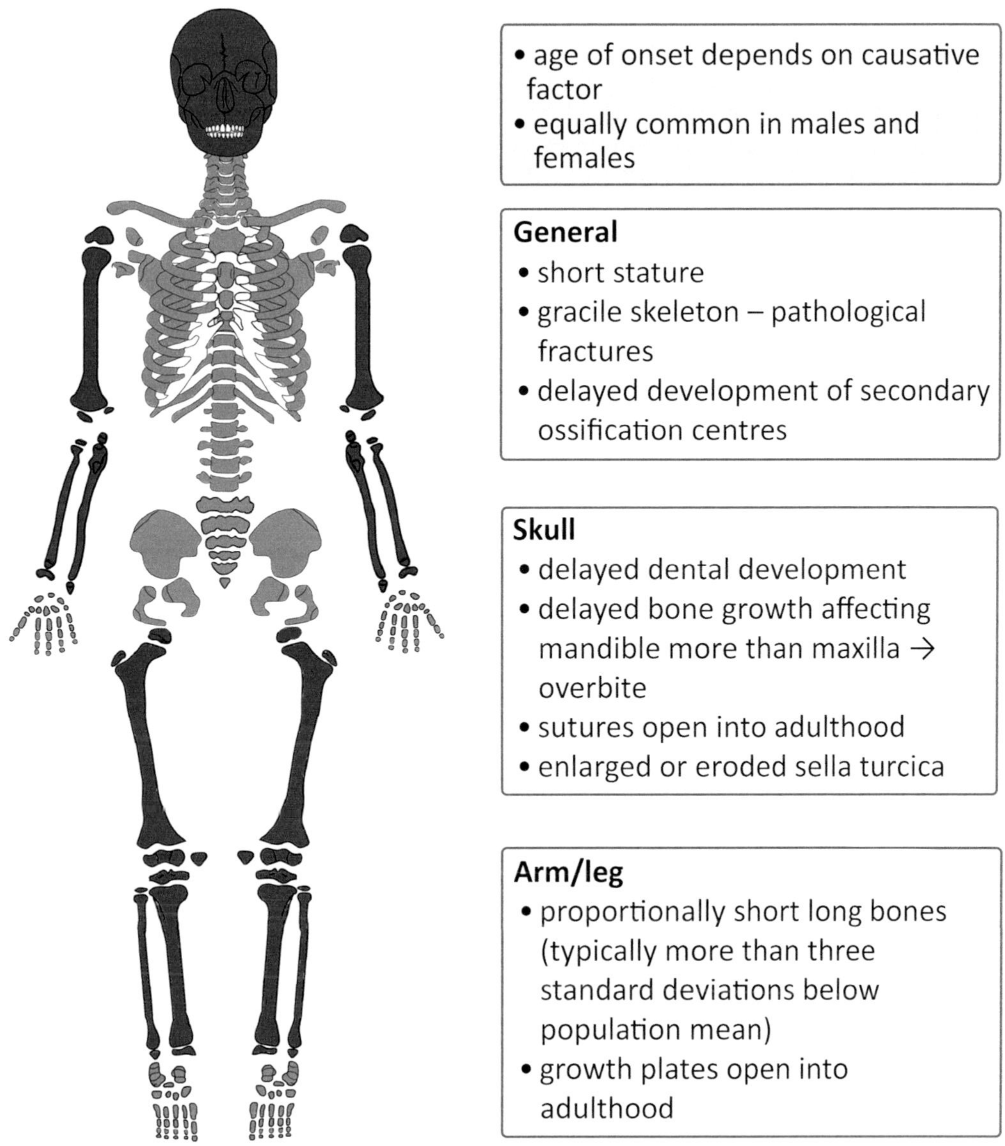

Figure 6.5 Skeletal manifestation of pituitary dwarfism. (Data from Lewis 2019; Waldron 2020; Wójcik and Beń-Skowronek 2020)

Parathyroid disturbances

The parathyroid glands are located posterior to the thyroid gland. They synthesise and secrete the parathyroid hormone (PTH), which is important for regulating blood calcium levels. PTH stimulates the release of calcium from the skeleton and facilitates its reabsorption by the kidneys. In addition, PTH enhances the absorption of calcium in the gastrointestinal tract by promoting the synthesis of calcitriol, the active form of vitamin D, in the kidneys.

Hyperparathyroidism

Hyperparathyroidism is characterised by elevated concentrations of parathyroid hormone due to the hyperactivity of one or more parathyroid glands. This condition promotes increased osteoclastic activity, which leads to bone resorption and demineralisation (Box 6.1, Figures 6.6 and 6.7). The term used to describe the deterioration of bone integrity associated with hyperparathyroidism is osteitis fibrosa cystica. Hyperparathyroidism may be primary or secondary. Primary hyperparathyroidism usually arises from a parathyroid adenoma, although it may result from glandular hyperplasia, and rarely from carcinoma. In contrast, secondary hyperparathyroidism is characterised by elevated parathyroid hormone secretion due to another disease, most commonly chronic kidney disease, which results in increased phosphate and decreased calcium in the blood.

Box 6.1 Skeletal manifestation of hyperparathyroidism

General

- diffuse cortical bone demineralisation
- brown tumours (well-defined, lytic lesions with minimal reactive bone formation, caused by localised, rapid osteoclastic turnover)
- pathological fractures

Skull

- brown tumour formation in mandible
- trabecular bone resorption

Shoulder girdle

- brown tumour formation in clavicle
- bone resorption at insertion of conoid ligament

Thorax

- brown tumour formation in ribs

Vertebrae

- subchondral bone resorption
- vertebral collapse → kyphosis

Pelvic girdle

- bone resorption at ischial tuberosity and pubic symphysis
- sacroiliac joint erosion
- brown tumour formation

Arm/leg

- bone resorption at ligament attachment sites (e.g. trochanters, deltoid tuberosity)
- cortical thinning
- brown tumour formation

Hand/foot

- phalangeal tuft osteolysis
- bone resorption at insertion of plantar fascia on calcaneus
- brown tumour formation in tubular bones
- gout

(Data from Jaffe 1940; Khan and Bilezikian 2000; Lewis 2019; Mays and Turner-Walker 2008; Mays et al. 2001)

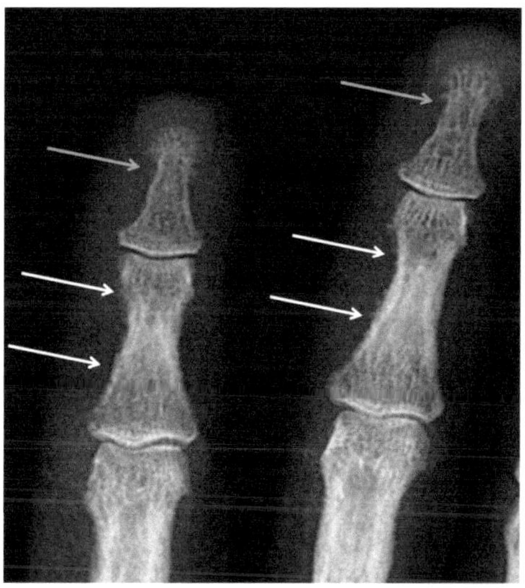

Figure 6.6 Bone resorption at the phalanges of the second and third fingers, and early tufts resorption-acroosteolysis in individual with primary hyperparathyroidism. (Figure 1 in Bennett et al. 2020; article licensed under a Creative Commons Attribution 4.0 International License)

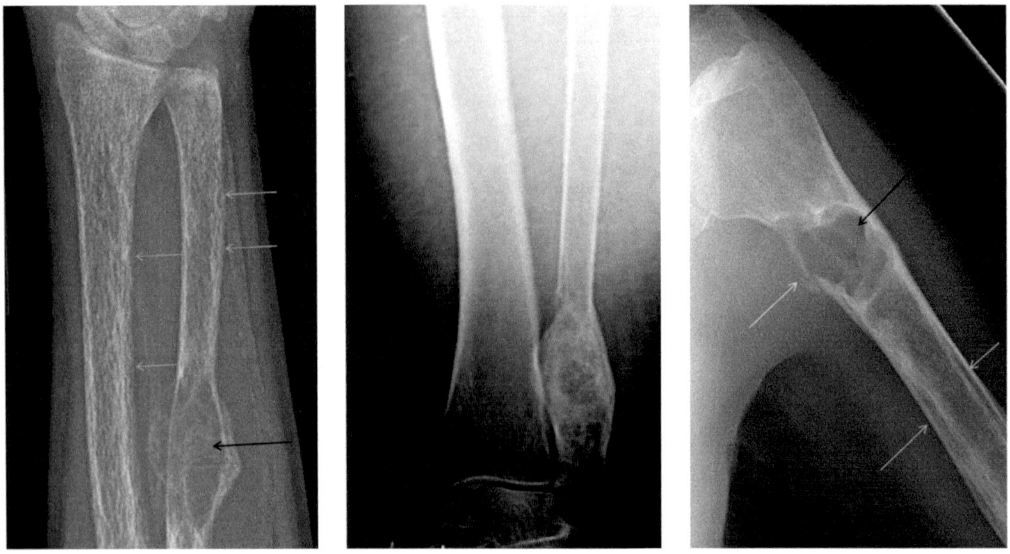

(a) (b) (c)

Figure 6.7 Brown tumours in the ulna, fibula, and humerus, demineralisation and bone resorption, and pathological fracture at the humerus brown tumour in individual with primary hyperparathyroidism. (Figure 3 in Bennett et al. 2020; article licensed under a Creative Commons Attribution 4.0 International License)

Box 6.2 Skeletal manifestation of hypoparathyroidism

- osteosclerosis
- thickened cranium
- enamel hypoplasia
- ossification of spinal ligaments and bridging osteophytes
- enthesopathy

(Data from John and Suthar 2016; Levine 2001; Lewis 2019)

Hypoparathyroidism

Hypoparathyroidism is characterised by insufficient production of parathyroid hormone by one or more parathyroid glands. This condition has various aetiologies, including trauma, autoimmune disorders, hypomagnesaemia (abnormally low levels of magnesium in the blood), or agenesis of the parathyroid glands. The deficiency in parathyroid hormone leads to reduced osteoclastic activity, thus to a reduced release of calcium from the bone matrix (Box 6.2).

Thyroid disturbances

The thyroid is a small gland at the front of the neck; it has two lobes that are positioned bilaterally to the trachea. This gland regulates numerous body functions by secreting thyroxine (T4), triiodothyronine (T3), and calcitonin into the bloodstream. Thyroxine and triiodothyronine are collectively referred to as the thyroid hormone; they regulate the metabolic rate, brain development, heart and digestive functions, as well as bone maintenance. In addition, calcitonin regulates blood calcium and phosphate concentrations by blocking osteoclast activity.

The function of the thyroid gland may also be disturbed by a malfunction of the pituitary gland. For example, specific pituitary adenomas may secrete thyroid-stimulating hormone (TSH). This leads to the continuous stimulation of the thyroid gland, resulting in hyperthyroidism. Similarly, damage to the pituitary gland can result in the cessation of TSH production, causing hypothyroidism. Note that several hormones secreted by the pituitary, including TSH, are under the regulation of the hypothalamus; thus, disturbances of the hypothalamus can also ultimately interfere with the functioning of the thyroid.

Hyperthyroidism

Hyperthyroidism is characterised by the overproduction of thyroid hormone (Box 6.3). It is more common in females, and may result from several factors, such as autoimmune diseases (e.g. Graves' disease), inflammation, neoplasms of the thyroid gland, pituitary gland, testes or ovaries, as well as excessive iodine intake.

Hypothyroidism

In hypothyroidism there is inadequate thyroid hormone synthesis (Box 6.4). This may arise from autoimmune diseases (e.g. Hashimoto's disease) or dietary iodine deficiency, which is often associated with certain ecological settings, such as elevated mountainous regions where there is limited natural availability of iodide. In addition, hypothyroidism may result from

Box 6.3 Skeletal manifestation of hyperthyroidism

- osteoporosis (mostly in cervical vertebrae, hands, feet, pelvis)
- pathological fractures (mostly in vertebrae and femoral neck)
- early closure of epiphyses and sutures
- cysts in frontal bone (rare and may mimic multiple myeloma)

(Data from Cardoso et al. 2014; Lewis 2019)

Box 6.4 Skeletal manifestation of hypothyroidism

General

- expression ranges from no skeletal effect to severe dwarfism
- within a patient some bones may be severely affected and others normal
- multifocal irregular ossification centres at epiphyses
- secondary osteoarthritis

Skull

- brachycephaly
- prognathism
- subnormal cranial base growth
- misshaped foramen magnum
- delayed closure of cranial sutures and fontanels
- wormian bones
- enlarged sella turcica

Thorax

- underdeveloped ribs

Vertebrae

- shortened vertebral bodies (bullet-shaped, particularly in T12 and L1) → kyphosis
- wedged-shaped lumbar vertebrae → spondylolisthesis

Arm/leg

- poor epiphyseal mineralisation
- diminished long bone growth → dwarfism
- growth in length affected more than growth in width
- lower extremities affected more than upper ones
- mushroom-like deformity of femoral head → early-onset and severe osteoarthritis; similar deformities possible on humeral head
- delayed epiphyseal and apophyseal union

(Data from Andersen 1975; Lewis 2017, 2019; Ortner and Hotz 2005)

genetic abnormalities affecting the development of the thyroid, as well as from infections, neoplasms, and other factors that can impair the function of the thyroid gland. The condition is more common in females.

Adrenal disturbances

The adrenal glands are small glands located atop each kidney. They play an important role in the secretion of hormones, including adrenaline, aldosterone, and cortisol. These hormones are instrumental in the regulation of the metabolism, immune responses, blood pressure, as well as responses to stress, among other functions.

Cushing's syndrome

Cushing's syndrome is characterised by elevated cortisol levels in the body. It may be caused by steroid use or by the overproduction of cortisol, usually due to a neoplasm. This syndrome is associated with hyperglycemia (elevated glucose levels in the blood), reduced protein synthesis, bone loss (Figures 6.8 and 6.9), suppression of the immune system, high blood pressure, weight gain, as well as depression.

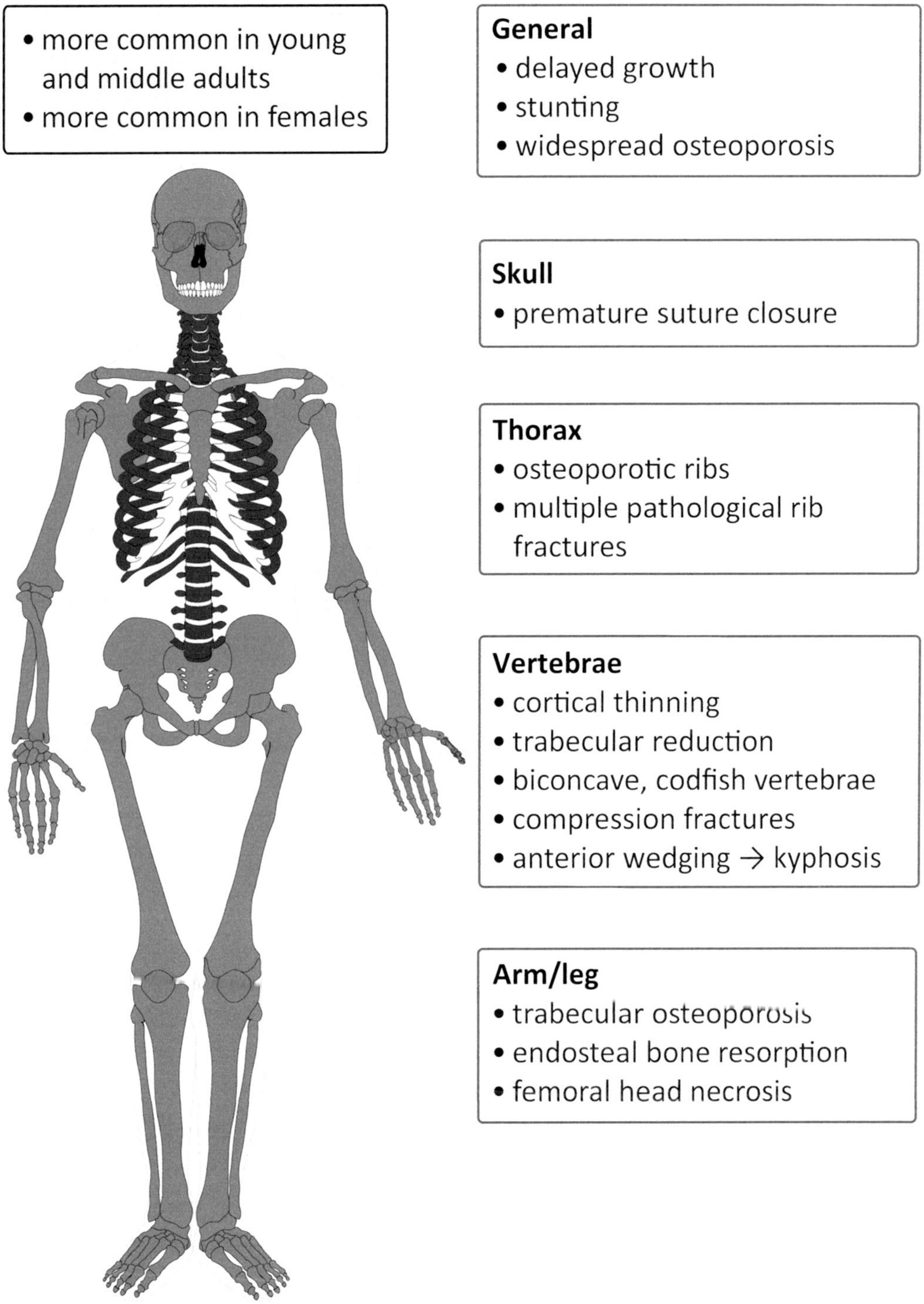

Figure 6.8 Skeletal manifestation of Cushing's syndrome. (Data from Aufderheide and Rodríguez-Martín 1998; Lewis 2019; Sissons 1956)

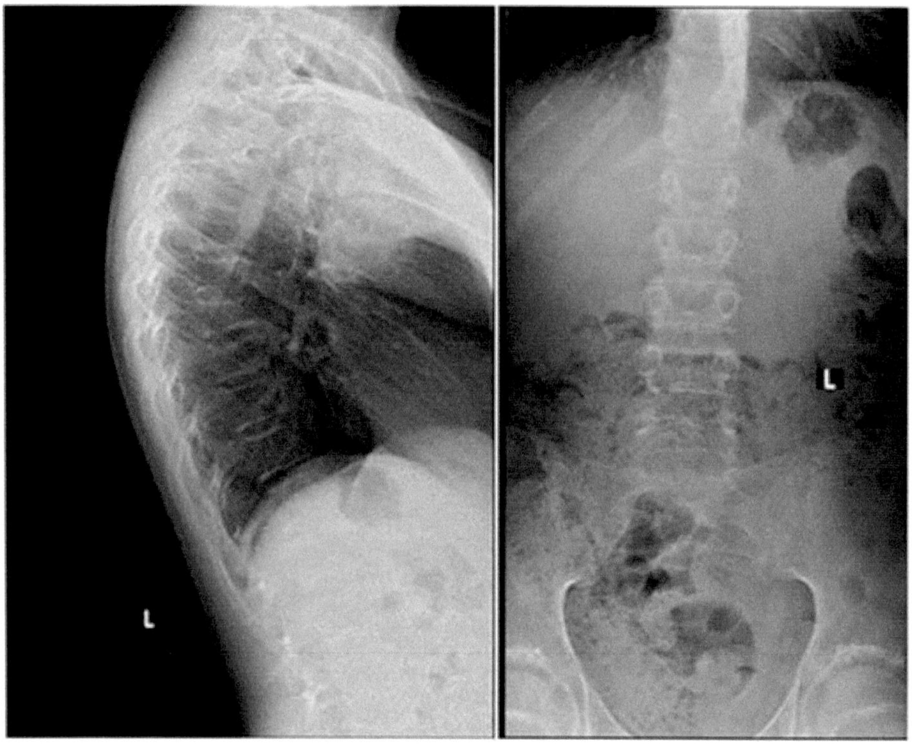

Figure 6.9 Radiograph of the thoracolumbar spine of individual with Cushing's syndrome. Note the vertebral fractures and decreased height of the T5–9. (Figure 2 in Łupińska et al. 2023; article licensed under a Creative Commons Attribution 4.0 International License)

Gonadal disturbances

The gonads are the glands that synthesise hormones important for reproduction and other functions. Key hormones produced by these glands are oestrogen, progesterone, and testosterone. The ovaries are the female gonads, while the testes are the male gonads. While both the ovaries and testes synthesise some of the same hormones, they do so in different concentrations. There are several gonadal disorders that manifest differently in males and females.

Hypergonadism

Hypergonadism appears when there is overactivity of the gonads, resulting in an abnormally high synthesis of sex hormones. This condition is less common than hypogonadism and causes precocious puberty. Skeletally, it manifests as a short and robust skeleton due to the premature fusion of the epiphyseal growth plates.

Hypogonadism

Primary hypogonadism is due to a malfunction of the testes or the ovaries; it can be linked to various genetic disorders that affect the sex chromosomes (e.g. Turner's syndrome), as well as to infectious diseases, trauma, kidney or liver disorders, or hemochromatosis. Medical procedures, such as radiation therapy or surgery, which involve the gonads, may also cause hypogonadism. In contrast, secondary hypogonadism results from a dysfunction in the pituitary gland, while tertiary hypogonadism results from hypothalamic dysfunction. The dysfunction in the pituitary or hypothalamus may be caused by genetic disorders, infections, nutritional deficiencies, drug use, surgical interventions, radiation exposure, or trauma. Oestrogen and testosterone are important in endochondral growth, secondary ossification centre formation, and puberty onset. Thus, a deficiency in these hormones can lead to delayed skeletal maturation, resulting in tall, elongated, and gracile skeletons with reduced cortical bone thickness.

References and suggested readings

Andersen, H. (1975). Hypothyroidism. In *Endocrine and Genetic Diseases of Childhood and Adolescence*, edited by Gardner, L., 2nd edition, pp. 234–238. Philadelphia: Saunders.

Aufderheide, A.C., Rodríguez-Martín, C. (1998). *The Cambridge Encyclopedia of Human Paleopathology*. Cambridge: Cambridge University Press.

Baptista, L.C., Martins, M.M., Marcos, V.N. (2023). Radiographic findings in acromegaly: pictorial essay. *Radiologia Brasileira* 56:110–115. https://doi.org/10.1590/0100-3984.2022.0083-en

Bennett, J., Suliburk, J.W., Moron, F.E. (2020). Osseous manifestations of primary hyperparathyroidism: imaging findings. *International Journal of Endocrinology* 2020:3146535. https://doi.org/10.1155/2020/3146535

Cardoso, L.F., Maciel, L.M., de Paula, F.J. (2014). The multiple effects of thyroid disorders on bone and mineral metabolism. *Arquivos Brasileiros de Endocrinologia & Metabologia* 58:452–463. https://doi.org/10.1590/0004-2730000003311

Claessen, K.M.J.A., Mazziotti, G., Biermasz, N.R., Giustina, A. (2016). Bone and joint disorders in acromegaly. *Neuroendocrinology* 103:86–95. https://doi.org/10.1159/000375450

Cordero, R.A., Barkan, A.L. (2008). Current diagnosis of acromegaly. *Review in Endocrine and Metabolic Disorders* 9:13–19. https://doi.org/10.1007/s11154-007-9060-2

Golds, G., Houdek, D., Arnason, T. (2017). Male hypogonadism and osteoporosis: the effects, clinical consequences, and treatment of testosterone deficiency in bone health. *International Journal of Endocrinology* 2017:4602129. https://doi.org/10.1155/2017/4602129

Hawkins, D. (1992). The diagnosis of pituitary disease from human skeletal remains. *International Journal of Osteoarchaeology* 2:51–64. https://doi.org/10.1002/oa.1390020108

Jaffe, H.L. (1940). Hyperparathyroidism. *Bulletin of the New York Academy of Medicine* 16:291–311.

John, D.R., Suthar, P.P. (2016). Radiological features of long-standing hypoparathyroidism. *Polish Journal of Radiology* 81:42–45

Kaltsas, G., Makras, P. (2010). Skeletal diseases in Cushing's syndrome: osteoporosis versus arthropathy. *Neuroendocrinology* 92:60–64. https://doi.org/10.1159/000314298

Karga, H., Papapetrou, P.D., Korakovouni, A., Papandroulaki, F., Polymeris, A., Pampouras, G. (2004). Bone mineral density in hyperthyroidism. *Clinical Endocrinology* 61:466–472. https://doi.org/10.1111/j.1365-2265.2004.02110.x

Khan, A., Bilezikian, J. (2000). Primary hyperparathyroidism: pathophysiology and impact on bone. *Canadian Medical Association Journal* 163:184–187.

Kozłowski, T., Witas, H.W. (2012). Metabolic and endocrine diseases. In *A Companion to Paleopathology*, edited by Grauer A.L., pp. 401–419. Hoboken, NJ: Wiley-Blackwell.

Levine, M.A. (2001). Hypoparathyroidism and pseudohypoparathyroidism. In *Endocrinology*, edited by DeGroot, L., Jameson, J., pp. 1133–1153. Philadelphia: Saunders.

Lewis, M. (2017). *Paleopathology of Children: Identification of Pathological Conditions in the Human Skeletal Remains of Non-Adults*. San Diego: Academic Press.

Lewis, M. (2019). Endocrine disturbances. In *Ortner's Identification of Pathological Conditions in Human Skeletal Remains*, edited by Buikstra, J., pp. 567–584. San Diego: Academic Press.

Łupińska, A., Aszkiełowicz, S., Zieliński, G., Stawerska, R., Lewiński, A. (2023). Osteoporosis as the first sign of Cushing's disease in a thin 16-year-old boy—A case report. *Journal of Clinical Medicine* 12:5967. https://doi.org/10.3390/jcm12185967

Mays, S., Turner-Walker, G. (2008). A possible case of renal osteodystrophy in a skeleton from medieval Wharram Percy, England. *International Journal of Osteoarchaeology* 18:307–316. https://doi.org/10.1002/oa.941

Mays, S., Rogers, J., Watt, I. (2001). A possible case of hyperparathyroidism in a burial of 15–17th century AD date from Wharram Percy, England. *International Journal of Osteoarchaeology* 11:329–335. https://doi.org/10.1002/oa.569

Ortner, D., Hotz, G. (2005). Skeletal manifestations of hypothyroidism from Switzerland. *American Journal of Physical Anthropology* 127:1–6. https://doi.org/10.1002/ajpa.20033

Reeves, G.D., Gibbs, M., Paulshock, B.Z., Rosenblum, H. (1978). Gigantism with slipped capital femoral epiphysis. *American Journal of Diseases of Children* 132:529–530.

Sissons, H. (1956). The osteoporosis of Cushing's syndrome. *The Journal of Bone & Joint Surgery* 38:418–433. https://doi.org/10.1302/0301-620X.38B1.418

van der Lely, A.J., Beckers, A., Daly, A.F., Lamberts, S.W.J., Clemmons, D.R. (2005). *Acromegaly: Pathology, Diagnosis and Treatment*. Milton Park: Taylor & Francis.

Waldron, T. (2020). *Palaeopathology*, 2nd edition. Cambridge: Cambridge University Press.

Wójcik, D., Beń-Skowronek, I. (2020). Craniofacial morphology in children with growth hormone deficiency and Turner syndrome. *Diagnostics* 10:88. https://doi.org/10.3390/diagnostics10020088

Chapter 7

Infectious disease

Infectious diseases may be caused by various pathogens, such as bacteria, viruses, fungi, or parasites. These diseases can be transmitted between individuals, from animals to humans, through the ingestion of contaminated food or water, or via exposure to pathogens present in the environment. An individual's susceptibility to infection is influenced by sex, age, genetic predisposition, dietary quality, immune system status, environmental conditions, hygiene, and other factors.

Infectious diseases have played a major role in the evolution of modern humans. Nonetheless, direct evidence of infection in skeletal remains is rare. Many infections will either heal or lead to death before identifiable skeletal lesions develop; thus, individuals with a strong immune system, but also individuals who succumb quickly to the disease, may not display skeletal changes. As a result, only a small number of individuals afflicted by disease will be visible in the bioarchaeological record.

This chapter will focus primarily on infections of non-specific origin, as well as bacterial infections, which have been more commonly reported in the palaeopathological record. Among the conditions that can be caused by other groups of pathogens, we only focus on smallpox and poliomyelitis, as viral infections, and malaria as a parasitic infection. Readers are advised to consult Grauer and Roberts (2019) for an overview of fungal, viral, and parasitic infections that may affect the human skeleton.

Infections of non-specific origin

Periostitis/periostosis

Periostitis (or periostosis) is characterised by periosteal new bone formation (Box 7.1, Figures 7.1–7.3). Periosteal new bone formation may occur in response to various stimuli. When it

Box 7.1 Skeletal manifestation of periostitis/periostosis

- periosteal new bone formation (woven bone gradually remodelling into lamellar bone)
- mostly on long bones (especially tibiae), but may affect any bone
- focal or diffuse pattern

(Data from Weston 2008, 2012)

DOI: 10.4324/9781003475026-7

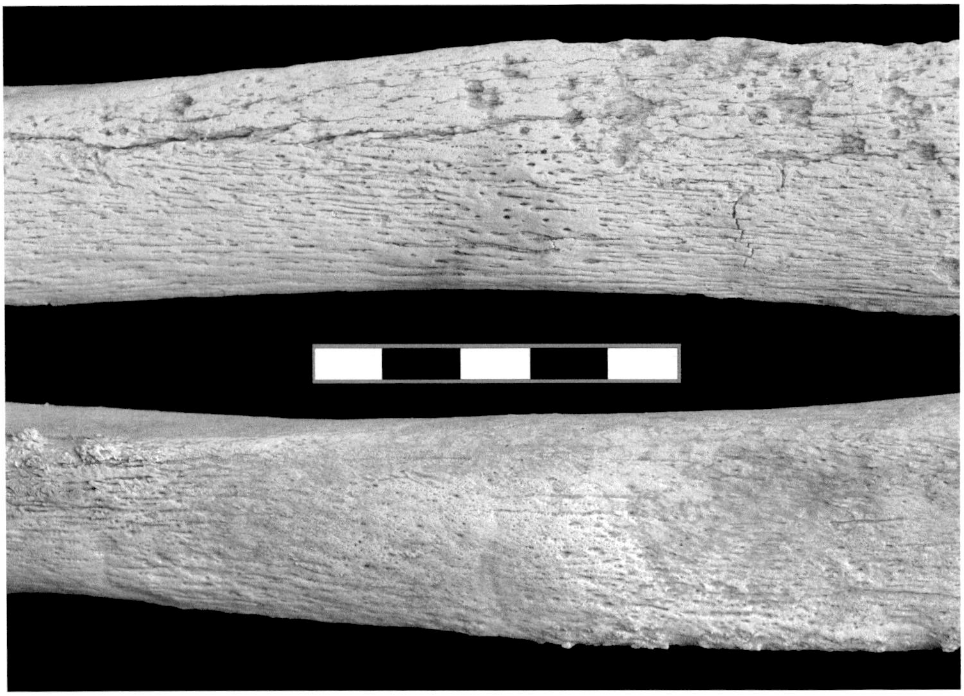

Figure 7.1 Periosteal new bone formation on tibial shafts. In both cases, the new bone formation is diffuse and consists of lamellar bone. (Sbide, Roman/Byzantine; photos by Efthymia Nikita, with the kind permission of Dr. Ahmet Ihsan Aytek, Burdur Mehmet Akif Ersoy University)

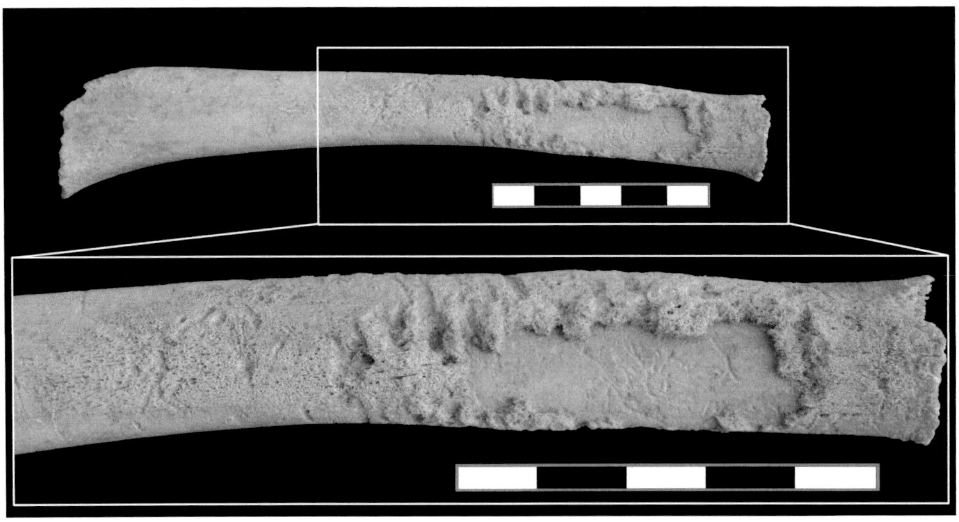

Figure 7.2 Periosteal new bone formation on the tibial shaft of a juvenile. The new bone is woven, and the underlying cortex is visible as part of the new bone was broken away postmortem. (Philadelphia, Roman/Byzantine; photo by Efthymia Nikita, with the kind permission of Dr. Ahmet Ihsan Aytek, Burdur Mehmet Akif Ersoy University)

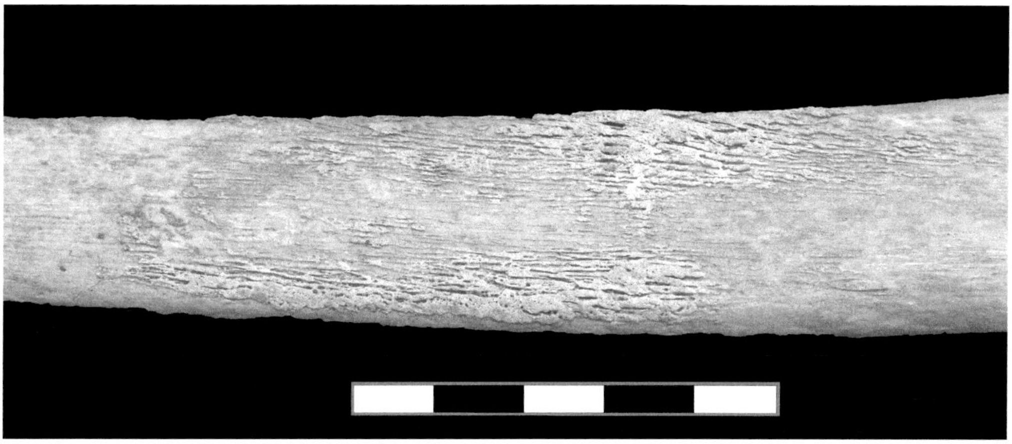

Figure 7.3 Periosteal new bone formation on a tibial diaphysis. (Male, 35–45 years old, Diever, Reformed Church graveyard, Collection NAD Nuis inv. Nr. D 2019-III.472; photo by Efthymia Nikita, with permission from the Noordelijk Archeologisch Depot)

results from inflammation, typically of infectious origin, the term *periostitis* is appropriate. In cases where the cause is uncertain, the broader term *periostosis* is preferred.

The stimuli that may cause new bone formation include infectious, metabolic, circulatory, or neoplastic disorders, as well as trauma and skeletal dysplasias. Inflammation is a major cause of periosteal new bone formation (Box 7.2). The inflammatory response is initially an acute process, localised to the area of the stimulus, and characterised by vasodilation, increased blood flow to the affected area, exudation of fluid, and recruitment of phagocytic cells. If the causative agent persists, the inflammatory response may become chronic. During bone healing, dead tissues are scavenged by macrophages and osteoclasts, and granulation tissue is formed. The granulation tissue provides the scaffold for periosteal new bone formation. This new bone is initially woven and, over time, it is remodelled into lamellar bone.

Several bioarchaeological studies utilise periostitis/periostosis as an indicator of "nonspecific infection." However, periosteal new bone formation is also linked to several specific infections, as well as a range of other pathological conditions, as briefly mentioned above.

Box 7.2 Inflammation and infection

Inflammation is the body's immune response to pathogens and other irritants. In contrast, infection is the invasion of pathogenic organisms in the body. Therefore, while infections are major triggers of inflammatory responses, not all inflammatory responses are due to infectious agents.

Osteomyelitis

Osteomyelitis is a bone infection that may be limited to a specific area or involve several parts, including the bone marrow, cortical bone, periosteum, and adjacent soft tissues (Boxes 7.3 and 7.4, Figures 7.4 and 7.5). The pathogen most often associated with this condition is *Staphylococcus aureus*; however, osteomyelitis has also been linked to many other bacteria, including streptococci and enterococci. While rare, osteomyelitis may also be caused by fungi and, less commonly, by viruses or parasites.

Box 7.3 Skeletal manifestation of osteomyelitis

Non-haematogenous osteomyelitis

- infection of periosteum and cortex but not necessarily spreading to medullary cavity
- cortical defect, possible sequestrum formation, focal periosteal new bone formation, and some adjacent sclerotic response

Haematogenous osteomyelitis

- medullary cavity affected
- mostly in long bone metaphyses-diaphyses in juveniles; mostly in axial skeleton in adults
- sequestrum: necrotic bone (small sequestra may be removed through cloacae, thus be missed)
- cloaca: draining abscess releasing necrotic bone and pus
- involucrum: new bone enclosing the sequestrum; perforated by cloaca; forms quickly and has irregular surface

(Data from Labbé et al. 2010; Lew and Waldvogel 1997; Ortner 2008; Roberts 2019)

Box 7.4 Osteomyelitis expression per age

Infantile osteomyelitis

- multiple bones affected
- extensive involucrum formation
- rare sequestra and cloacae
- joint involvement → growth deformity, bone atrophy, limb shortening, joint dislocation

Juvenile osteomyelitis

- sequestrum may be present
- involucrum and cloaca usually absent
- epiphyses usually spared; in prolonged/recurring cases, the joints may be involved → ankyloses
- pathological fractures

Adult osteomyelitis

- mostly in metaphyses (especially femur/tibia)
- involvement of epiphyses and joints
- small sequestra
- involucrum and cloacae
- common in spine and pelvis

(Data from Lewis 2017; Roberts 2019)

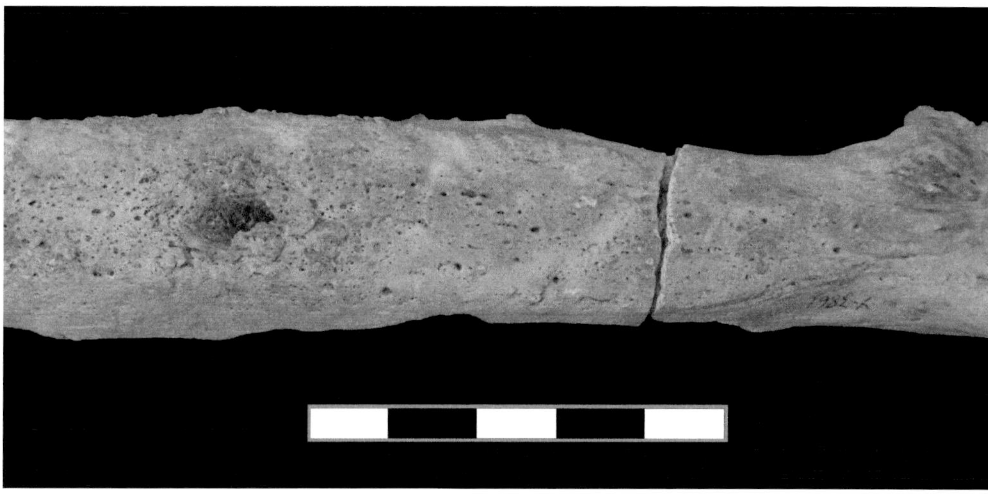

Figure 7.4 Fibular diaphysis with new bone formation and cloacal opening. (Male, 23–39 years old, All Saints Church, Fishergate, York, Medieval, Y-3861; photo by Efthymia Nikita; copyright: Human Skeletal Collection, University of Sheffield)

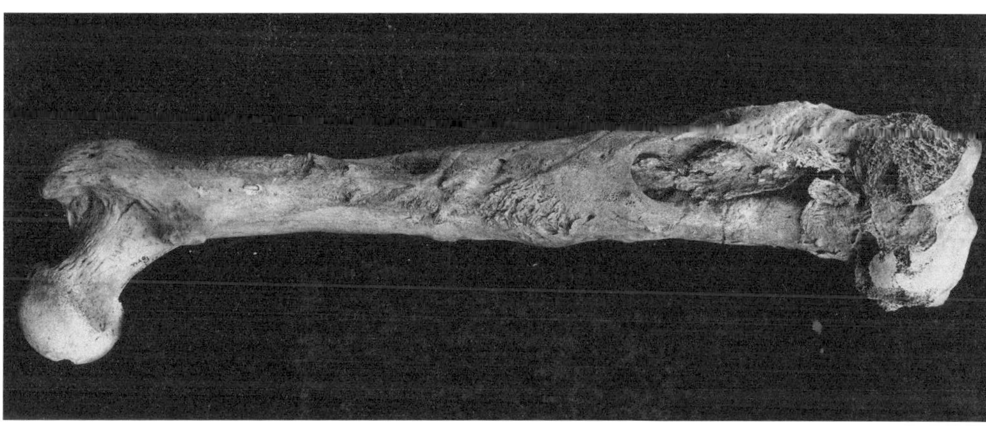

Figure 7.5 Femur osteomyelitis; individual from ancient cemetery at Chicama Valley, Peru. (National Museum of Health and Medicine Series number 14195, Code: 152.616; figure uploaded to Wikimedia Commons by the Otis Historical Archives Nat'l Museum of Health & Medicine USA; licensed under a Creative Commons Attribution 2.0 Generic license)

Infectious agents can reach the skeleton through direct infection as a result of trauma or surgical procedures, extension from adjacent soft tissue infections, or dissemination from a remote site of infection through the haematogenous route. In addition, osteomyelitis may arise secondarily to vascular insufficiency, particularly in individuals with diabetes mellitus.

Osteomyelitis may be acute or chronic. Acute osteomyelitis usually appears within a two-week period following disease onset. Individuals may experience redness, swelling, and increased warmth at the infection site, as well as bone pain, fever, and sweating. Chronic osteomyelitis may develop over a long period, ranging from months to years, and is characterised by the ongoing presence of microorganisms, low-grade inflammation, and necrosis of the cortical bone due to compromised vascular supply, leading to the formation of a sequestrum (i.e. necrotic bone). In addition, chronic osteomyelitis is characterised by the formation of new bone around the sequestrum (involucrum), as well as the development of sinus tracts that allow the drainage of pus from the infected bone to adjacent soft tissues (cloacae). However, chronic osteomyelitis does not necessarily result in the formation of a sequestrum or cloacae, as the infection may spread extensively throughout the bone and stimulate osteoblastic activity. This process results in the expansion of the bone's external contours and a decrease in the dimensions of the medullary cavity (Garré's sclerosing osteomyelitis). Moreover, in some juvenile cases, osteomyelitis may not produce an involucrum or a clearly discernible cloaca, as pus can permeate the bone rather easily. However, extensive involucrum formation is also frequently observed in children, as the periosteum may be detached along the entire shaft, producing hypertrophic changes in the affected bone.

In children, osteomyelitis is mostly an acute condition, disseminated through the haematogenous route. In contrast, in adults, osteomyelitis is most often a chronic condition that arises as a secondary complication following an open injury to the bone and adjacent soft tissues.

Sinusitis

Sinusitis is the inflammation of the mucous membrane lining the paranasal sinuses (Figures 7.6–7.8). These sinuses are found within the ethmoid, sphenoid, maxillary, and frontal bones, and they are lined by the mucous membrane (mucosa). The mucosa is very important for the immune system as it forms a protective barrier against exogenous particles. It captures these particles with its viscous mucus and facilitates their removal. The cilia, which are hairlike structures of the mucosa, beat in a coordinated and directional fashion to transport mucus along with trapped pathogens and inhaled particles through drainage pathways. Mucus is expelled from the sinus through the ostium. The ostia associated with the maxillary, frontal, and anterior ethmoidal sinuses drain into the ostiomeatal complex. If either the ostium or the ostiomeatal complex is obstructed, mucociliary flow is interrupted, so pathogens and other inhaled particles cannot be expelled, causing sinus inflammation.

Inflammation is often initiated by infections. Ostial obstruction and subsequent inflammation can also result from craniofacial anomalies or variations, trauma to the nasal region, immunodeficiency, and metabolic syndrome. Furthermore, hormonal fluctuations associated with pregnancy and menopause also increase susceptibility to sinusitis.

Environmental factors are also important in the development of sinusitis. Air pollutants, especially fine particulate matter, can induce oxidative stress and inflammation in the respiratory system, if inhaled. The inhalation of particulate matter can also impede immune response and render individuals more vulnerable to respiratory infections. Furthermore, exposure to

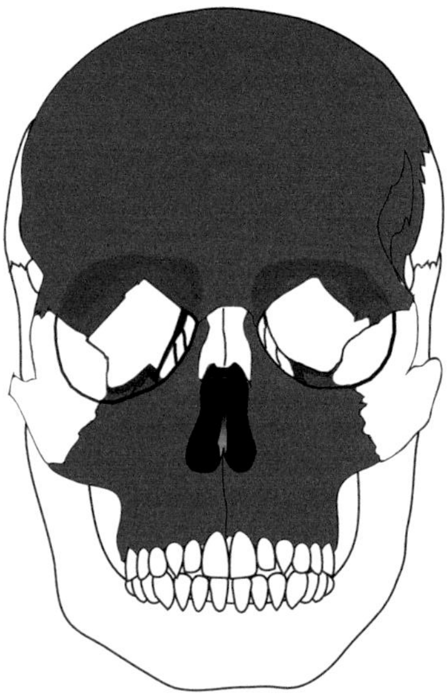

- more common in middle and old adulthood
- more common in females

General

- bone resorption*
  - cysts (hemispherical lesions with smooth walls and rim of new bone deposition)
  - pits (holes < 1 mm in diameter; adjacent pits may fuse → holes 3–5 mm in diameter)
- new bone formation**
  - spicules (isolated osseous spikes projecting from the bone surface; may form small groups and bridge; in severe expressions they create several partially overlapping bone discs)
  - remodelled spicules (spicules in the course of remodelling into the sinus walls; as they merge, they may have a plaque-like or molten wax appearance)
  - plaque (variable thickness; dense or porous bone)
  - lobules (rounded osseous masses on sinus surface)

Figure 7.6 Skeletal manifestation of sinusitis

*In juveniles, sinusitis-related pitting may be misinterpreted as developmental pitting, as the expansion of the maxillary alveolar bone to accommodate the emergence of developing teeth can influence the morphology of the sinus floor.

**An additional often-used category of bony lesion is white pitted bone. However, due to possible taphonomic discolouration and morphological similarity to other categories (e.g. pits or plaque), we do not use it here. (Data from Boocock et al. 1995; Mays et al. 2024; Merrett and Pfeiffer 2000; Sundman and Kjellström 2011)

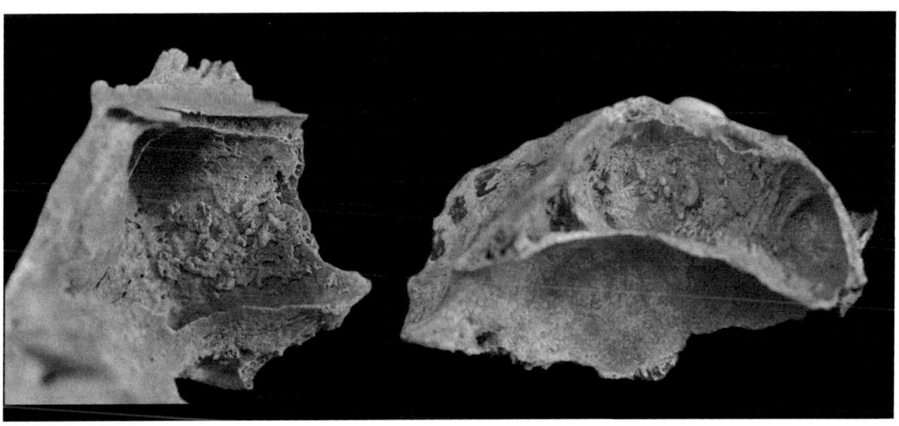

Figure 7.7 Maxillary sinusitis. Spicules/remodelled spicules and lobules of new bone on the maxillary sinus walls. (Left: University of Sheffield Teaching Collection, BAII W2 3219; right: Black Gate cemetery, Newcastle Upon-Tyne, 8th-12th c. CE, BG 3285; photos by Efthymia Nikita; copyright: Human Skeletal Collection, University of Sheffield)

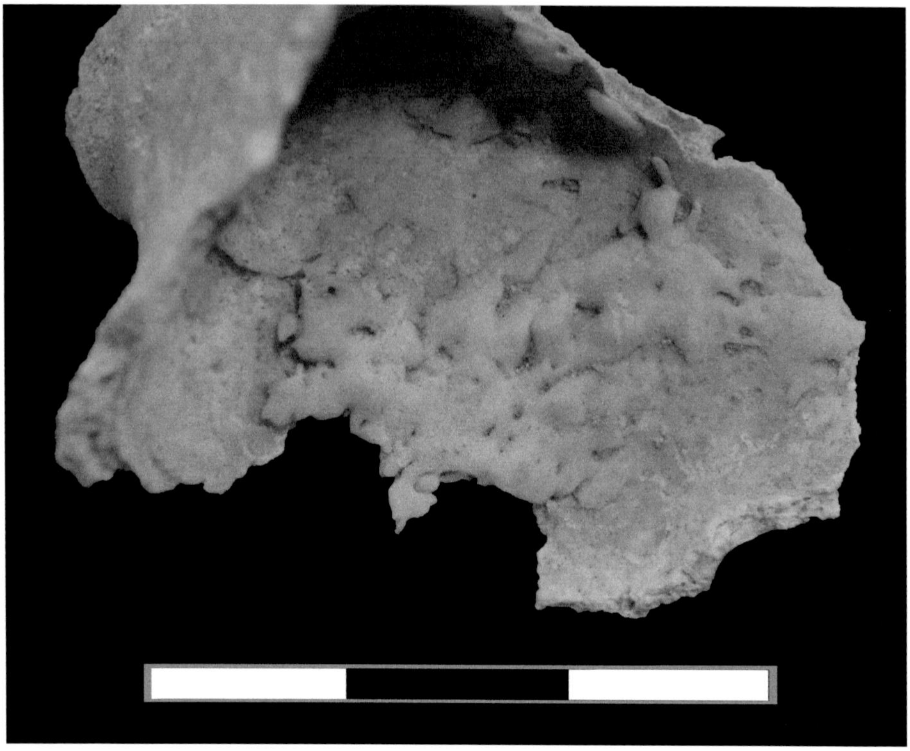

Figure 7.8 Maxillary sinusitis. Remodelled spicules covering the sinus wall; the spicules have merged and have a molten wax appearance. (Probable female, Adolescent/Young adult, Ayia Napa Monastery, Cyprus, B352; photo by Anna Karligkioti; permission to use this image has been granted by the Director of the Department of Antiquities, Cyprus)

cold and dry winds may dry the mucous membrane, thus potentially reducing the mucosa's resistance to infectious agents.

Maxillary sinusitis can also have a secondary aetiology. The molar roots often extend into the sinus cavity; thus, infections affecting these teeth can disseminate to the sinus cavity, causing sinusitis (Box 7.5).

Box 7.5 Different types of bone formation, different aetiologies

Mays et al. (2024) suggest that porous new bone formation within the maxillary sinuses is associated with diseased posterior maxillary teeth, which in turn is a cause of maxillary sinusitis; however, this did not apply to spicules or lobules of bone. Thus, these different types of bone formation within the sinuses should be analysed separately and keeping in mind that spicules and lobules may not indicate sinusitis.

Sinusitis may be acute, subacute, or chronic depending on the host's immune response and the virulence of the causative pathogens. Acute sinusitis is characterised by symptoms that last for less than four weeks and typically improve without treatment. In contrast, in subacute sinusitis, symptoms last for four to twelve weeks. In cases of chronic sinusitis, the symptoms persist for twelve weeks or longer, and in some cases, the condition may last for years. The initial phase of an acute sinus infection is often associated with viruses, particularly rhinoviruses, influenza viruses, and parainfluenza viruses. In some cases, a bacterial infection may follow the viral one. In contrast, most cases of chronic sinusitis are associated with bacterial infections. Fungal sinusitis may also appear when an individual inhales specific mould spores.

Septic arthritis

Septic arthritis is an infection of the joints caused by bacteria, viruses, or fungi. The pathogen most commonly associated with septic arthritis is *Staphylococcus aureus*. Infections leading to septic arthritis may reach the joints through four routes. Haematogenous spread, where pathogens disseminate through the bloodstream, is the most common. The second route involves direct extension from adjacent infected tissues. The third route is the direct introduction of infectious agents during trauma that compromises the integrity of the joint capsule. Lastly, the fourth route, a subtype of direct introduction, covers the postoperative onset of infection, which occurs as a result of contamination during surgical procedures. Septic arthritis may involve any joint, but haematogenous dissemination most frequently involves the joints of the lower limbs, particularly the hip and knee. The pathogens invade the joint space, triggering inflammation. The inflammatory response leads to the degradation of articular cartilage, followed by the destruction of subchondral and perichondral bone (Box 7.6, Figures 7.9–7.11).

Box 7.6 Skeletal manifestation of septic arthritis

- any synovial joint may be affected; haematogenous spread mostly seen in large weight-bearing joints (especially knee and hip), penetrating trauma most often resulting in small hand/foot joint involvement
- mostly monoarticular (polyarticular associated with immunocompromise)
- asymmetric lytic lesions
- bone erosion starts at joint surface margin but may spread to entire joint surface
- joint fusion if unrelieved

(Data from Burt et al. 2013; Del Val Del et al. 1997; Nade 2003; Waldron 2020)

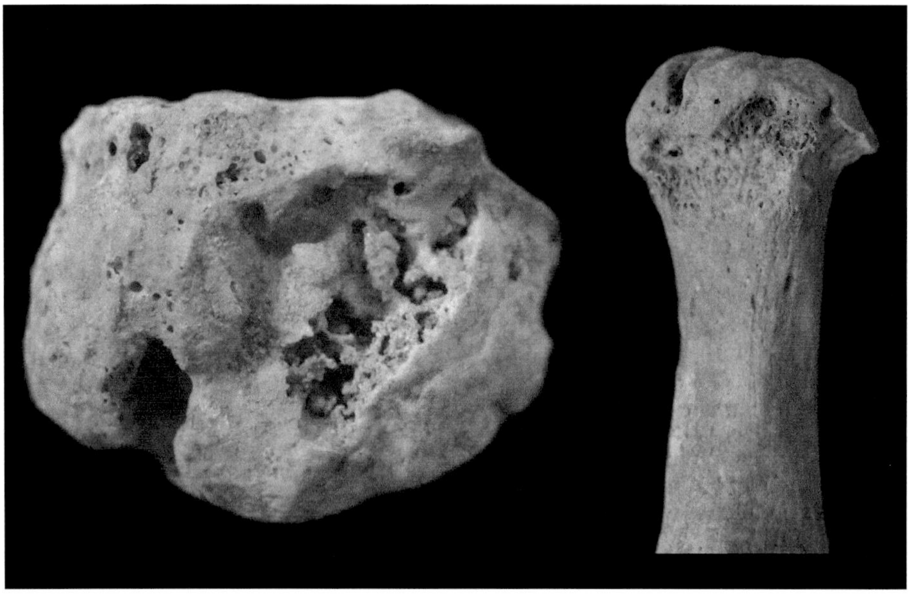

Figure 7.9 Septic arthritis of the first metatarsophalangeal joint. Note the extensive lytic lesions on the metatarsal head. (Female, 30–40 years old, St Hilda's Church, Coronation Street, South Shields, Newcastle, 19th c., CS06 564; photos by Efthymia Nikita; copyright: Human Skeletal Collection, University of Sheffield)

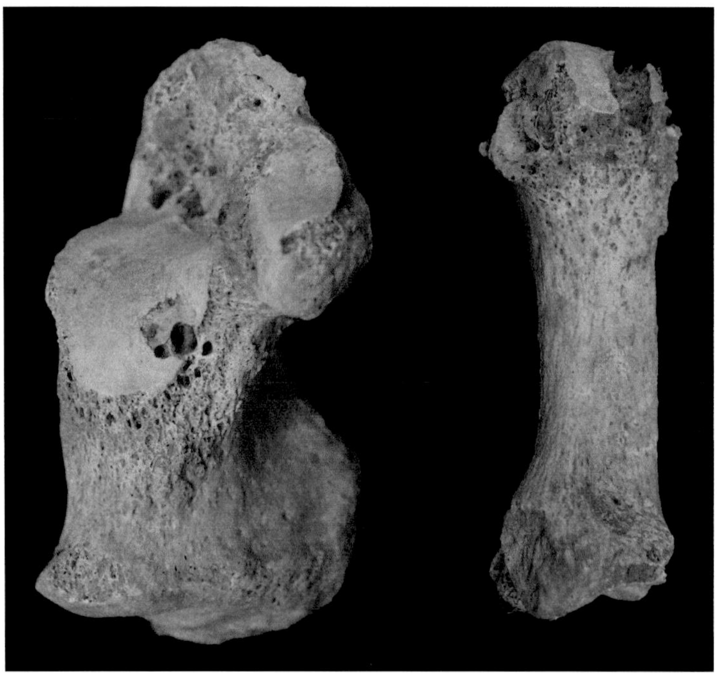

Figure 7.10 Septic arthritis of the left foot. Note the lytic lesions on the posterior facet of the calcaneus and the head of the first metatarsal, coupled with porosity and new bone formation in the periarticular area. (Grafton Regis GR65 SK9; photos by Efthymia Nikita; copyright: Duckworth Laboratory, University of Cambridge)

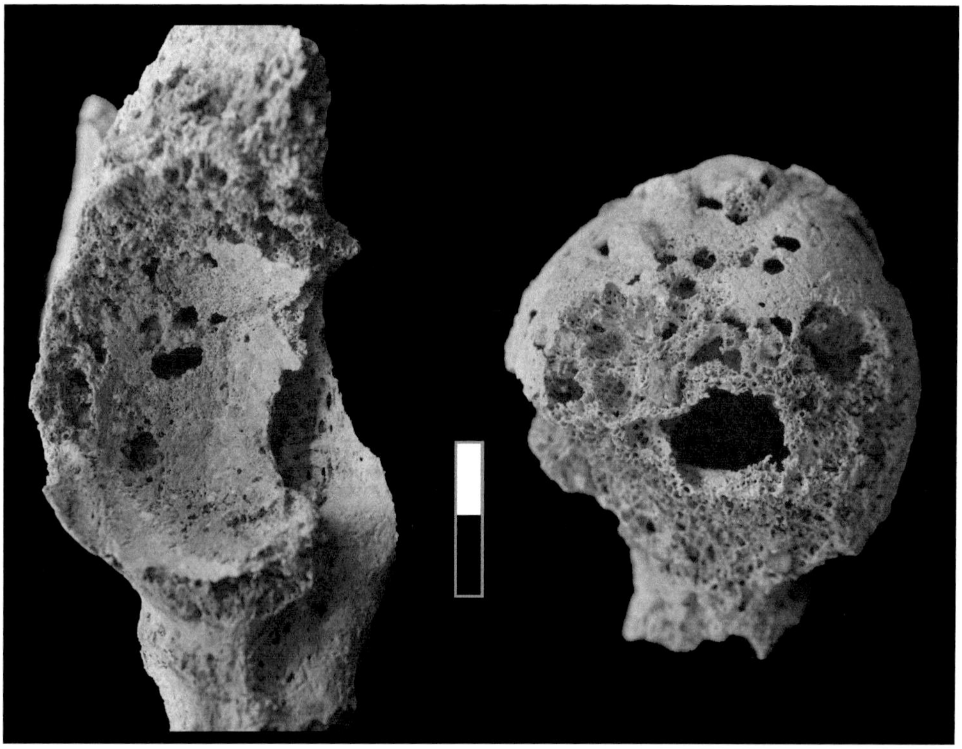

Figure 7.11 Septic arthritis of the right hip. Note the extensive lytic lesions on the femoral head and the acetabulum. (Finglesham 1965, Grave 188; photos by Efthymia Nikita; copyright: Duckworth Laboratory, University of Cambridge)

Bacterial infections

Tuberculosis

Tuberculosis is an infectious disease caused by species of the *Mycobacterium tuberculosis* complex. Among these species, *M. tuberculosis*, *M. africanum*, and *M. canettii* affect primarily humans but may also infect animals (humans are the primary hosts), while *M. bovis*, *M. caprae*, *M. microti*, and *M. pinnipedii* infect primarily domesticated and wild animals, but they may spread to humans (humans are the secondary hosts). The risk factors associated with tuberculosis include malnutrition, smoking, diabetes mellitus, alcohol abuse, exposure to indoor and outdoor air pollutants, and various other conditions that weaken the immune system.

The infection is usually transmitted through the respiratory system when individuals inhale respiratory droplets released by infected individuals or contaminated aerosols from infected animals. In addition, transmission may occur via the gastrointestinal route through the consumption of contaminated animal products. Upon entering the lungs or gastrointestinal tract, the bacteria disseminate through the circulatory and lymphatic systems to the skeleton and other parts of the body. While congenital transmission is rare, it is possible and occurs either haematogenously via the placenta or during childbirth through the inhalation or ingestion of infected amniotic fluid.

Tuberculosis develops in two phases: a) primary infection and b) reinfection or reactivation. Primary infection most commonly occurs in childhood and tends to be asymptomatic, often resolving spontaneously without further dissemination of the infection. In contrast, secondary infections are mostly found in adults and may arise from the reactivation of a latent infection or from reinfection after new exposure to pathogens. Older individuals and those with a compromised immune system are particularly vulnerable to disease reactivation.

The clinical manifestations of tuberculosis depend on the initial site of infection. In cases of pulmonary tuberculosis, the symptoms include dyspnoea, fatigue, night sweats, persistent cough, chest pain, haemoptysis, significant weight loss, and fever. Gastrointestinal tuberculosis is characterised by abdominal pain, diarrhoea (though constipation may also occur), gastrointestinal bleeding, fever, fatigue, vomiting, and loss of appetite. Depending on the parts of the body where tuberculosis may spread (e.g. lymph nodes, brain), other symptoms may emerge. Skeletal tuberculosis arises from the lymphohaematogenous dissemination of bacilli following a secondary infection, but only approximately 3–5% of individuals diagnosed with tuberculosis will exhibit skeletal changes (Box 7.7, Figures 7.12–7.15).

Brucellosis

Brucellosis is an infectious disease caused by bacteria belonging to the genus *Brucella*, and is transmitted from animals to humans (zoonosis). Four species of *Brucella* – *B. melitensis* (mostly affecting goats and sheep), *B. suis* (mostly affecting pigs), *B. abortus* (mostly affecting cattle), and *B. canis* (mostly affecting dogs) – are associated with almost all reported cases of brucellosis in humans across the world. Specifically, most cases of brucellosis in humans are due to *Brucella melitensis*. Brucellosis can be transmitted to humans through the ingestion of

Box 7.7 Diagnosing tuberculosis

Some authors consider Pott's disease to be pathognomonic of tuberculosis, while smooth-walled lytic lesions on the anterior part of the vertebral bodies with lack of lesions at the neural arch and anterior wedging is seen as indicative of tuberculosis (e.g. Mosher et al. 2015). Nonetheless, the prevailing opinion is that no skeletal lesions can be considered pathognomonic for this disease. Recent research has focused on evaluating the sensitivity and specificity of various skeletal lesions in the accurate diagnosis of TB. Masiu et al. (2023) found vertebral lesions to be far more prevalent in individuals with TB compared to controls; however, such lesions were also often seen in other types of pulmonary disease. In addition, new bone formation on the visceral rib surfaces was much more common in the TB cohort, while lesions in the anterior and middle cranial fossae were possibly associated with TB meningitis. However, the authors emphasise the need to evaluate the diagnostic value of TB skeletal markers across different assemblages. Dangvard Pedersen et al. (2019) found that lesions on the visceral rib surface, the ventral aspects of the vertebral bodies, the lateral part of the ilium, the iliac auricular surface, the acetabular fossa, and the ulnar olecranon process were much more prevalent in confirmed TB cases compared to control groups, and these lesions were also associated with each other.

- more common in infants and young children, adolescents and young adults, as well as older adults
- more common in males

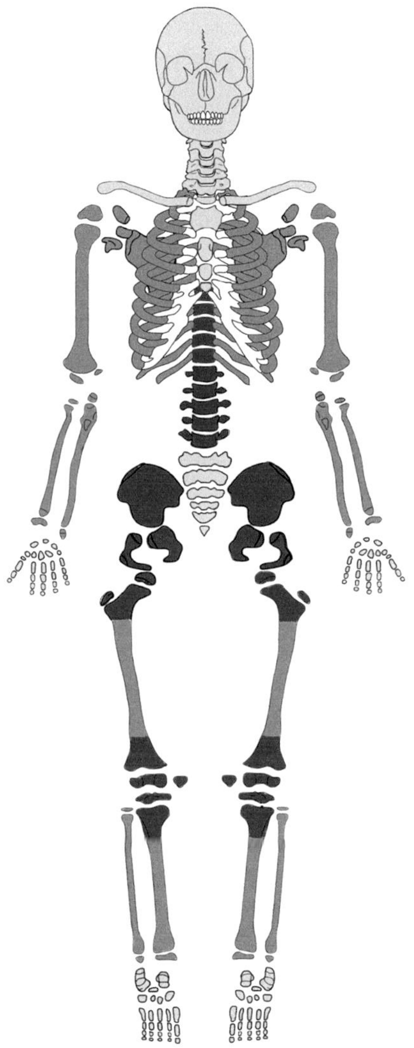

Skull
- rare involvement in adults but not uncommon in children
- lytic lesions with moth-eaten appearance (inner and outer table destruction; lesions greater in diameter endocranially)
- multiple round lesions < 2 cm in children; one large lesion in adults
- mostly affecting frontal and parietal bones; may involve lateral orbit, maxilla, zygomatic and nasal bones (facial bone involvement, lupus vulgaris, more common in young children)
- endocranial lesions linked to tuberculous meningitis (granular impressions, abnormal blood vessel impressions, periosteal apositions or abnormally pronounced digital impressions)*
- otitis media secondary to TB → lytic lesions on petrous bone and mastoid process
- porotic hyperostosis
- cribra orbitalia
- mandibular osteomyelitis

Shoulder girdle
- lytic lesions and new bone formation on clavicle and scapula

Figure 7.12 Skeletal manifestation of tuberculosis.

*Based on sensitivity and specificity estimate values by Spekker et al. (2022), granular impressions are sufficient for a definitive diagnosis of tuberculous meningitis, whereas the remaining lesions are not specific to this condition, though they may have a tuberculous origin. (Data from Arriaza et al. 1995; Aufderheide and Rodríguez-Martín 1998; Cruz and Starke 2007; Dangvard Pedersen et al. 2019; Lewis 2017; Masiu et al. 2023; Masson et al. 2013; Matos and Santos 2006; Meng and Wu 1942; Mosher et al. 2015; Pigrau-Serrallach and Rodríguez-Pardo 2013; Roberts and Buikstra 2003, 2019; Santos and Roberts 2006; Spekker et al. 2022; Steyn et al. 2013; Teo and Peh 2004; Turunc et al. 2007)

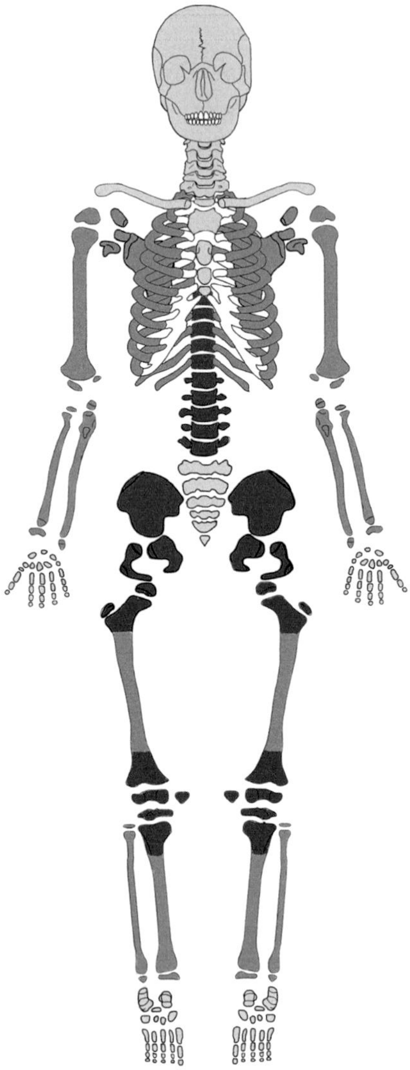

Thorax

- lytic lesions on manubrium or corpus sterni
- new bone formation on sternum
- bone formation on visceral rib surface
- lytic lesions on visceral rib surface

Vertebrae (tuberculous spondylitis)

- most distinctly affected anatomical area
- bone destruction (abscess/cavitation) of vertebral bodies (mostly on ventral part of lower thoracic and upper lumbar bodies but entire body may be gradually involved) → vertebral collapse resulting in kyphosis and ankylosis (Pott's disease)
- very limited new bone formation
- neural arch usually spared
- typically 1-4 contiguous vertebrae involved (rarely the lesions will "skip" vertebrae)
- extravertebral cold (tuberculous) abscesses → variable skeletal manifestations, e.g. concavity on anterior part of adjacent vertebrae, sacroiliac lesions etc.

Figure 7.12 (Continued)

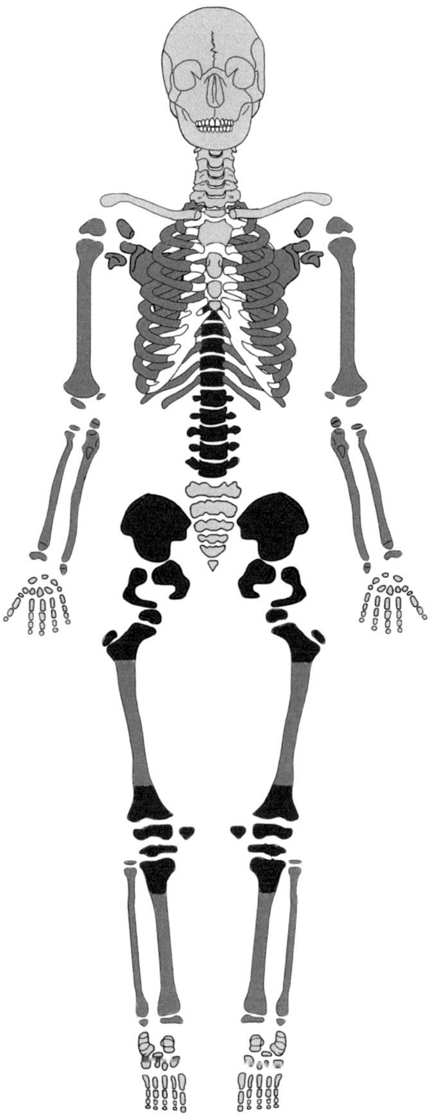

Pelvic girdle

- bone loss or formation on lateral body of ilium, adjacent to acetabulum
- pitting/cavitation on acetabular articular surface
- cavitation on acetabular fossa with minimal, if any, reactive bone formation
- pitting/cavitation on iliac auricular surface
- bilateral involvement of sacroiliac joint

Hand/foot

- mostly involved in children
- inflammation of tubular bones, osteolysis, cyst-like swelling, involucrum (tuberculous dactylitis/spina ventosa)
- symmetric periostitis on tubular bones
- shortened digits
- abscesses in talus and calcaneus

Arm/leg

- lytic lesions mostly in metaphyses and epiphyses (diaphysis may be affected through nutrient canals or infected metaphysis)
- growth plate destruction → growth deficit, limb shortening and/or bone deformity
- central sequestrum, endosteal lytic lesions and periosteal new bone formation
- hypertrophic pulmonary osteoarthropathy (widespread symmetric periostitis)
- tuberculous arthritis initially manifesting as erosive lesions at the joint margin with little new bone formation and later fibrous ankylosis
- mostly monoarticular and unilateral joint affliction
- in severe cases, the femoral or humeral head may be destroyed

Figure 7.12 (Continued)

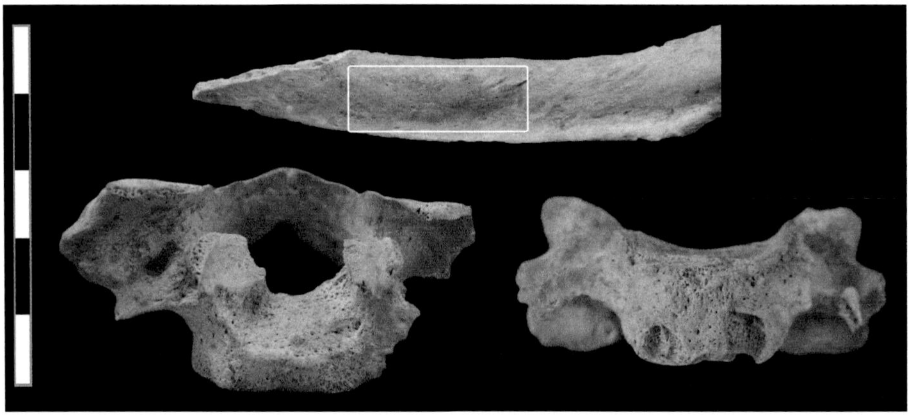

Figure 7.13 Probable tuberculosis. Top: New bone formation on the visceral rib surface. Bottom: Cervical vertebrae with lytic lesions in the body. (Male, 25–28 years old, Methodist Chapel, Carver Street, 19th c., CAR99 1286; photos by Efthymia Nikita; copyright: Human Skeletal Collection, University of Sheffield)

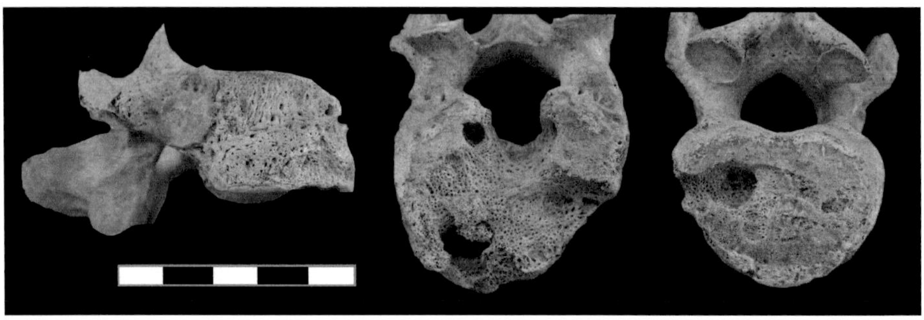

Figure 7.14 Probable tuberculosis. Left: New bone formation on the lateral surface of a thoracic vertebral body. Middle: Extensive destruction of the superior surface of a vertebral body. Right: Lytic lesions on the inferior surface of a vertebral body. (Same individual as in Figure 7.13; photos by Efthymia Nikita; copyright: Human Skeletal Collection, University of Sheffield)

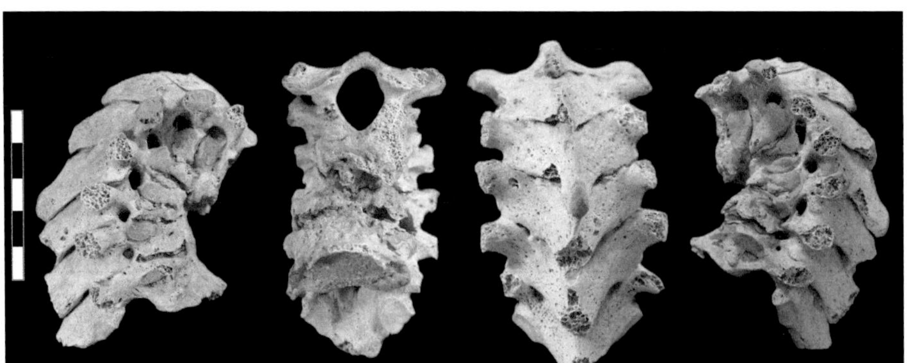

Figure 7.15 Probable tuberculosis. Note the collapse and ankylosis of the spine, resulting in kyphosis. (11 ± 1 years old, Stratford Road, Warwick, Medieval, WR15 34; photos by Efthymia Nikita; copyright: Human Skeletal Collection, University of Sheffield)

contaminated meat and dairy products, direct handling of infected animals, or inhalation of respiratory droplets during contact with infected animals. The condition has an incubation period of two to four weeks. Its symptoms include fever, headache, joint and muscle pain, as well as fatigue, while infection of the skeleton can arise when the bacteria disseminate via a haematogenous route (Figures 7.16 and 7.17).

Hansen's disease

Hansen's disease, or leprosy, is an infectious disease caused by *Mycobacterium leprae* and *Mycobacterium lepromatosis*. It is transmitted primarily through the inhalation of respiratory droplets released by an infected person when coughing or sneezing. The infection may also spread through prolonged direct contact with an affected individual's open lesions. However, the condition is not highly contagious, thus it does not spread through casual contact with an infected person.

Although much is known about Hansen's disease, its epidemiology is not fully clear. The typical incubation period is about five years; however, as much as two decades may pass before symptoms become visible. The manifestation of the disease depends on the host's immune response. At one extreme of the spectrum lies lepromatous leprosy (LL), which is characterised by low resistance, while at the opposite end is tuberculoid leprosy (TL), which is associated with high resistance. Many patients show borderline leprosy, which has a wide range of symptoms that lie between the extremes of TL and LL.

Individuals with the tuberculoid type of leprosy exhibit a strong cellular immune response, which can limit the disease to a small number of discoloured and thickened skin lesions (dry, scaly patches or plaques). In addition, peripheral nerves may be affected, resulting in sensory, motor, and autonomic loss of function. The damage to autonomic nerves can restrict the skin's ability to sweat, resulting in dryness and cracking, and increasing susceptibility to secondary infections. Involvement of the motor nerves can cause paralysis, manifesting, for example, as "claw hand" and "claw foot" deformities. The involvement of sensory nerves in the extremities makes individuals susceptible to trauma, as they cannot perceive pain. However, the reduced bacterial load in cases of TL results in an overall less severe manifestation of the disease.

LL is characterised by impaired cell-mediated immune response. Multiple organs may be exposed to the bacilli, but because the bacillus prefers cooler parts of the body, the most severe pathological alterations are usually found in the superficial subcutaneous tissues. Nodules and papules form in the skin and mucous membranes of the face and harbour a significant bacterial load. In the early stages of the disease, patients may show nasal symptoms consistent with chronic rhinitis, but gradually, the bones of the nasal cavity and adjacent structures will be destroyed. The heavy bacterial load also promotes more extensive peripheral nerve involvement.

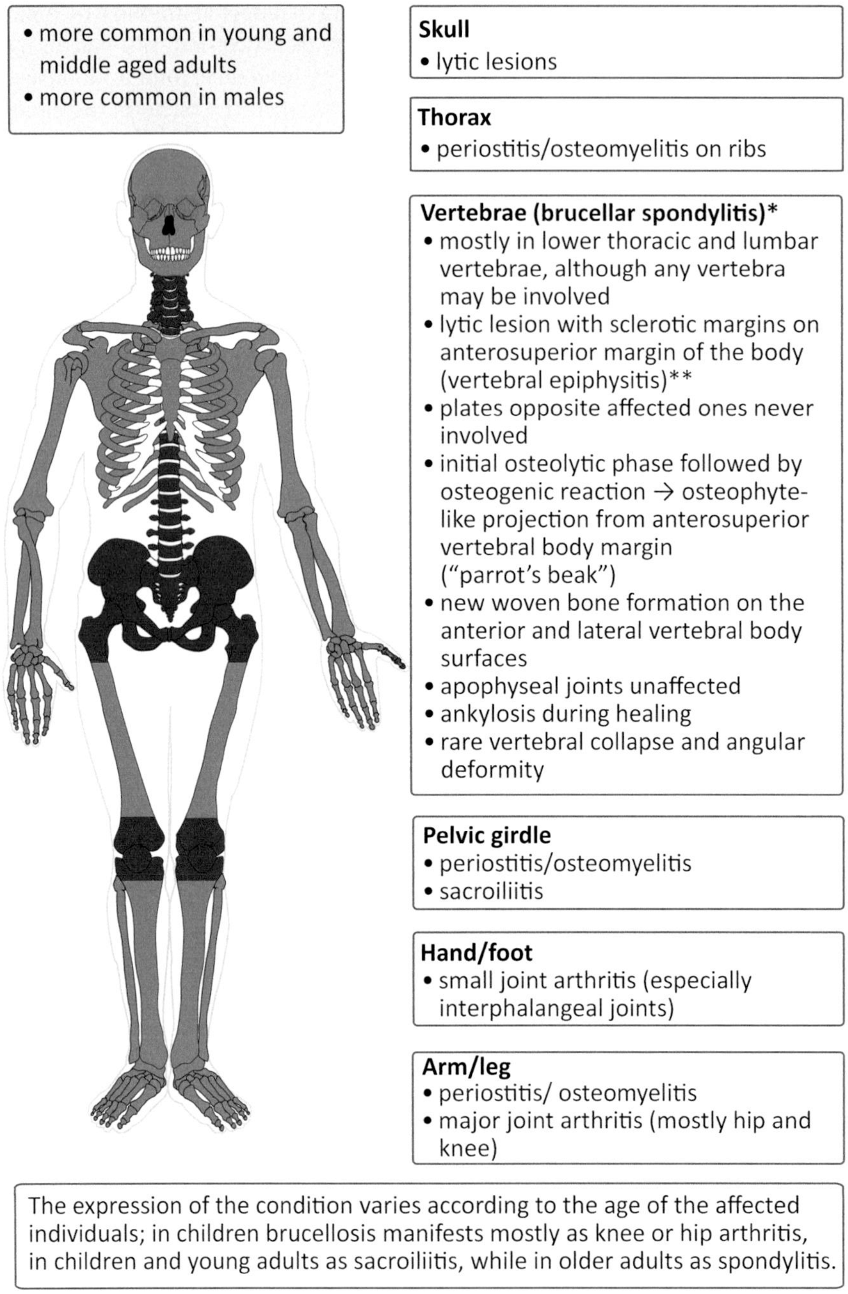

Figure 7.16 Skeletal manifestation of brucellosis.

*Two forms of spinal brucellosis:

focal pattern: one vertebra affected; lesions mostly on superior edge

diffuse pattern: lesions distributed throughout a vertebra; infection disseminating to adjacent vertebrae

**The radiological expression of epiphysitis of the anterosuperior angle of lumbar vertebrae (Pedro Pons' sign) is considered diagnostic of brucellosis (D'Anastasio et al. 2011)

(Data from Aufderheide and Rodríguez-Martín 1998; Chelli Bouaziz et al. 2008; D'Anastasio et al. 2011; Esmaeilnejad-Ganji and Esmaeilnejad-Ganji 2019; Khateeb et al. 1990; Madkour 1989; Ortner 2008; Sohn et al. 2010; Yuan et al. 2020)

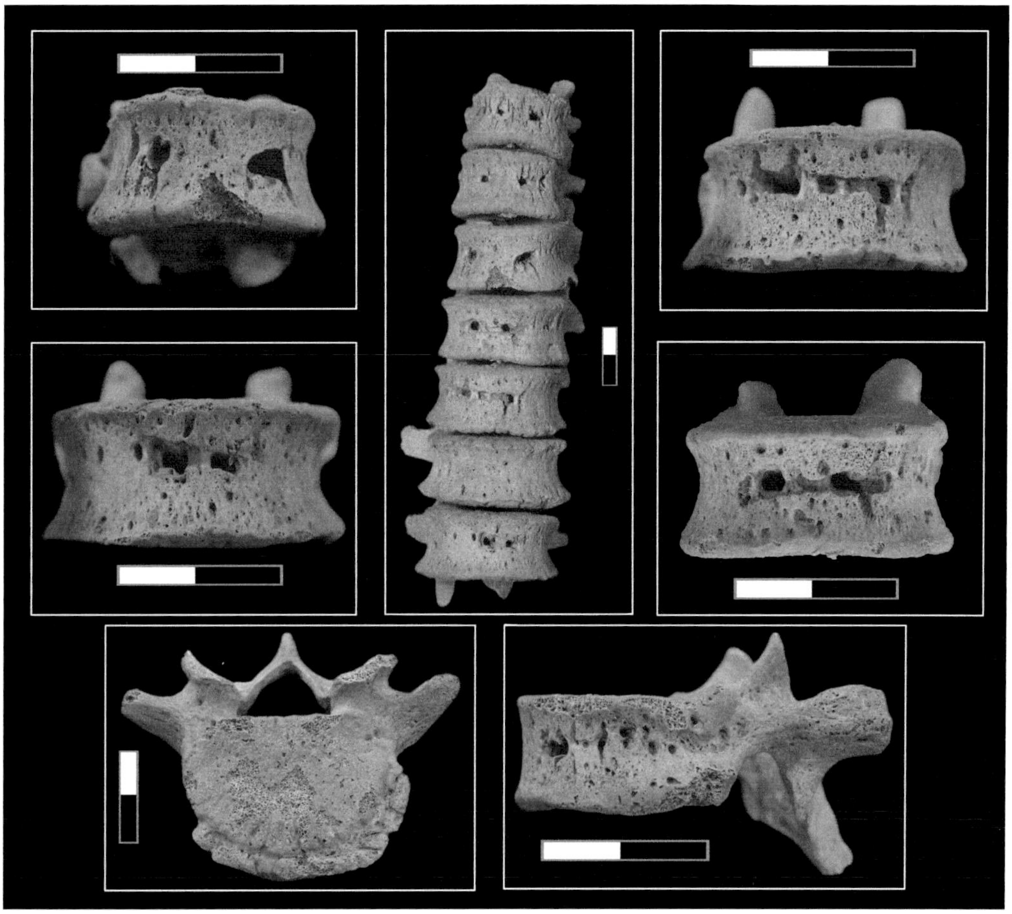

Figure 7.17 Probable brucellosis. Note the lytic lesions and woven bone formation on the anterior and lateral lower thoracic and lumbar vertebral bodies, as well as the marginal osteophytic formation on the anterosuperior body of a lumbar vertebra. (15–18 years old, Parish Church of St Mary and St Lawrence, Bolsover, 13th c CE, BOL 037/038; photos by Efthymia Nikita; copyright: Human Skeletal Collection, University of Sheffield)

Hansen's disease primarily affects the nervous system and the skin; the skeleton can be involved directly or indirectly. The pathogenic bacteria have a direct effect on the craniofacial region, while indirect effects arise from the involvement of sensory, motor, and autonomic nerves, as described above. Skeletal changes are mostly seen in individuals with LL or long-standing TL; however, not all patients with this condition will develop skeletal lesions (Figures 7.18–7.27).

- may affect individuals of all ages
- more common in males

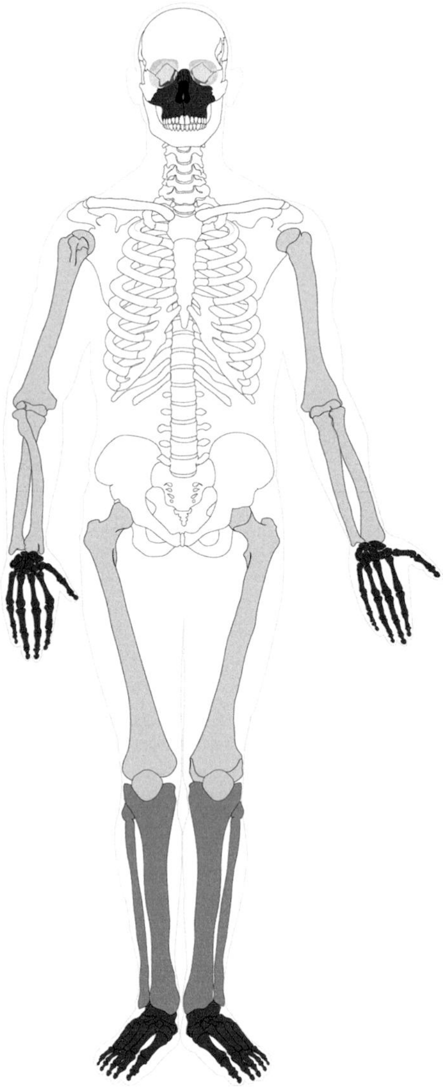

General

- specific osseous changes due to bacterial load; non-specific osseous changes resulting from recurrent injuries, chronic infection, lack of sensation and ulcerations

Skull (rhinomaxillary syndrome)

- mixed bone erosion and new bone formation
- maxillary alveolar process resorption, starting from the prosthion and progressing to the rest of the maxilla → antemortem loss of incisors (in advanced stages teeth beyond the lateral incisors may be affected)
- anterior nasal spine pitting and resorption (until the spine is eliminated)
- resorption and remodelling of lateral and inferior nasal aperture margins (bilateral and symmetric)
- nasal surface of maxillary palatine process: a) fine pitting followed by plaques of subperiosteal new bone and, finally, a relatively smooth surface, b) discrete lytic lesions, smaller than 0.5cm in diameter, single or multiple
- oral surface of maxillary palatine process: small erosive pits towards the palatine suture, gradual confluence of the pits and possible perforation of the hard palate
- pitting and resorption of nasal septum and nasal conchae
- leprogenic odontodysplasia (stunted roots in permanent maxillary incisors)

Figure 7.18 Skeletal manifestation of Hansen's disease. (Data from Andersen and Manchester 1987, 1988, 1992; Andersen et al. 1992, 1994; Danielsen 1968; Lewis 2017; Møller-Christensen 1961, 1978; Roberts and Buikstra 2019)

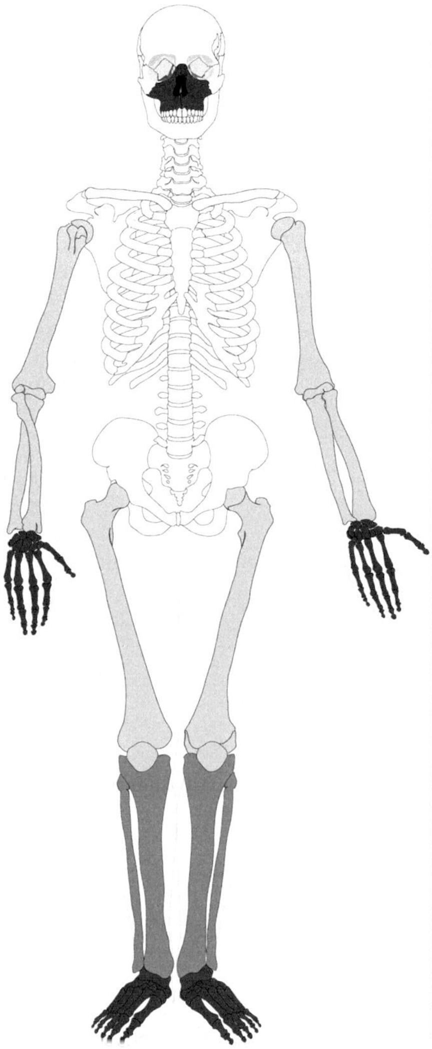

Hand/foot

- in hands, osseous involvement rare beyond the metacarpophalangeal joints, except for thumb; in feet, all bones may be affected
- atrophy and concentric bone loss starting from distal manual phalanges and metatarsophalangeal joint in the hands and feet, respectively
- diaphyseal remodelling commences at midshaft in phalanges, but in distal third in metatarsals and metacarpals
- diaphyseal remodelling in metatarsals may be concentric or medio-lateral (leading to knife-edge deformity)
- most distally affected bone may be tapered ("pencil ends")
- cup-shaped proximal phalangeal articular surfaces due to subluxation and osteophytes
- osteophyte formation circumferentially at proximal ends and bone resorption at distal ends ("shark-tooth" deformity)
- volar grooves on proximal manual phalanges (due to finger contractures)
- osteomyelitis
- destruction of foot and ankle joints (Charcot joints)
- subluxation or dislocation
- ankylosed metacarpophalangeal, metatarsophalangeal and interphalangeal joints
- transverse hypertrophic bone bridges/bars across dorsal tarsal surface
- carpal and tarsal erosion/destruction
- enlarged nutrient foramina

Figure 7.18 (Continued)

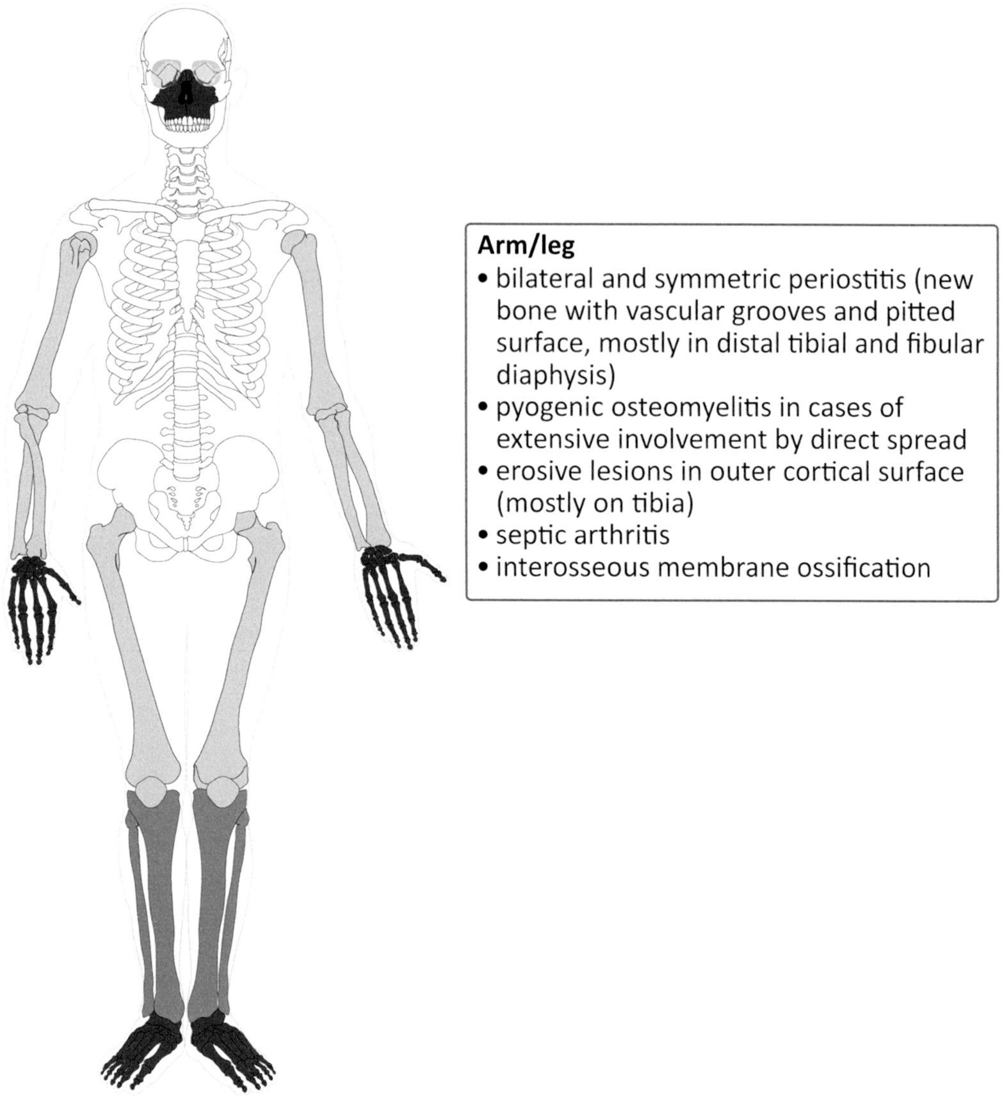

Figure 7.18 (Continued)

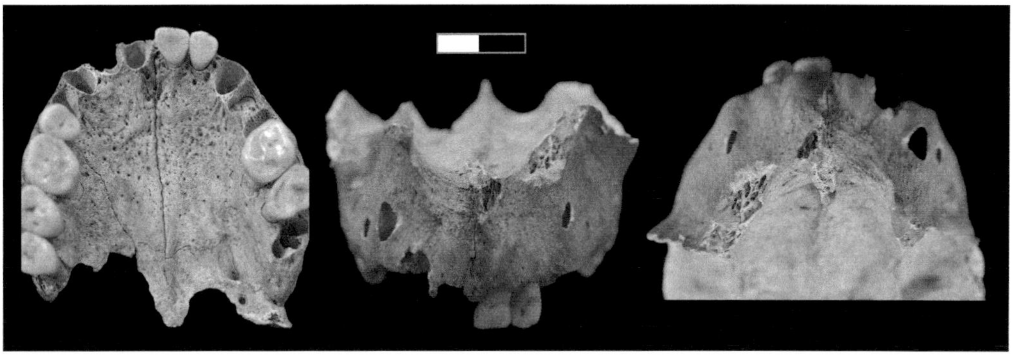

Figure 7.19 Hansen's disease. Note the porosity on the oral surface of the hard palate (left), the resorption of the anterior nasal spine (middle), and the bilateral and symmetric resorption and remodelling of the inferior nasal aperture margins (right). (Male, 20–40 years old, London Road, Grantham, 12th-15th c. CE, GLR 40; photos by Efthymia Nikita; copyright: Human Skeletal Collection, University of Sheffield)

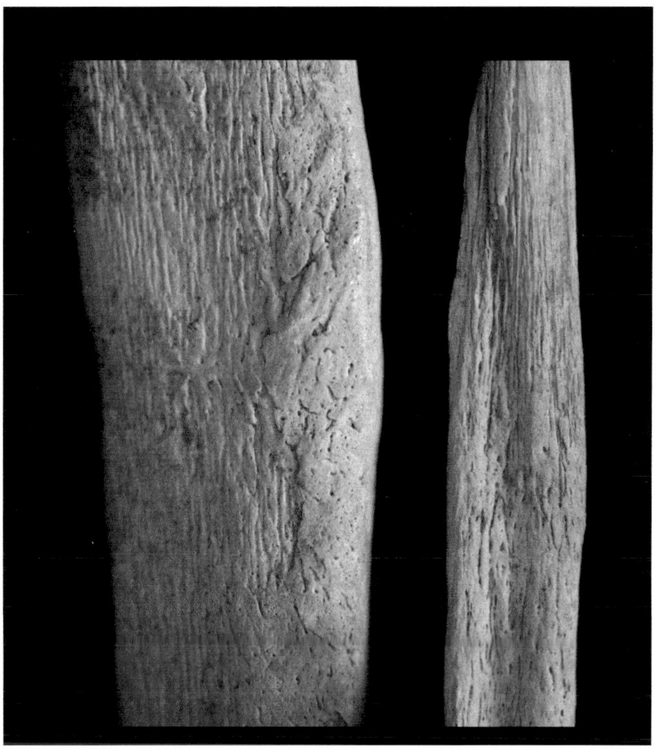

Figure 7.20 Hansen's disease. Periosteal new bone formation on tibial and fibular diaphyses. (Same individual as in Figure 7.19; photos by Efthymia Nikita; copyright: Human Skeletal Collection, University of Sheffield)

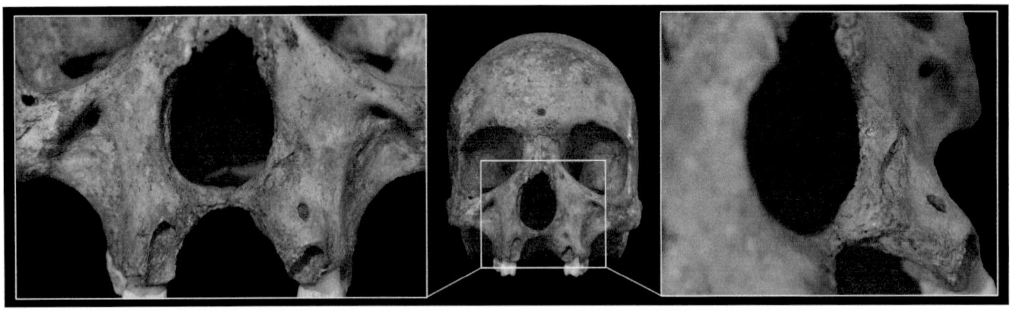

Figure 7.21 Hansen's disease. Note the maxillary alveolar process resorption that has resulted in the antemortem loss of the incisors. Also note the extensive remodelling (rounding) of the lateral and inferior nasal aperture margins. (Photos by Efthymia Nikita; copyright: Duckworth Laboratory, University of Cambridge)

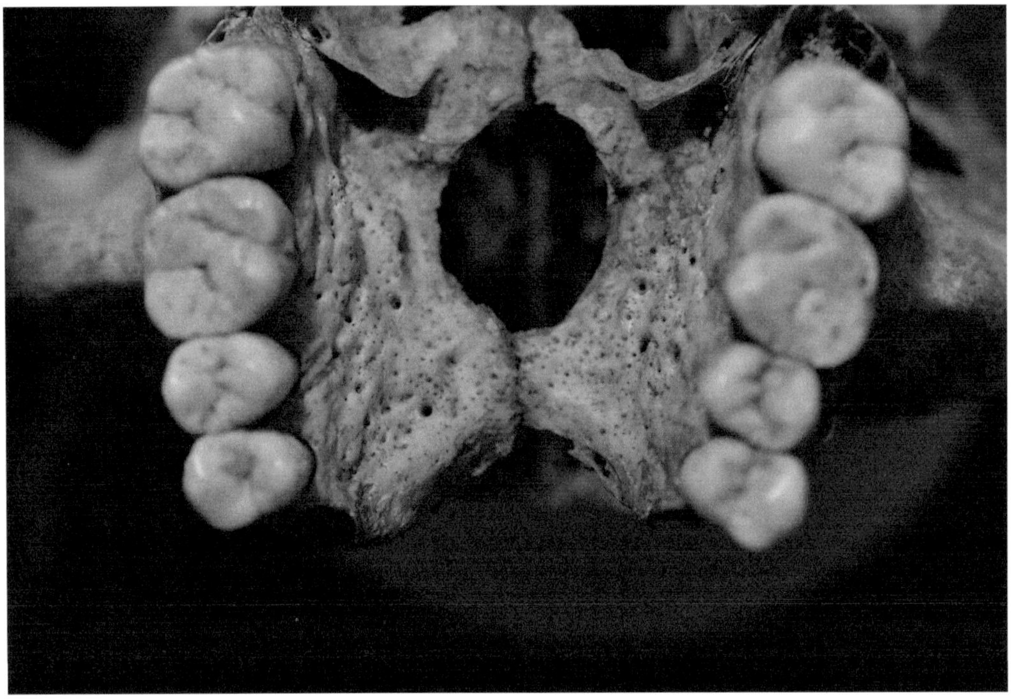

Figure 7.22 Hansen's disease. Note the maxillary alveolar process resorption that has resulted in the antemortem loss of the incisors and the perforation of the hard palate. (Same individual as in Figure 7.21; photo by Efthymia Nikita; copyright: Duckworth Laboratory, University of Cambridge)

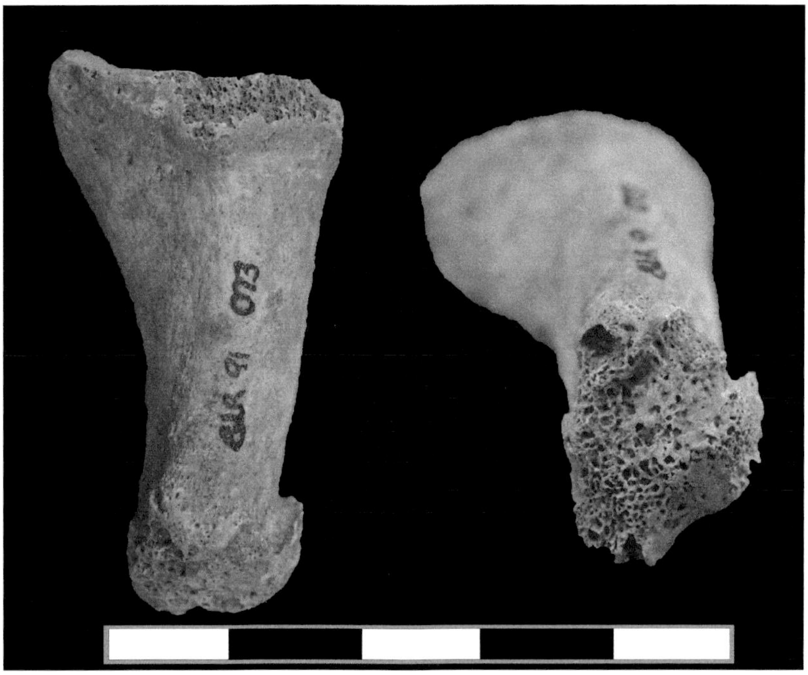

Figure 7.23 Hansen's disease. Note the bone loss at the head of the first metatarsal. (Female, 40–80 years old, London Road, Grantham, 12th-15th c. CE, GLR91-73; photos by Efthymia Nikita; copyright: Human Skeletal Collection, University of Sheffield)

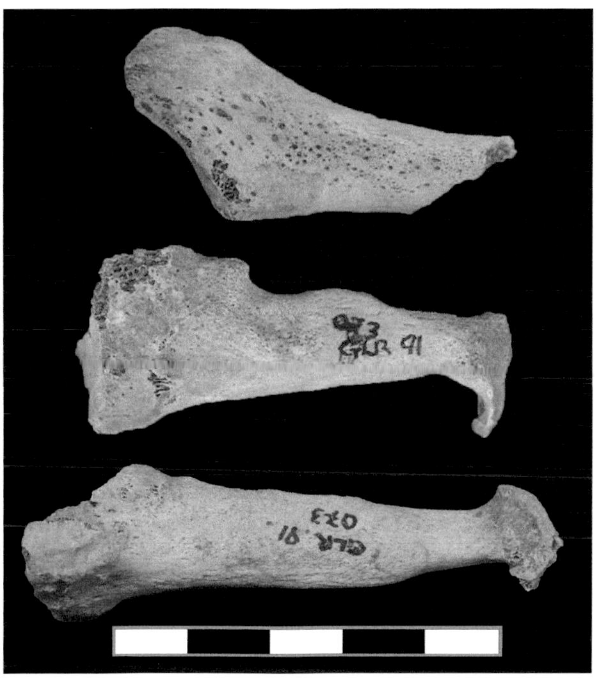

Figure 7.24 Hansen's disease. Note the bone loss at the distal part (head) of the metatarsals, as well as the diffuse porosity, particularly visible on the shaft of the fifth metatarsal (top). (Same individual as in Figure 7.23; photos by Efthymia Nikita; copyright: Human Skeletal Collection, University of Sheffield)

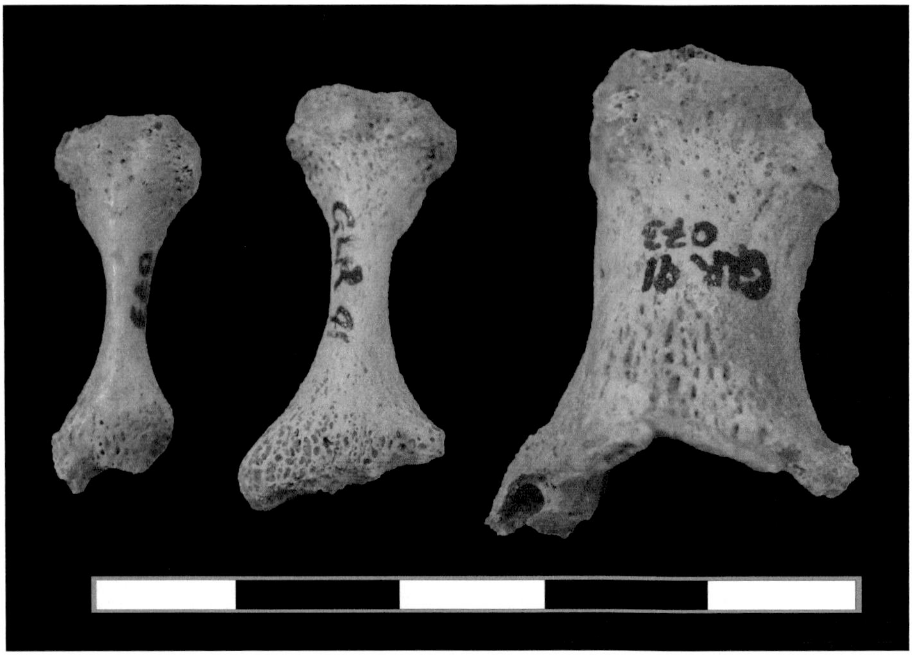

Figure 7.25 Hansen's disease. Note the remodelling of the base of the pedal phalanges (cup-shaped deformity), as well as the concentric bone loss in the midshaft of the same bones. (Same individual as in Figures 7.23 and 7.24; photos by Efthymia Nikita; copyright: Human Skeletal Collection, University of Sheffield)

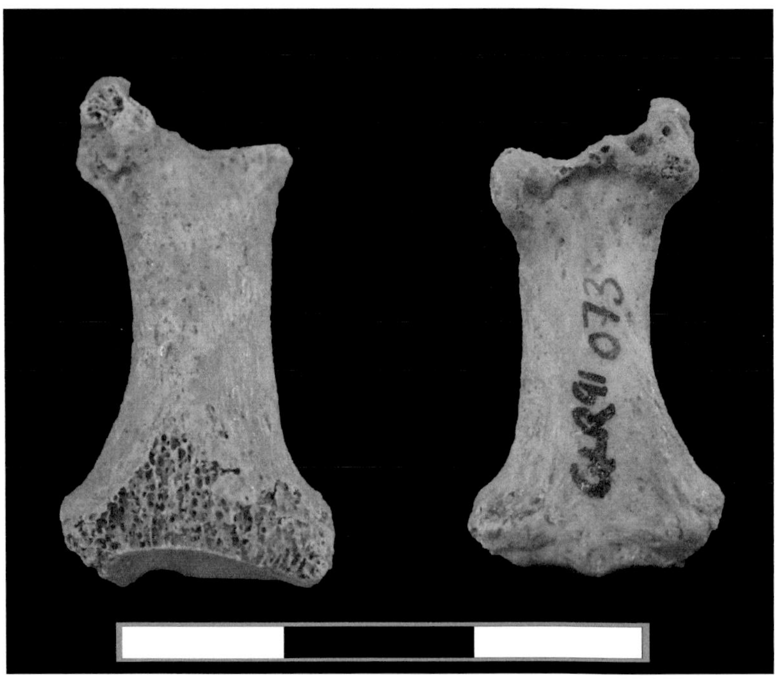

Figure 7.26 Hansen's disease. Note the destruction of the head of the manual phalanx. (Same individual as in Figures 7.23–7.25; photos by Efthymia Nikita; copyright: Human Skeletal Collection, University of Sheffield)

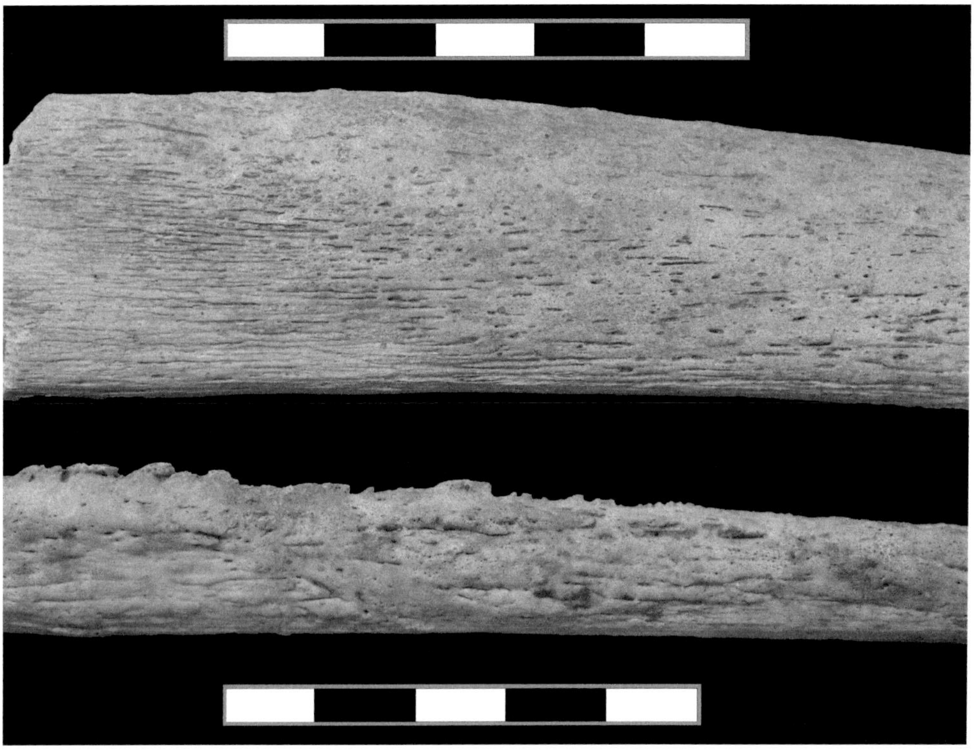

Figure 7.27 Hansen's disease. Periosteal new bone formation on tibial and fibular diaphyses. (Same individual as in Figures 7.23–7.26; photos by Efthymia Nikita; copyright: Human Skeletal Collection, University of Sheffield)

Treponemal disease

Treponemal disease is caused by spirochetes (spiral-shaped bacteria) of the genus *Treponema*. Treponemes can survive within the host organism for long periods by evading detection and subsequent immune responses. Four treponematoses have been identified: pinta, yaws, bejel, and venereal syphilis. Pinta is caused by *Treponema carateum* and predominantly occurs in Central and South America. In contrast, yaws is associated with *Treponema pallidum* subsp. *pertenue* and is mostly found in warm, humid, tropical regions. Bejel, also known as endemic syphilis, is caused by *Treponema pallidum* subsp. *endemicum* and primarily affects individuals in warm, arid to semiarid regions. Finally, venereal (acquired) syphilis is a sexually transmitted disease caused by *Treponema pallidum* subsp. *pallidum*, and it is distributed globally.

Pinta does not cause skeletal lesions; therefore, it will not be further considered in this chapter. In all remaining conditions, spirochetes enter the host organism through the mucous membranes or a skin lesion. Bejel and yaws usually appear during childhood. In contrast, syphilis mostly afflicts sexually active adults, as well as infants who may be infected transplacentally (congenital syphilis). In all cases (yaws, bejel, syphilis), the pathogens spread throughout the body and eventually reach the skeleton through the haematogenous route (Box 7.8, Figures 7.28–7.44).

Box 7.8 Diagnosing treponemal disease

According to Baker et al. (2020) and references therein, the sequence of lesions from serpiginous cavities to *caries sicca* is considered pathognomonic for treponemal disease, as is the occurrence of extensive bone resorption in the palatal and nasal bones, which may exhibit signs of healing, the presence of bilateral nodes with rugose surface and focal superficial cavitation in the long bones, as well as the presence of Hutchinson's incisors and Moon's molars (for cases of congenital syphilis). Skeletal changes strongly suggestive of treponemal disease include cranial lesions that range from clustered pits to radial scarring, dactylitis, saber shins, bilateral enlargement of the long bones featuring smooth lamellar bone alongside a combination of striations and rippling, bilateral nodes on the long bones associated with a rugose surface but without bone destruction, as well as unilateral nodes on the long bones associated with a rugose surface and focal superficial cavitation. However, somewhat different criteria have been used by other scholars (see, e.g., Harper et al. 2011).

The course of treponemal diseases, except for congenital syphilis, has three active stages. The primary stage usually lasts a few weeks and is characterised by the formation of an initial lesion (chancre) at the site of infection. The symptoms during this stage are typically painless and often resolve even without treatment. This stage rarely affects the skeleton; if any lesions develop, they appear as nonspecific periosteal new bone formation. In the secondary stage, the spirochete spreads through the bloodstream and causes extensive rashes and other mucocutaneous lesions. Other symptoms during this stage include lymph node enlargement, fever, alopecia, and fatigue, and usually appear four to ten weeks following the appearance of the primary chancre. During this stage, individuals may experience bone pain, but skeletal changes are generally minimal and usually resolve spontaneously. In the absence of treatment, although lesions will ultimately resolve, the infection will enter a latent phase, which may then lead to the tertiary stage. The latent stage varies greatly in duration, and it may last for years. Finally, the tertiary stage is characterised by destructive lesions in cutaneous and osseous tissues. A typical trait of the tertiary stage is the gumma, a granulomatous lesion that can appear in the skin, bones, and other parts of the body.

As mentioned above, pinta causes no skeletal lesions. Yaws, bejel, and venereal syphilis produce lesions that are very similar. Attempts have been made to differentiate skeletally these syndromes (e.g. SPIRAL criteria by Rothschild and Rothschild 1995); however, most scholars avoid any finer diagnosis beyond treponemal disease based on skeletal markers.

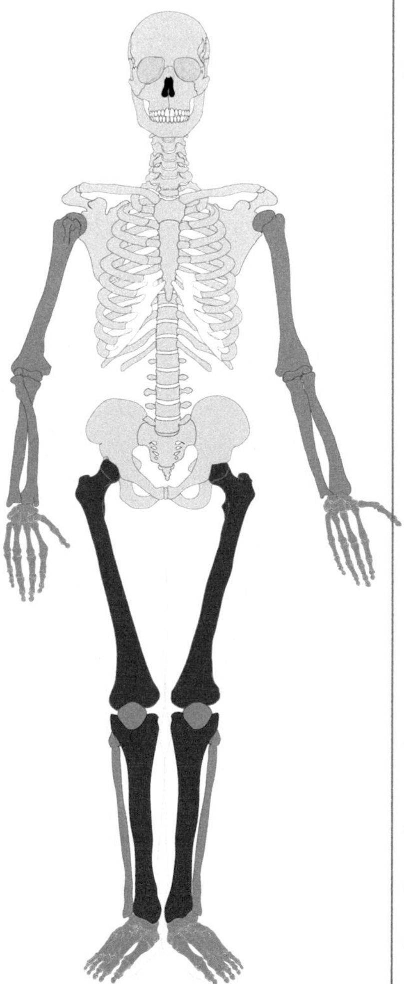

Skull
progressive changes of lesions on frontal and parietal bones (caries sicca sequence) – different stages may coexist on same cranium:

- stage 1: clustered pits (clearly delineated area measuring 10 to 15mm in diameter, characterised by pits approximately 1mm in diameter; zone of increased bone density around each cluster of pits; minimal or no involvement of inner table; lesions generally not involving the sutures)
- stage 2: confluent clustered pits (pits enlarged and coalescing → central erosion or pitted osseous plug with peripheral erosion)
- stage 3: focal superficial cavitation (superficial cavities with concave walls and sharp edges; diploë visible on floor; slightly pitted endocranial surface and thin new bone layer)
- stage 4: circumvallate cavitation (lesion surrounded by osseous rim; lesion margins rolled and grooved by small blood vessels (stellate lesion); adjacent cavities may coalesce; minor endocranial changes)
- stage 5: radial scarring (new bone fills in the cavity, leaving behind shallow depression; initial configuration consisting of a radial arrangement of thin lines, encircled by rimmed margin; gradual flattening of the margin, but residual depression; possible endocranial bone formation)
- stage 6: serpiginous cavitation (confluence of clustered pits; snake-like cavities with sharp irregular margins and diploë visible at the floor)
- stage 7: nodular cavitation (cavities with rounded margins; nodule formation)
- stage 8: caries sicca (nodule enlargement, stellate depressions between nodules; thickened inner table)
- goundou: periosteal new bone formation on rhino-maxillary area
- gangosa: nasal cavity resorption/smooth lateral walls ("saddle nose" but nasal spine usually spared) and hard palate abnormal porosity, resorption/penetration

Figure 7.28 Skeletal manifestation of treponemal disease. (Data from Baker et al. 2020; Castro et al. 2016; Hackett 1975, 1976, 1981, 1983; Harper et al. 2011; Lefort and Bennike 2007; Mitchell 2003; Powell and Cook 2005; Roberts and Buikstra 2019; Rothschild and Rothschild 1995; Waldron 2020)

*True bowing characterises juvenile treponemal disease and pseudo-bowing adult cases

Note: The distribution of lesions shown in the skeleton diagram broadly reflects yaws; in syphilis and bejel, the lower limb long bones are also the most commonly affected elements, the cranium is often affected in syphilis, followed by the humeri and ribs, while the rest of the skeleton is rarely involved in both conditions.

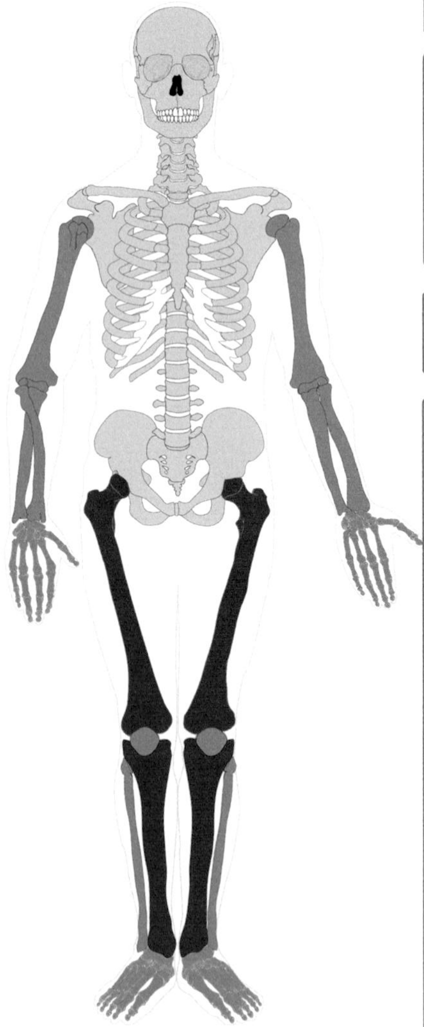

Thorax
- lytic lesions and new bone formation on ribs

Vertebrae
- mostly in cervical vertebrae
- lytic lesions and new bone formation on bodies (rare involvement of neural arch)
- aortic aneurysm: resorptive lesion on lateral side (usually left) of one or adjacent thoracic or lumbar vertebrae

Hand/foot
- dactylitis

Arm/leg
- anterior tibial bowing (boomerang leg) or pseudobowing (saber shin, where tibiae appear bowed but their long axis is straight and the bowing is due to periosteal new bone accumulation)*
- non-gummatous lesions (thickened bone due to periosteal bone formation; small osseous nodes; new bone may gradually remodel and the end result can be an abnormally enlarged element)
- gummatous lesions (lytic foci of necrotic bone surrounded by reactive new bone) in the cortex and medullary cavity
- enlargement and thickening of trabeculae
- narrowed medullary cavity
- osteomyelitis
- joint lesions
  - o Charcot joint (loss of sensation leads to repeated trauma and infection → articular surface destruction, eburnation and new bone formation; usually bilateral; most often in hip)
  - o gummatous arthritis: gumma may perforate a joint (usually a single joint)

Figure 7.28 (Continued)

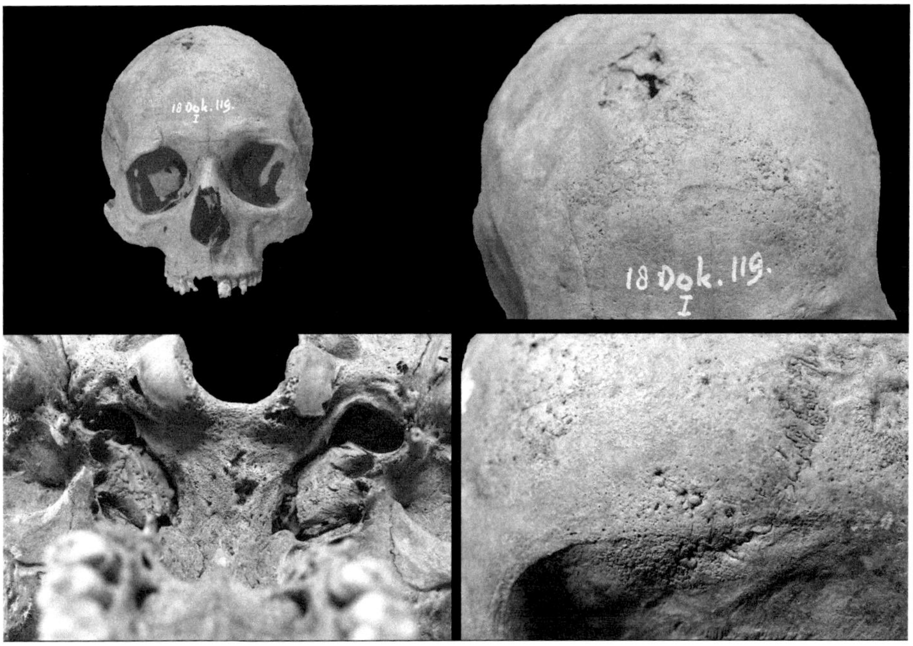

Figure 7.29 Treponemal disease. Note the active, healing, and healed destructive lesions throughout the cranium, including on the cranial base. (Probable male, Dokkum Marktplein, Collection NAD Nuis inv. Nr. F 2021-X-18; photos by Efthymia Nikita, with permission from the Noordelijk Archeologisch Depot)

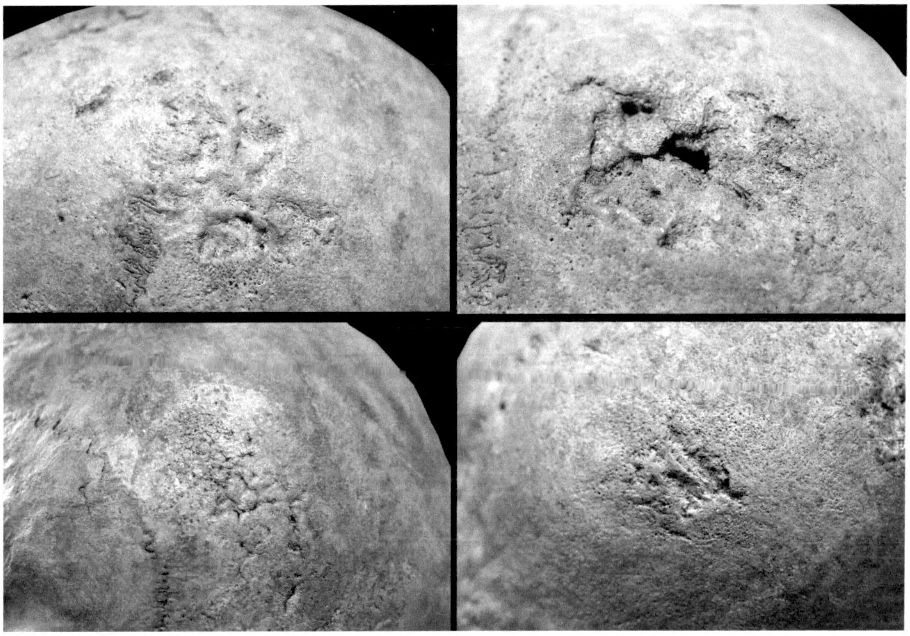

Figure 7.30 Treponemal disease. Note the cranial lesions at different states of the disease: active/healing (right top and bottom) and advanced healing/healed (left top and bottom). (Same individual as in Figure 7.29; photos by Efthymia Nikita, with permission from the Noordelijk Archeologisch Depot)

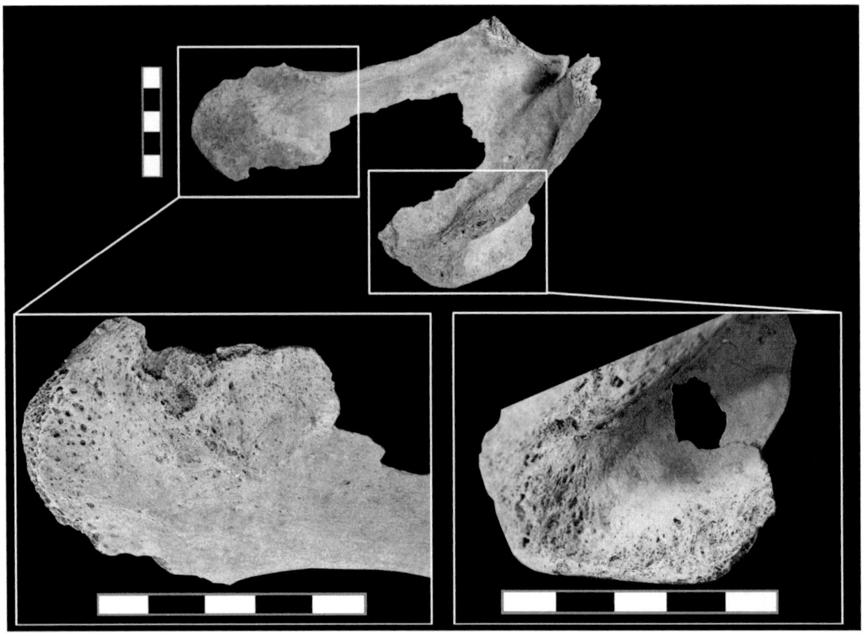

Figure 7.31 Treponemal disease. Note the diffuse erosive lesions at the inferior part of the body of the left scapula, as well as at the medial end of the scapular spine. (Same individual as in Figures 7.29 and 7.30; photos by Efthymia Nikita, with permission from the Noordelijk Archeologisch Depot)

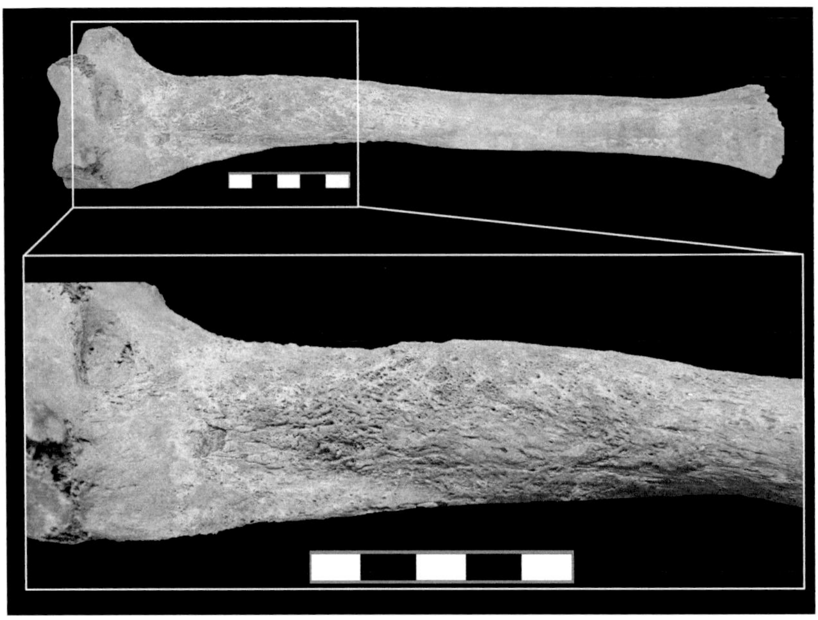

Figure 7.32 Treponemal disease. Note the nongummatous lesions (bone thickening due to periosteal new bone formation) on the distal diaphysis of the left humerus. (Same individual as in Figures 7.29–7.31; photos by Efthymia Nikita, with permission from the Noordelijk Archeologisch Depot)

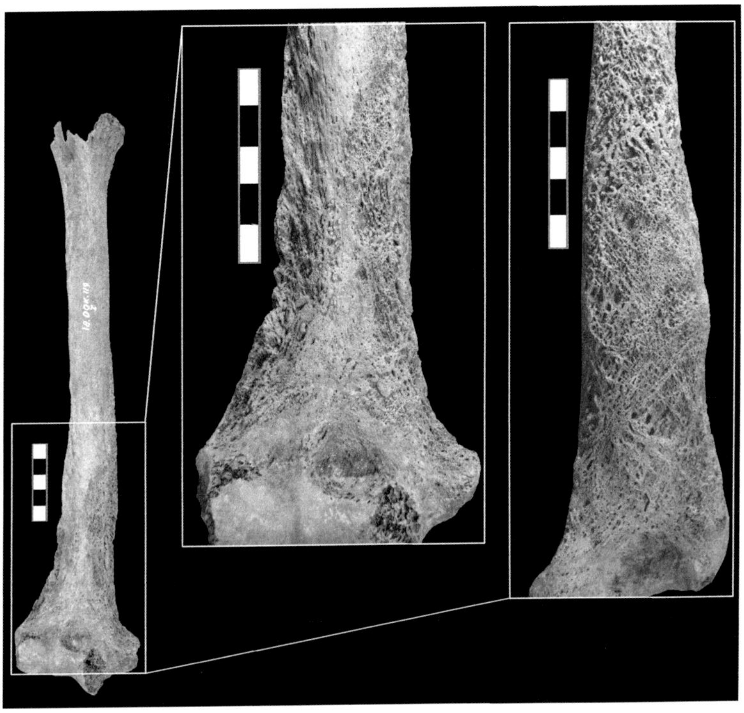

Figure 7.33 Treponemal disease. Note the extensive periosteal new bone formation as well as bone resorption at the distal diaphysis and metaphysis of the right humerus. Note also the disorganised nature of the newly formed bone. (Same individual as in Figures 7.29–7.32; photos by Efthymia Nikita, with permission from the Noordelijk Archeologisch Depot)

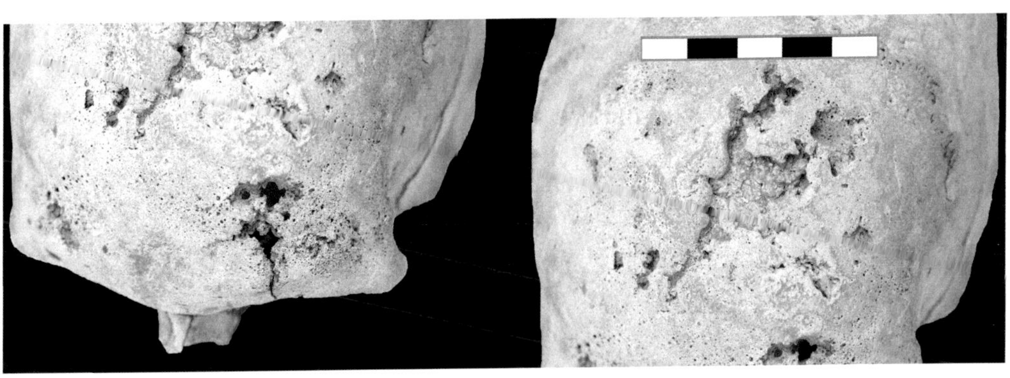

Figure 7.34 Probable treponemal disease. Note the extensive lytic lesions on the frontal bone, whereby active lesions coexist with advanced sclerotic healing. (Probable male, 31–65 years old, 5217; photos by Efthymia Nikita, from the reference collection of the Cultural Heritage Agency of the Netherlands)

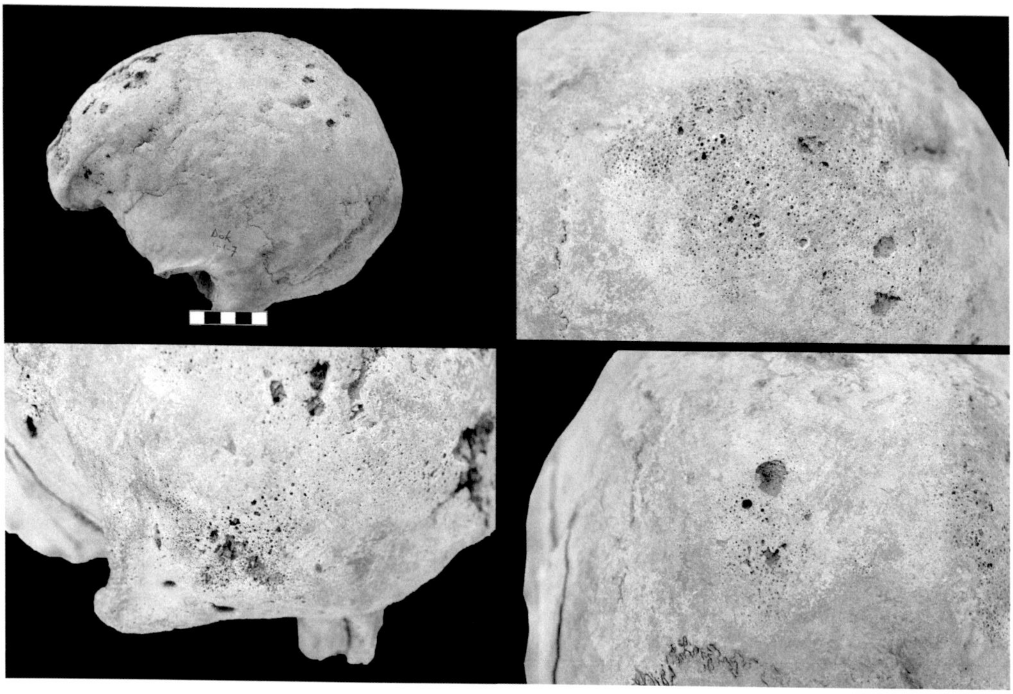

Figure 7.35 Probable treponemal disease. Note the lytic lesions throughout the cranium but at different stages. Overview of the cranium (upper left) showing lytic lesions with and without sclerotic margin in the frontal and left parietal bones. Pitting and cavitations shown in the remaining three images. (Same individual as in Figure 7.34; photos by Efthymia Nikita, from the reference collection of the Cultural Heritage Agency of the Netherlands)

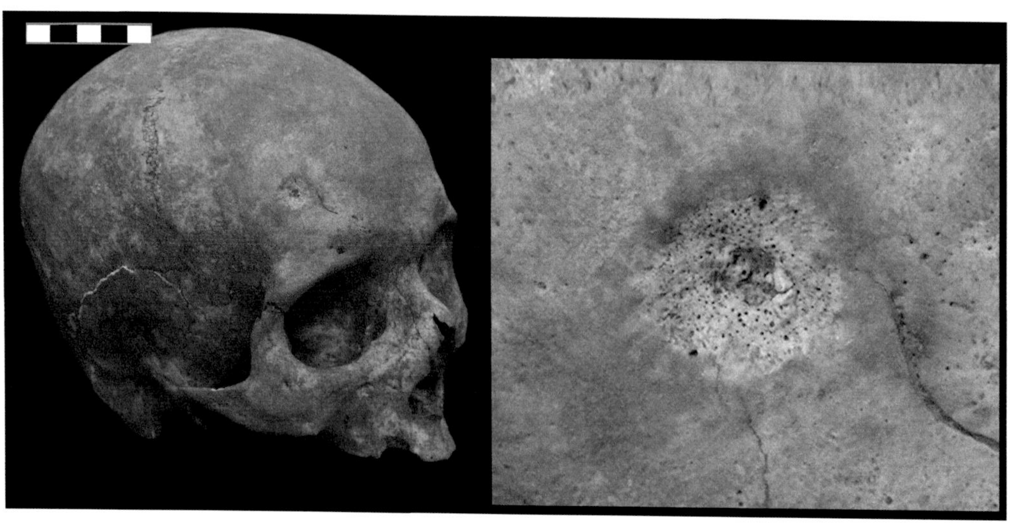

Figure 7.36 Lytic lesion with peripheral erosion on the frontal bone. (Male, 30–40 years old, St Hilda's Church, Coronation Street, South Shields, Newcastle, 19th c., CS06-62; photos by Efthymia Nikita; copyright: Human Skeletal Collection, University of Sheffield)

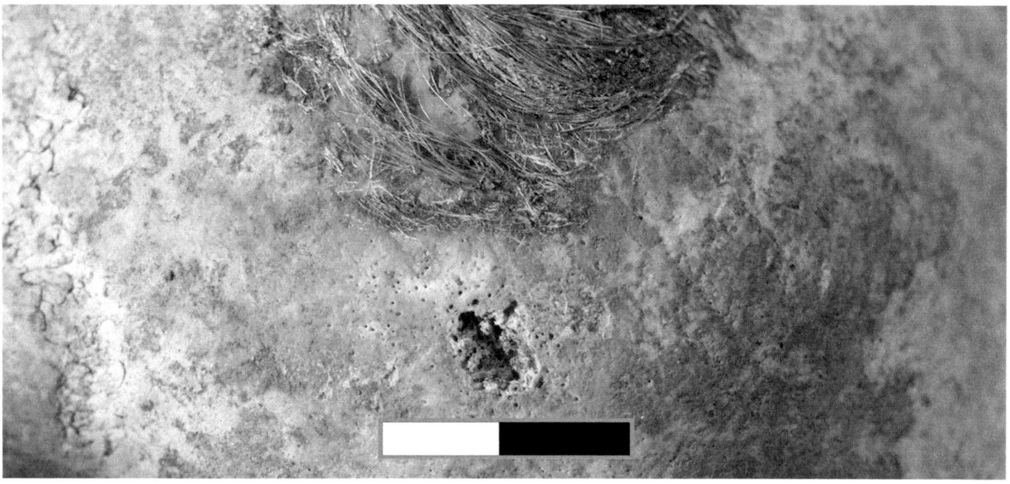

Figure 7.37 Focal superficial cavitation and fine pitting on the frontal bone. (Female, 50–70 years old, St Hilda's Church, Coronation Street, South Shields, Newcastle, 19th c., CS06-507; photo by Efthymia Nikita; copyright: Human Skeletal Collection, University of Sheffield)

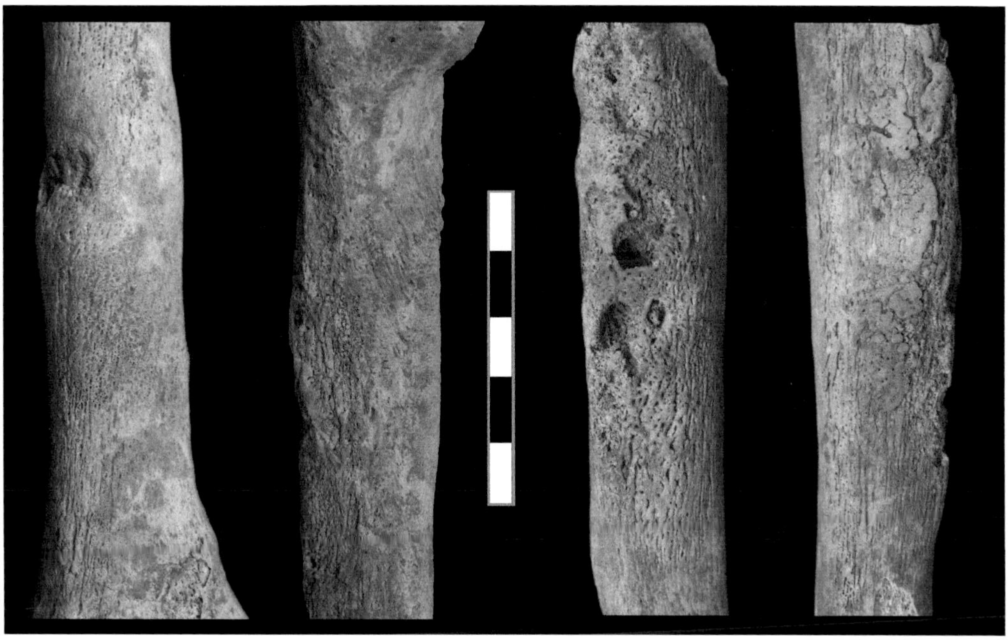

Figure 7.38 Probable treponemal disease. Note the new bone formation (woven bone) on the distal epiphysis and metaphysis, as well as the lytic lesion with remodelled margins of the left femur (left); the sclerotic bone formation on the proximal epiphysis of the left femur (second from left); the lytic foci surrounded by periosteal new bone at the left tibial diaphysis (second from right), and the sclerotic new bone formation on the left tibial diaphysis (right). (Female, 35–55 years old, All Saints Church, Fishergate, York, Y-3870; photos by Efthymia Nikita; copyright: Human Skeletal Collection, University of Sheffield)

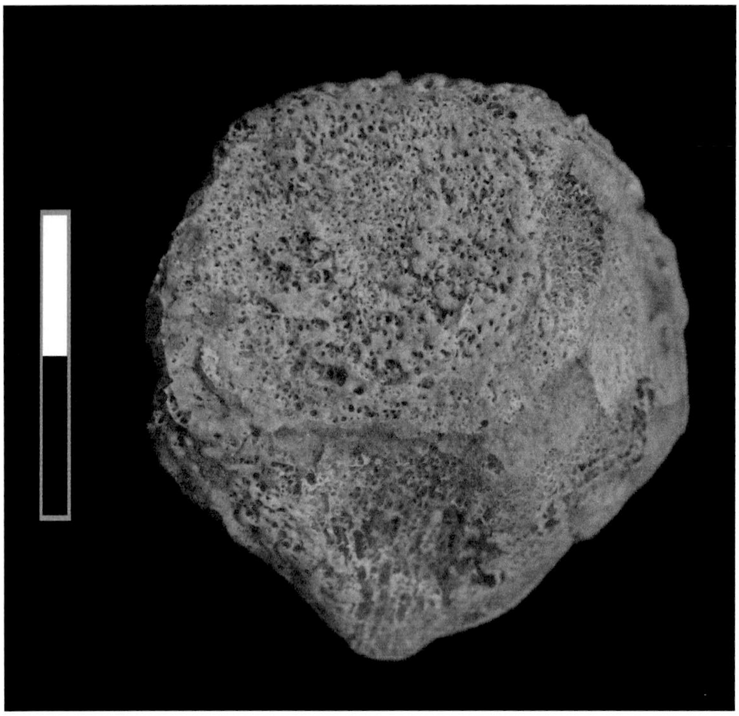

Figure 7.39 Probable treponemal disease. Note extensive porosity and new bone formation on the articular facet of the left patella. (Same individual as in Figure 7.38; photo by Efthymia Nikita; copyright: Human Skeletal Collection, University of Sheffield)

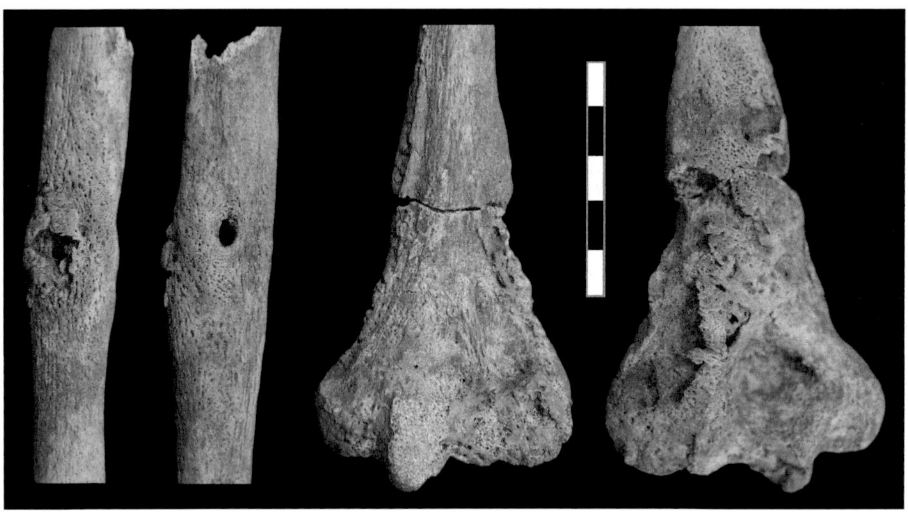

Figure 7.40 Probable treponemal disease. Note the lytic foci and mixed woven and sclerotic bone surrounding them in the humeral diaphysis (left), as well as the extensive deformity of the distal left humerus appearing mostly as sclerotic new bone on the anterior aspect and as large lytic defects with new bone formation on the posterior aspect (right). (Same individual as in Figures 7.38 and 7.39; photos by Efthymia Nikita; copyright: Human Skeletal Collection, University of Sheffield)

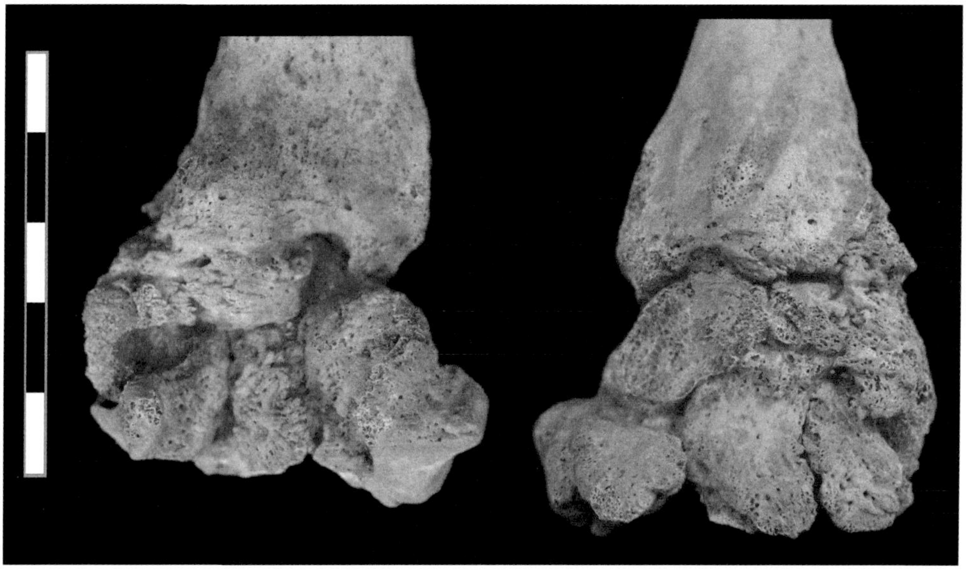

Figure 7.41 Probable treponemal disease. Note the fusion of the left radius with the carpal bones due to extensive new bone formation. (Same individual as in Figures 7.38–7.40; photos by Efthymia Nikita; copyright: Human Skeletal Collection, University of Sheffield)

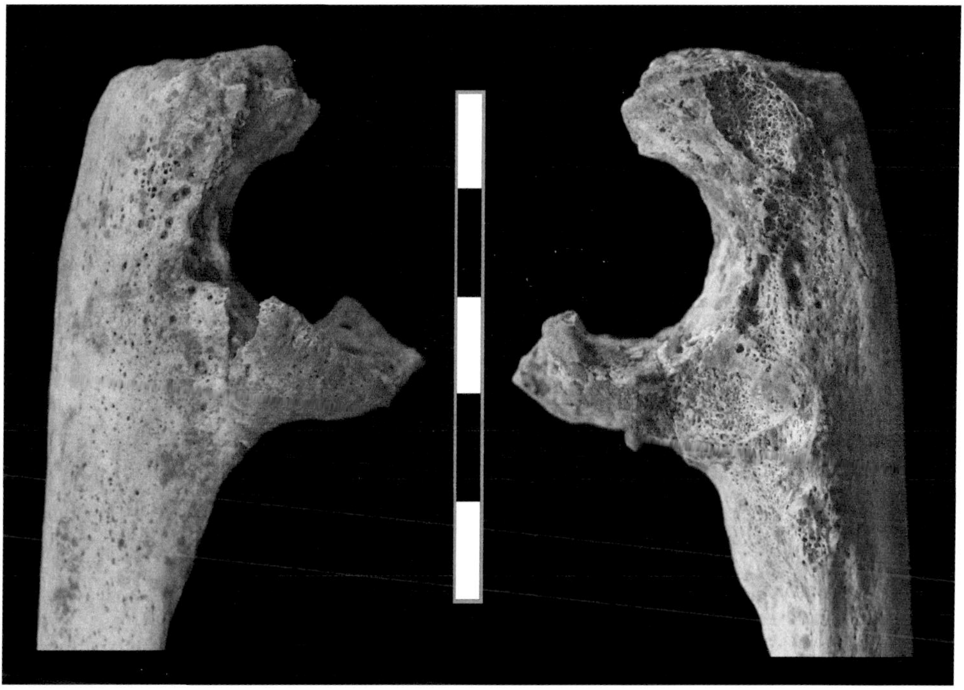

Figure 7.42 Probable treponemal disease. Note the lytic lesions and new bone formation in the upper left ulna. (Same individual as in Figures 7.38–7.41 photos by Efthymia Nikita; copyright: Human Skeletal Collection, University of Sheffield)

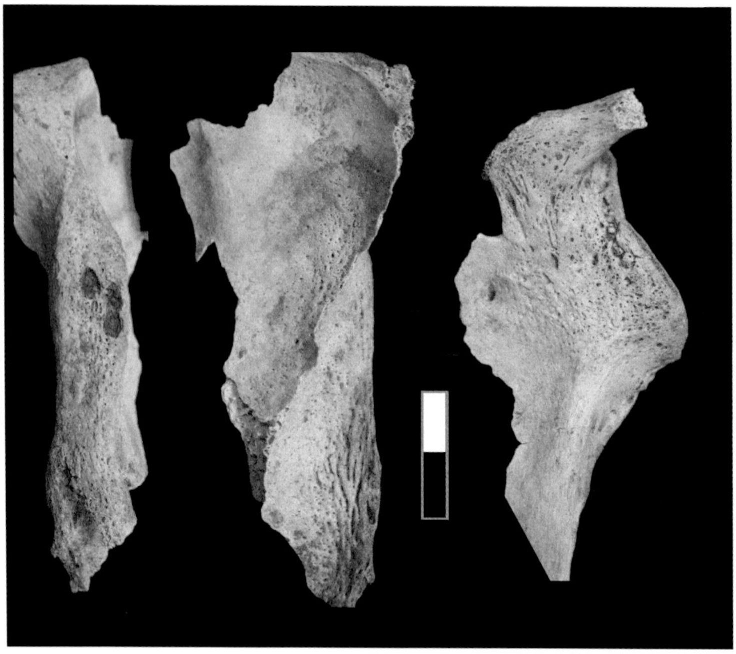

Figure 7.43 Lytic foci and new bone formation on the scapular spine, the neck of the scapula, and the coracoid process. (Same individual as in Figures 7.38–7.42; photos by Efthymia Nikita; copyright: Human Skeletal Collection, University of Sheffield)

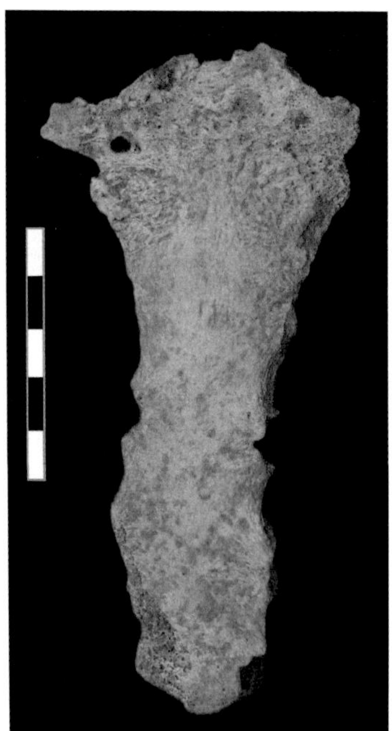

Figure 7.44 Sclerotic new bone formation on the manubrium, coupled with a lytic focus. (Same individual as in Figures 7.38–7.43; photo by Efthymia Nikita; copyright: Human Skeletal Collection, University of Sheffield)

Congenital syphilis

In cases of congenital syphilis[1] *Treponema pallidum* is transmitted from an infected mother to her fetus. This infection can cause miscarriage, stillbirth, neonatal death, or the birth of an infected child. While many infants born with congenital syphilis may initially appear healthy, symptoms will appear over time. In cases of so-called early congenital syphilis, symptoms typically manifest in infants under the age of two, and may include enlarged liver and spleen (hepatosplenomegaly), failure to thrive, fever, irritability, respiratory tract infections, convulsions, skin rashes, mucopurulent or blood-tinged nasal discharge, and skeletal abnormalities (Box 7.9). Late congenital syphilis generally appears after the age of two years and is characterised by gummatous lesions, especially in the nose and hard palate, as well as periosteal new bone, particularly in the tibiae, and other skeletal lesions (Box 7.10). Other clinical manifestations can include eye disorders (e.g. interstitial keratitis), hearing loss, dental anomalies, and skin lesions.

Box 7.9 Skeletal manifestation of early congenital syphilis

Osteochondritis

- mostly in fastest-growing bones (distal femur/proximal tibia, but also the rest of the long bones)
- symmetric lesions
- jagged metaphyses (in serious cases)
- displaced epiphysis or crushed inside deformed metaphysis (in severe cases)

Osteomyelitis

- usually at or near long bone metaphyses
- dactylitis in hand bones

Periostitis

- diffuse, symmetric, and/or layered deposition of new bone

Skull

- rare involvement
- bone necrosis affecting both tables
- syphilitic rhinitis (perforated nasal elements)

(Data from Baker et al. 2020; Caffey 1939; Frangos et al. 2011; Hillson et al. 1998; Ioannou et al. 2016, 2017; Lewis 2017; Rasool and Govender 1989; Robinson 2009)

Box 7.10 Skeletal manifestation of late congenital syphilis

Skull

- gummatous lesions
- collapsed nasal bridge ("saddle nose")
- frontal and parietal bossing
- high, arched palate
- disproportionate maxillae and mandible
- hydrocephaly

Teeth (Figures 7.45–7.47)

- Moon's molars (or bud molars): permanent upper or lower first molars dome-shaped, with several closely positioned small knobs representing atrophied cusps
- Fournier's (or mulberry) molars: first upper or lower permanent molars with hypoplastic occlusal third of the crown
- Hutchinson's incisors: maxillary permanent central incisors with peg-like or "screwdriver" appearance, convergence of mesial and distal margins, presence of central notch at incisal edge
- circumferential groove-like hypoplastic defect in occlusal third of permanent upper or lower canine crown ("fanged" canines)
- darkened enamel
- reduced tooth size
- incisors, canines, and first molars may exhibit pitted, rugged, or missing enamel due to mercury treatment of syphilis if treatment occurred during enamel formation

Shoulder girdle

- sternoclavicular thickening (Higoumenakis' sign)
- flared scapulae

Hand/foot

- dactylitis

Arm/leg

- nongummatous periostitis (true tibial bowing or pseudobowing)
- gummatous lesions
- syphilitic arthritis

(Data from Baker et al. 2020; Fiumara and Lessel 1970; Frangos et al. 2011; Hillson et al. 1998; Ioannou et al. 2016, 2017; Lewis 2017; Rasool and Govender 1989; Robinson 2009)

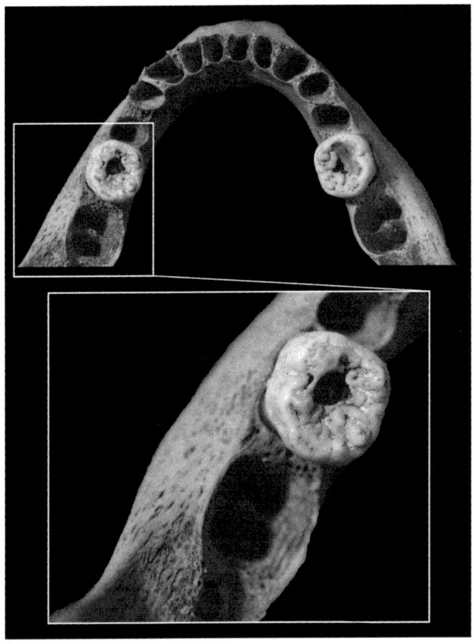

Figure 7.45 Mulberry (Fournier) first mandibular permanent molars; note the hypoplastic shape of the occlusal third of the crown. (Photo by Efthymia Nikita; copyright: Duckworth Laboratory, University of Cambridge)

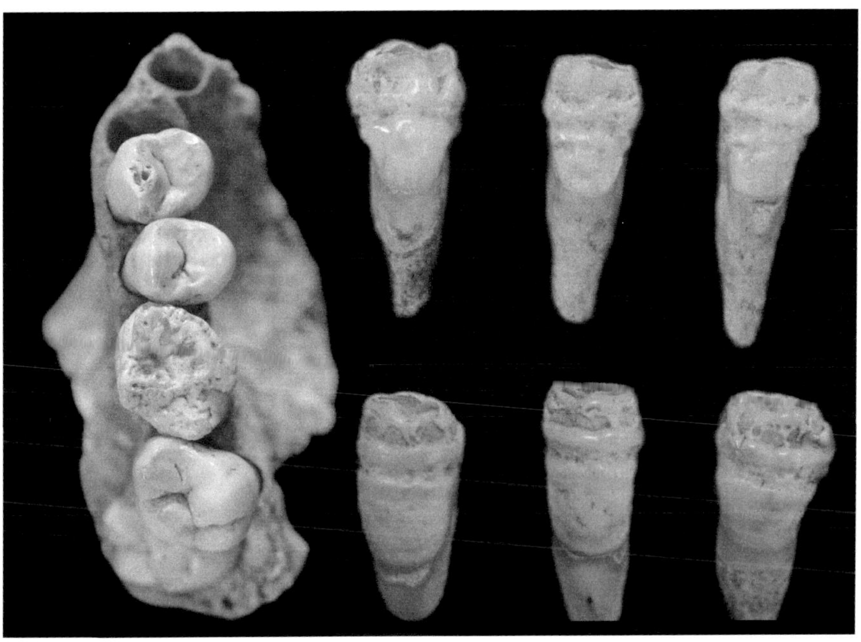

Figure 7.46 Mulberry (Fournier) right maxillary first permanent molar and pronounced linear hypoplastic defects on the maxillary and mandibular incisors and canines. (Sheffield Cathedral, 19th c., ARCUS 546d Sk 2101; photos by Efthymia Nikita; copyright: Human Skeletal Collection, University of Sheffield)

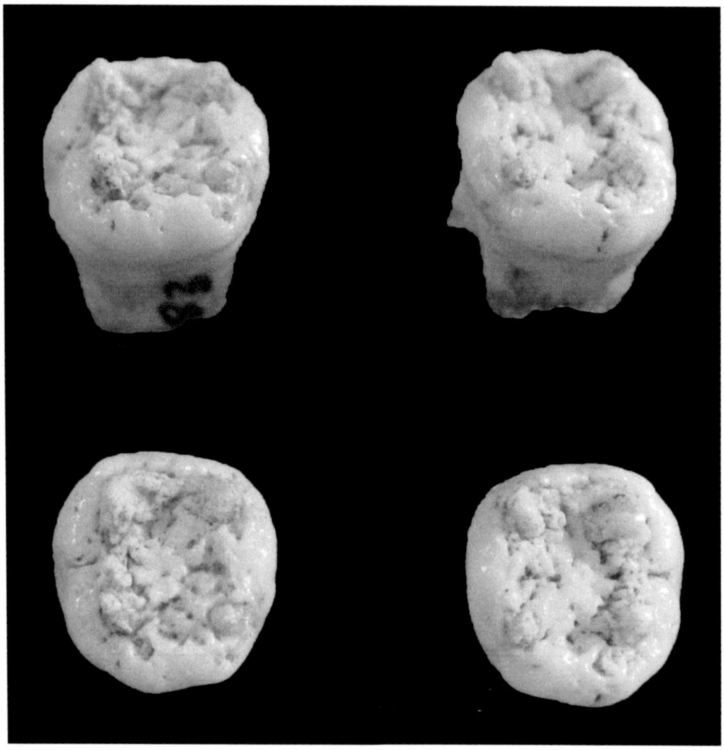

Figure 7.47 Mulberry (Fournier) first mandibular permanent molars. (5–7 years old, Methodist Chapel, Carver Street, 19th c., CS 1283; photos by Efthymia Nikita; copyright: Human Skeletal Collection, University of Sheffield)

Viral infections

Smallpox (osteomyelitis variolosa)

Smallpox, an infectious disease that has now been eradicated, is caused by the variola virus, which belongs to the genus *Orthopoxvirus*. This virus was primarily transmitted through direct contact, mostly via respiratory droplets. Transmission required direct and rather extended face-to-face interaction between individuals. In rare cases, smallpox could also spread through the air in enclosed spaces, such as within buildings or airplanes. Furthermore, the virus could spread through contact with infected bodily fluids or with contaminated objects, since the virus could stay viable outside the human body for up to several days under favourable conditions.

The condition had two main variants: variola major, which had greater prevalence and severity, and variola minor, which was less common and had milder symptoms. In variola major cases, the symptoms included fever, headache, back, and abdominal pain. Within a few days, a rash appeared initially in the oral cavity and on the face, and then spread to other parts of the body. Shortly after, blisters filled with pus formed in the skin, and eventually they crusted. The infection could affect various organs, including the lungs, brain, and bones. When the variola major virus affected bone tissue, the condition was called osteomyelitis variolosa (Box 7.11, Figures 7.48 and 7.49). Almost one-third of the individuals infected with

Box 7.11 Diagnosing smallpox

The primary skeletal markers of smallpox infection include bilateral involvement of the elbow joints and the engagement of all three major bones of the arm, with the earliest signs of involvement observed in the proximal radius and ulna (Crawford et al. 2024, and references therein).

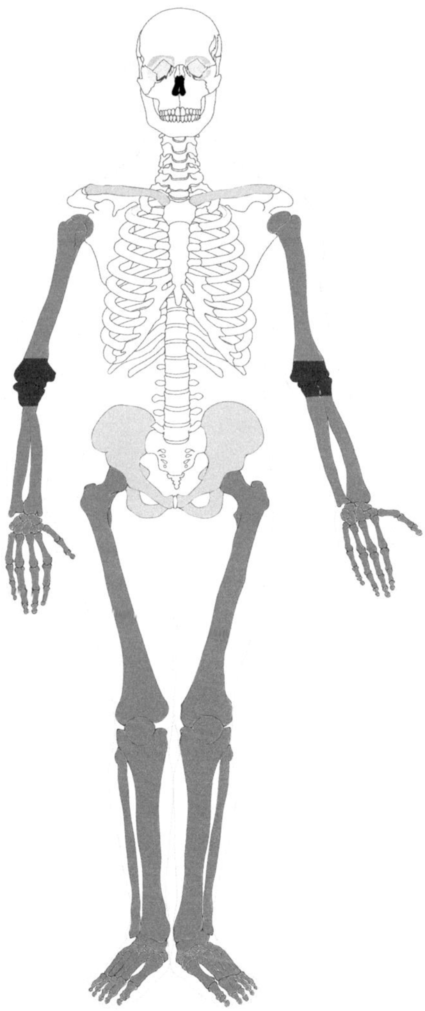

- no age or sex predilection

General
- bilateral lesions, often affecting multiple bones
- extensive periosteal new bone formation (possible involucrum)
- growth reduction and/or bending deformities in children
- pathological fractures

Hand/foot
- distorted calcaneus (flattening and shortening)
- epiphyseal destruction and arrested growth
- lytic lesions
- short, stunted digits
- bilateral and symmetric involvement

Arm/leg
- common involvement of arm bones (mostly of elbow joint); often involvement of all three arm bones (earliest involvement in proximal radius and ulna)
- lower limb involvement not always secondary to arm involvement
- bilateral bone involvement
- lesions start in metaphyses and spread to epiphyses and diaphysis
- diaphyseal osteomyelitis
- epiphyseal destruction, deformity, and premature fusion

Figure 7.48 Skeletal manifestation of smallpox. (Data from Arora et al. 2008; Crawford et al. 2024; Jackes 1983; Lentz and Noyes 1979)

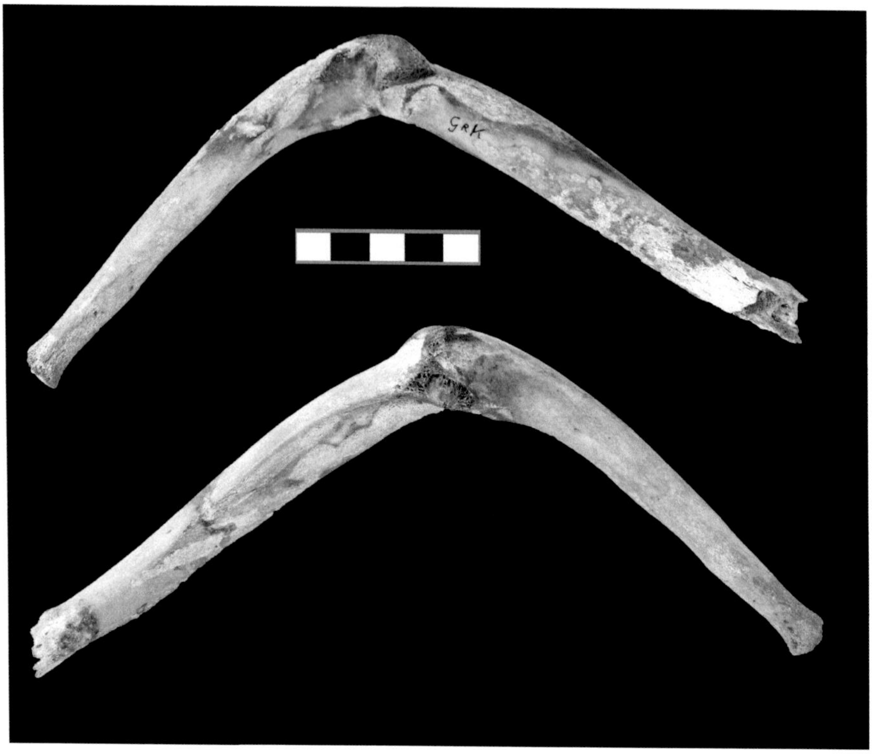

Figure 7.49 Possible smallpox. Note the ankylosis of the elbow joint. (3 years old, Alkmaar-Grote Kerk, Medieval-Modern, 5054; photos by Efthymia Nikita, from the reference collection of the Cultural Heritage Agency of the Netherlands)

variola major would die, while the survivors often had to live with extensive scars. A rare and severe form of smallpox was haemorrhagic smallpox; this was characterised by bleeding in the skin, mucous membranes, and gastrointestinal tract, and resulted in death in almost all cases. In contrast, variola minor had milder symptoms that included headache, backache, sweating, fever, vomiting, and a rash mostly confined to the face and extremities. In cases of variola minor, the mortality rate was very low, below 1%.

Poliomyelitis

Poliomyelitis is a highly contagious disease caused by poliovirus; it spreads through the faecal-oral route in cases of faecal contamination of the hands, utensils, food, and water, as well as through inhalation of respiratory droplets emitted by infected individuals (e.g. during coughing or sneezing). Most individuals with poliovirus are asymptomatic or experience symptoms resembling those of influenza (e.g. fever, headache, vomiting, diarrhoea). In about 5% of the cases, individuals may develop nonparalytic aseptic meningitis, while even fewer (less than 1%) may experience paralytic poliomyelitis if the virus invades the central nervous system (Figure 7.50).

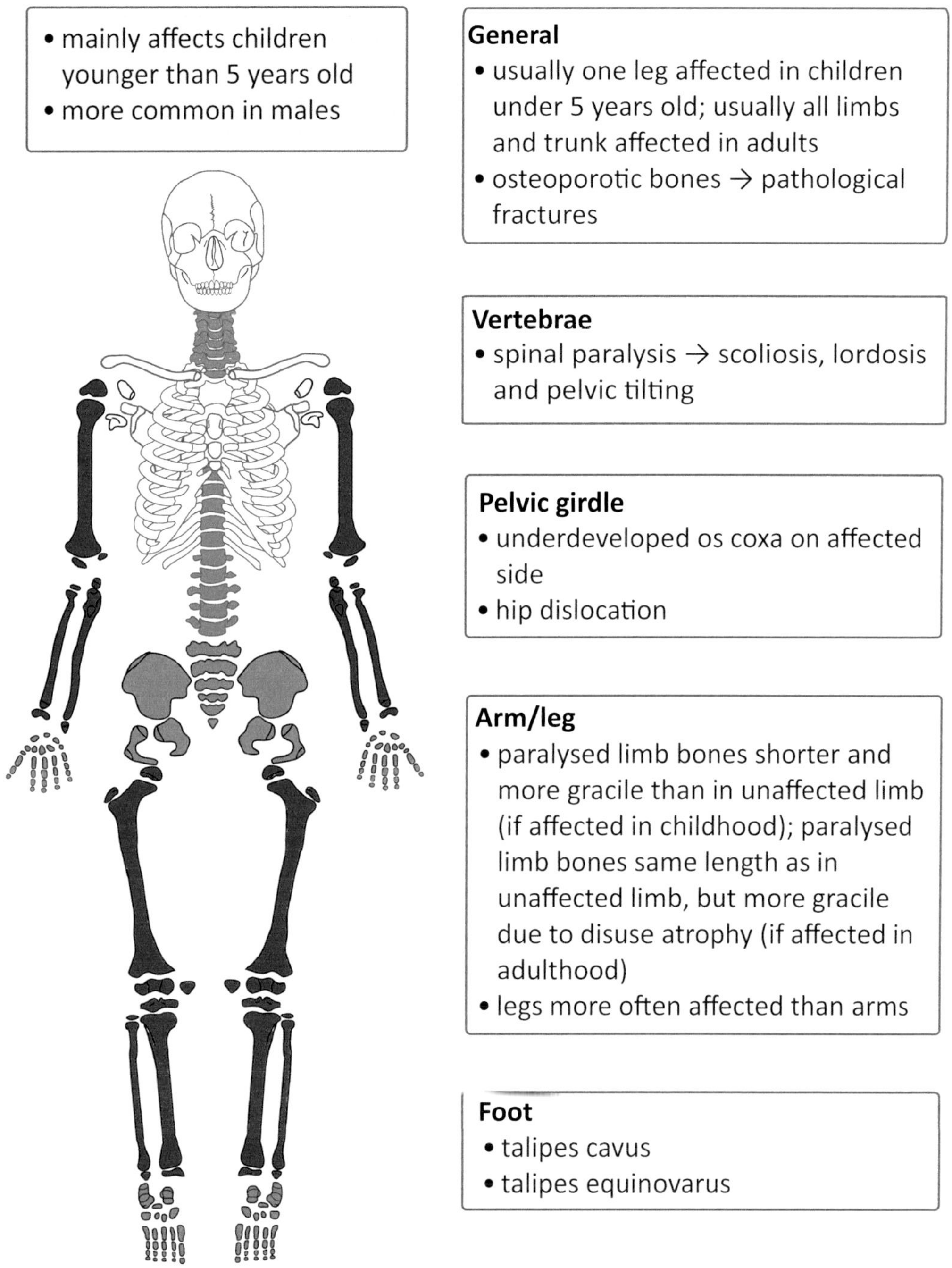

Figure 7.50 Skeletal manifestation of poliomyelitis. (Data from Berner et al. 2021; Lewis 2017; Nathanson and Kew 2010; Thompson 2014; Waldron 2020)

Parasitic infections

Malaria

Malaria is an infectious disease caused by protozoan parasites of the genus *Plasmodium*. Four *Plasmodium* species naturally infect humans: *P. falciparum*, *P. vivax*, *P. ovale*, and *P. malariae*. However, a simian malaria parasite – *P. knowlesi* – may also infect humans.

The primary defence against malaria is naturally acquired immunity in individuals who have previously survived the infection. As a result, individuals arriving from nonendemic regions to endemic areas are more likely to experience severe malaria due to their lack of acquired immunity. Moreover, in endemic regions, malaria poses a significant threat to vulnerable individuals, like children, pregnant women, and individuals with compromised immune system.

Malaria parasites infect humans via the bite of infected female *Anopheles* mosquitoes; however, transmission can also occur through blood transfusions and the use of contaminated needles. Following transmission, the parasites enter the bloodstream and reach the liver. There they multiply and mature, and then they enter the bloodstream and infect the red blood cells. Patients typically experience fever, chills, fatigue, malaise, sweating, cough, diarrhoea, vomiting, muscle ache, and headache. Many of these symptoms appear every two or three days, in association with the rupture of the infected red blood cells and the release of cell and parasite debris into the bloodstream. More serious complications include haemolytic anaemia, respiratory distress, acute kidney injury, and cerebral malaria.

Malaria does not produce any pathognomonic skeletal lesions; however, it has a complex relationship with anaemia, which does affect the skeleton (see Chapter 4). Malaria can lead to haemolytic anaemia, as briefly mentioned above, while genetic blood disorders, such as thalassemia and sickle cell anaemia, offer some resistance to malaria. Anaemic individuals may show porous bone surfaces (e.g. porotic hyperostosis, cribra orbitalia, cribra humeralis, cribra femoralis) (Figures 7.51 and 7.52). Nevertheless, several pathological processes can result in bone porosity, while studies have also indicated that cribra orbitalia and porotic hyperostosis may arise from distinct pathological conditions. In addition, clinical studies have shown that the relationship between malaria, other infectious diseases, and nutritional disorders is complex, and all these conditions may cause bone porosity. As a result, bone porosity cannot be used to securely diagnose malaria without additional lines of evidence. Besides macroscopic analyses, the detection of malaria in palaeopathological contexts has employed ancient DNA analysis, immunological techniques, and the identification of haemozoin.

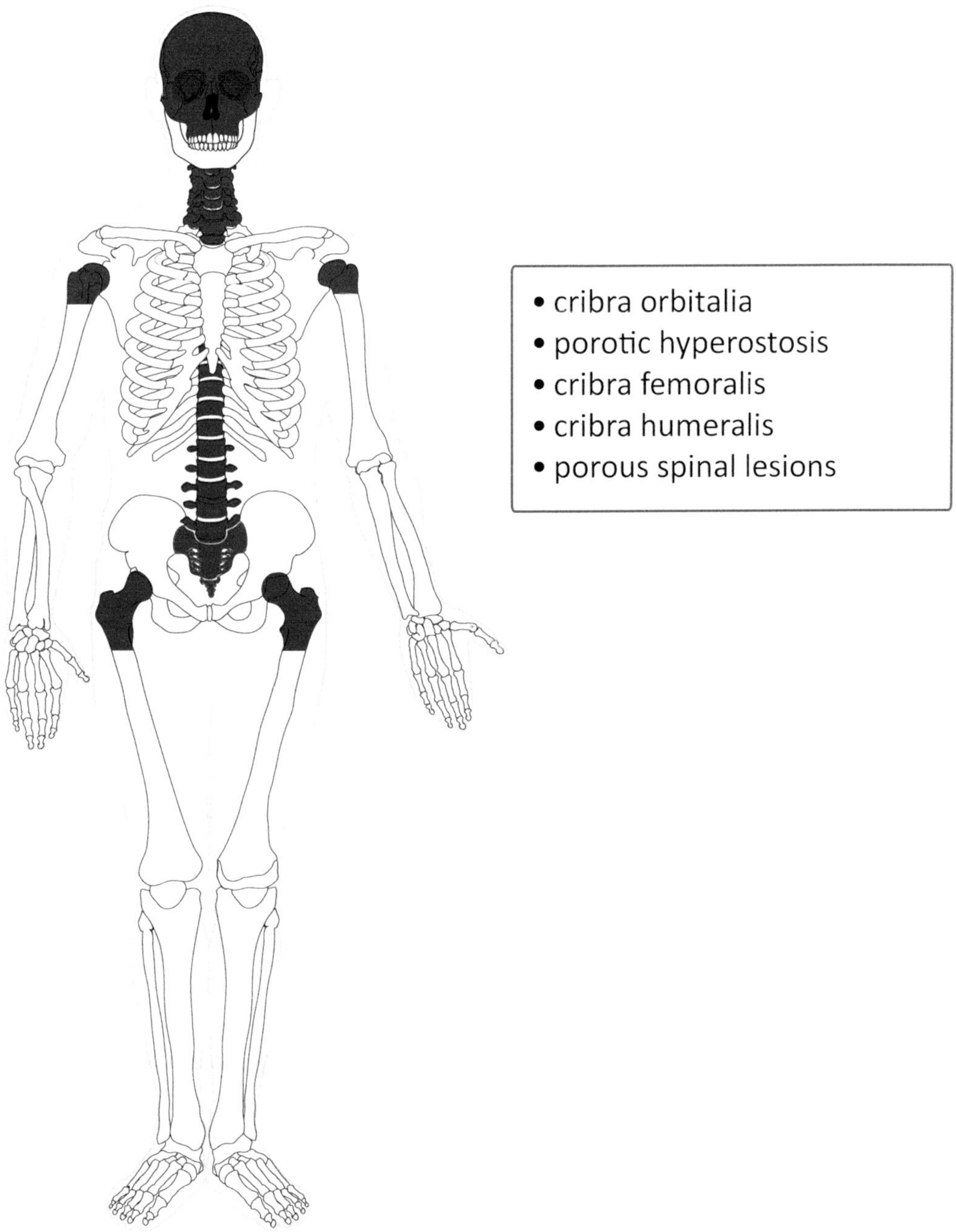

Figure 7.51 Skeletal manifestation of malaria. (Data from Schats 2023; Setzer 2014; Smith-Guzmán 2015)

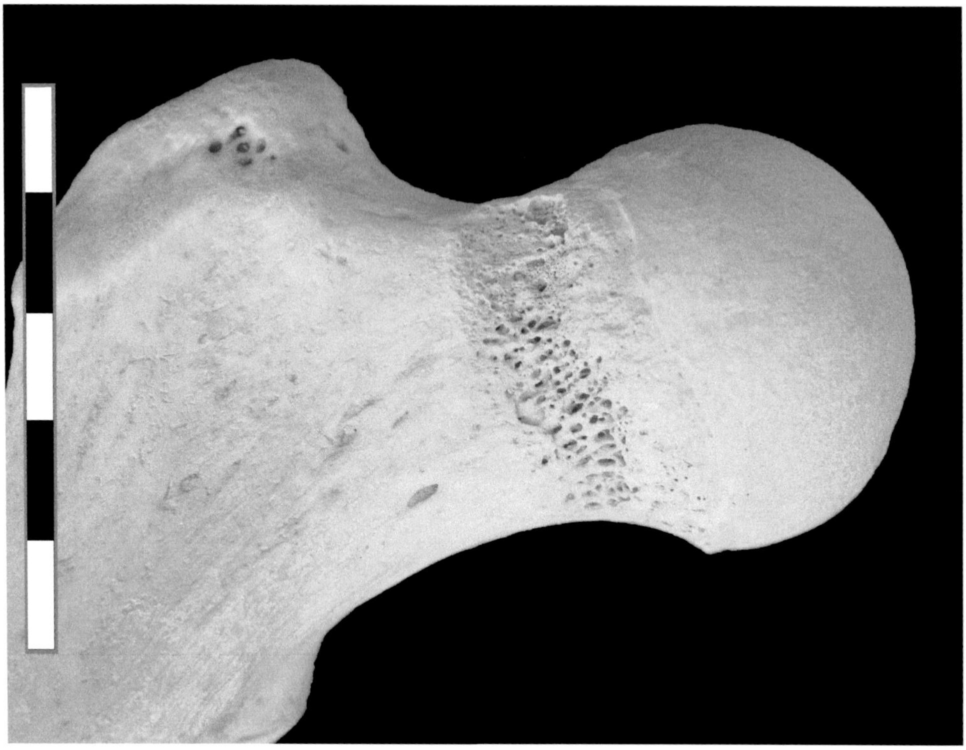

Figure 7.52 Cribra femoralis. (Sbide, Roman/Byzantine; photo by Efthymia Nikita, with the kind permission of Dr. Ahmet Ihsan Aytek, Burdur Mehmet Akif Ersoy University)

Note

1 The congenital form of treponemal disease is associated with venereal syphilis; nevertheless, there are anecdotal accounts supporting the congenital transmission of yaws and bejel.

References and suggested readings

Andersen, J.G., Manchester, K. (1987). Grooving of the proximal phalanx in leprosy: A palaeopathological and radiological study. *Journal of Archaeological Science* 14:77–82. https://doi.org/10.1016/S0305-4403(87)80007-9

Andersen, J.G., Manchester, K. (1988). Dorsal tarsal exostoses in leprosy: A palaeopathological and radiological study. *Journal of Archaeological Science* 15:51–56. https://doi.org/10.1016/0305-4403(88)90018-0

Andersen, J.G., Manchester, K. (1992). The rhinomaxillary syndrome in leprosy: A clinical, radiological and palaeopathological study. *International Journal of Osteoarchaeology* 2:121–129. https://doi.org/10.1002/oa.1390020204

Andersen, J.G., Manchester, K., Ali, R.S. (1992). Diaphyseal remodelling in leprosy: A radiological and palaeopathological study. *International Journal of Osteoarchaeology* 2:211–219. https://doi.org/10.1002/oa.1390020305

Andersen, J.G., Manchester, K., Roberts, C. (1994). Septic bone changes in leprosy: A clinical, radiological and palaeopathological review. *International Journal of Osteoarchaeology* 4:21–30. https://doi.org/10.1002/oa.1390040105

Anstey, N.M., Russell, B., Yeo, T.W., Price, R.N. (2009). The pathophysiology of vivax malaria. *Trends in Parasitology* 25:220–227. https://doi.org/10.1016/j.pt.2009.02.003

Arora, A., Agarwal, A., Kumar, S. (2008). Osteomyelitis variolosa: A report of two cases. *Journal of Orthopaedic Surgery* 16:355–358.

Arriaza, B.T., Salo, W., Aufderheide, A.C., Holcomb, T.A. (1995). Pre-Columbian tuberculosis in Northern Chile: Molecular and skeletal evidence. *American Journal of Physical Anthropology* 98:37–45. https://doi.org/10.1002/ajpa.1330980104

Aufderheide, A.C., Rodríguez-Martín, C. (1998). *The Cambridge Encyclopedia of Human Paleopathology*. Cambridge: Cambridge University Press.

Baker, B.J. (2023). Treponemal infection. In *The Routledge Handbook of Paleopathology*, edited by Grauer, A.L., pp. 292–305. London: Routledge.

Baker, B.J., Crane-Kramer, G., Dee, M.W., Gregoricka, L.A., Henneberg, M., Lee, C., Lukehart, S.A., Mabey, D.C., Roberts, C.A., Stodder, A.L.W., Stone, A.C., Winingear, S. (2020). Advancing the understanding of treponemal disease in the past and present. *American Journal of Physical Anthropology* 171:5–41. https://doi.org/10.1002/ajpa.23988

Belli, E., Matteini, C., Andreano, T. (2002). Sclerosing osteomyelitis of Garré periostitis ossificans. *The Journal of Craniofacial Surgery* 13:765–768.

Berner, M., Pany-Kucera, D., Doneus, N., Sladek, V., Gamble, M., Eggers, S. (2021). Challenging definitions and diagnostic approaches for ancient rare diseases: The case of poliomyelitis. *International Journal of Paleopathology* 33:113–127. https://doi.org/10.1016/j.ijpp.2021.04.003

Bianucci, R., Araujo, A., Pusch, C.M., Nerlich, A.G. (2015). The identification of malaria in paleopathology – an in-depth assessment of the strategies to detect malaria in ancient remains. *Acta Tropica* 152:176–180. https://doi.org/10.1016/j.actatropica.2015.09.002

Boldsen, J.L. (2001). Epidemiological approach to the paleopathological diagnosis of leprosy. *American Journal of Physical Anthropology* 115:380–387. https://doi.org/10.1002/ajpa.1094

Boocock, P., Roberts, C.A., Manchester, K. (1995). Maxillary sinusitis in medieval Chichester, England. *American Journal of Physical Anthropology* 98:483–495. https://doi.org/10.1002/ajpa.1330980408

Buckley, H.R., Dias, G.J. (2002). The distribution of skeletal lesions in treponemal disease: Is the lymphatic system responsible? *International Journal of Osteoarchaeology* 12:178–188. https://doi.org/10.1002/oa.606

Burt, N.M., Semple, D., Waterhouse, K., Lovell, N.C. (2013). *Identification and Interpretation of Joint Disease in Paleopathology and Forensic Anthropology*. Springfield, IL: Charles C. Thomas.

Caffey, J. (1939). Syphilis of the skeleton in early infancy: The non-specificity of many of the roentgenographic changes. *American Journal of Roentgenology* 42:637–655.

Castro, M.M., Benavente, M.A., Ortega, J., Acuna, R., Montero, C., Thomas, C., Castro, N. (2016). Thoracic aortic aneurysm in a pre-Columbian (210 BC) inhabitant of Northern Chile: Implications for the origins of syphilis. *International Journal of Paleopathology* 13:20–26. https://doi.org/10.1016/j.ijpp.2016.01.002

Chelli Bouaziz, M., Ladeb, M.F., Chakroun, M., Chaabane, S. (2008). Spinal brucellosis: A review. *Skeletal Radiology* 37:785–790. https://doi.org/10.1007/s00256-007-0371-x

Cook, D.C., Powell, M.L. (2012). Treponematosis: Past, present, and future. In *A Companion to Paleopathology*, edited by Grauer, A.L., pp. 472–491. Hoboken, NJ: Wiley Blackwell.

Crawford, R.R., Hodson, C.M., Errickson, D. (2024). Guidance for the identification of bony lesions related to smallpox. *International Journal of Paleopathology* 44:65–77. https://doi.org/10.1016/j.ijpp.2023.12.002

Crespo, F. (2020). Reconstructing immune competence in skeletal samples. A theoretical and methodological approach. In: *Theoretical Approaches in Bioarchaeology*, edited by Cheverko, C.M., Prince-Buitenhuys, J.R., Hubbe, M., pp. 76–92. London: Routledge.

Crespo, F., White, J., Roberts, C. (2019). Revisiting the tuberculosis and leprosy cross-immunity hypothesis: Expanding the dialogue between immunology and paleopathology. *International Journal of Paleopathology* 26:37–47. https://doi.org/10.1016/j.ijpp.2019.05.005

Cruz, A.T., Starke, J.R. (2007). Clinical manifestations of tuberculosis in children. *Paediatric Respiratory Reviews* 8:107–117. https://doi.org/10.1016/j.prrv.2007.04.008

D'Anastasio, R., Staniscia, T., Milia, M.L., Manzoli, L., Capasso, L. (2011). Origin, evolution and paleoepidemiology of brucellosis. *Epidemiology and Infection* 139:149–156. https://doi.org/10.1017/S095026881000097X

Dangvard Pedersen, D., Milner, G.R., Kolmos, H.J., Boldsen, J.L. (2019). The association between skeletal lesions and tuberculosis diagnosis using a probabilistic approach. *International Journal of Paleopathology* 27:88–100. https://doi.org/10.1016/j.ijpp.2019.01.001

Danielsen, K. (1968). Leprogenic odontodysplasia. *International Journal of Leprosy* 36:552–666.

Davies-Barrett, A.M., Antoine, D., Roberts, C.A. (2019). Inflammatory periosteal reaction on ribs associated with lower respiratory tract disease: A method for recording prevalence from sites with differing preservation. *American Journal of Physical Anthropology* 168:530–542. https://doi.org/10.1002/ajpa.23769

Del Val Del, A.N., Erausquin, A.C., Blanco, R., Pinillos, A.V. (1997). Study of 112 patients with septic arthritis caused by pyogenic organisms and fungi: Changes in the clinical spectrum during the last two decades. *Revista Clinica Espanola* 197:540–544.

DeWitte, S.N., Stojanowski, C.M. (2015). The osteological paradox 20 years later: Past perspectives, future directions. *Journal of Archaeological Research* 23:397–450. https://doi.org/10.1007/s10814-015-9084-1

Dutour, O. (2023). Paleopathology of infectious diseases. In *The Routledge Handbook of Paleopathology*, edited by Grauer, A.L., pp. 324–337. London: Routledge.

Esmaeilnejad-Ganji, S.M., Esmaeilnejad-Ganji, S.M.R. (2019). Osteoarticular manifestations of human brucellosis: A review. *World Journal of Orthopedics* 18:54–62.

Fiumara, N.J., Lessell, S. (1970). Manifestations of late congenital syphilis: An analysis of 271 patients. *Archives of Dermatology* 102:78–83. https://doi.org/10.1001/archderm.1970.04000070080012

Frangos, C.C., Lavranos, G.M., Frangos, C.C. (2011). Higoumenakis' sign in the diagnosis of congenital syphilis in anthropological specimens. *Medical Hypotheses* 77:128–131. https://doi.org/10.1016/j.mehy.2011.03.044

Grauer, A.L., Roberts, C.A. (2019). Fungal, viral, multicelled parasitic, and protozoan infections. In *Ortner's Identification of Pathological Conditions in Human Skeletal Remains*, edited by Buikstra, J., pp. 441–478. San Diego: Academic Press.

Hackett, C.J. (1975). An introduction to diagnostic criteria of syphilis, treponarid and yaws (treponematoses) in dry bones, and some implications. *Virchows Archiv* 368:229–241. https://doi.org/10.1007/BF00432525

Hackett, C.J. (1976). *Diagnostic Criteria of Syphilis, Yaws and Treponarid (Treponematoses) and of Some Other Diseases in Dry Bones*. Berlin: Springer-Verlag.

Hackett, C.J. (1981). Development of caries sicca in a dry calvaria. *Virchows Archiv* 391:53–79. https://doi.org/10.1007/BF00589795

Hackett, C.J. (1983). Problems in the paleopathology of the human treponematoses. In *Disease in Ancient Man*, edited by Hart, G.D., pp. 106–128. Toronto: Clarke Irwin.

Harper, K.N., Zuckerman, M.K., Harper, M.L., Kingston, J.D., Armelagos, G.J. (2011). The origin and antiquity of syphilis revisited: An appraisal of Old World pre-Columbian evidence for treponemal infection. *Yearbook of Physical Anthropology* 54:99–133. https://doi.org/10.1002/ajpa.21613

Hillson, S., Grigson, C., Bond, S. (1998). Dental defects of congenital syphilis. *American Journal of Physical Anthropology* 107:25–40. https://doi.org/10.1002/(sici)1096-8644(199809)107:1%3C25::aid-ajpa3%3E3.0.co;2-c

Holloway, K.L., Henneberg, R.J., de Barros Lopes, M., Henneberg, M. (2011). Evolution of human tuberculosis: A systematic review and meta-analysis of paleopathological evidence. *HOMO-Journal of Comparative Human Biology* 62:402–458. https://doi.org/10.1016/j.jchb.2011.10.001

Holloway, K.L., Link, K., Rühli, F., Henneberg, M. (2013). Skeletal lesions in human tuberculosis may sometimes heal: An aid to palaeopathological diagnoses. *PLoS One* 8:e62798. https://doi.org/10.1371/journal.pone.0062798

Ioannou, S., Sassani, S., Henneberg, M., Henneberg, R.J. (2016). Diagnosing congenital syphilis using Hutchinson's method: Differentiating between syphilitic, mercurial, and syphilitic-mercurial dental defects. *American Journal of Physical Anthropology* 159:617–629. https://doi.org/10.1002/ajpa.22924

Ioannou, S., Henneberg, R.J., Henneberg, M. (2017). Presence of dental signs of congenital syphilis in pre-modern specimens. *Archives of Oral Biology* 85:192–200. https://doi.org/10.1016/j.archoralbio.2017.10.017

Jackes, M.K. (1983). Osteological evidence for smallpox: A possible case from seventeenth century Ontario. *American Journal of Physical Anthropology* 60:75–81. https://doi.org/10.1002/ajpa.1330600112

Jaffe, H.J. (1972). *Metabolic, Degenerative and Inflammatory Diseases of Bones and Joints*. Philadelphia: Lea & Febiger.

Khateeb, M.I., Araj, G.F., Majeed, S.A., Lulu, A.R. (1990). Brucella arthritis: A study of 96 cases in Kuwait. *Annals of the Rheumatic Diseases* 49:994–998. https://doi.org/10.1136/ard.49.12.994

Kumpitak, C., Duangmanee, A., Thongyod, W., Rachaphaew, N., Suansomjit, C., Manopwisedjaroen, K., Aung, P.L., Imad, H.A., Cui, L., Sattabongkot, J., Nguitragool, W., Bantuchai, S. (2024). Human-to-*Anopheles dirus* mosquito transmission of the anthropozoonotic malaria parasite, *Plasmodium knowlesi*. *Parasites & Vectors* 17:415. https://doi.org/10.1186/s13071-024-06500-5

Labbé, J.L., Peres, O., Leclair, O., Goulon, R., Scemama, P., Jourdel, F., Menager, C., Duparc, B, Lacassin, F. (2010). Acute osteomyelitis in children: The pathogenesis revisited? *Orthopaedics & Traumatology, Surgery & Research* 96:268–275. https://doi.org/10.1016/j.otsr.2009.12.012

Lee, M.J., Siek, T.J., Hirst, C.S. (2024). Chronic maxillary sinusitis in palaeopathology: A review of methods. *International Journal of Paleopathology* 44:51–64. https://doi.org/10.1016/j.ijpp.2023.11.005

Lefort, M., Bennike, P. (2007). A case study of possible differential diagnoses of a medieval skeleton from Denmark: Leprosy, ergotism, treponematosis, sarcoidosis or smallpox? *International Journal of Osteoarchaeology* 17:337–349. https://doi.org/10.1002/oa.905

Lentz, M.W., Noyes, F.R. (1979). Osseous deformity from osteomyelitis variolosa. *Clinical Orthopaedics and Related Research* 143:155–157.

Lew, D.P., Waldvogel, F.A. (1997). Osteomyelitis. *The New England Journal of Medicine* 336:999–1007. https://doi.org/10.1056/NEJM199704033361406

Lewis, M. (2004). Endocranial lesions in non-adult skeletons: Understanding their aetiology. *International Journal of Osteoarchaeology* 14:82–97. https://doi.org/10.1002/oa.713

Lewis, M. (2017). *Paleopathology of Children: Identification of Pathological Conditions in the Human Skeletal Remains of Non-Adults*. San Diego: Academic Press.

Lynnerup, N., Boldsen, J.L. (2012). Leprosy (Hansen's disease). In *A Companion to Paleopathology*, edited by Grauer, A.L., pp. 458–471. Hoboken, NJ: John Wiley & Sons.

Madkour, M.M. (1989). Bone and joint brucellosis. In *Brucellosis*, edited by Madkour, M.M., pp. 90–104. London: Butterworths.

Masiu, R., Pedersen, D.D., Hill, L., Steyn, M. (2023). The association between skeletal lesions and tuberculosis in a pre-antibiotic South African sample. *International Journal of Paleopathology* 40:20–32. https://doi.org/10.1016/j.ijpp.2022.11.001

Masson, M., Molnár, E., Donoghue, H.D., Besra, G.S., Minnikin, D.E., Wu, H.H.T., Lee, O.Y.-C., Bull, I.D., Pálfi, G. (2013). Osteological and biomolecular evidence of a 7000-year old case of hypertrophic pulmonary osteopathy secondary to tuberculosis from Neolithic Hungary. *PLoS One* 8:e78252. https://doi.org/10.1371/journal.pone.0078252

Matos, V., Santos, A.L. (2006). On the trail of pulmonary tuberculosis based on rib lesions: Results from the human identified skeletal collection from the Museu Bocage (Lisbon, Portugal). *American Journal of Physical Anthropology* 130:190–200. https://doi.org/10.1002/ajpa.20309

Mays, S., Stark, S., Zakrzewski, S., Vekony, A. (2024). Which types of bony changes in the maxillary sinus indicate chronic sinusitis? *International Journal of Paleopathology* 46:16–23. https://doi.org/10.1016/j.ijpp.2024.05.003

Meng, C., Wu, Y. (1942). Tuberculosis of the flat bones of the vault of the skull: A study of 40 cases. *The Journal of Bone & Joint Surgery* 24:341–353.

Merrett, D.C., Pfeiffer, S. (2000). Maxillary sinusitis as an indicator of respiratory health in past populations. *American Journal of Physical Anthropology* 111:301–318. https://doi.org/10.1002/(SICI)1096-8644(200003)111:3<301::AID-AJPA2>3.0.CO;2-0

Mitchell, P.D. (2003). Pre-Columbian treponemal disease from 14th century AD Safed, Israel, and implications for the medieval eastern Mediterranean. *American Journal of Physical Anthropology* 121:117–124. https://doi.org/10.1002/ajpa.10205

Møller-Christensen, V. (1961). *Bone Changes in Leprosy*. Bristol: John Wright & Sons.

Møller-Christensen, V. (1978). *Leprosy Changes of the Skull*. Odense: Odense University Press.

Mosher, G.M., Smith, M.O., Albrecht, J.L., Salaka, V.P. (2015). Treponemal disease, tuberculosis and subsistence-settlement pattern in the Late Woodland period West-central Illinois. *International Journal of Osteoarchaeology* 25:776–787. https://doi.org/10.1002/oa.2344

Nade, S. (2003). Septic arthritis. *Best Practice & Research Clinical Rheumatology* 17:183–200.

Nathanson, N., Kew, O.M. (2010). From emergence to eradication: The epidemiology of poliomyelitis deconstructed. *American Journal of Epidemiology* 172:1213–1229. https://doi.org/10.1093/aje/kwq320

Ortner, D.J. (2008). Differential diagnosis of skeletal lesions in infectious disease. In *Advances in Human Palaeopathology*, edited by Pinhasi, R., Mays, S., pp. 191–214. Hoboken, NJ: John Wiley & Sons.

Paica, I.C., Rusu, I., Popescu, O., Brînzan, A., Pencea, I., Dobrinescu, C., Kelemen, B. (2023). Tentative indicators of malaria in archaeological skeletal samples, a pilot study testing different methods. *International Journal of Paleopathology* 40:109–116. https://doi.org/10.1016/j.ijpp.2023.01.004

Pigrau-Serrallach, C., Rodríguez-Pardo, D. (2013). Bone and joint tuberculosis. *European Spine Journal* 22:S556–S566. https://doi.org/10.1007/s00586-012-2331-y

Powell, M.L., Cook, D.C. (2005). *The Myth of Syphilis: The Natural History of Treponematosis in North America*. Gainesville, FL: University Press of Florida.

Rasool, M.N., Govender, S. (1989). The skeletal manifestations of congenital syphilis. A review of 197 cases. *The Journal of Bone & Joint Surgery* 71:752–755. https://doi.org/10.1302/0301-620X.71B5.2584243

Resnick, D.J. (2002). *Diagnosis of Bone and Joint Disorders*, 4th edition. Philadelphia: Saunders.

Resnick, M., Jacobson, J.A., Chung, C.B., Kransdorf, M.J., Pathria, M.N. (2024). *Resnick's Bone and Joint Imaging*, 4th edition. Philadelphia: Saunders.

Roberts, C.A. (2007). A bioarcheological study of maxillary sinusitis. *American Journal of Physical Anthropology* 133:792–807. https://doi.org/10.1002/ajpa.20601

Roberts, C.A. (2012). Re-emerging infections: Developments in boarchaeological contributions to understanding tuberculosis today. In *A Companion to Paleopathology*, edited by Grauer, A.L., pp. 434–457. Hoboken, NJ: John Wiley & Sons.

Roberts, C.A. (2019). Infectious disease: Introduction, periostosis, periostitis, osteomyelitis, and septic arthritis. In *Ortner's Identification of Pathological Conditions in Human Skeletal Remains*, edited by Buikstra, J., pp. 285–319. San Diego: Academic Press.

Roberts, C.A. (2020). *Leprosy: Past and Present*. Gainesville, FL: University Press of Florida.

Roberts, C.A., Buikstra, J.E. (2003). *The Bioarchaeology of Tuberculosis. A Global View on a Reemerging Disease*. Gainesville, FL: University Press of Florida.

Roberts, C.A., Buikstra, J. (2019). Bacterial infections. In *Ortner's Identification of Pathological Conditions in Human Skeletal Remains*, edited by Buikstra, J., pp. 321–439. San Diego: Academic Press.

Roberts, C.A., Blevins, K.E., Filipek, K.L., Miranda, A.P. (2023). Here and now, there and then: Two Mycobacterial diseases still with us today. In *The Routledge Handbook of Paleopathology*, edited by Grauer, A.L., pp. 306–323. London: Routledge.

Robinson, J.L. (2009). Congenital syphilis: No longer just of historical interest. *Paediatrics & Child Health* 14:337–344. https://doi.org/10.1093/pch/14.5.337

Rogers, J., Waldron, T. (1989). Infections in palaeopathology: The basis of classification according to most probable cause. *Journal of Archaeological Science* 16:611–625. https://doi.org/10.1016/0305-4403(89)90026-5

Rogers, J., Waldron, T. (1995). *A Field Guide to Joint Disease in Archaeology*. Hoboken, NJ: John Wiley & Sons.

Rothschild, B., Rothschild, C. (1995). Treponemal disease revisited: Skeletal discriminators for yaws, bejel, and venereal syphilis. *Clinical Infectious Diseases* 20:1402–1408.

Rothschild, B.M., Rothschild, C. (1997). Congenital syphilis in the archaeological record: Diagnostic insensitivity of osseous lesions. *International Journal of Osteoarchaeology* 7:39–42. https://doi.org/10.1002/(SICI)1099-1212(199701)7:1%3C39::AID-OA313%3E3.0.CO;2-J

Santos, A.L., Roberts, C.A. (2006). Anatomy of a serial killer: Differential diagnosis of tuberculosis based on rib lesions of adult individuals from the Coimbra identified skeletal collection, Portugal. *American Journal of Physical Anthropology* 130:38–49. https://doi.org/10.1002/ajpa.20160

Santos, A.L., Suby, J.A. (2015). Skeletal and surgical evidence for acute osteomyelitis in non-adult individuals. *International Journal of Osteoarchaeology* 25:110–118. https://doi.org/10.1002/oa.2276

Schats, R. (2023). Developing an archaeology of malaria. A critical review of current approaches and a discussion on ways forward. *International Journal of Paleopathology* 41:32–42. https://doi.org/10.1016/j.ijpp.2023.03.002

Setzer, T.J. (2014). Malaria detection in the field of paleopathology: A meta-analysis of the state of the art. *Acta Tropica* 140:97–104. https://doi.org/10.1016/j.actatropica.2014.08.010

Singh, H., Bhatt, A., Kumar, M., Deshmukh, P. (2023). Tonsillitis and sinusitis: A narrative review of pathogenesis, diagnosis, and management. *Cureus* 15:e47192. https://doi.org/10.7759/cureus.47192

Smith-Guzmán, N.E. (2015). The skeletal manifestation of malaria: An epidemiological approach using documented skeletal collections. *American Journal of Physical Anthropology* 158:624–635. https://doi.org/10.1002/ajpa.22819

Sohn, M.H., Lim, S.T., Jeong, Y.J., Kim, D.W., Jeong, H.J., Lee, C.S. (2010). Unusual case of occult Brucella osteomyelitis in the skull detected by bone scintigraphy. *Nuclear Medicine and Molecular Imaging* 44:161–163. https://doi.org/10.1007/s13139-010-0023-2

Spekker, O., Hunt, D.R., Váradi, O.A., Berthon, W., Molnár, E., Pálfi, G. (2018). Rare manifestations of spinal tuberculosis in the Robert J. Terry anatomical skeletal collection (National Museum of Natural History, Smithsonian Institution, Washington, DC, USA). *International Journal of Osteoarchaeology* 28:343–353. https://doi.org/10.1002/oa.2658

Spekker, O., Hunt, D.R., Berthon, W., Molnár, E., Pálfi, G. (2022). Insights into the diagnostic efficacy and macroscopic appearance of endocranial bony changes indicative of tuberculous meningitis: Three example cases from the Robert J. Terry Anatomical Skeletal Collection. *International Journal of Osteoarchaeology* 32:444–456. https://doi.org/10.1002/oa.3079

Steinbock, R. (1976). *Paleopathological Diagnosis and Interpretation: Bone Diseases in Ancient Human Populations*. Springfield, IL: Charles C. Thomas.

Steyn, M., Scholtz, Y., Botha, D., Pretorius, S. (2013). The changing face of tuberculosis: Trends in tuberculosis-associated skeletal changes. *Tuberculosis* 93:467–474. https://doi.org/10.1016/j.tube.2013.04.003

Stone, A.C., Wilbur, A.K., Buikstra, J.E., Roberts, C.A. (2009). Tuberculosis and leprosy in perspective. *American Journal of Physical Anthropology* 140:66–94. https://doi.org/10.1002/ajpa.21185

Sundman, E.A., Kjellström, A. (2011). Chronic maxillary sinusitis in Medieval Sigtuna, Sweden: A study of sinus health and effects on bone preservation. *International Journal of Osteoarchaeology* 23:447–458. https://doi.org/10.1002/oa.1268

Teo, H.E., Peh, W.C. (2004). Skeletal tuberculosis in children. *Pediatric Radiology* 34:853–860. https://doi.org/10.1007/s00247-004-1223-7

Thomas, J. (2017). Osteomyelitis variolosa. *Journal of Clinical Rheumatology* 23:114. https://doi.org/10.1097/RHU.0000000000000517

Thompson, A.R. (2014). Differential diagnosis of limb length discrepancy in a 19th century burial from Southwest Mississippi. *International Journal of Osteoarchaeology* 24:517–530. https://doi.org/10.1002/oa.2238

Tschinkel, K., Verano, J., Prieto, G. (2024). Two cases of smallpox from 1540 CE circum-contact (early colonial) Northern Coastal Peru. *International Journal of Paleopathology* 45:35–45. https://doi.org/10.1016/j.ijpp.2024.04.002

Turunc, T., Demiroglu, Y.Z., Uncu, H., Colakoglu, S., Arslan, H. (2007). A comparative analysis of tuberculous, brucellar and pyogenic spontaneous spondylodiscitis patients. *Journal of Infection* 55:158–163. https://doi.org/10.1016/j.jinf.2007.04.002

Vannet, N.B., Williams, H.L., Healy, B., Morgan-Jones, R. (2014). Sclerosing osteomyelitis of Garré: Management of femoral pain by intramedullary nailing. *BMJ Case Reports 2014*:bcr2014206533. https://doi.org/10.1136/bcr-2014-206533

Waldron, T. (2020). *Palaeopathology*, 2nd edition. Cambridge: Cambridge University Press.

Weston, D.A. (2008). Investigating the specificity of periosteal reactions in pathology museum specimens. *American Journal of Physical Anthropology* 137:48–59. https://doi.org/10.1002/ajpa.20839

Weston, D.A. (2012). Nonspecific infection in paleopathology: Interpreting periosteal reactions. In *A Companion to Paleopathology*, edited by Grauer, A.L., pp. 492–512. Hoboken, NJ: John Wiley & Sons.

Wood, J.W., Milner, G.R., Harpending, H.C., Weiss, K.M. (1992). The osteological paradox: Problems of inferring prehistoric health from skeletal samples. *Current Anthropology* 33:343–370.

Wright, L.E., Yoder, C.J. (2003). Recent progress in bioarchaeology: Approaches to the osteological paradox. *Journal of Archaeological Research* 11:43–70. https://doi.org/10.1023/A:1021200925063

Yuan, H.T., Wang, C.L., Liu, L.N., Wang, D., Li, D., Li, Z.J., Liu, Z.G. (2020). Epidemiologically characteristics of human brucellosis and antimicrobial susceptibility pattern of *Brucella melitensis* in Hinggan League of the Inner Mongolia Autonomous Region, China. *Infectious Diseases of Poverty* 9:1–9.

Chapter 8

Neoplastic disease

Neoplastic disease is characterised by an uncontrolled proliferation of cells. The terms "neoplasm" and "tumour" are often used interchangeably to refer to the result of this proliferation, and this will be the practice also adopted in this chapter. However, these terms do not have exactly the same meaning. The term "neoplasm" is broader and expresses an abnormal cell growth, while a "tumour" appears when the abnormal cells grow enough and aggregate to form a distinct mass. Whereas most neoplastic diseases result in the formation of a tumour, not all do. For example, leukaemia is a malignant neoplastic disease but it does not form tumours.

Neoplastic disease results from an interplay of several risk factors, including aspects of the cultural environment (e.g. manmade carcinogens), exposure to naturally occurring carcinogens (e.g. ultraviolet radiation), and genetic susceptibility.

Bone tumours may be primary or secondary. Primary bone tumours originate from the skeletal tissue and may be benign or malignant. Secondary bone tumours originate in other parts of the body and metastasise to the skeleton; thus, they are always malignant. Benign tumours are typically solitary, have a slow growth rate, and cannot metastasise, that is, they do not spread beyond their site of origin. These tumours are composed of well-differentiated and well-organised cells. Individuals with benign tumours may remain asymptomatic, but they may also experience serious health issues when the tumours exert pressure on adjacent organs or tissues. Furthermore, some benign tumours may become malignant over time. Malignant neoplasms, commonly called cancers, show a rapid and uncontrolled growth and can metastasise to distant parts of the body. Cancer cells can spread from a primary site to the bone through haematogenous, lymphatic, or cerebrospinal fluid routes, or through direct extension from adjacent soft tissues.

Bone changes due to neoplastic disease include new bone formation, bone resorption, or both. Moreover, certain soft tissue neoplasms, such as tumours of the urinary bladder, can lead to the formation of calcifications, but these are easily missed during excavation. Finally, soft tissue tumours affecting various endocrine glands, such as the pituitary, parathyroid, and thyroid glands, can influence skeletal morphology, as discussed in Chapter 6.

DOI: 10.4324/9781003475026-8

The following sections of this chapter offer a brief overview of selected bone tumours and how they affect the skeleton. In the organisation of the chapter, we broadly follow Waldron (2020) and Marques (2019). We start with benign bone tumours, covering osteoid osteoma, osteoblastoma, chondroma, osteochondroma, chondroblastoma, chondromyxoid fibroma, haemangioma, meningioma, giant cell tumour, and Langerhans cell histiocytosis. Then we proceed to malignant bone tumours, starting with primary malignant bone tumours (osteosarcoma, Ewing's sarcoma, chondrosarcoma, chordoma, fibrosarcoma, angiosarcoma) and then covering metastatic bone disease. Finally, we discuss lesions of undefined or nonneoplastic nature, which are often categorised together with neoplastic disease in the literature (bone cysts, osteoma, nonossifying fibroma). Note that leukaemia and multiple myeloma have been covered in the haematopoietic diseases chapter (Chapter 4), but they are also neoplastic diseases.

The diagnosis of neoplastic disease in bones usually relies on the integrated analysis of histological, clinical, radiological, and molecular data. Such data are rarely available to palaeopathologists; thus, it is advisable to be cautious when performing differential diagnosis of neoplastic conditions, and to favour broader disease classifications. Moreover, it is strongly recommended to collaborate with other experts (e.g. radiologists) when examining potential neoplastic disease in archaeological remains.

Benign bone tumours

Osteoid osteoma

The osteoid osteoma is a small osteoblastic tumour (Figures 8.1 and 8.2). The central part, or nidus, of this tumour is composed of osteoid, surrounded by a zone of reactive bone. Radiographically, the lesion appears as a radiolucent core with a sclerotic margin. Individuals with osteoid osteoma often experience pain that intensifies at night.

Osteoblastoma

Osteoblastoma is an osteoid-forming tumour. Histologically, it is similar to osteoid osteoma, but it has a larger size. It may cause pain, swelling, and tenderness, and is associated with an elevated risk of fractures because osteoid has inferior mechanical properties compared to normal bone. If the tumour is in the arms or legs, individuals may show limping, while if it affects the spine, neurological symptoms may appear (Figures 8.3 and 8.4).

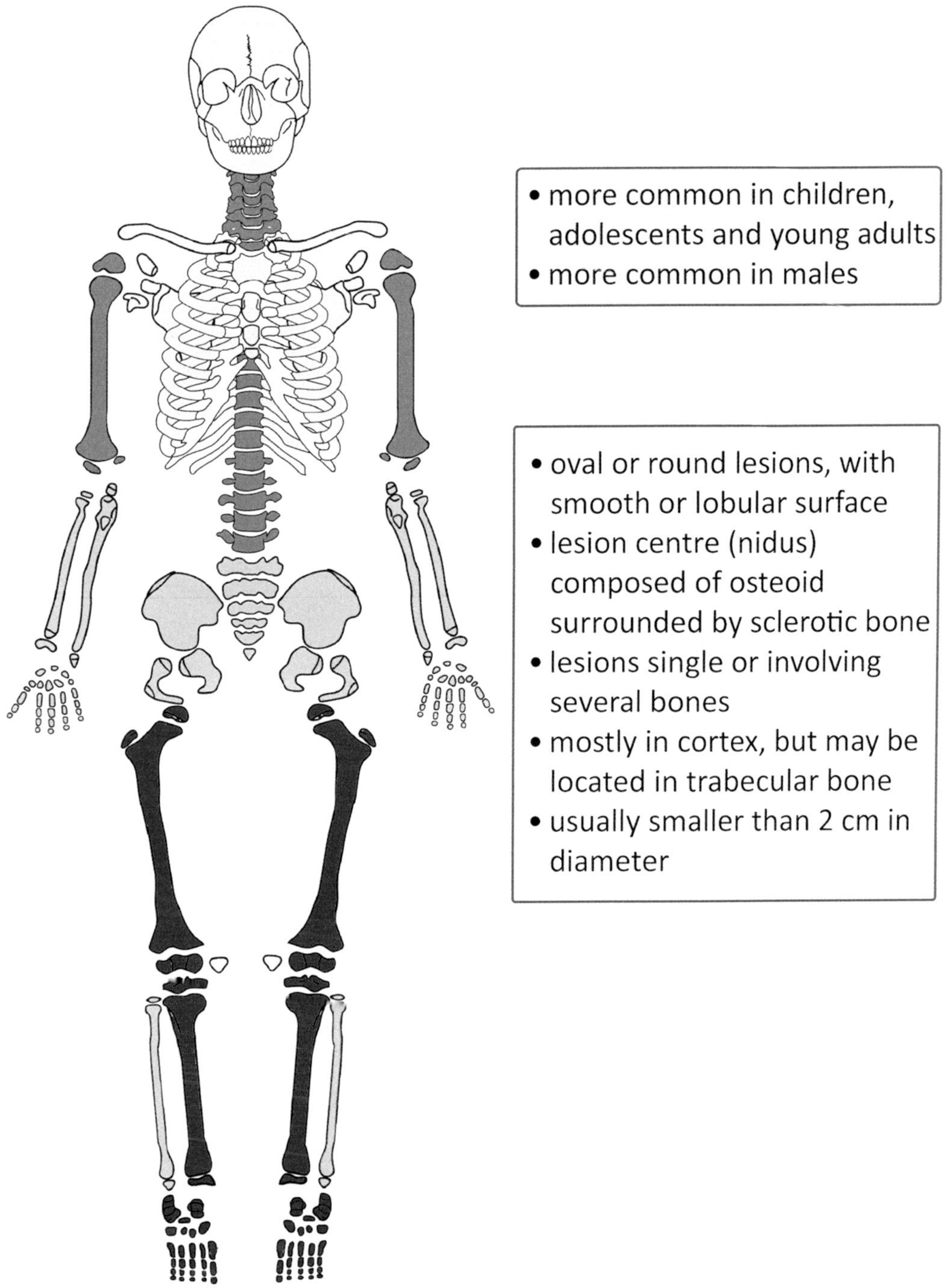

Figure 8.1 Skeletal manifestation of osteoid osteoma. (Data from Atesok et al. 2011; Bhure et al. 2019; Campanacci 2020a; Isler and Turcotte 2003; Marques 2019; Nielsen and Rosenberg 2010; Stoker 1986; Waldron 2020)

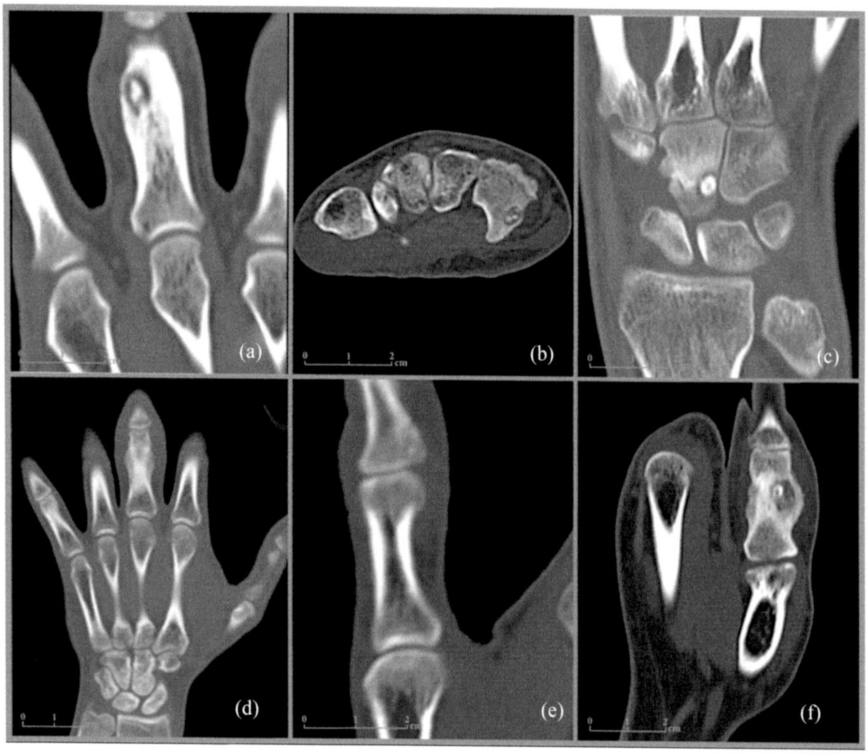

Figure 8.2 CT scans of osteoid osteomata in hand bones. In all cases (except (d)), note the central nidus with surrounding sclerosis; in (d) note the enlarged proximal phalanx of the middle finger. (Figure 2 in Meyer et al. 2023; article licensed under a Creative Commons Attribution 4.0 International License)

Chondroma

Chondromas are tumours composed of cartilage (Figures 8.5–8.7). When these tumours are located within the bone, usually in the medullary cavity, they are called enchondromas. In contrast, the tumours that develop on the surface of the bone are called periosteal or juxtacortical chondromas. Some chondromas can transform into malignant chondrosarcomas. Enchondromas typically cause no symptoms; however, they can lead to pain or localised swelling, and increased fracture risk. Although periosteal chondromas may also be asymptomatic, they frequently cause pain, tenderness, and swelling.

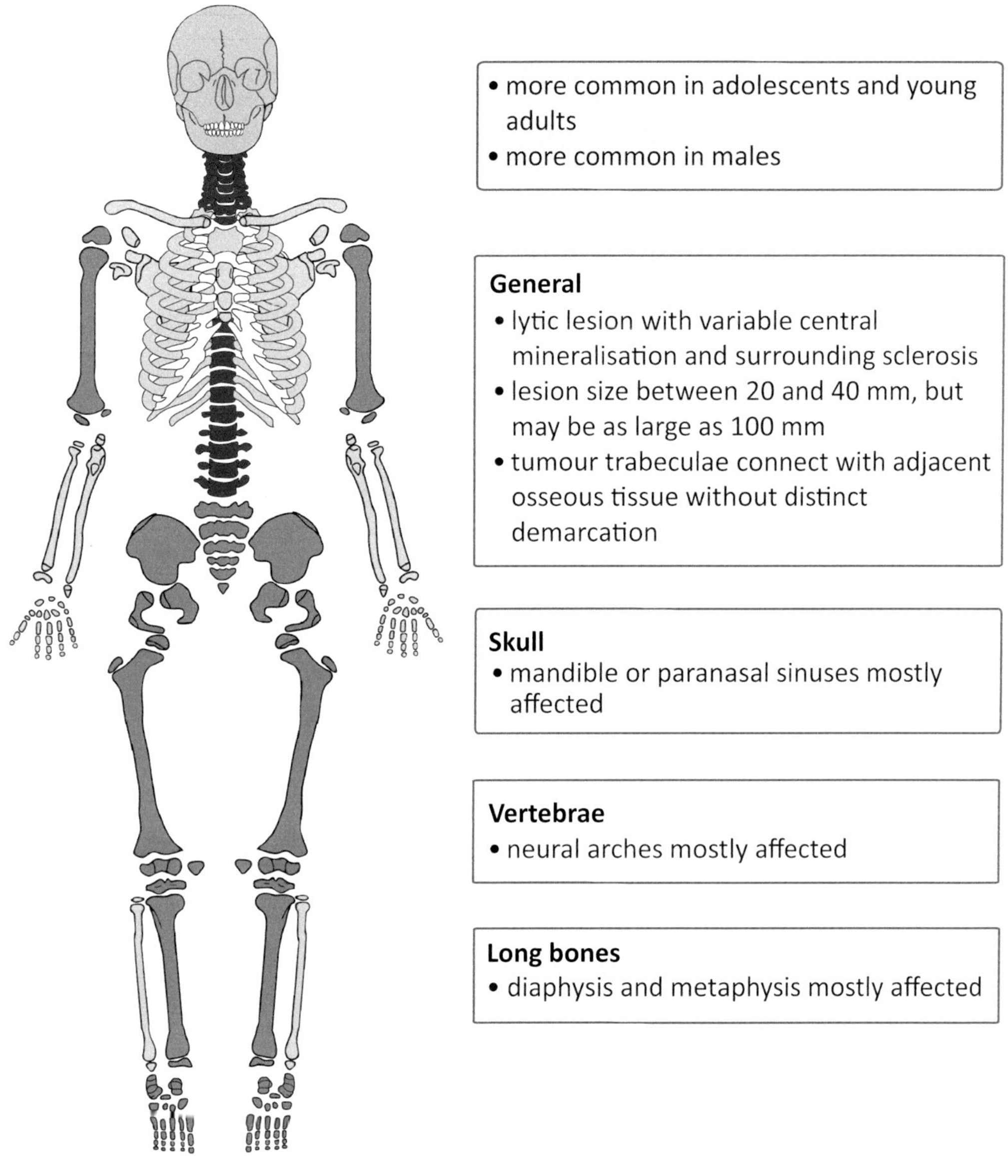

Figure 8.3 Skeletal manifestation of osteoblastoma. (Data from Atesok et al. 2011; Campanacci 2020b; Hakim et al. 2015; Moon et al. 2006; Ohkawa et al. 1997; Stoker 1986)

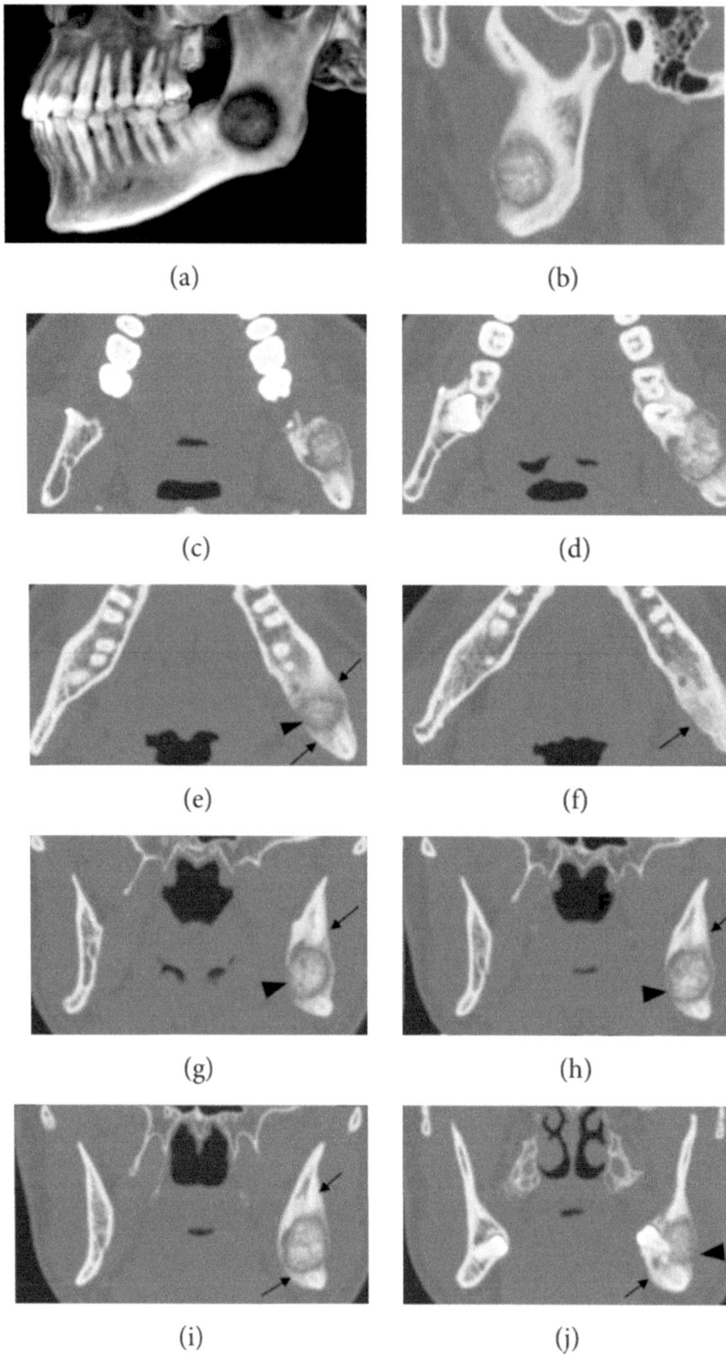

Figure 8.4 3D CT scans of mandible with osteoblastoma. Note the lytic lesion with sclerotic rim and expansion of the bone contour. (Figure 1 in Ellingsen et al. 2022; article licensed under a Creative Commons Attribution 4.0 International License)

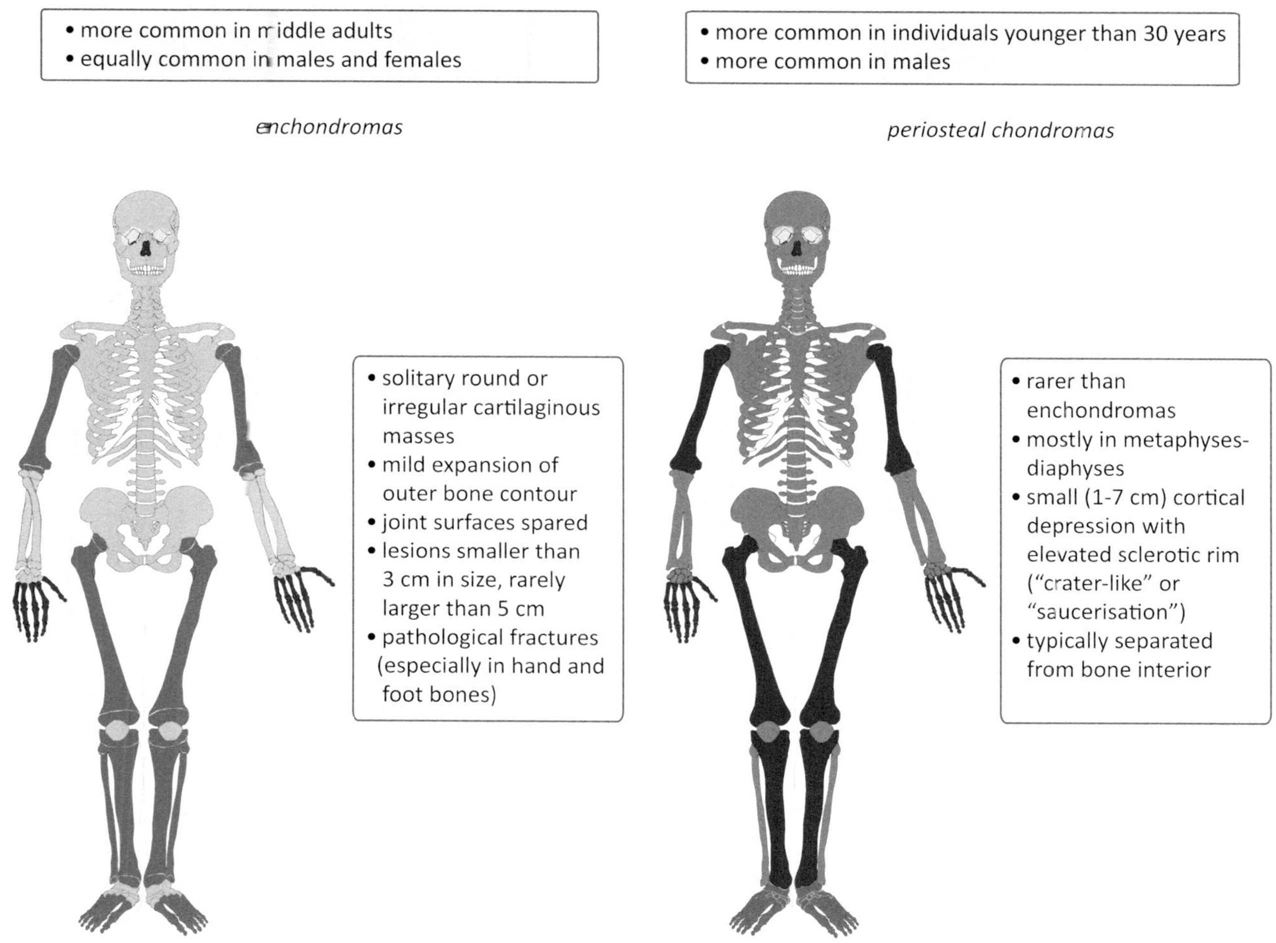

Figure 8.5 Skeletal manifestation of enchondromas and periosteal chondromas. (Data from Donati and Staals 2020a; Jaffe 1958; Khurana and Unni 2003; Lucas and Bridge 2002; Marques 2019; Stoker 1986; Waldron 2020)

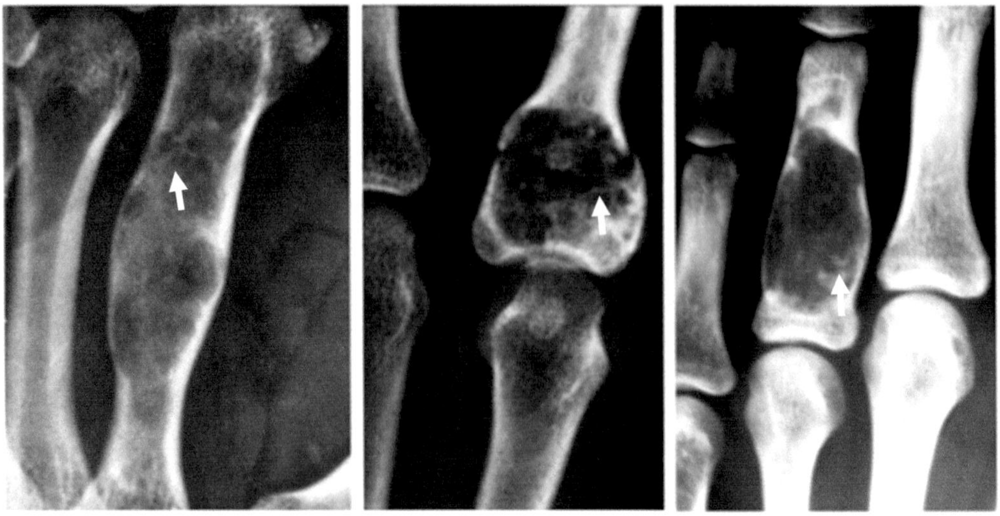

Figure 8.6 Radiographs of enchondromas. Note the intramedullary lytic lesions and expansion of the bone contours. (Figure 1 in Pietramala et al. 2025; article licensed under a Creative Commons Attribution 4.0 International License)

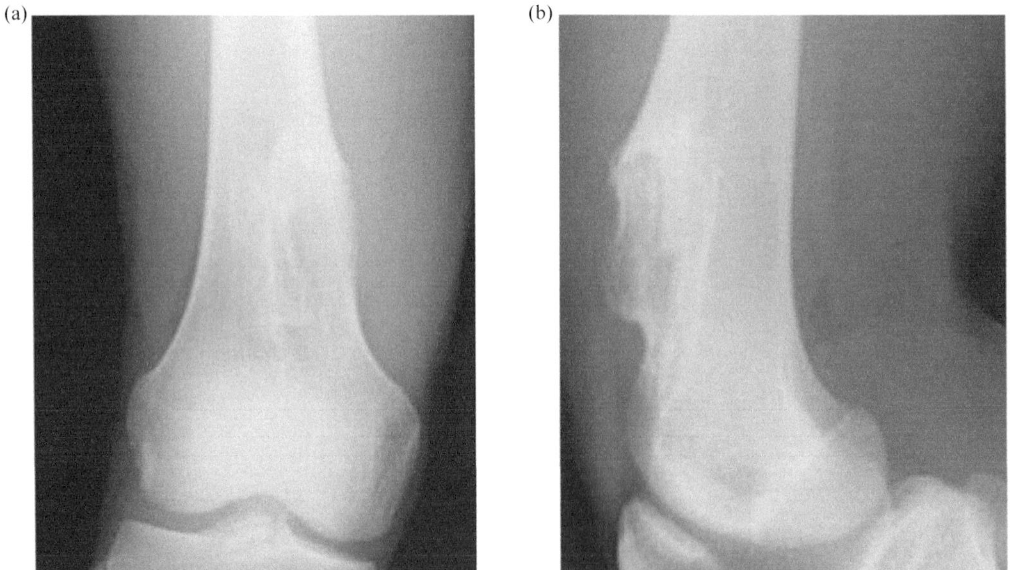

Figure 8.7 Radiographs of distal femur with periosteal chondroma. Note the cortical erosion with sclerotic rim, and saucerisation of the underlying cortex. (Figure 1 in Imura et al. 2014; article licensed under a Creative Commons Attribution 4.0 International License)

Enchondromatosis is the presence of multiple enchondromas, asymmetrically distributed. The condition appears in childhood. The lesions vary in terms of size, number, and anatomical location. The most common skeletal deformities associated with enchondromatosis include phalangeal enlargement, limb shortening, long bone bowing, wrist and elbow deformities, and genu valgum. However, the severity of the skeletal manifestation of enchondromatosis is highly variable, ranging from asymptomatic lesions to severe disability.

Osteochondroma

Osteochondromas appear as cartilage-capped exostoses, that is, they consist of trabecular bone covered by hyaline cartilage (Figures 8.8–8.10). Osteochondromas may be solitary or multiple. Solitary osteochondromas are more common; their precise aetiology remains unclear, and in many cases, they are asymptomatic. In contrast, multiple osteochondromas is an autosomal dominant disorder whereby two or more osteochondromas are present. Multiple osteochondromas may cause various complications, as they can disrupt normal bone growth and produce skeletal deformities. In addition, they have been associated with pain and potential impingement on adjacent tendons, nerves, and vessels.

Chondroblastoma

Chondroblastoma is a benign tumour, though it may rarely metastasise. It is characterised by the proliferation of chondroblasts, which are important cartilage-forming cells. Chondroblastomas predominantly form in the long bone epiphyses (Figures 8.11 and 8.12). Their aetiology remains unclear. The most frequently reported symptoms include localised pain, joint stiffness and swelling, muscle atrophy, restricted mobility of the adjacent joint, and the presence of a limp.

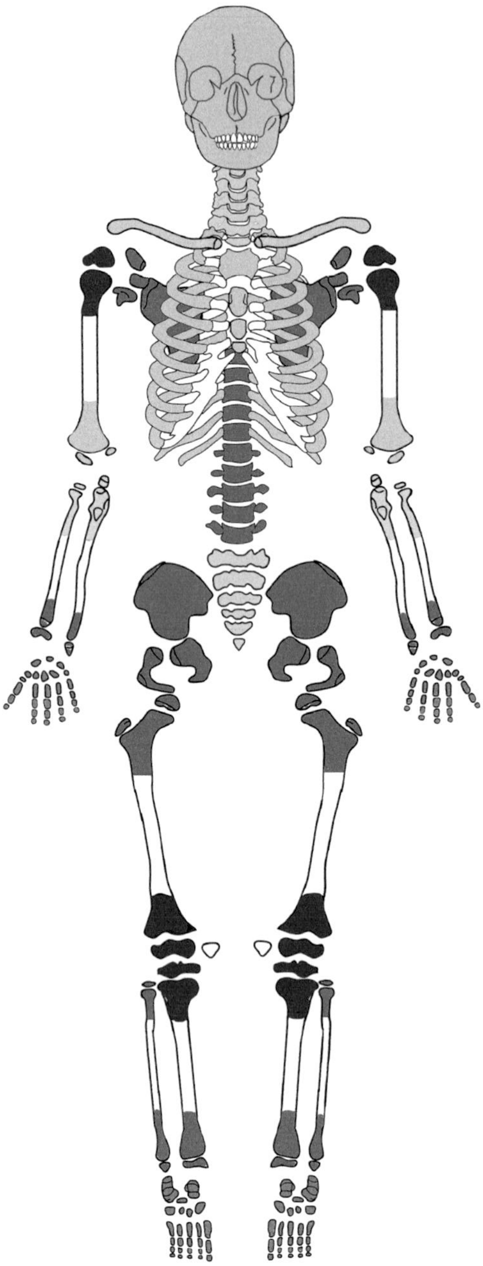

- onset in first decade of life and continued growth until skeletal maturity
- more common in males

- bony outgrowth capped with cartilage, which is not preserved in dry bone
- usually solitary; when multiple, the condition has autosomal dominant inheritance
- cortex and medullary cavity continuous with the bone from which osteochondromas arise
- two forms of exostoses:
  - o sessile (broad and bulbous)
  - o pedunculated (spur-like)
- size ranges from 1 to 10 cm
- skeletal deformities due to osteochondromas in juveniles: widening and irregularity of metaphyses and delayed bone growth → bowing and shortening of affected bones, reduced stature, limb-length discrepancies, coxa vara, knee and ankle valgus deformities, shortened hand and foot bones, asymmetric pectoral and pelvic girdles, scoliosis
- in paired bones of lower and upper extremities, large osteochondromas may cause erosions in adjacent bones ("kissing osteochondroma"); synostoses between two opposite bones are possible

Figure 8.8 Skeletal manifestation of osteochondroma. (Data from Bessler et al. 1997; Donati and Staals 2020b; Jaffe 1958; Khurana et al. 2002; Marques 2019; Murphey et al. 2000; Murphy and McKenzie 2010; Stieber and Dormans 2005; Stoker 1986)

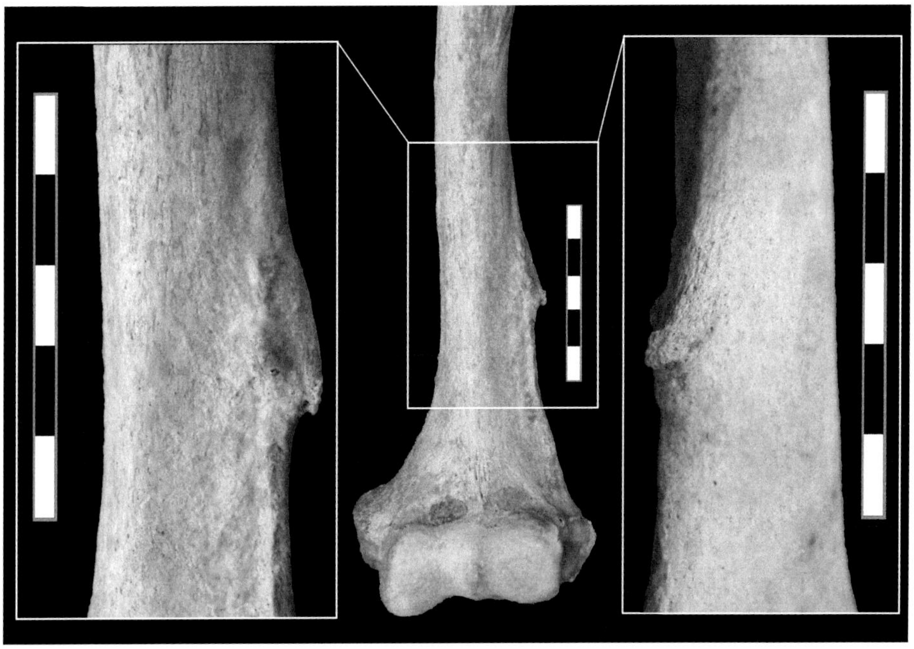

Figure 8.9 Possible osteochondroma. Note the solitary pedunculated bony outgrowth on the lateral part of the distal left humerus. (Male, 40–55 years old, All Saints Church, Fishergate, York, Medieval, Y-2066; photos by Efthymia Nikita; copyright: Human Skeletal Collection, University of Sheffield)

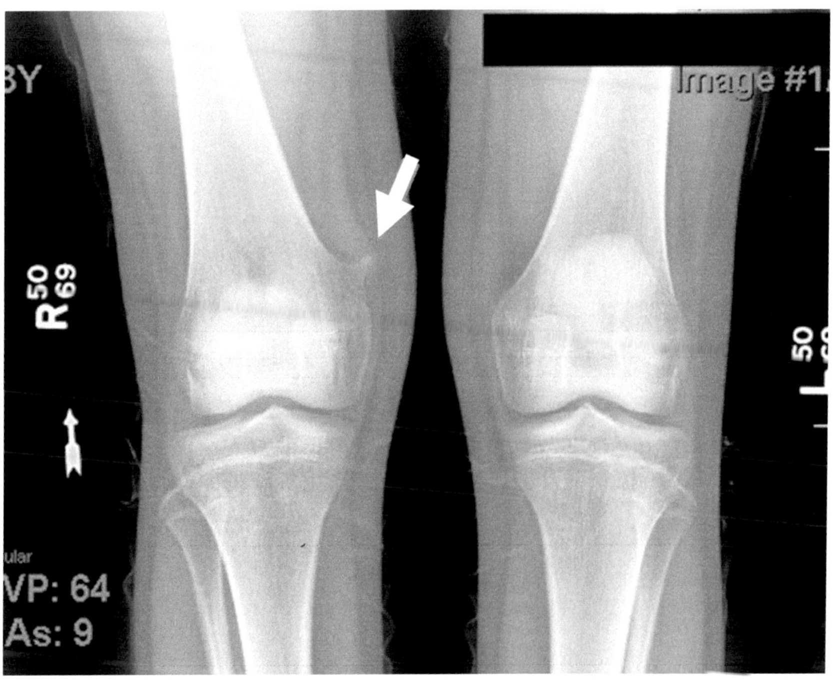

Figure 8.10 Radiograph of the knees of individual with osteochondroma. Note the osseous projection at the right medial femoral condyle. (Figure 1 in Badders and Carmichael 2023; article licensed under a Creative Commons Attribution 4.0 International License)

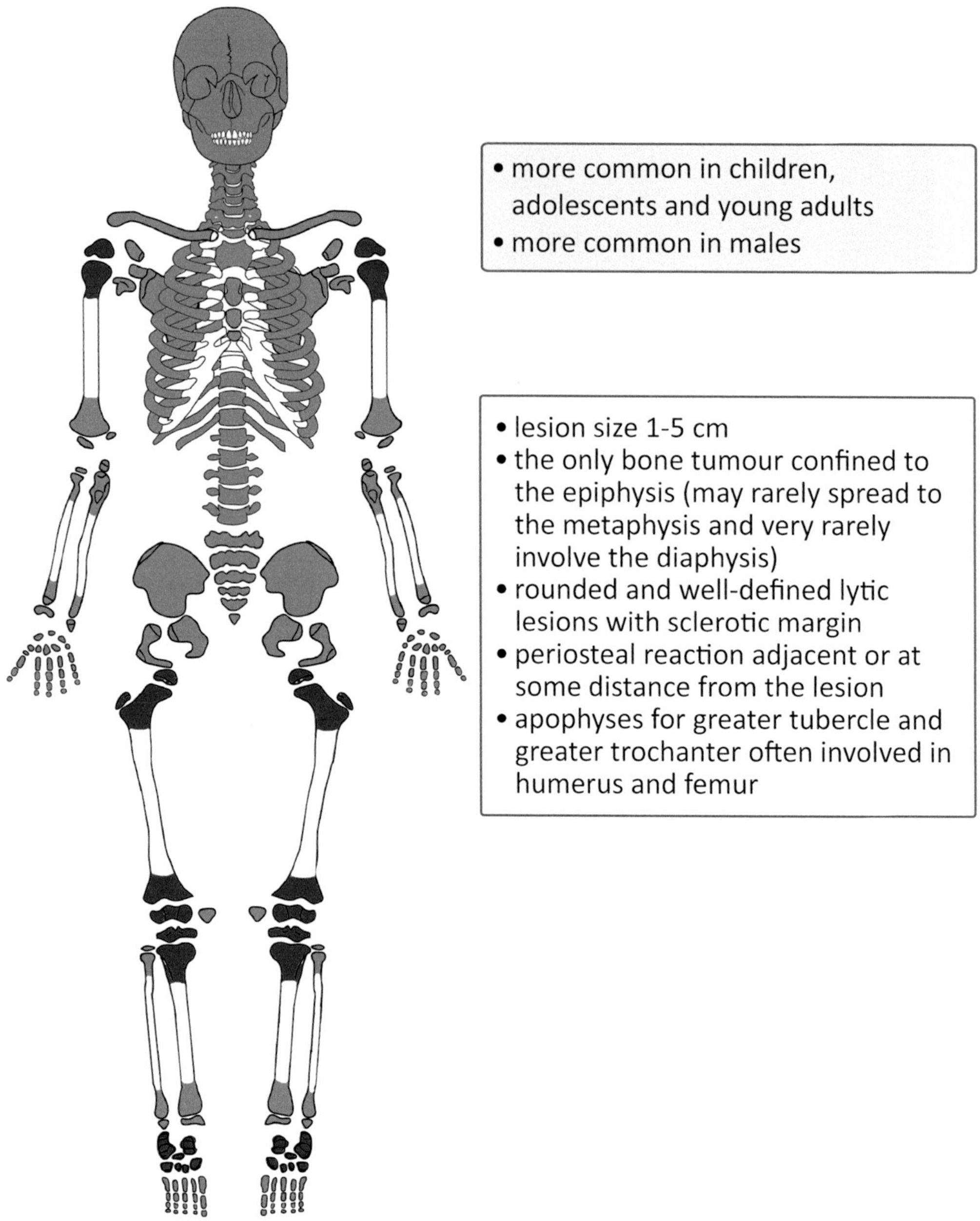

Figure 8.11 Skeletal manifestation of chondroblastoma. (Data from Douis and Saifuddin 2012; Erickson et al. 2001; Marques 2019; Staals 2020a; Stoker 1986; Unni and Inwards 2010; Waldron 2020)

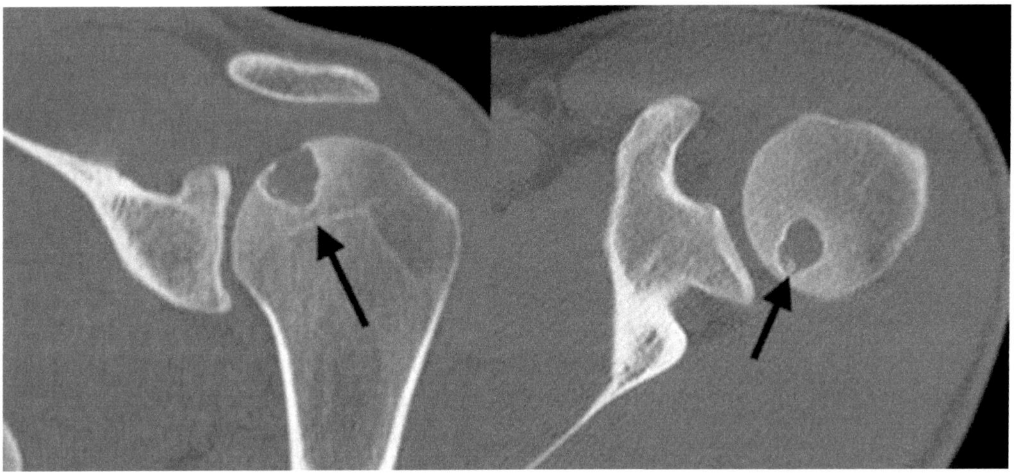

Figure 8.12 CT scan of the left shoulder of individual with chondroblastoma. Note that the lesion does not involve the growth plate. (Figure 3 in Lambert et al. 2016; article licensed under a Creative Commons Attribution 4.0 International License)

Chondromyxoid fibroma

Chondromyxoid fibroma is a rare cartilaginous tumour, consisting of chondroid, myxoid, and fibrous tissues (Figures 8.13 and 8.14). While it cannot metastasise, it can invade surrounding tissues. Its aetiology remains unknown, and the symptoms may include persistent pain, swelling, stiffness, tenderness, and the presence of a palpable mass beneath the skin.

Haemangioma

Haemangiomas are benign tumours characterised by a proliferation of capillary endothelial cells (Figures 8.15 and 8.16). Their aetiology is largely unknown, but they have been linked to ectopic placental tissue. Endothelial progenitor cells may also contribute to haemangioma formation, as do various enzymes, such as matrix metalloproteinases and proangiogenic factors. Haemangiomas appear as red or purple marks or bulges on the skin, often located on the face, scalp, chest, or back, although they can occur in any part of the body. They mostly appear at birth or during infancy, and often regress over time. Nonetheless, some haemangiomas may affect important functions such as breathing, eating, and vision. While haemangiomas predominantly appear in infants, they can also affect adults, particularly older individuals. Haemangiomas are mostly found in the skin, but they can also appear in other tissues, including bone.

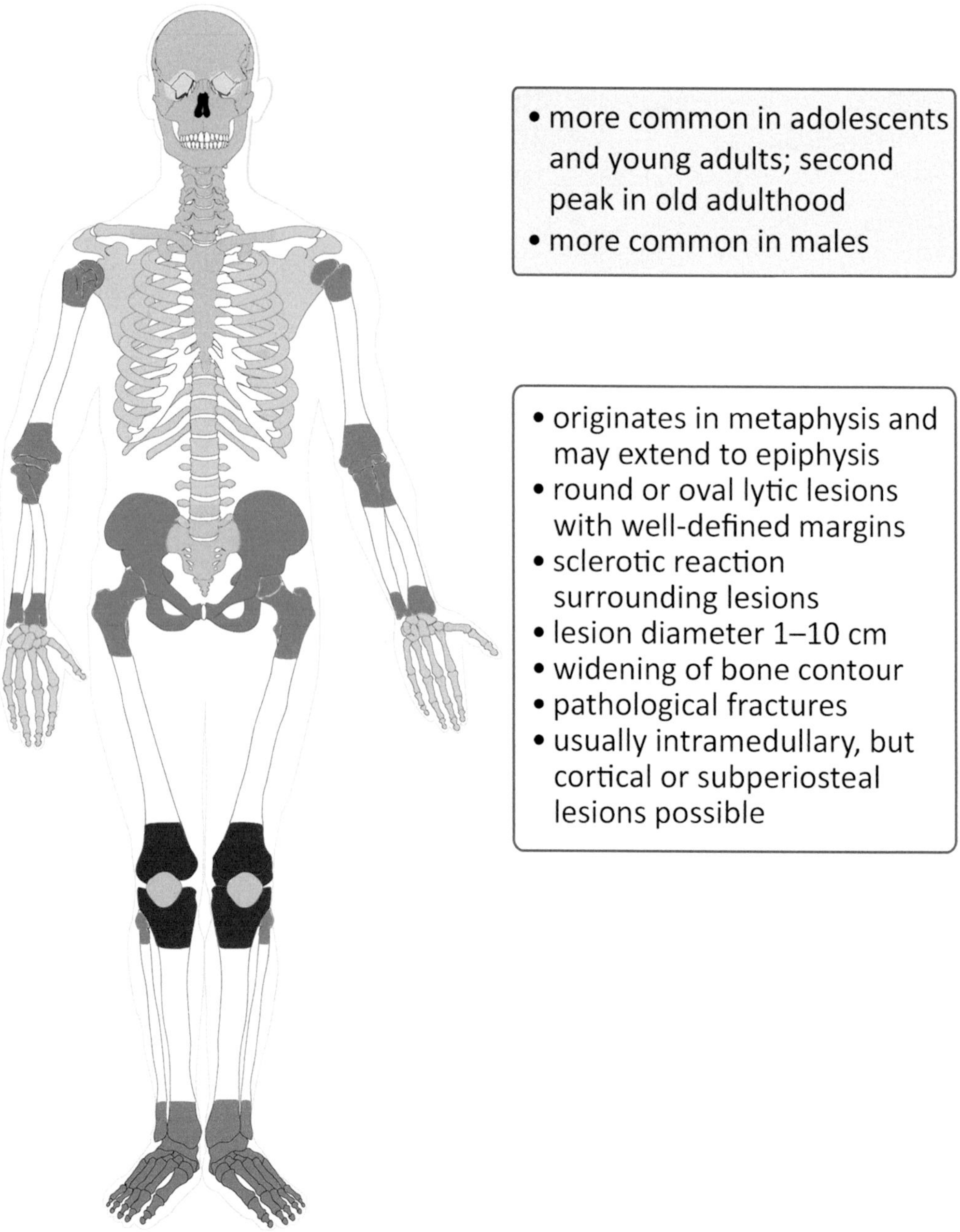

Figure 8.13 Skeletal manifestation of chondromyxoid fibroma. (Data from Cappelle et al. 2016; Douis and Saifuddin 2012; Isler and Turcotte 2003; Marques 2019; Schajowicz and Gallardo 1971; Staals 2020b; Stoker 1986; Unni and Inwards 2010)

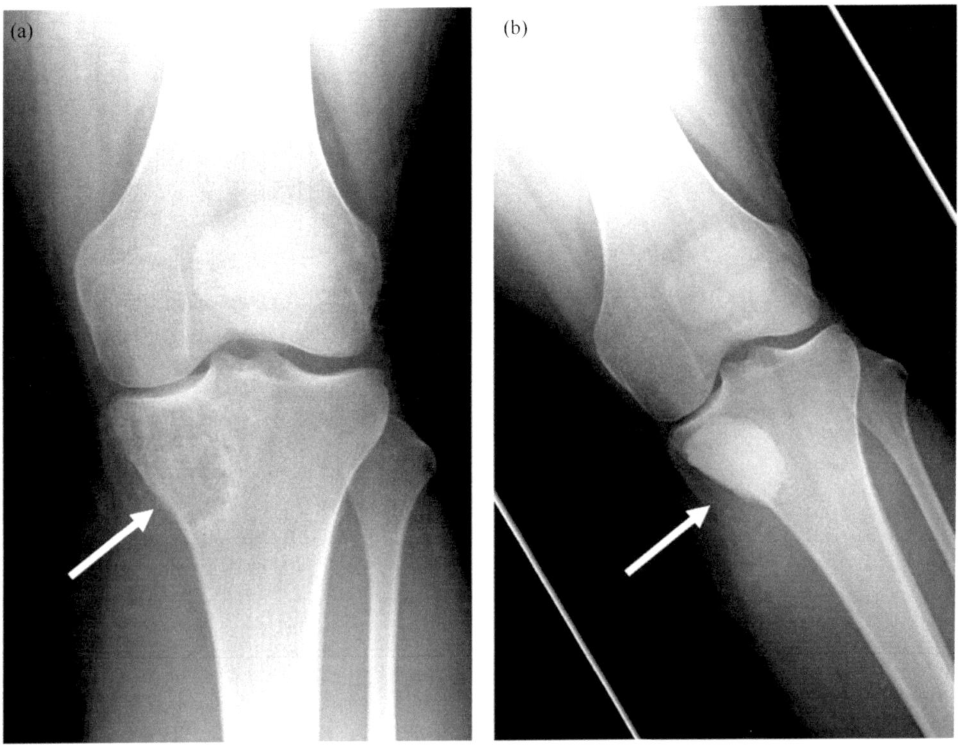

Figure 8.14 Radiographs showing chondromyxoid fibroma of the tibia ((a) preoperative, (b) post-operative). Note the lytic lesion in the medial tibial plateau in the preoperative figure. (Figure 2 in Bhamra et al. 2014; article licensed under a Creative Commons Attribution 2.0 Generic License)

- more common in middle aged individuals
- more common in females

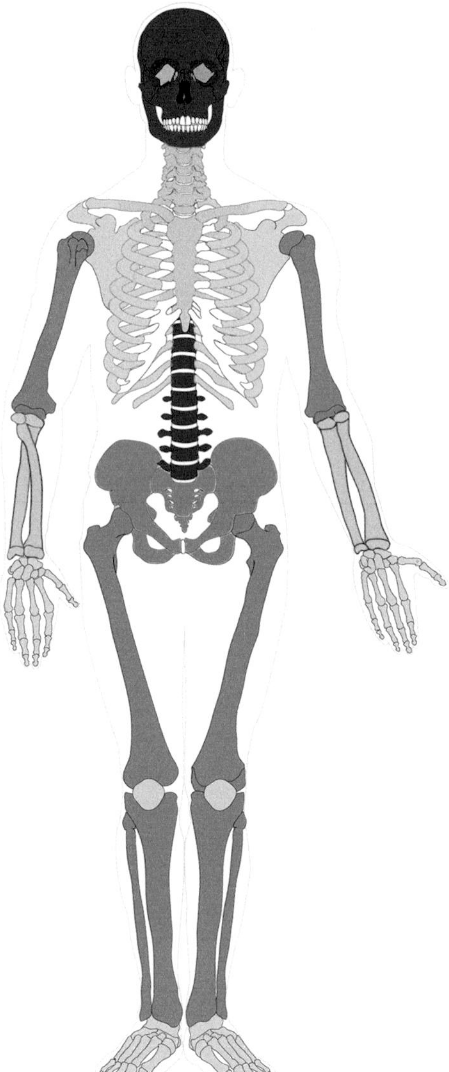

General

- solitary lytic lesion
- lesions mostly in intramedullary spaces, but also periosteal and intracortical

Skull

- mostly in frontal and parietal bones, and rarely in mandible
- round lytic lesions, several centimetres in diameter
- destruction of inner and outer tables
- pronounced vascular grooves
- coarse diplöic trabeculae
- may cause "sunburst" type of periosteal reaction

Thorax

- destruction of trabecular bone and coarsening of remaining trabeculae
- thinning and expansion of cortex

Vertebrae

- mostly affects lower spine
- trabecular bone destruction
- compression fractures
- usually monostotic but several vertebrae (usually noncontiguous) may be involved

Arm/leg

- lytic and sometimes sclerotic lesions

Figure 8.15 Skeletal manifestation of haemangioma. (Data from Bastug et al. 1995; Fox and Onofrio 1993; Marques 2019; Righi 2020)

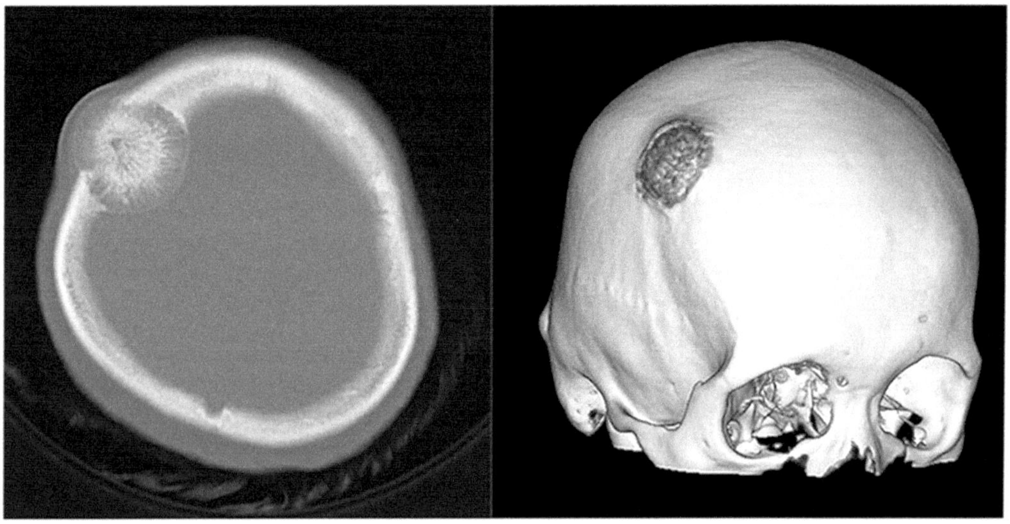

(a) (b)

Figure 8.16 Cranial CT scan (a) and CT 3D reconstruction of cranium (b) with haemangioma. Note the mass on the right frontoparietal junction area, accompanied by osteolytic changes. (Figure 1 in Cao et al. 2022; article licensed under a Creative Commons Attribution 4.0 International License)

Meningioma

Meningiomas are benign tumours that originate from arachnoid cap cells within the leptomeninges (i.e. the pia mater and arachnoid mater) (Figures 8.17 and 8.18). Although most meningiomas are benign, they can rarely metastasise. Large meningiomas can exert pressure on adjacent brain tissue, leading to neurological complications, or increased intracranial pressure. Certain meningiomas may be more aggressive and grow rapidly. Several factors can increase the risk of developing meningioma, including the presence of the genetic disorder neurofibromatosis type 2 and exposure to ionising radiation. Hormonal factors, especially elevated levels of progesterone, may also contribute to the aetiology of meningiomas. Finally, viral infections, such as those caused by human papillomavirus, might be linked to this tumour.

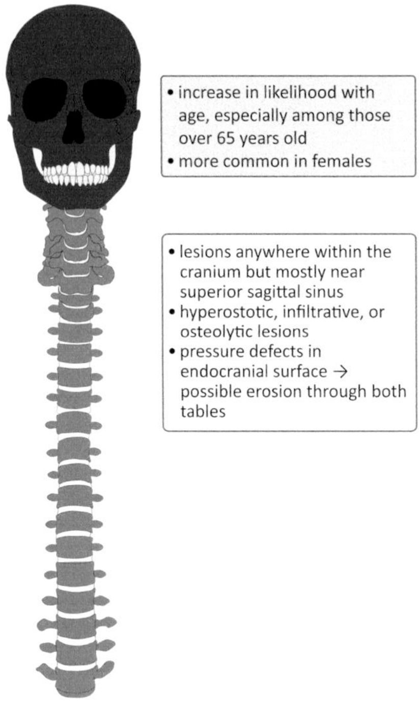

Figure 8.17 Skeletal manifestation of meningioma. (Data from Brkić et al. 2013; Campillo 1991; Di Cristofori et al. 2018; Marques 2019; Mehta et al. 2009; Menon et al. 2009; Waldron 1998)

Note: The expression of meningiomas in juveniles is different to that seen in adults: meningiomas are rare in juveniles, they affect mostly males, the lesions are larger, cystic changes are more frequent, and the tumours are more aggressive.

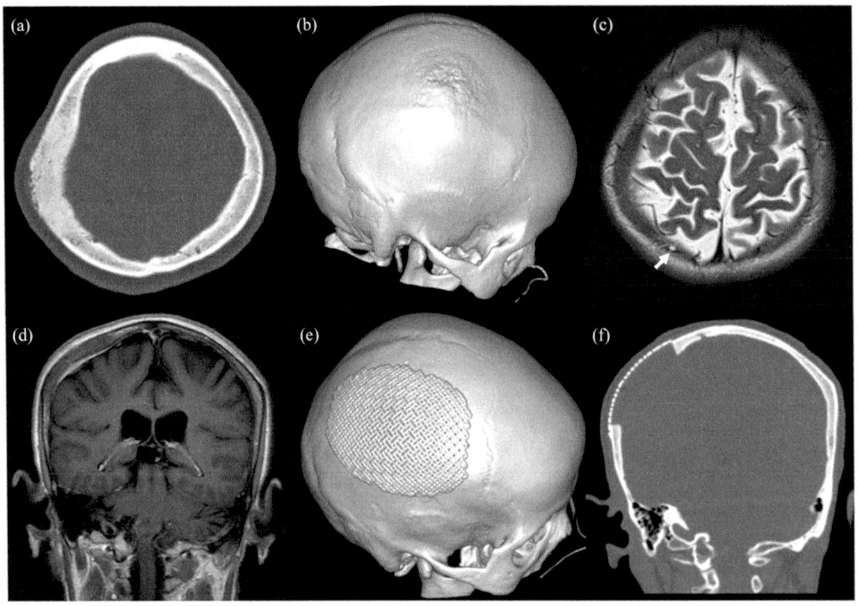

Figure 8.18 Preoperative CT showing meningioma in the right parietal bone (a), 3D-CT showing lesion in the ectocranial surface (b), axial T2 imaging revealing an intraosseous lesion and arachnoid granulations protruding into the affected bone (c), MRI showing intense dural reaction (d), and postoperative 3D-CT and CT (e, f). (Figure 1 in Zou et al. 2022; article licensed under a Creative Commons Attribution 4.0 International License)

Giant cell tumour

Giant cell tumours are characterised by a proliferation of stromal cells and the presence of multinucleated giant cells (Figures 8.19 and 8.20). Although they are benign, they can become malignant and metastasise. Their aetiology is unclear, but there is a possible association between giant cell tumours and Paget's disease of bone. Symptoms of giant cell tumours may

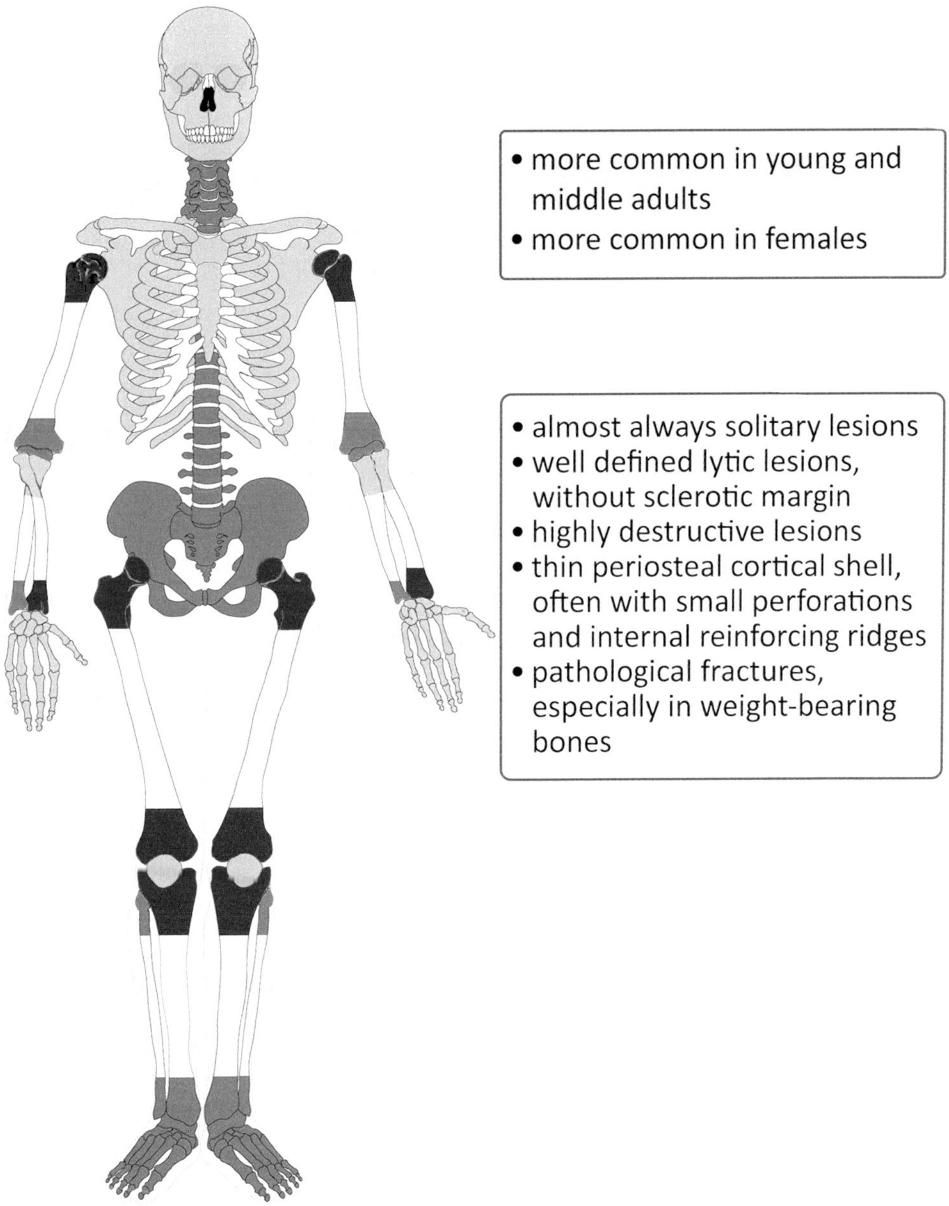

Figure 8.19 Skeletal manifestation of giant cell tumour. (Data from Gadelha Vasconcelos et al. 2013; Isler and Turcotte 2003; Manfrini 2020; Marques 2019; Sobti et al. 2016; Stoker 1986; Waldron 2020)

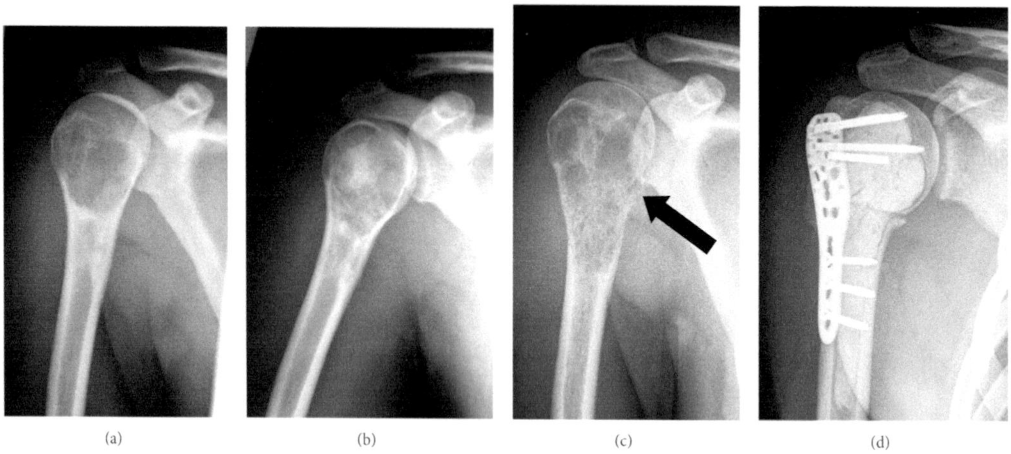

Figure 8.20 Radiographs of the proximal right humerus in individual with giant cell tumour. Note the lytic lesion before (a) and after treatment (b), the pathological fracture four months later (c), and additional treatment (d). (Figure 1 in Wirbel et al. 2013; article licensed under a Creative Commons Attribution 3.0 Unported License)

include pain, swelling, a visible mass under the skin, pathological bone fractures, muscle atrophy, stiffness in the joint near the affected site, and limited mobility.

Langerhans cell histiocytosis

Langerhans cell histiocytosis (LCH) is characterised by an overproduction of cells with a Langerhans cells phenotype (Figures 8.21 and 8.22). Langerhans cells have an important immune function and are found in several tissues of the body, particularly in the skin, but also in the bone marrow and elsewhere. The aetiology of LCH is unclear. While several researchers classify it as a neoplastic disorder, others consider it an inflammatory disease.

LCH manifests in distinct clinical syndromes: Letterer–Siwe disease, Hand–Schüller–Christian disease, and eosinophilic granuloma. Letterer–Siwe disease predominantly affects children younger than three years and has high mortality rates. Hand–Schüller–Christian disease is seen mostly in children aged 3–6 years, but it can occur in individuals of any age. This syndrome manifests as diabetes insipidus (i.e. the body produces excessive urine), exophthalmos (bulging eyes), and lytic bone lesions. Finally, eosinophilic granuloma primarily occurs in individuals younger than 15 years, but cases in adults have also been documented. It usually involves a single bone, and patients require minimal treatment, as the lesion often heals on its own.

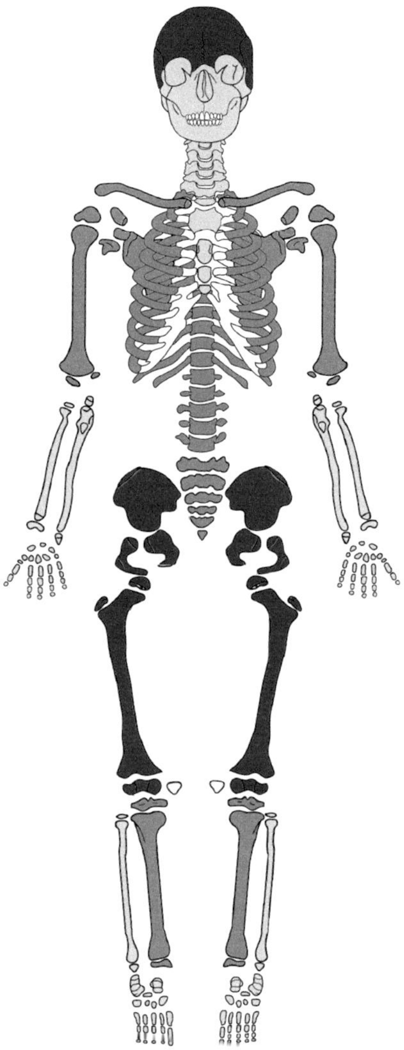

General

- destructive lesions, sharply circumscribed and punched out
- limited osteoblastic response
- mostly solitary lesions; multifocal lesions also possible and may coalesce into large areas of destruction with undulating margins (geographic or map-like lesions)

Skull

- sharply defined, round or oval lytic lesions in vault, with bevelled appearance
- lesions may coalesce and produce geographic pattern
- more common in frontal and parietal bones
- no periosteal reaction

Thorax

- eroded rib cortex
- expanded rib diameter
- sclerotic reactive bone formation
- pathological fractures

Vertebrae

- lytic lesions on bodies
- vertebral collapse
- rare involvement of neural arches

Arm/leg

- pathological fractures
- lytic lesions mostly in metaphyses, followed by mid-diaphyses, and rarely epiphyses
- periosteal and endosteal bone formation

Figure 8.21 Skeletal manifestation of Langerhans cell histiocytosis. (Data from Azouz et al. 2005; Grauer 2019; Lieberman 1975; Papadopoulou et al. 2018; Robert et al. 1987)

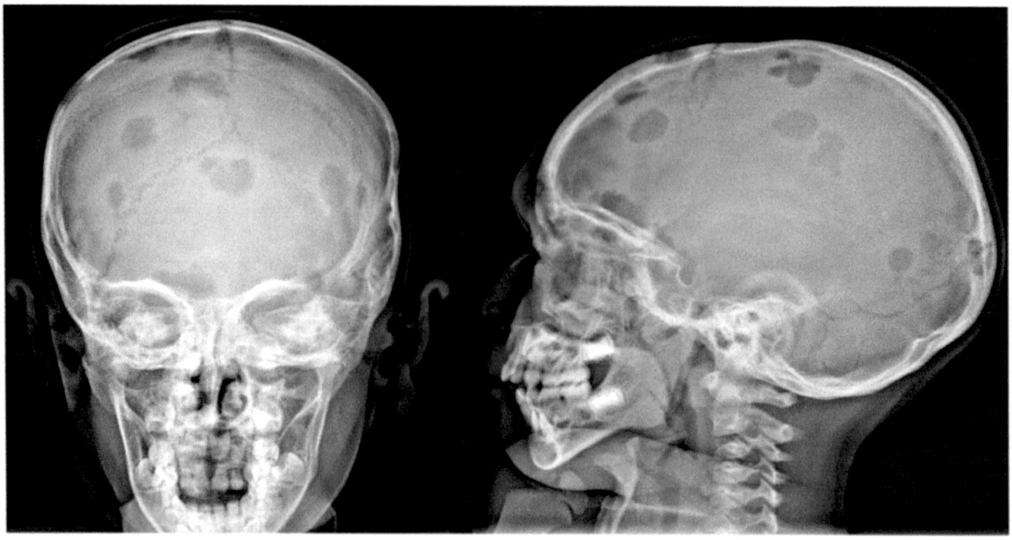

Figure 8.22 Radiograph of skull of individual with Langerhans cell histiocytosis. Note the multiple osteolytic lesions in the calvaria. (Figure 2 in Leenknegt et al. 2020; article licensed under a Creative Commons Attribution 4.0 International License)

Malignant bone tumours

Osteosarcoma

Osteosarcoma is a bone tumour of mesenchymal origin, characterised by the production of malignant osteoid (Box 8.1, Figures 8.23 and 8.24). Osteosarcoma can develop as a primary malignancy, especially in individuals aged 10–20 years, a period marked by active bone growth. Alternatively, it may develop as a secondary malignancy in older adults, frequently associated with conditions such as Paget's disease or as a consequence of radiotherapy for other conditions. According to their location in the bones, osteosarcomas may be intraosseous or surface. Intraosseous osteosarcomas are the most common type; these tumours arise within the medullary cavity and are typically located close to the metaphyses. Surface osteosarcomas are divided into three subtypes: parosteal, periosteal or high-grade surface osteosarcomas, depending on whether they originate from the outer or inner layer of the periosteum, or arise from the bone surface.

Box 8.1 Skeletal manifestation of osteosarcomas

Intraosseous osteosarcomas

- more common in adolescents and young adults; second peak in old adulthood
- more common in males
- may cause lytic, sclerotic, or mixed bone lesions (e.g. "sunburst," "onion skin," "cauliflower," "moth-eaten")
- Codman's triangle (elevation of the periosteum, marginal to the tumour)
- single lesion (rare metastasis to other bones)

- extensive medullary involvement
- pathological fractures

Parosteal osteosarcomas

- more common in the third and fourth decade of life
- more common in females
- mostly on long bone metaphyses/diaphysis
- large masses of dense bone
- rare penetration into medullary cavity

Periosteal osteosarcomas

- onset in puberty or late adulthood
- more common in males
- extensive periosteal new bone formation
- rare spiculated reaction ("sunburst"), cortical erosion of underlying cortex ("saucerisation")
- rare extension into medullary cavity

(Data from Aufderheide and Rodríguez-Martín 1998; Brothwell 2012; di Ruffano and Waldron 2018; Gorlick and Khanna 2010; Kundu 2014; Lindsey et al. 2017; Marques 2019; Murphey et al. 2004; Ottaviani and Jaffe 2009; Steinbock 1976; Stoker 1986; Waldron 2020)

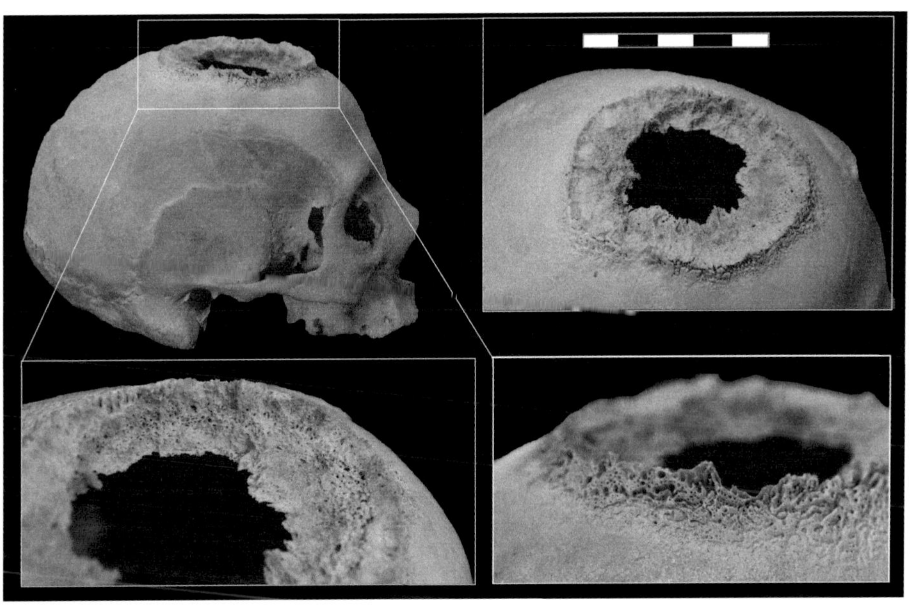

Figure 8.23 Probable osteosarcoma. Note the massive lytic lesion with perimetric new bone formation between the frontal and parietal bones. The lesion may instead represent a meningioma, but a differential diagnosis supporting a more likely osteosarcoma aetiology is provided at Tondini et al. (2024). (Gizeh E270; photos by Efthymia Nikita; copyright: Duckworth Laboratory, University of Cambridge)

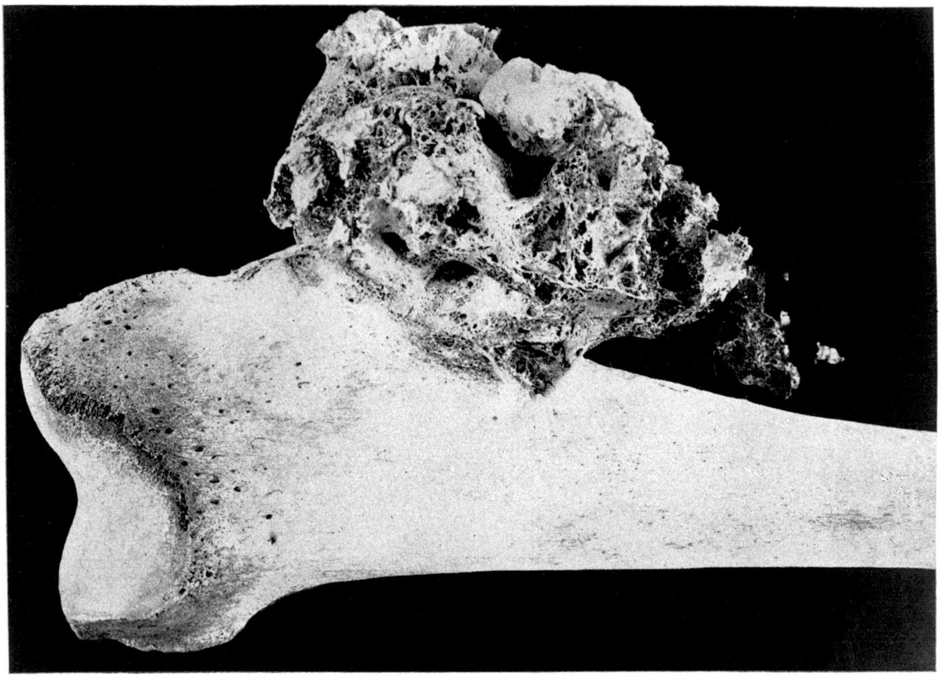

FIG. 64.—OSTEO-SARCOMA OF THE THIGH-BONE. (Vth DYNASTY)

Figure 8.24 Osteosarcoma of the distal femur, Egyptian, 5th Dynasty. (Egyptian mummies by G. Elliot Smith and Warren R. Dawson; with woodcuts by A. Horace Gerrard and K. Leigh-Pemberton and other illustrations. Source: Wellcome Collection; licensed under a Creative Commons Attribution 4.0 International License)

Ewing's sarcoma

Ewing's sarcoma is a bone tumour arising from mesenchymal stem cells (Figure 8.25). In some cases, it may not develop within the bones but in soft tissues (extraosseous Ewing's sarcoma). The aetiology of Ewing's sarcoma remains unknown. Specific genetic changes have been associated with this condition; however, they are not heritable. A rapid growth spurt may also make certain individuals more susceptible to Ewing's sarcoma, while a larger birthweight is another potentially important risk factor. In rare cases, Ewing's sarcoma can develop as a secondary malignancy in patients who have already received treatment for a different neoplastic condition.

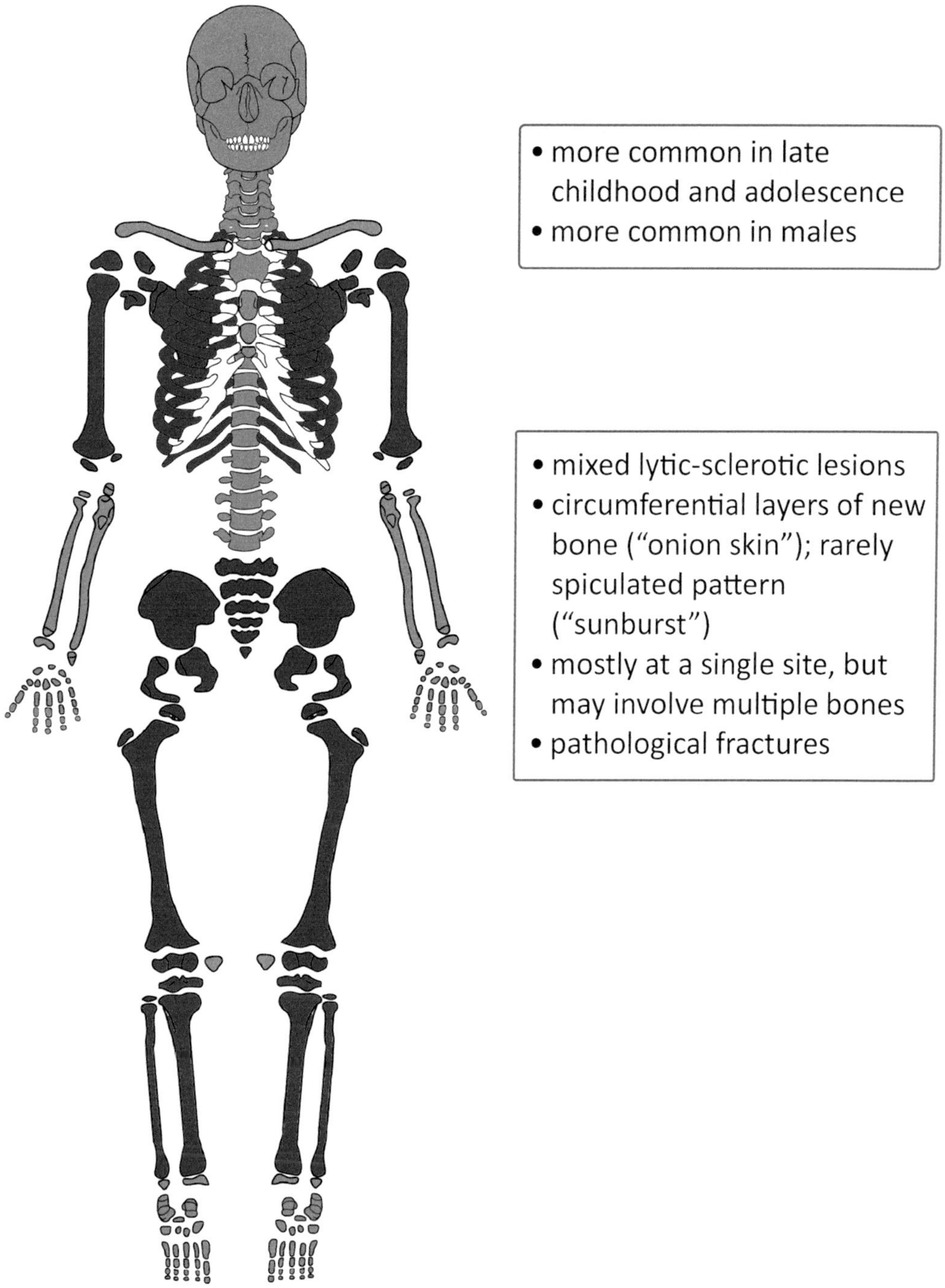

Figure 8.25 Skeletal manifestation of Ewing's sarcoma. (Data from Aufderheide and Rodríguez-Martín 1998, Peersman et al. 2007, Stoker 1986)

Chondrosarcoma

Chondrosarcoma is a neoplasm characterised by cartilage production (Figures 8.26 and 8.27). It may be primary or secondary. Primary chondrosarcomas appear in previously healthy bone tissue, whereas secondary chondrosarcomas develop from the malignant transformation of

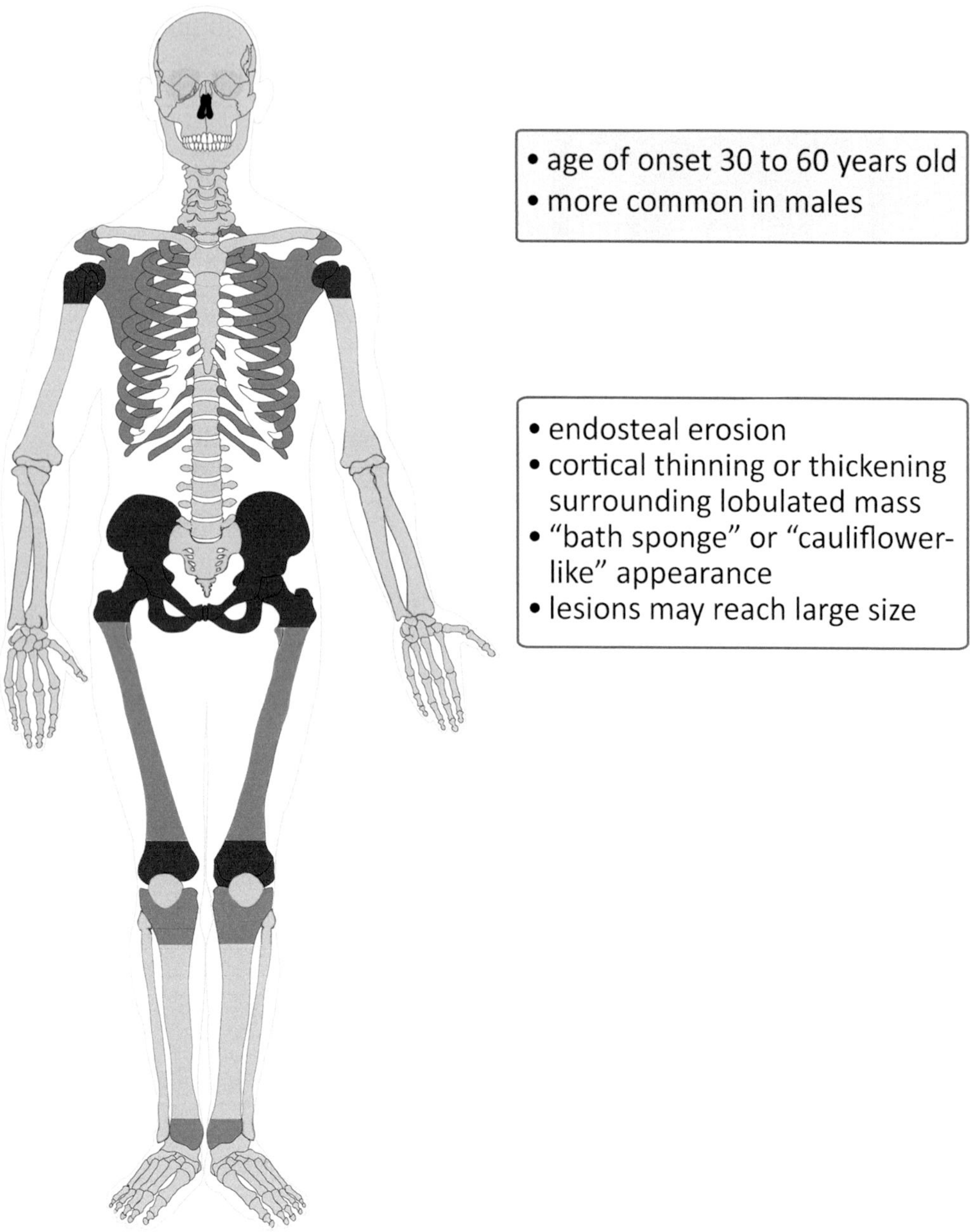

Figure 8.26 Skeletal manifestation of chondrosarcoma. (Data from Brothwell 2012; Chaabane et al. 2009; Donati and Bianchi 2020; Stoker 1986; Unni and Inwards 2010; Waldron 2020)

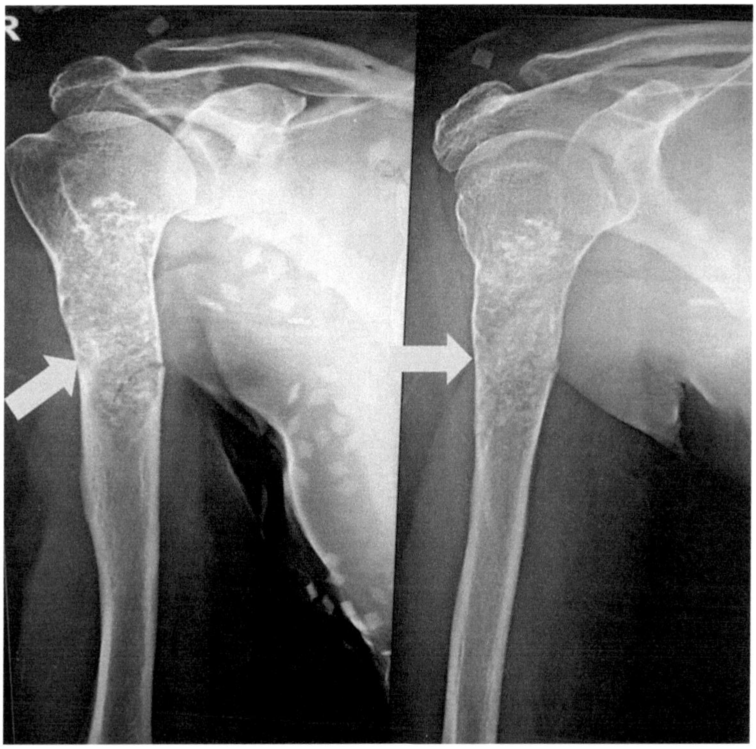

Figure 8.27 Radiographs showing chondrosarcoma in the proximal humerus. Note the thinned cortical bone and enlarged bone contour. (Figure 1 in Sarin et al. 2024; article licensed under a Creative Commons Attribution 4.0 International License)

pre-existing benign tumours, such as osteochondromas. Chondrosarcomas may develop within the medullary cavity of the bone (central chondrosarcomas) or on the bone surface (peripheral chondrosarcomas).

Chordoma

Chordomas are tumours that arise from notochordal cells that fail to regress completely during embryonic development (Figures 8.28 and 8.29). Although chordomas grow slowly, they can be aggressive and increase considerably in size, exerting pressure on adjacent tissues and organs. The aetiology of chordomas remains unclear; however, certain genetic changes have been associated with their development.

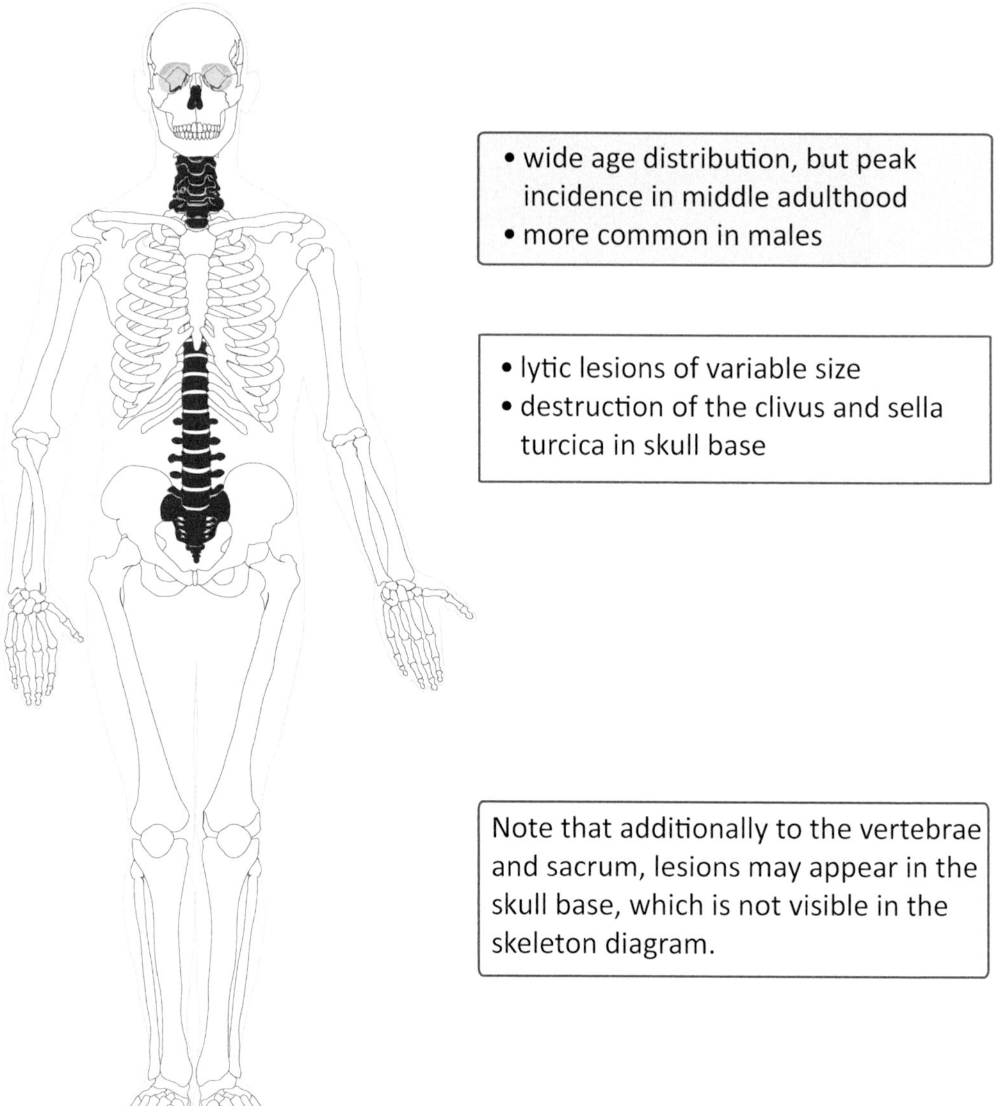

Figure 8.28 Skeletal manifestation of chordoma. (Data from Marques 2019; Ulici and Hart 2022; Unni and Inwards 2010)

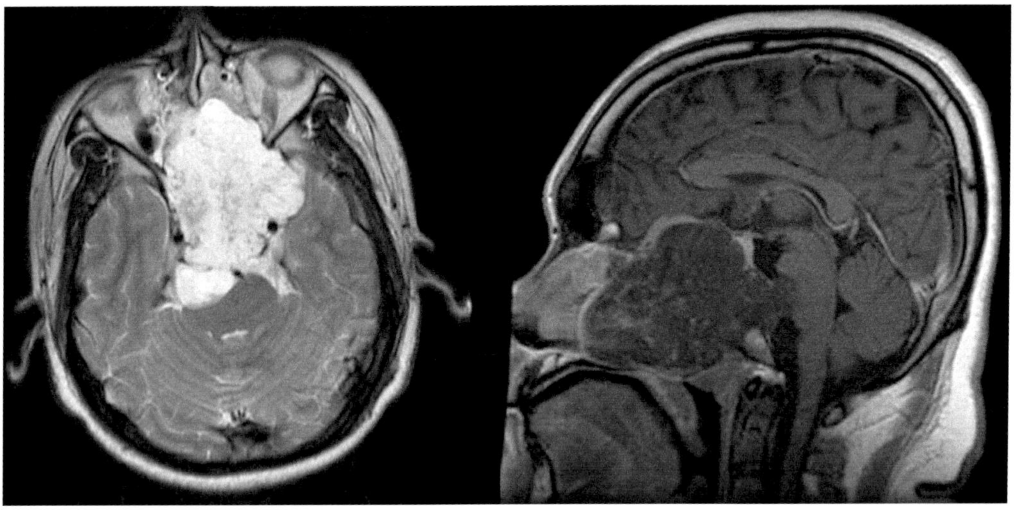

Figure 8.29 Brain MRI scan showing chordoma in the nasopharynx. (Figure 1 in Hassan et al. 2008; article licensed under a Creative Commons Attribution 2.0 Generic License)

Fibrosarcoma

Fibrosarcoma is a mesenchymal tumour, composed of fibroblasts. It may arise in the skeleton or in the soft tissues (Figure 8.30). According to its location on the bones, fibrosarcoma can be classified as central, when it develops within the medullary canal, or peripheral, when it originates from the periosteum. In addition, fibrosarcoma may be primary or secondary; secondary fibrosarcoma typically develops from an existing lesion or as a consequence of radiotherapy.

Depending on the age of onset, fibrosarcoma can be infantile (congenital) or adult-type. Infantile fibrosarcoma usually appears at birth or shortly after; it is unlikely to metastasise, and has a high probability of long-term survival. In contrast, adult-type fibrosarcoma is mostly found in adults but may also appear in children, and it is highly malignant.

The precise aetiology of fibrosarcoma remains undetermined; however, genetic mutations may contribute to its development. Moreover, fibrosarcoma has been associated with conditions such as bone infarction, chronic osteomyelitis, fibrous dysplasia, and Paget's disease of bone. Environmental risk factors have also been linked to this condition, including prior radiation therapy, severe burns, and exposure to specific metals found in orthopaedic implants.

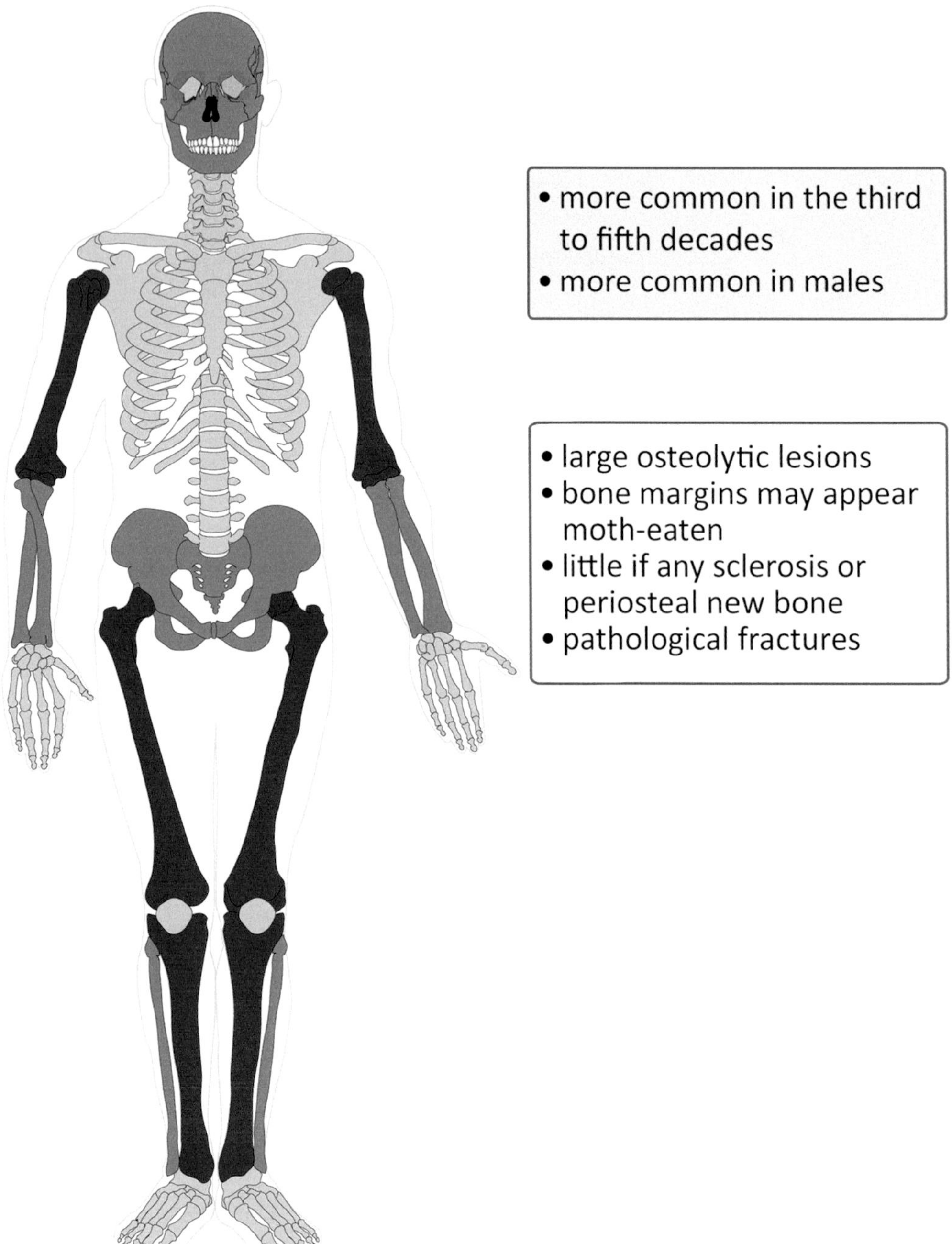

Figure 8.30 Skeletal manifestation of fibrosarcoma. (Data from Brothwell 2012; Dahlin and Ivins 1969; Huvos and Higinbotham 1975; Stoker 1986; Waldron 2020)

Angiosarcoma

Angiosarcomas are rare neoplasms that originate from the endothelial cells lining the walls of blood or lymph vessels (Figures 8.31 and 8.32). These tumours can appear throughout the body; however, they are more common in the skin of the head and neck, as well as in the liver, spleen, and breast. Angiosarcomas are aggressive tumours; they grow rapidly, tend to recur

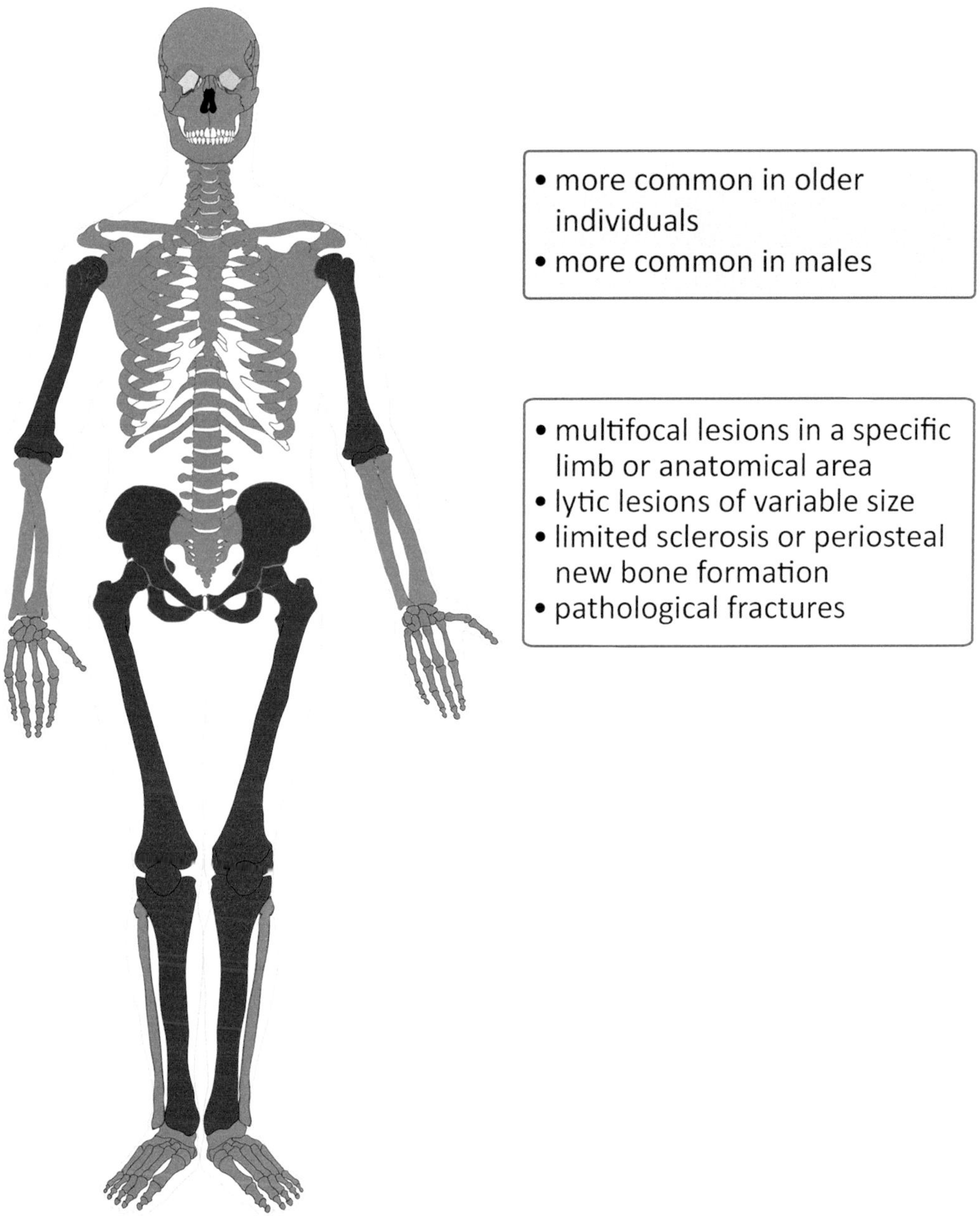

Figure 8.31 Skeletal manifestation of angiosarcoma. (Data from Chugh et al. 2014; Righi 2020; Roessner and Boehling 2002; Waldron 2020)

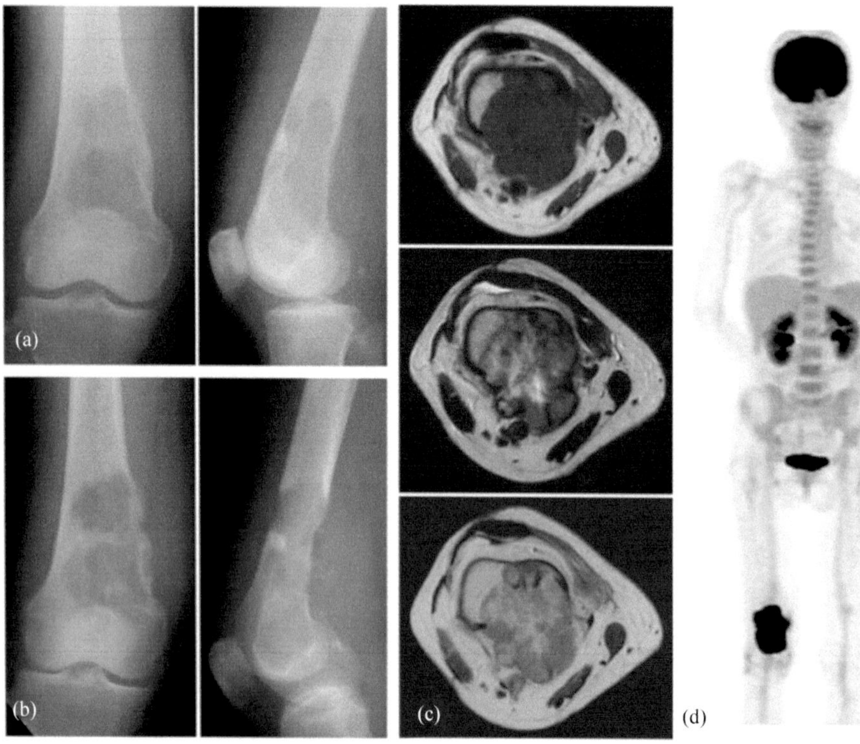

Figure 8.32 Imaging of individual with angiosarcoma. Note the lytic lesion in the distal femur (a), lesion enlargement after one month (b), lobulated lesion in MRI (c), and lesion in the distal femur in [18F]-2-fluoro-2-deoxy-D-glucose positron emission tomography (d). (Figure 1 in Sakamoto et al. 2014; article licensed under a Creative Commons Attribution 2.0 Generic License)

after treatment, and metastasise extensively. Their aetiology remains unknown; however, they have been associated with prior radiation therapy, chronic lymphedema, exposure to certain chemical toxins, familial syndromes (e.g. Maffucci syndrome), reaction to foreign bodies (e.g. synthetic materials used in prostheses), bone infarcts, Paget's disease of bone, and chronic osteomyelitis.

Metastatic bone disease

Skeletal metastases are malignant and spread to the skeleton through haematogenous, lymphatic, and cerebrospinal fluid routes, or via direct extension from the primary tumour site. Bone tissue is frequently targeted for tumour metastasis. This phenomenon can be attributed to the extensive vascular network of the skeletal system, alongside the skeleton's role as a reservoir of minerals and growth factors that facilitate the survival and proliferation of metastatic tumour cells.

Bone metastases predominantly arise through haematogenous dissemination. The vertebral column, femur, ribs, sternum, skull, pelvis, humerus, and shoulder girdle are frequently involved in metastases due to their important function in haematopoiesis. However, any skeletal element may be affected (Figures 8.33–8.50). While all types of cancer can metastasise to bone, breast, prostate, thyroid, lung, and kidney cancers are particularly likely to do so.

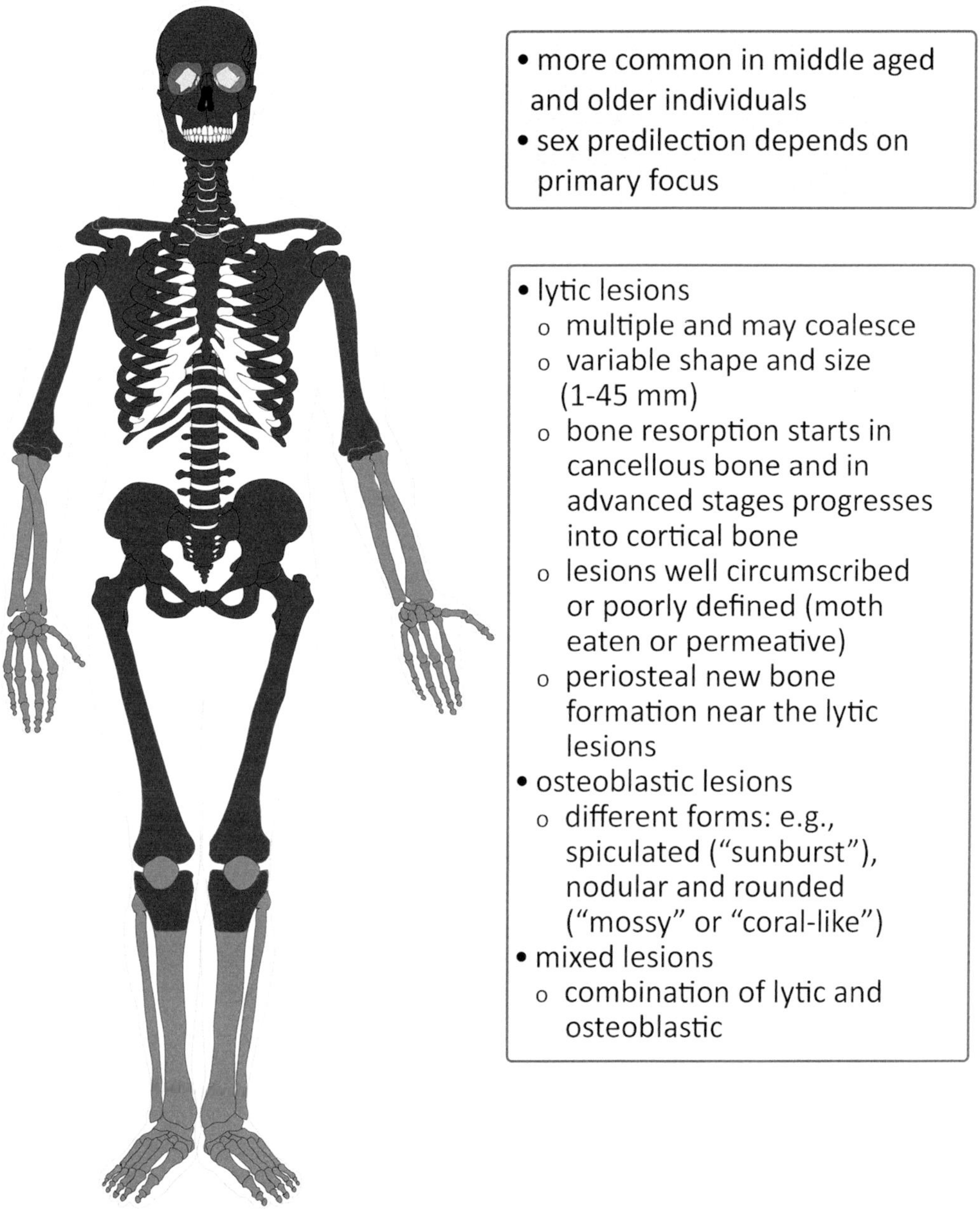

Figure 8.33 Skeletal manifestation of metastatic bone disease. (Data from Gambarotti and Sbaraglia 2020; Marks and Hamilton 2007; Mundy 1997; Ragsdale et al. 2018; Reith 2016; Rothschild and Rothschild 1995; Rothschild et al. 1998; Steinbock 1976; Strouhal 1991)

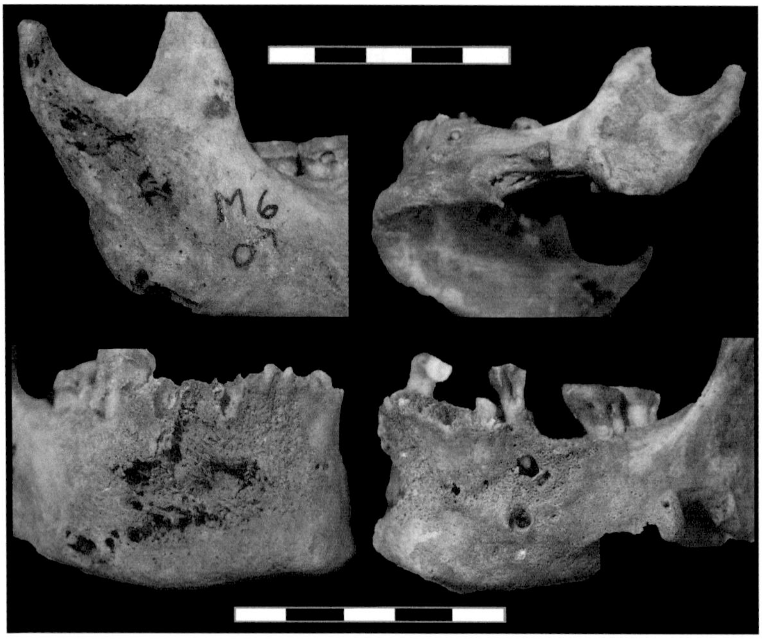

Figure 8.34 Predominantly osteolytic lesions of the mandible due to metastatic bone disease. Note the extensive lytic lesions of variable shape and size throughout this element; the bone surrounding them is heavily pitted, while new bone formation is seen at the inferior border of the corpus (upper and lower right). (Haya Af.23.0.114 AF 264; photos by Efthymia Nikita; copyright: Duckworth Laboratory, University of Cambridge)

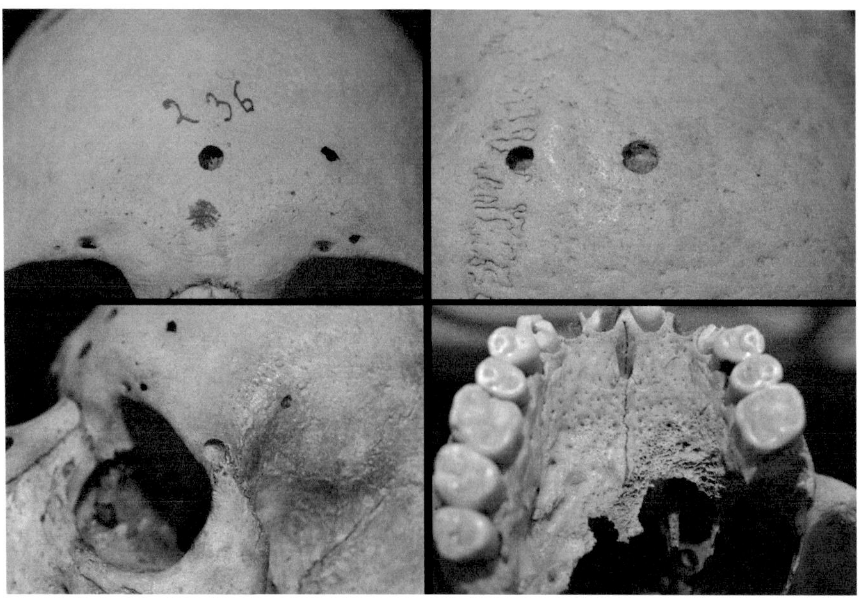

Figure 8.35 Metastatic bone disease in the cranium. Note the multiple lytic lesions on the frontal and parietal bones as well as the destruction of the hard palate. (Duckworth Laboratory EDN 236; photos by Efthymia Nikita; copyright: Duckworth Laboratory, University of Cambridge)

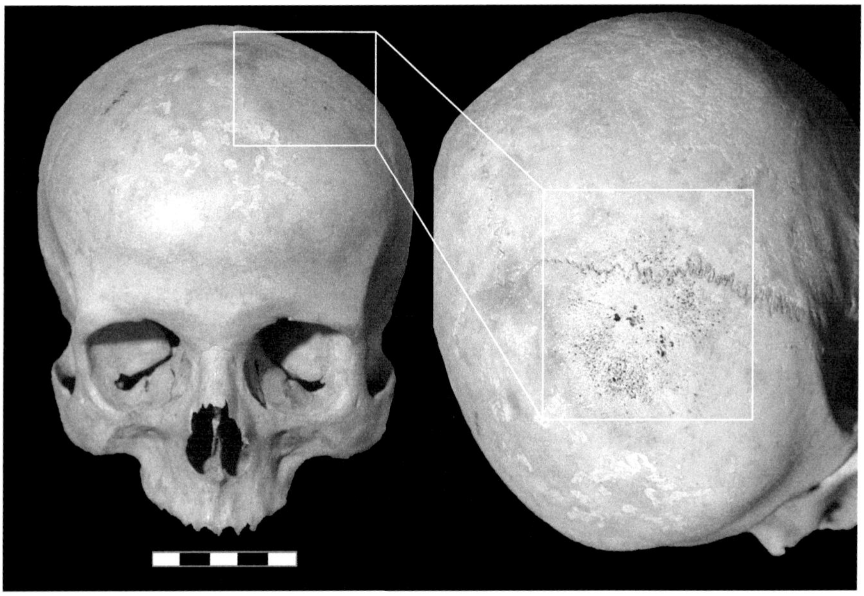

Figure 8.36 Metastatic bone disease. Note the wide area of coalescent porosity on the left part of the frontal bone. (Female, 49 years old, Athens Collection, WLH13, cause of death: lung cancer; photos by Efthymia Nikita, copyright: Athens Collection, Department of Animal and Human Physiology of the National and Kapodistrian University of Athens)

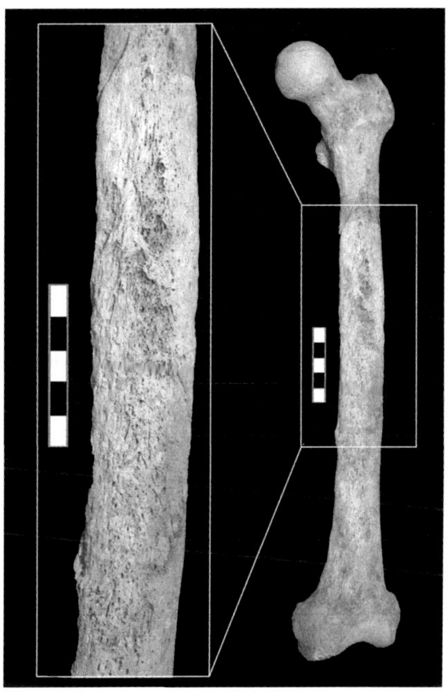

Figure 8.37 Metastatic bone disease. Note the extensive mixed (osteoblastic and osteolytic) lesion across the anterior of the diaphysis of the left femur. (Same individual as in Figure 8.36; photo by Efthymia Nikita; copyright: Athens Collection, Department of Animal and Human Physiology of the National and Kapodistrian University of Athens)

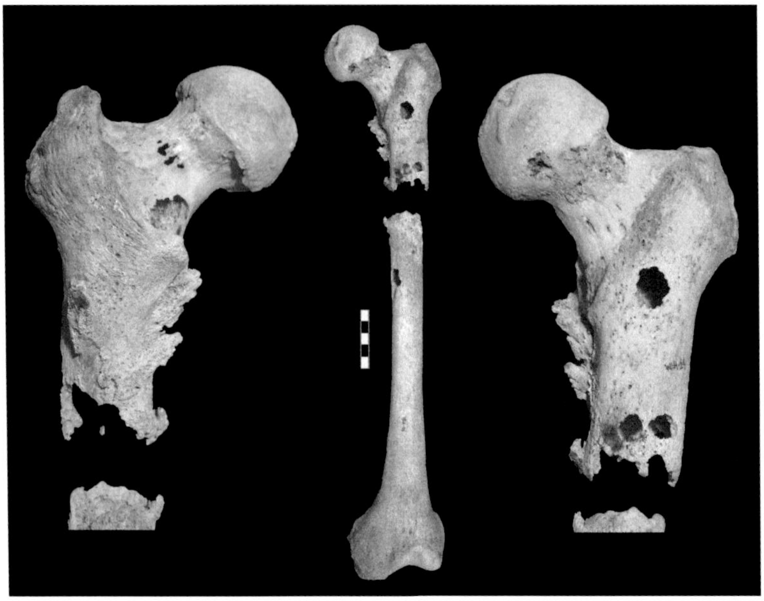

Figure 8.38 Metastatic bone disease. Note the extensive lytic lesions in the proximal half of the left femur, coupled with new bone formation. The lytic lesions are mostly circular or oval and of different sizes, and the bone has been weakened to the point that a transverse fracture has separated the proximal part from the rest of the element. (Male, 65 years old, Athens Collection, WLH14, cause of death: brain cancer; photos by Efthymia Nikita; copyright: Athens Collection, Department of Animal and Human Physiology of the National and Kapodistrian University of Athens)

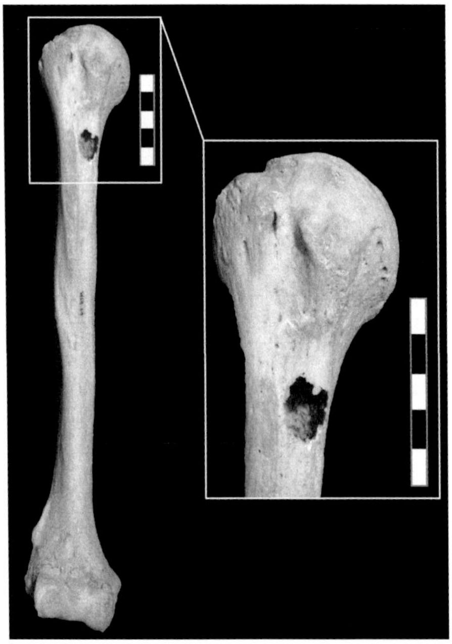

Figure 8.39 Metastatic bone disease. Note the solitary lytic lesion in the proximal right humerus. (Same individual as in Figure 8.38; photos by Efthymia Nikita; copyright: Athens Collection, Department of Animal and Human Physiology of the National and Kapodistrian University of Athens)

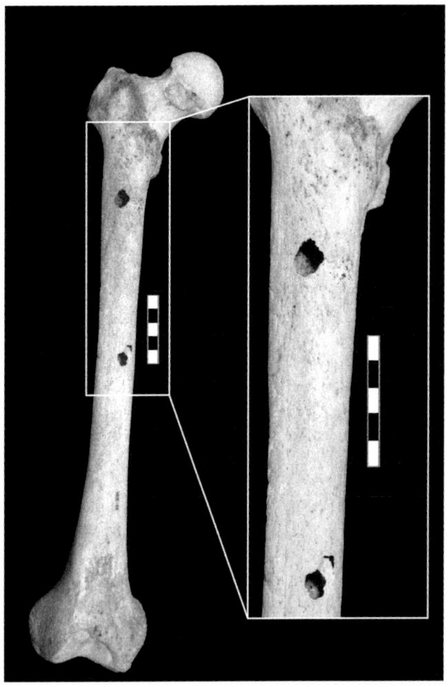

Figure 8.40 Metastatic bone disease. Note the two osteolytic lesions in the midshaft and proximal diaphysis of the right femur. (Same individual as in Figures 8.38 and 8.39; photos by Efthymia Nikita; copyright: Athens Collection, Department of Animal and Human Physiology of the National and Kapodistrian University of Athens)

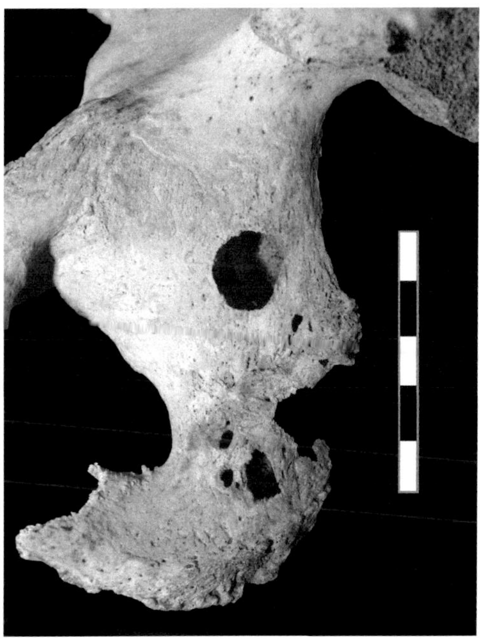

Figure 8.41 Metastatic bone disease. Note the predominantly osteolytic lesions of different shapes and sizes on the right os coxa. (Same individual as in Figures 8.38–8.40; photo by Efthymia Nikita; copyright: Athens Collection, Department of Animal and Human Physiology of the National and Kapodistrian University of Athens)

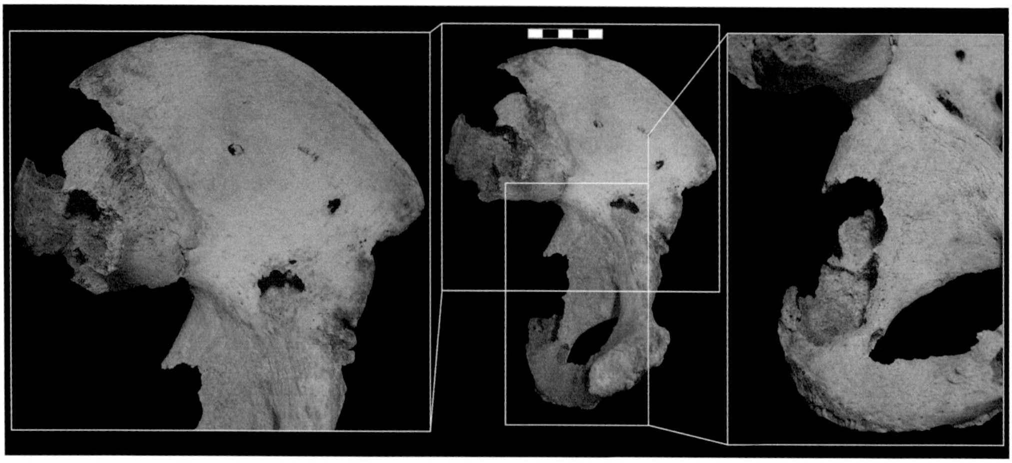

Figure 8.42 Metastatic bone disease. Note the osteolytic lesions of different shapes and sizes on the left os coxa. (Same individual as in Figures 8.38–8.41; photos by Efthymia Nikita; copyright: Athens Collection, Department of Animal and Human Physiology of the National and Kapodistrian University of Athens)

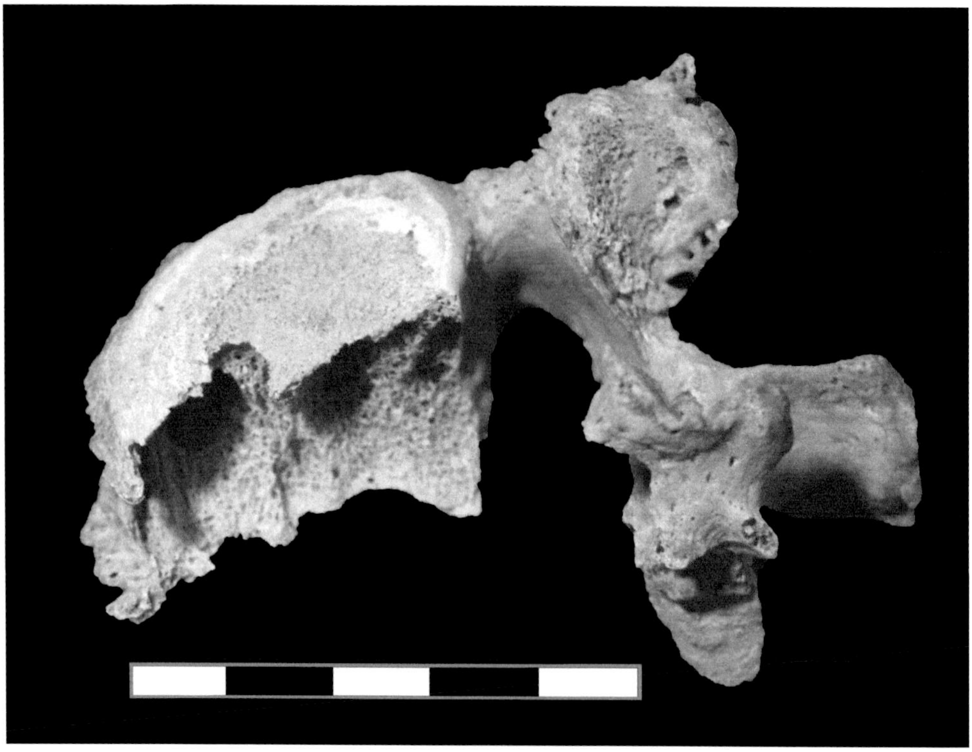

Figure 8.43 Metastatic bone disease. Note the lytic lesion that has resulted in the destruction of half of the vertebral body. (Same individual as in Figures 8.38–8.42; photo by Efthymia Nikita; copyright: Athens Collection, Department of Animal and Human Physiology of the National and Kapodistrian University of Athens)

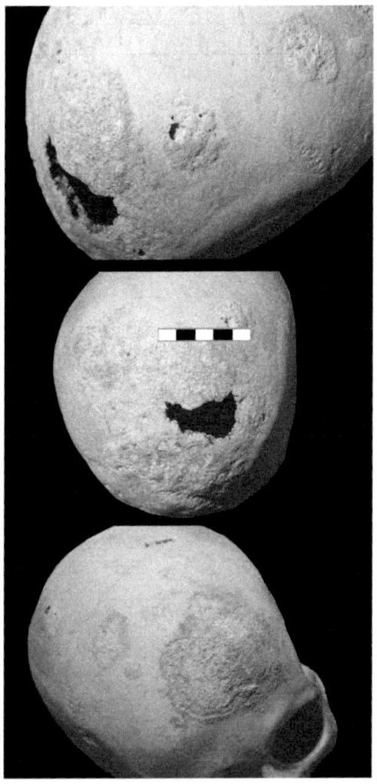

Figure 8.44 Metastatic bone disease. Note the mixed osteoblastic and osteolytic lesions of different sizes and shapes throughout the frontal and parietal bones. (Female, 68 years old, Athens Collection, WLH4; photos by Efthymia Nikita; copyright: Athens Collection, Department of Animal and Human Physiology of the National and Kapodistrian University of Athens)

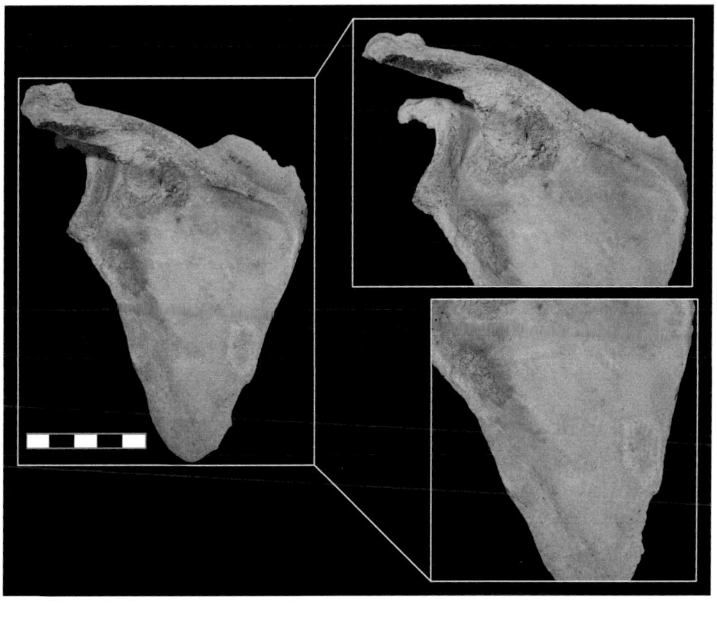

Figure 8.45 Metastatic bone disease. Note the nodular new bone formation throughout the left scapula. (Same individual as in Figure 8.44; photos by Efthymia Nikita; copyright: Athens Collection, Department of Animal and Human Physiology of the National and Kapodistrian University of Athens)

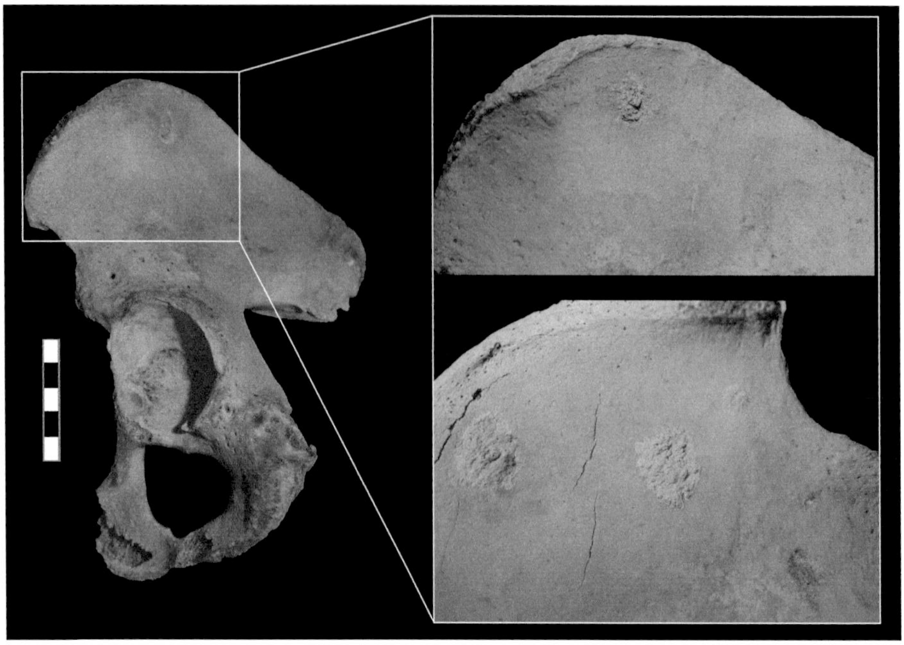

Figure 8.46 Metastatic bone disease. Note the osteoblastic lesions throughout the left ilium. (Same individual as in Figures 8.44 and 8.45; photos by Efthymia Nikita; copyright: Athens Collection, Department of Animal and Human Physiology of the National and Kapodistrian University of Athens)

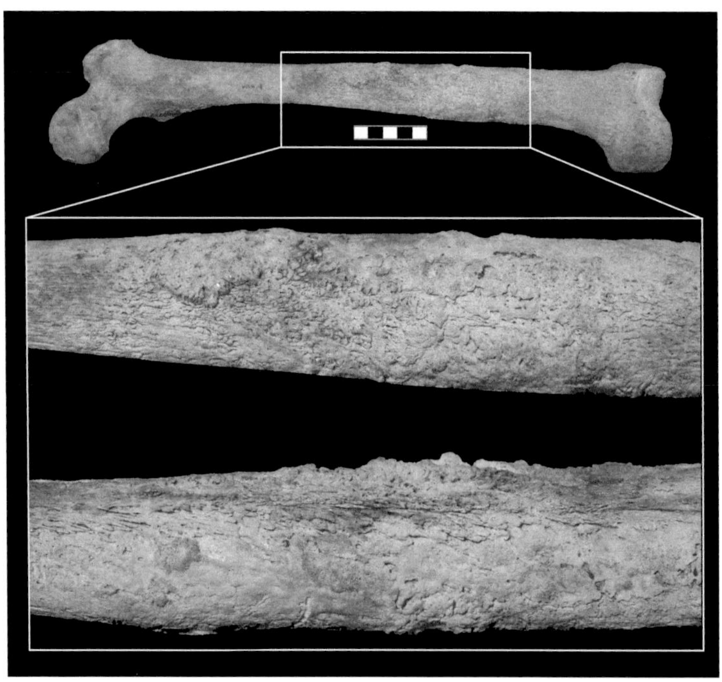

Figure 8.47 Metastatic bone disease. Note the nodular new bone formation throughout the left femoral diaphysis. (Same individual as in Figures 8.44–8.46; photos by Efthymia Nikita; copyright: Athens Collection, Department of Animal and Human Physiology of the National and Kapodistrian University of Athens)

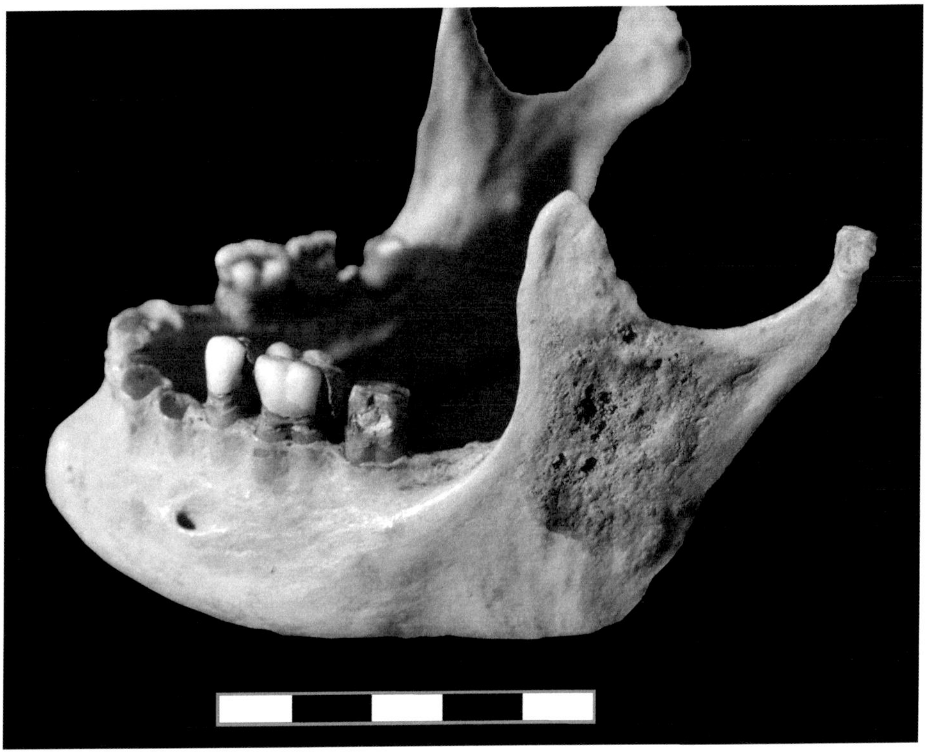

Figure 8.48 Metastatic bone disease. Note the lytic lesion on the left mandibular ramus, with minimal new bone formation surrounding it. (Same individual as in Figures 8.44–8.47; photo by Efthymia Nikita; copyright: Athens Collection, Department of Animal and Human Physiology of the National and Kapodistrian University of Athens)

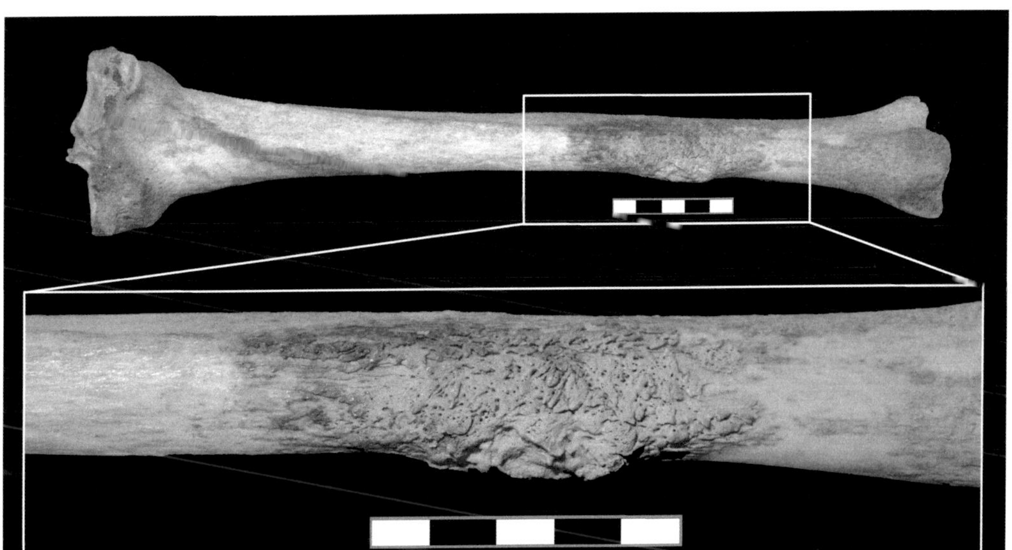

Figure 8.49 Metastatic bone disease. Note the nodular new bone formation at the distal part of the diaphysis of the right tibia. (Same individual as in Figures 8.44–8.48; photos by Efthymia Nikita; copyright: Athens Collection, Department of Animal and Human Physiology of the National and Kapodistrian University of Athens)

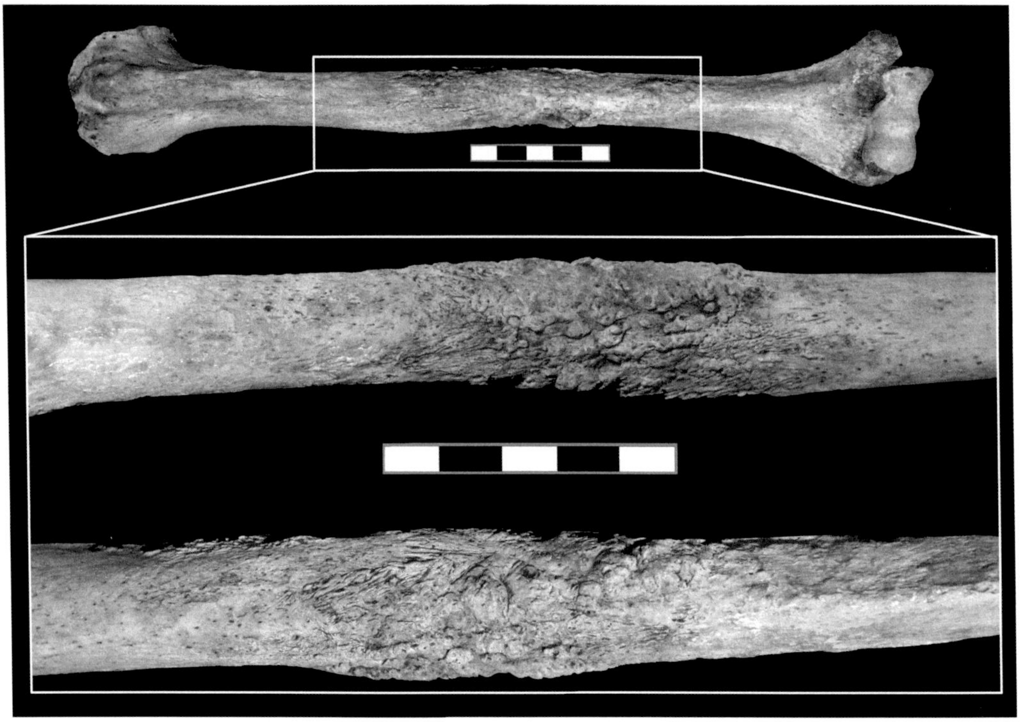

Figure 8.50 Metastatic bone disease. Note the nodular new bone formation at the midshaft of the right humerus. (Same individual as in Figures 8.44–8.49; photos by Efthymia Nikita; copyright: Athens Collection, Department of Animal and Human Physiology of the National and Kapodistrian University of Athens)

Metastatic lesions on the skeleton depend on the origin of the primary tumour, the duration of the disease, and the age of the patient. Metastases originating from kidney, thyroid, lung, and breast cancers are mostly osteolytic, whereas osteoblastic lesions are typically associated with prostate cancer and a small percentage of breast cancers.

Bone metastases tend to occur in highly vascularised parts of bone, specifically within trabecular bone. Therefore, they are often undetectable through macroscopic examination, and radiographic evaluation is essential for the identification of metastatic bone disease and for assessing its extent and severity. Moreover, metastatic bone disease is often confused with multiple myeloma, though various criteria have been proposed for the distinction of the two (Box 8.2).

Box 8.2 Differential diagnosis between multiple myeloma and metastatic bone disease

Multiple myeloma (MM) and metastatic bone disease (MBD) have several common characteristics. Both conditions principally affect individuals over 40 years old and involve multiple skeletal elements, particularly the axial skeleton, as well as the proximal femur and humerus. In addition, the lesions associated with these diseases are either exclusively or predominantly lytic. However, the following criteria may be used for their differentiation:

- lesion outline is regular and round, with sharp, punched-out edges in MM, while lesions are more irregular with denticulations and scallops in MBD
- lesion size is more consistent and ranges from small to medium in MM (unless different lesions have coalesced), while it is more variable and ranging from small to large in MBD
- lesions are more numerous and scattered through the skeleton in MM, but usually fewer and more localised in MBD
- surrounding bone surface is smooth in MM, but pitted in MBD
- osteoblastic reaction at the lesion edges or in the observable trabeculae is absent or minimal in MM, but slight or substantial in MBD
- obliteration of cortical and trabecular bone is seen in MM, but some cortical bone is preserved in MBD

Source: From Rothschild et al. (1998); Strouhal (1991)

Lesions of undefined or nonneoplastic nature

Bone cysts

Cysts are sacs containing air, fluid, or other substances; they can develop in various locations throughout the body. Most cysts are benign and often resolve without treatment. Their aetiology is multifactorial, with infections, obstructions in ducts, genetic conditions, developmental abnormalities, and chronic inflammation implicated in their development. The size of the cysts can vary substantially, and they may remain asymptomatic until they enlarge and cause discomfort.

Unicameral bone cyst

Unicameral bone cysts, often called simple or solitary bone cysts, are benign tumour-like lesions (Figures 8.51 and 8.52). They typically appear near the growth plates (active lesions;

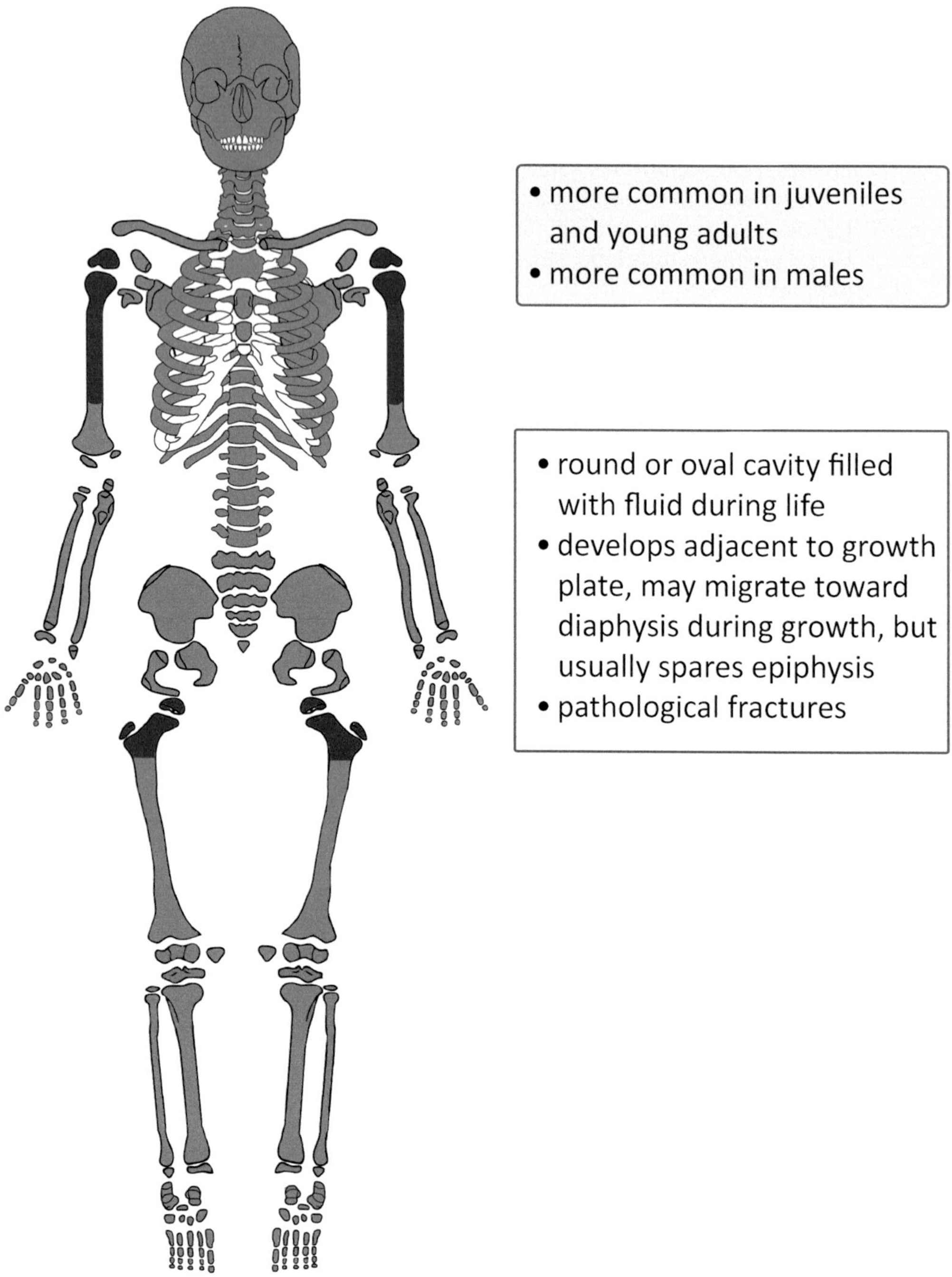

Figure 8.51 Skeletal manifestation of unicameral bone cyst. (Data from Campanacci 2020c; Isler and Turcotte 2003; Lenze et al. 2015; Marques 2019; Mascard et al. 2015; Waldron 2020)

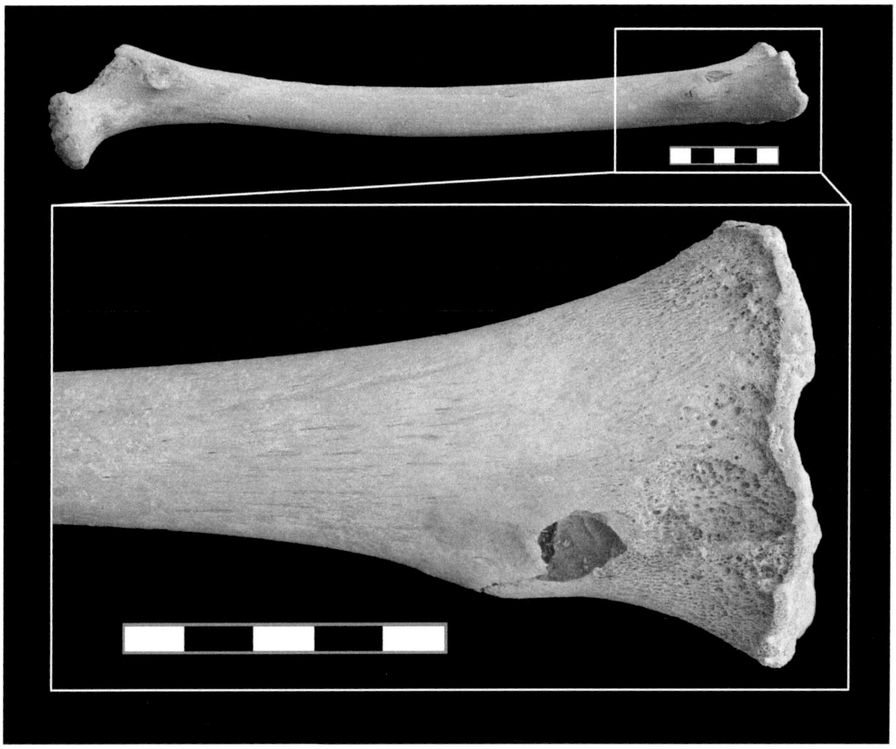

Figure 8.52 Possible unicameral bone cyst at the distal metaphysis of the right femur. Note the oval shape of the cavity where the bone cortex has been broken, and the expansion of the bone contour adjacent to this cavity. (Juvenile, Sbide, Roman/Byzantine; photos by Efthymia Nikita, with the kind permission of Dr. Ahmet Ihsan Aytek, Burdur Mehmet Akif Ersoy University)

usually uniloculated); however, as a child's skeleton grows, the cysts migrate away from these growth areas (latent lesions; maybe multiloculated). Unicameral bone cysts are mostly asymptomatic, but symptoms may appear, especially if the cysts result in pathological fractures.

Aneurysmal bone cyst

Aneurysmal bone cysts are benign, tumour-like, vascular lesions (Figure 8.53). They can be aggressive and locally destructive, compromising bone integrity and leading to pathological fractures. Such cysts may be primary or secondary, with secondary lesions arising as a consequence of a primary bone pathology, such as chondroblastoma, giant cell tumour, LCH, osteoblastoma, and osteosarcoma.

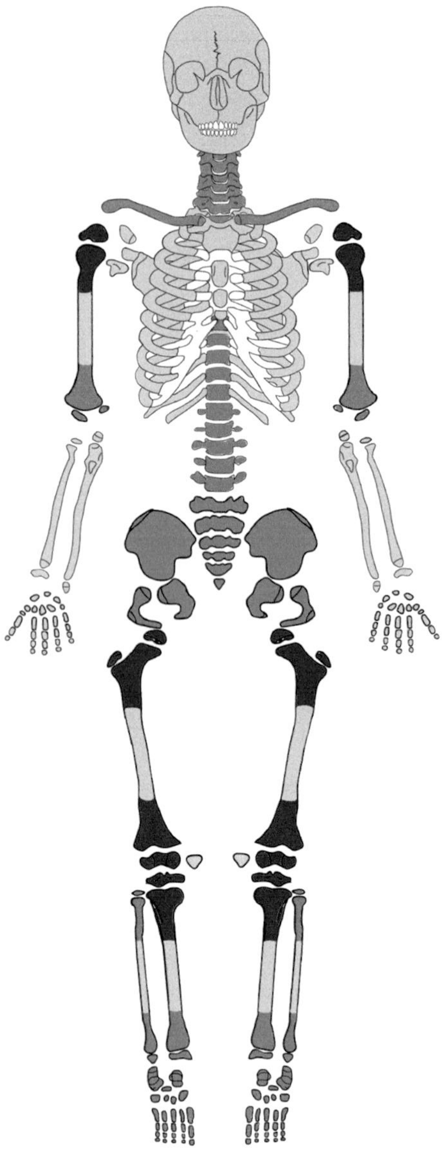

- more common in juveniles and young adults
- equally common in males and females

General
- small lytic lesion → gradually grows to distinct bulge (thin shell over eroded cortex) → progressive ossification and formation of bony mass

Skull
- lesions mostly on frontal bone

Vertebrae
- transverse processes and neural arches mostly affected
- large lesions → pressure defects on adjacent vertebrae

Arm/leg
- distal femur and proximal tibia mostly affected
- lesions usually in metaphysis, seldom in diaphysis or epiphysis
- widened bone contour

Figure 8.53 Skeletal manifestation of aneurysmal cyst. (Data from Campanacci 2020d; Khurana and Unni 2003; Mankin et al. 2005; Marques 2019; Mascard et al. 2015; Waldron 2020)

Osteoma

Osteomata are slow-growing bone-forming lesions (Box 8.3, Figures 8.54 and 8.55). Although they are generally asymptomatic, they may cause complications depending on their size and anatomical location. For example, an osteoma located close to the orbit may cause visual disturbances if it exerts pressure on the optic nerve.

Box 8.3 Skeletal manifestation of osteoma

- mostly found on frontal and parietal bones but can be present in paranasal sinuses and endocranial surface
- osseous mass made of compact and cancellous bone in different proportions
- small (up to 2 cm), but may grow large
- mostly solitary
- well-defined borders

(Data from Eshed et al. 2002, Larrea-Oyarbide et al. 2008, Marques 2019, Stoker 1986, Tarsitano et al. 2021)

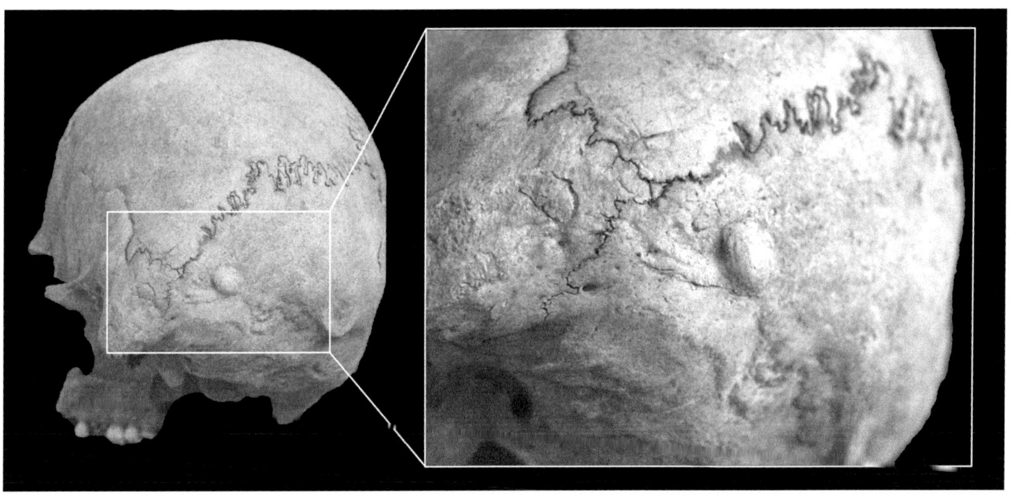

Figure 8.54 Well-defined and circumscribed "button" osteoma on the left side of the occipital bone. (Alanya Castle, Ottoman; photos by Efthymia Nikita, with the kind permission of Dr. Ahmet Ihsan Aytek, Burdur Mehmet Akif Ersoy University)

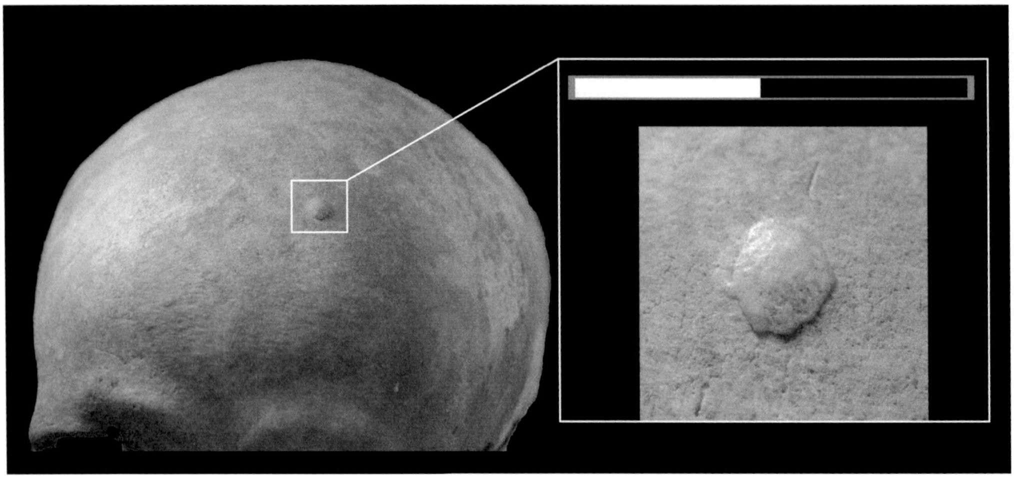

Figure 8.55 Well-defined and circumscribed "button" osteoma on the left side of the frontal bone. (Female, Older adult, St Hilda's Church, Coronation Street, South Shields, Newcastle, 19th c., CS06 952; photos by Efthymia Nikita; copyright: Human Skeletal Collection, University of Sheffield)

Whether osteomata are true neoplasms is a subject of debate given their unclear aetiology (Box 8.4). Three predominant theories have been proposed to explain their formation. The embryologic theory supports that osteomata arise from developmental anomalies occurring in the fronto-ethmoid region, but does not account for the high prevalence of osteomata away from this anatomical area. The traumatic theory posits that osteomata form due to prior trauma, but it cannot explain the great number of individuals who have osteomata but no documented history of trauma. The infectious theory suggests that osteomata arise from chronic inflammation that may trigger a proliferation of osteogenic cells within the periosteum. More recently, osteomata have been associated with mutations in the *CTNNB1* gene (Baumhoer et al. 2022).

Box 8.4 Button osteoma

Eshed et al. (2002) support that the circumscribed bony overgrowths observed on the cranial vault, commonly called button osteomas, should be classified as hamartomas based on their macrostructural and microstructural characteristics. This phenomenon, coupled with their high prevalence in both ancient and contemporary populations, their occurrence irrespective of sex and ancestry, and their rarity among other primate species, led the authors to further propose that these lesions may result from the accelerated growth of the human skull, particularly the calvarium, during foetal development and early life.

Nonossifying fibroma

The nonossifying fibroma is a benign proliferation of fibrous tissue (Figure 8.56). It is most likely to be a developmental abnormality rather than a true neoplasm. In the literature, nonossifying fibromas are frequently referred to as fibrous cortical defects; however, the two may be distinguished based on their size and progression. In specific, fibrous cortical defects are typically smaller than 3 cm and tend to heal spontaneously, although there are cases where they may enlarge and progress into nonossifying fibromas.

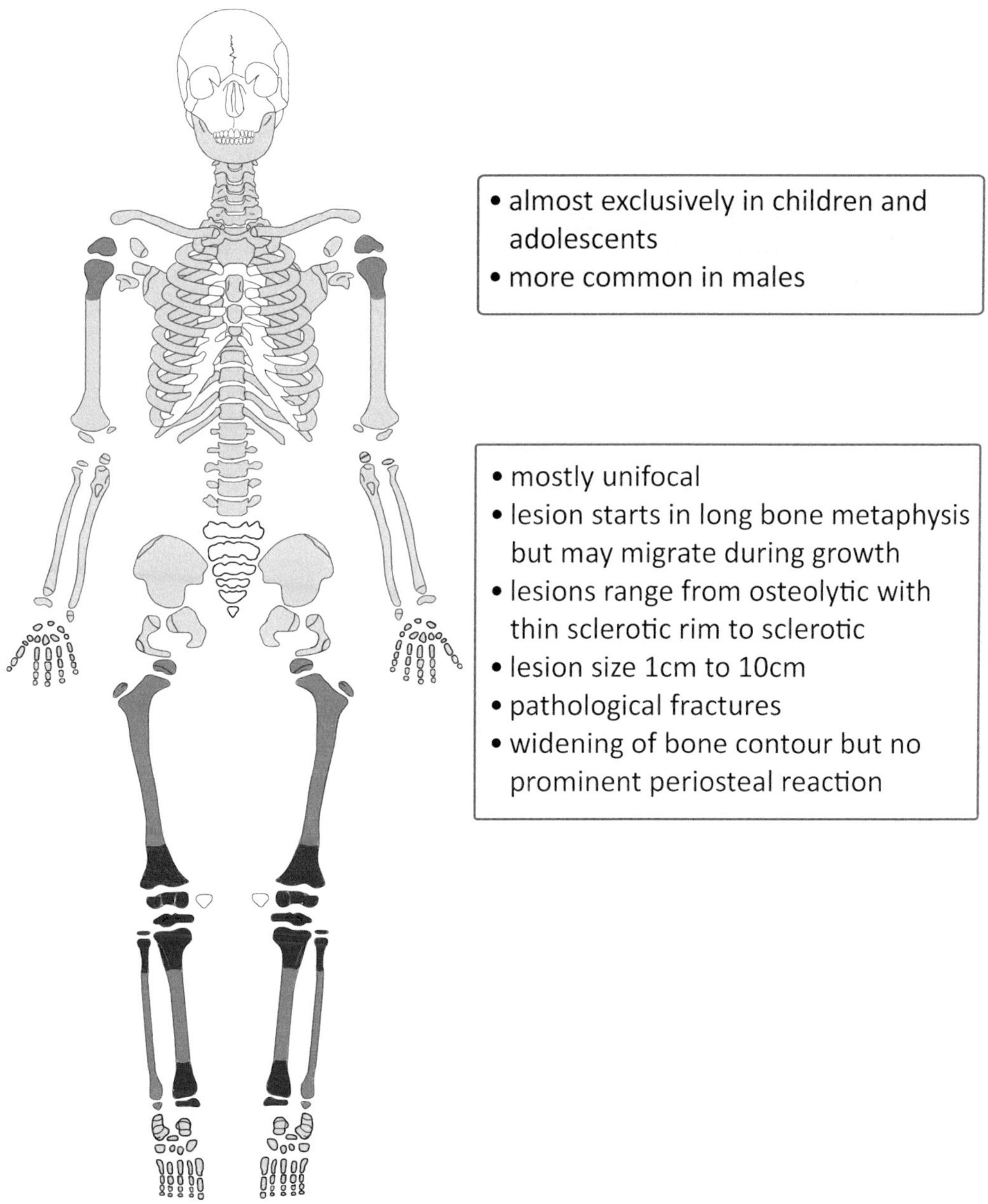

Figure 8.56 Skeletal manifestation of nonossifying fibroma. (Data from Błaż et al. 2011; Caffey 1955; Campanacci 2020e; Herget et al. 2016; Marques 2019; Stoker 1986)

References and suggested readings

Atesok, K.I., Alman, B.A., Schemitsch, E.H. (2011). Osteoid osteoma and osteoblastoma. *Journal of the American Academy of Orthopaedic Surgeons* 19:678–689.

Aufderheide, A.C., Rodríguez-Martín, C. (1998). *The Cambridge Encyclopedia of Human Paleopathology*. Cambridge: Cambridge University Press.

Azouz, E.M., Saigal, G., Rodriguez, M.M., Podda, A. (2005). Langerhans' cell histiocytosis: Pathology, imaging and treatment of skeletal involvement. *Pediatric Radiology* 35:103–115. https://doi.org/10.1007/s00247-004-1262-0

Badders, J.D., Carmichael, K.D. (2023). Spontaneous resolution of an osteochondroma. *Cureus* 15:e37565. https://doi.org/10.7759/cureus.37565

Bastug, D., Ortiz, O., Schochet, S.S. (1995). Haemangiomas in the calvaria: Imaging findings. *American Journal of Roentgenology* 164:683–687. https://doi.org/10.2214/ajr.164.3.7863894

Baumhoer, D., Berthold, R., Isfort, I., Heinst, L., Ameline, B. Grünewald, I., Thieringer, F.M., Rudack, C., Wardelmann, E., Vieth, V., Sperveslage, J.,Trautmann, M., Hartmann, W. (2022). Recurrent *CTNNB1* mutations in craniofacial osteomas. *Modern Pathology* 35:489–494. https://doi.org/10.1038/s41379-021-00956-x

Bessler, W., Eich, G., Stuckmann, G., Zollikofer, Ch. (1997). Kissing osteochondromata leading to synostoses. *European Radiology* 7:480–485. https://doi.org/10.1007/s003300050188

Bhamra, J.S., Al-Khateeb, H., Dhinsa, B.S., Gikas, P.D., Tirabosco, R., Pollock, R.C., Skinner, J.A., Aston, W.J., Saifuddin, A., Briggs, T.W. (2014). Chondromyxoid fibroma management: A single institution experience of 22 cases. *World Journal of Surgical Oncology* 12:283. https://doi.org/10.1186/1477-7819-12-283

Bhure, U., Roos, J. E., & Strobel, K. (2019). Osteoid osteoma: Multimodality imaging with focus on hybrid imaging. *European Journal of Nuclear Medicine and Molecular Imaging* 46:1019–1036. https://doi.org/10.1007/s00259-018-4181-2

Błaż, M., Palczewski, P., Świątkowski, J., Gołębiowski, M. (2011). Cortical fibrous defects and non-ossifying fibromas in children and young adults: The analysis of radiological features in 28 cases and a review of literature. *Polish Journal of Radiology* 76:32–39.

Brkić, H., Hodžić, M., Moranjkić, M. (2013). Intracranial meningioma--ten-year evaluation. *Medicinski Glasnik (Zenica)* 10:157–160.

Brothwell, D. (2012). Tumors: Problems of differential diagnosis in paleopathology. In *A Companion to Paleopathology*, edited by Grauer, A.L., pp. 420–433. Hoboken, NJ: John Wiley & Sons.

Caffey, J. (1955). On fibrous defects in cortical walls of growing tubular bones: Their radiologic appearance, structure, prevalence, natural course, and diagnostic significance. *Advances in Pediatrics* 7:13–15. https://doi.org/10.1016/S0065-3101(22)00436-4

Campanacci, L. (2020a). Osteoid osteoma. In *Diagnosis of Musculoskeletal Tumors and Tumor-like Conditions*, edited by Picci, P., Manfrini, M., Donati, D.M., Gambarotti, M., Righi, A., Vanel, D., Dei Tos, A.P., *2nd edition*, pp. 89–92. Berlin: Springer.

Campanacci, L. (2020b). Osteoblastoma. In *Diagnosis of Musculoskeletal Tumors and Tumor-like Conditions*, edited by Picci, P., Manfrini, M., Donati, D.M., Gambarotti, M., Righi, A., Vanel, D., Dei Tos, A.P., 2nd edition, pp. 93–96. Berlin: Springer.

Campanacci, L. (2020c). Simple bone cyst (unicameral bone cyst). In *Diagnosis of Musculoskeletal Tumors and Tumor-like Conditions*, edited by Picci, P., Manfrini, M., Donati, D.M., Gambarotti, M., Righi, A., Vanel, D., Dei Tos, A.P., 2nd edition, pp. 37–40. Berlin: Springer.

Campanacci, L. (2020d). Aneurysmal bone cyst (ABC). In *Diagnosis of Musculoskeletal Tumors and Tumor-like Conditions*, edited by Picci, P., Manfrini, M., Donati, D.M., Gambarotti, M., Righi, A., Vanel, D., Dei Tos, A.P., 2nd edition, pp. 97–100. Berlin: Springer.

Campanacci, L. (2020e). Histiocytic fibroma. In *Diagnosis of Musculoskeletal Tumors and Tumor-like Conditions*, edited by Picci, P., Manfrini, M., Donati, D.M., Gambarotti, M., Righi, A., Vanel, D., Dei Tos, A.P., 2nd edition, pp. 47–50. Berlin: Springer.

Campillo, D. (1991). The possibility of diagnosing meningiomas in palaeopathology. *International Journal of Osteoarchaeology* 1:225–230. https://doi.org/10.1002/oa.1390010315

Cao, X., Chen, X., Wang, Y., Feng, S., Wang, Z. (2022). Case report: Cavernous hemangioma in the right frontoparietal junction. *Frontiers in Surgery* 9:972641. https://doi.org/10.3389/fsurg.2022.972641

Cappelle, S., Pans, S., Sciot, R. (2016). Imaging features of chondromyxoid fibroma: Report of 15 cases and literature review. *British Journal of Radiology* 89:20160088. https://doi.org/10.1259/bjr.20160088

Chaabane, S., Bouaziz, M.C., Drissi, C., Abid, L., Ladeb, M.F. (2009). Periosteal chondrosarcoma. *American Journal of Roentgenology* 192:W1–W6. https://doi.org/10.2214/AJR.08.1159

Chugh, A.P., Gandhoke, C.S., Mohite, A.G., Khedkar, B.V. (2014). Primary angiosarcoma of the skull: A rare case report. *Surgical Neurology International* 5:92. https://doi.org/10.4103/2152-7806.134365

Dahlin, D.C., Ivins, J.C. (1969). Fibrosarcoma of bone: A study of 114 cases. *Cancer* 23:35–41. https://doi.org/10.1002/1097-0142(196901)23:1<35::aid-cncr2820230104>3.0.co;2-v

Di Cristofori, A., Del Bene, M., Locatelli, M., Boggio, F., Ercoli, G., Ferrero, S., Del Gobbo, A. (2018). Meningioma and bone hyperostosis: Expression of bone stimulating factors and review of the literature. *World Neurosurgery* 115:e774–e781. https://doi.org/10.1016/j.wneu.2018.04.176

Di Ruffano, L.F., Waldron, T. (2018). On the importance of considering disease subtypes: Earliest detection of a parosteal osteosarcoma? Differential diagnosis of an osteosarcoma in an Anglo–Saxon female. *International Journal of Paleopathology* 21:128–137. https://doi.org/10.1016/j.ijpp.2016.12.001

Donati, D.M., Bianchi, G. (2020). Chondrosarcomas. In *Diagnosis of Musculoskeletal Tumors and Tumor-like Conditions*, edited by Picci, P., Manfrini, M., Donati, D.M., Gambarotti, M., Righi, A., Vanel, D., Dei Tos, A.P., 2nd edition, pp. 157–180. Berlin: Springer.

Donati, D.M., Staals, E.L. (2020a). Chondromas. In *Diagnosis of Musculoskeletal Tumors and Tumor-like Conditions*, edited by Picci, P., Manfrini, M., Donati, D.M., Gambarotti, M., Righi, A., Vanel, D., Dei Tos, A.P., 2nd edition, pp. 65–74. Berlin: Springer.

Donati, D.M., Staals, E.L. (2020b). Osteochondromas. In *Diagnosis of Musculoskeletal Tumors and Tumor-like Conditions*, edited by Picci, P., Manfrini, M., Donati, D.M., Gambarotti, M., Righi, A., Vanel, D., Dei Tos, A.P., 2nd edition, pp. 75–81. Berlin: Springer.

Douis, H., Saifuddin, A. (2012). The imaging of cartilaginous bone tumours. I. Benign lesions. *Skeletal Radiology* 41:1195–1212. https://doi.org/10.1007/s00256-012-1427-0

Dudley, R.W., Torok, M.R., Randall, S., Béland, B., Handler, M.H., Mulcahy-Levy, J.M., Liu, A.K., Hankinson, T. C. (2018). Pediatric versus adult meningioma: Comparison of epidemiology, treatments, and outcomes using the Surveillance, Epidemiology, and End Results database. *Journal of Neuro-Oncology* 137:621–629. https://doi.org/10.1007/s11060-018-2756-1

Ellingsen, T., Nalley, A., Oda, D., Dodson, T.B., Lee, P.P. (2022). Osteoblastoma and osteoid osteoma of the mandible: Review of the literature and report of two cases. *Case Reports in Dentistry* 2022:7623855. https://doi.org/10.1155/2022/7623855

Erickson, K., Rosenthal, J., Rosenthal, I., Zaleske, J.D., Gebhardt, M.D., Cates, M.J. (2001). Primary treatment of chondroblastoma with percutaneous radio-frequency heat ablation: Report of three cases. *Radiology* 221:463–468. https://doi.org/10.1148/radiol.2212010262

Eshed, V., Latimer, B., Greenwald, C.M., Jellema, L.M., Rothschild, B.M., Wish-Baratz, S., Hershkovitz, I. (2002). Button osteoma: Its etiology and pathophysiology. *American Journal of Physical Anthropology* 118:217–230. https://doi.org/10.1002/ajpa.10087

Ewald, P.W. (2018). Ancient cancers and infection-induced oncogenesis. *International Journal of Paleopathology* 21:178–185. https://doi.org/10.1016/j.ijpp.2017.08.007

Fatula, S. (2021). Detection of cancerous lesions in skeletal remains using visual methods and radiographs. *International Journal of Osteoarchaeology* 31:916–925. https://doi.org/10.1002/oa.3008

Fox, M.W., Onofrio, B.M. (1993). The natural history and management of symptomatic and asymptomatic vertebral hemangiomas. *Journal of Neurosurgery* 78:36–45. https://doi.org/10.3171/jns.1993.78.1.0036

Gadelha Vasconcelos, R., Gadelha Vasconcelos, M., Guedes Queiroz, L.M. (2013). Peripheral and central giant cell lesions: Etiology, origin of giant cells, diagnosis and treatment. *Jornal Brasileiro de Patologia e Medicina Laboratorial* 49:446–452. https://doi.org/10.1590/S1676-24442013000600011

Gambarotti, M., Sbaraglia, M. (2020). Metastatic lesions. In *Diagnosis of Musculoskeletal Tumors and Tumor-like Conditions*, edited by Picci, P., Manfrini, M., Donati, D.M., Gambarotti, M., Righi, A., Vanel, D., Dei Tos, A.P., 2nd edition, pp. 357–362. Berlin: Springer.

Gorlick, R., Khanna, C. (2010). Osteosarcoma. *Journal of Bone and Mineral Research* 25:683–691. https://doi.org/10.1002/jbmr.77

Grauer, A.L. (2019). Circulatory, reticuloendothelial, and hematopoietic disorders. In *Ortner's Identification of Pathological Conditions in Human Skeletal Remains*, edited by Buikstra, J., pp. 491–530. San Diego: Academic Press.

Hakim, D.N., Pelly, T., Kulendran, M., Caris, J.A. (2015). Benign tumours of the bone: A review. *Journal of Bone Oncology* 4:37–41. https://doi.org/10.1016/j.jbo.2015.02.001

Hassan, S., Abdullah, J.M., Wan Din, S.J., Idris, Z. (2008). Combined use of maxillomandibular swing approach and neurosurgical ultrasonic aspirator in the management of extensive clival chordoma: A case report. *Journal of Medical Case Reports* 2:49. https://doi.org/10.1186/1752-1947-2-49

Herget, G.W., Mauer, D., Krauss, T., El Tayeh, A., Uhl, M., Südkamp, N.P., Hauschild, O. (2016). Non-ossifying fibroma: Natural history with an emphasis on astage-related growth, fracture risk and the need for follow-up. *BMC Musculoskeletal Disorders* 17:147. https://doi.org/10.1186/s12891-016-1004-0

Hunt, K.J., Roberts, C., Kirkpatrick, C. (2018). Taking stock: A systematic review of archaeological evidence of cancers in human and early hominin remains. *International Journal of Paleopathology* 21:12–26. https://doi.org/10.1016/j.ijpp.2018.03.002

Huvos, A.G., Higinbotham, N.L. (1975). Primary fibrosarcoma of bone. A clinicopathologic study of 130 patients. *Cancer* 35:837–847.

Imura, Y., Shigi, A., Outani, H., Hamada, K., Tamura, H., Morii, E., Myoui, A., Yoshikawa, H., Naka, N. (2014). A giant periosteal chondroma of the distal femur successfully reconstructed with synthetic bone grafts and a bioresorbable plate: A case report. *World Journal of Surgical Oncology* 12:354. https://doi.org/10.1186/1477-7819-12-354

Isler, M., Turcotte, R. (2003). Bone tumors in children. In *Pediatric Bone: Biology and Diseases*, edited by Glorieux, F., Pettifor, J., Jüppner, M., pp. 703–743. New York: Academic Press.

Jaffe, H.L. (1958). *Tumors and Tumorous Conditions of the Bones and Joints*. Philadelphia: Lea and Febiger.

Khurana, J., Abdul-Karim, F., Bovée, J. (2002). Osteochondroma. In *Pathology and Genetics of Tumours of Soft Tissue and Bone*, edited by Fletcher, C., Unni, K., Mertens, F., 3rd edition, pp. 234–236. Lyon: International Agency for Research on Cancer.

Khurana, J., Unni, K. (2003). Pathological diagnosis of common tumours of bone and cartilage. In *Handbook of Histology Methods for Bone and Cartilage*, edited by Yuehuei, H., Martin, K., pp. 447–494. New Jersey: Humana Press.

Kirkpatrick, C.L. (2023). Tumors and neoplastic diseases: Assessing antiquity and pondering prevalence. In *Routledge Handbook of Paleopathology*, edited by Grauer, A.L., pp. 271–291. New York: Routledge.

Kissane, J.M., Askin, F.B., Foulkes, M., Stratton, L.B., Shirley, S.F. (1983). Ewing's sarcoma of bone: Clinicopathologic aspects of 303 cases from the Intergroup Ewing's Sarcoma Study. *Human Pathology* 14:773–779. https://doi.org/10.1016/S0046-8177(83)80300-1

Kundu, Z.S. (2014). Classification, imaging, biopsy and staging of osteosarcoma. *Indian Journal of Orthopaedics* 48:238–246. https://doi.org/10.4103/0019-5413.132491

Lambert, J., Verstraeten, T., Mermuys, K. (2016). Chondroblastoma: An unusual cause of shoulder pain in adolescence. *Journal of the Belgian Society of Radiology* 100:16. https://doi.org/10.5334/jbr-btr.1027

Larrea-Oyarbide, N., Valmaseda-Castello, E., Berini-Ayte, L., Gay-Escoda, C. (2008). Osteomas of the craniofacial region. Review of 106 cases. *Journal of Oral Pathology & Medicine* 37:38–42. https://doi.org/10.1111/j.1600-0714.2007.00590.x

Leddy, L.R., Holmes, R.E. (2014). Chondrosarcoma of bone. In *Orthopaedic Oncology: Primary and Metastatic Tumors of the Skeletal System*, edited by Peabody, T.D., Attar, S., pp. 117–130. Cham: Springer.

Leenknegt, B., Herregods, N., Lemmerling, M. (2020). Craniofacial and intracranial Langerhans cell histiocytosis. *Journal of the Belgian Society of Radiology* 104:57. https://doi.org/10.5334/jbsr.2245

Lenze, U., Stolberg-Stolberg, J., Pohlig, F., Lenze, F., von Eisenhart-Rothe, R., Rechl, H., Toepfer, A. (2015). Unicameral bone cyst in the calcaneus of mirror image twins. *The Journal of Foot and Ankle Surgery* 54:754–757. https://doi.org/10.1053/j.jfas.2014.09.017

Lewis, M. (2017). *Paleopathology of Children: Identification of Pathological Conditions in the Human Skeletal Remains of Non-Adults*. San Diego: Academic Press.

Lieberman, P.H. (1975). Eosinophilic granuloma and related syndromes. In *Textbook of Medicine*, edited by Beeson, P.A., McDermott, W., pp. 1529–1534. Philadelphia: W.B. Saunders.

Lindsey, B.A., Markel, J.E., Kleinerman, E.S. (2017). Osteosarcoma overview. *Rheumatology and Therapy* 4:25–43. https://doi.org/10.1007/s40744-016-0050-2

Lucas, D.R., Bridge, J.A. (2002). Chondromas: Enchondroma, periosteal chondroma, and enchondromatosis. In *Pathology and Genetics of Tumours of Soft Tissue and Bone*, edited by Fletcher, C.D.M., Unni, K.K., Mertens, F., 3rd edition, pp. 237–240. Lyon: International Agency for Research on Cancer.

Manfrini, M. (2020). Giant cell tumor. In *Diagnosis of Musculoskeletal Tumors and Tumor-like Conditions*, edited by Picci, P., Manfrini, M., Donati, D.M., Gambarotti, M., Righi, A., Vanel, D., Dei Tos, A.P., 2nd edition, pp. 101–106. Berlin: Springer.

Mankin, H.J., Hornicek, F.J., Ortiz-Cruz, E., Villafuerte, J., Gebhardt, M.C. (2005). Aneurysmal bone cyst: A review of 150 patients. *Journal of Clinical Oncology* 20:6756–6762. https://doi.org/10.1200/JCO.2005.15.255

Marks, M.K., Hamilton, M.D. (2007). Metastatic carcinoma: Paleopathology and differential diagnosis. *International Journal of Osteoarchaeology* 17:217–234. https://doi.org/10.1002/oa.874

Marques, C. (2019). Tumors of bone. In *Ortner's Identification of Pathological Conditions in Human Skeletal Remains*, edited by Buikstra, J., pp. 639–717. San Diego: Academic Press.

Marques, C. (2021). Bioarchaeology of neoplasms: Lessons to learn from the past. In *Primary Bone Cancers and Bone Metastases: From Bench to Bedside*, edited by Heyman, D., 3rd edition, pp. 5–15. San Diego: Academic Press.

Marques, C., Roberts, C., Matos, V.M., Buikstra, J.E. (2021). Cancers as rare diseases: Terminological, theoretical, and methodological biases. *International Journal of Paleopathology* 32:111–122. https://doi.org/10.1016/j.ijpp.2020.12.005

Mascard, E., Gomez-Brouchet, A., Lambot, K. (2015). Bone cysts: Unicameral and aneurysmal bone cyst. *Orthopaedics & Traumatology: Surgery & Research* 101:S119–S127. https://doi.org/10.1016/j.otsr.2014.06.031

Mehra, P. (2009). Benign cysts and tumors of the jaw bones. In *Rhinology and Facial Plastic Surgery*, edited by Stucker, F.J., De Souza, C., Kenyon, G.S., Lian, T.S., Draf, W., Schick, B., pp. 395–429. Berlin: Springer.

Mehta, N., Bhagwati, S., Parulekar, G. (2009). Meningiomas in children: A study of 18 cases. *Journal of Pediatric Neurosciences* 4:61–65. https://doi.org/10.4103/1817-1745.57322

Menon, G., Nair, S., Sudhir, J., Rao, B.R., Mathew, A., Bahuleyan, B. (2009). Childhood and adolescent meningiomas: A report of 38 cases and review of literature. *Acta Neurochirurgica* 151:239–244. https://doi.org/10.1007/s00701-009-0206-8

Meyer, J., Priemel, M., Rolvien, T., Frosch, K.H., Schlickewei, C., Yarar-Schlickewei, S. (2023). The diagnostic challenge of osteoid osteoma in the bones of the hand—A case series. *Diagnostics* 13:1279. https://doi.org/10.3390/diagnostics13071279

Moon, K.-S., Jung, S., Lee, J.-H., Jung, T.-Y., Kim, I.-Y., Kim, S.-H., Kang, S.-S. (2006). Benign osteoblastoma of the occipital bone: Case report and literature review. *Neuropathology* 26:141–146. https://doi.org/10.1111/j.1440-1789.2006.00643.x

Mundy, G. (1997). Mechanisms of bone metastasis. *Cancer* 80:1546–1556. https://doi.org/10.1002/(SICI)1097-0142(19971015)80:8+<1546::AID-CNCR4>3.0.CO;2-I

Murphey, M., Choi, J., Kransdorf, M., Flemming, D., Gannon, F. (2000). Imaging of osteochondroma: Variants and complications with radiologic-pathologic correlation. *RadioGraphics* 20:1407–1434. https://doi.org/10.1148/radiographics.20.5.g00se171407

Murphey, M. D., Jelinek, J. S., Temple, H. T., Flemming, D. J., Gannon, F. H. (2004). Imaging of periosteal osteosarcoma: Radiologic-pathologic comparison. *Radiology*, *233*(1), 129–138. https://pubs.rsna.org/doi/abs/10.1148/radiol.2331030326

Murphy, E.M., McKenzie, C.J. (2010). Multiple osteochondromas in the archaeological record: A global review. *Journal of Archaeological Science* 37:2255–2264. https://doi.org/10.1016/j.jas.2010.03.023

Nielsen, G.P., Rosenberg, A.E. (2010). Bone-forming tumors. In *Bone and Soft Tissue Pathology*, edited by Folpe, A.L., Inwards, C.Y., pp. 309–329. Philadelphia: Saunders.

Ohkawa, M., Fujiwara, N., Tanabe, M., Takashima, H., Satoh, K., Mori, Y., Honjo, Y., Nagao, S. (1997). Benign osteoblastoma of the temporal bone. *American Journal of Neuroradiology* 18:324–326.

Ottaviani, G., Jaffe, N. (2009). The epidemiology of osteosarcoma. In *Pediatric and Adolescent Osteosarcoma*, edited by Jaffe, N., Bruland, O.S., Bielack, S., pp. 3–13. Berlin: Springer.

Papadopoulou, M., Panagopoulou, P., Papadopoulou, A., Hatzipantelis, E., Efstratiou, I., Galli-Tsinopoulou, A., Papadopoulou-Alataki, E. (2018). The multiple faces of Langerhans cell histiocytosis in childhood: A gentle reminder. *Molecular and Clinical Oncology* 8:489–492. https://doi.org/10.3892/mco.2017.1539

Peersman, B., Vanhoenacker, F.M., Heyman, S., Van Herendael, B., Stam, M., Brys, P., Verstraete, K.L., Samson, I. (2007). Ewing's sarcoma: Imaging features. *JBR-BTR* 90:368–376.

Pietramala, S., Rovere, G., Ravaioli, C., Mignano, C., Smakaj, A., Fidanza, A., Farsetti, P., Rocchi, L., Fulchignoni, C. (2025). Surgical treatment of enchondromas of the hand: Our experience in curettage only and early mobilization. *Diseases* 13:84. https://doi.org/10.3390/diseases13030084

Porter, D.E., Lonie, L., Fraser, M., Dobson-Stone, C., Porter, J.R., Monaco, A.P., Simpson, A.H. (2004). Severity of disease and risk of malignant change inhereditary multiple exostoses. A genotype-phenotype study. *The Journal of Bone & Joint Surgery* 86:1041–1046. https://doi.org/10.1302/0301-620x.86b7.14815

Ragsdale, B.D., Campbell, R.A., Kirkpatrick, C.L. (2018). Neoplasm or not? General principles of morphologic analysis of dry bone specimens. *International Journal of Paleopathology* 21:27–40. https://doi.org/10.1016/j.ijpp.2017.02.002

Reith, J.D. (2016). Metastatic tumors in bone. In *Dorfman and Czerniak's Bone Tumors*, edited by Czerniak, B., 2nd edition, pp. 1217–1258. Philadelphia: Elsevier.

Resnick, D.J. (2002). *Diagnosis of Bone and Joint Disorders*, 4th edition. Philadelphia: Saunders.

Resnick, M., Jacobson, J.A., Chung, C.B., Kransdorf, M.J., Pathria, M.N. (2024). *Resnick's Bone and Joint Imaging*, 4th edition. Philadelphia: Saunders.

Richter, G.T., Friedman, A.B. (2012). Hemangiomas and vascular malformations: Current theory and management. *International Journal of Pediatrics* 2012:645678. https://doi.org/10.1155/2012/645678

Righi, A. (2020). Vascular tumors. In *Diagnosis of Musculoskeletal Tumors and Tumor-like Conditions*, edited by Picci, P., Manfrini, M., Donati, D.M., Gambarotti, M., Righi, A., Vanel, D., Dei Tos, A.P., 2nd edition, pp. 299–316. Berlin: Springer.

Robert, H., Dubousset, J., Miladi, L. (1987). Histiocytosis X in the juvenile spine. *Spine* 12:167–172. https://doi.org/10.1097/00007632-198703000-00013

Roessner, A., Boehling, T. (2002). Angiosarcoma. In *Pathology and Genetics of Tumours of Soft Tissue and Bone*, edited by Fletcher, C.D.M., Unni, K., Mertens, F., 3rd edition, pp. 243–245. Lyon: International Agency for Research on Cancer.

Rothschild, B.M., Rothschild, C. (1995). Comparison of radiologic and gross examination for detection of cancer in defleshed skeletons. *American Journal of Physical Anthropology* 96:357–363. https://doi.org/10.1002/ajpa.1330960404

Rothschild, B., Hershkovitz, I., Dutour, O. (1998). Clues potentially distinguishing lytic lesions of multiple myeloma from those of metastatic carcinoma. *American Journal of Physical Anthropology* 105:241–250. https://doi.org/10.1002/(SICI)1096-8644(199802)105:2<241::AID-AJPA10>3.0.CO;2-0

Sakamoto, A., Takahashi, Y., Oda, Y., Iwamoto, Y. (2014). Aggressive clinical course of epithelioid angiosarcoma in the femur: A case report. *World Journal of Surgical Oncology* 12:281. https://doi.org/10.1186/1477-7819-12-281

Sarin, D., Bansal, K., Gupta, A. (2024). Limb salvage in chondrosarcoma of the proximal humerus: A case report. *Cureus* 16:e64266. https://doi.org/10.7759/cureus.64266

Schajowicz, F., Gallardo, H. (1971). Chondromyxoid fibroma (fibromyxoid chondroma) of bone. *The Journal of Bone & Joint Surgery* 53:198–216.

Shaheen, F., Ahmad, N., Gojwari, T., Teli, M.A., Resold, R., Singh, M. (2010). Multiple enchondromatosis: Ollier's disease. *JK Science* 12:207–209.

Siek, T. (2020). In defence of the osteoma: The relevance of benign tumours in bioarchaeology and palaeo-oncology. *International Journal of Osteoarchaeology* 30:281–283. https://doi.org/10.1002/oa.2839

Sobti, A., Agrawal, P., Agarwala, S, Agarwal, M. (2016). Giant cell tumor of bone – an overview. *The Archives of Bone and Joint Surgery* 20:2–9.

Staals, E.L. (2020a). Chondroblastoma. In *Diagnosis of Musculoskeletal Tumors and Tumor-like Conditions*, edited by Picci, P., Manfrini, M., Donati, D.M., Gambarotti, M., Righi, A., Vanel, D., Dei Tos, A.P., 2nd edition, pp. 81–84. Berlin: Springer.

Staals, E.L. (2020b). Chondromyxoid fibroma. In *Diagnosis of Musculoskeletal Tumors and Tumor-like Conditions*, edited by Picci, P., Manfrini, M., Donati, D.M., Gambarotti, M., Righi, A., Vanel, D., Dei Tos, A.P., 2nd edition, pp. 85–88. Berlin: Springer.

Steinbock, R. (1976). *Paleopathological Diagnosis and Interpretation. Bone Diseases in Ancient Human Populations*. Springfield, IL: Charles C. Thomas.

Stieber, J.R., Dormans, J.P. (2005). Manifestations of hereditary multiple exostoses. *Journal of the American Academy of Orthopaedic Surgeons* 13:110–120.

Stoker, D.J. (1986). Bone tumours. In *Diagnostic Radiology*, edited by Grainger R.G., Allison D.J., pp. 1273–1326. Edinburgh: Churchill Livingstone.

Strouhal, E. (1991). Myeloma multiplex versus osteolytic metastatic carcinoma: Differential diagnosis in dry bones. *International Journal of Osteoarchaeology* 1:219–224. https://doi.org/10.1002/oa.1390010314

Tarsitano, A., Ricotta, F., Spinnato, P., Chiesa, A.M., Di Carlo, M., Parmeggiani, A., Miceli, M., Facchini, G. (2021). Craniofacial osteomas: From diagnosis to therapy. *Journal of Clinical Medicine* 10:5584. https://doi.org/10.3390/jcm10235584

Tondini, T., Isidro, A., Camarós, E. (2024). Case report: Boundaries of oncological and traumatological medical care in ancient Egypt: New palaeopathological insights from two human skulls. *Frontiers in Medicine* 11:1371645. https://doi.org/10.3389/fmed.2024.1371645

Ulici, V., Hart, J. (2022). Chordoma: A review and differential diagnosis. *Archives of Pathology & Laboratory Medicine* 146:386–395. https://doi.org/10.5858/arpa.2020-0258-RA

Unni, K.K., Inwards, C.Y. (2010). *Dahlin's Bone Tumors: General Aspects and Data on 10,165 Cases*, 6th edition. Philadelphia: Lippincott Williams & Wilkins.

Waldron, T. (1996). What was the prevalence of malignant disease in the past? *International Journal of Osteoarchaeology* 6:463–470. https://doi.org/10.1002/(SICI)1099-1212(199612)6:5<463::AID-OA304>3.0.CO;2-Y

Waldron, T. (1998). An unusual cluster of meningiomas?. *International Journal of Osteoarchaeology* 8:213–217. https://doi.org/10.1002/(SICI)1099-1212(199805/06)8:3<213::AID-OA418>3.0.CO;2-A

Waldron, T. (2020). *Palaeopathology*, 2nd edition. Cambridge: Cambridge University Press.

Wirbel, R., Blümler, F., Lommel, D., Syré, G., Krenn, V. (2013). Multicentric giant cell tumor of bone: Synchronous and metachronous presentation. *Case Reports in Orthopedics* 2013:756723. https://doi.org/10.1155/2013/756723

Zhang, Y., Rosenberg, A.E. (2020). Angiosarcoma. In *Tumors and Tumor-Like Lesions of Bone. For Surgical Pathologists, Orthopedic Surgeons and Radiologists*, edited by Santini-Araujo, E., Kalil, R.K., Bertoni, F., Park, Y.-K. pp. 519–523. Cham: Springer.

Zou, M., Yang, R., Tang, Z., Luo, D., Jiang, Q. (2022). Primary intraosseous meningioma with subcutaneous and dural invasion: A case report and literature review. *Frontiers in Surgery* 9:995986. https://doi.org/10.3389/fsurg.2022.995986

Chapter 9

Joint disease

Joint diseases, also called arthropathies, are pathological conditions that affect the joints. Joint diseases are very common in both past and contemporary contexts. They can be categorised using different classification systems. This chapter will be structured in accordance with Burt et al. (2013), with minor adjustments. We will begin with an examination of osteoarthritis, followed by a discussion of erosive arthropathies, which include rheumatoid arthritis and seronegative spondyloarthritides. This will be followed by a presentation of less common forms of synovial joint disease, that is, gout and juvenile idiopathic arthritis. Finally, we will examine various conditions affecting the joints of the spine, specifically spinal osteophytosis, Schmorl's nodes, and diffuse idiopathic skeletal hyperostosis. Septic arthritis will not be addressed in this chapter, as it is covered in Chapter 7.

Osteoarthritis

Osteoarthritis is a chronic disorder that affects the synovial joints (Box 9.1, Figures 9.1–9.13). This condition is characterised by increased production of cartilage-degrading enzymes, such as metalloproteinases, due to an alteration in chondrocyte metabolism. This enzymatic activity causes the breakdown of cartilage and releases proteoglycans and collagen fragments into the synovial fluid. The accumulation of these breakdown products triggers an inflammatory response characterised by elevated synthesis of pro-inflammatory cytokines, which contribute

Box 9.1 Issues of terminology

In different works, different terms have been used for the condition described in this book as osteoarthritis. Terms such as degenerative joint disease or degenerative arthropathy have been proposed and stress the progressive deterioration of the joint. However, these terms have been criticised because the changes observed in dry bone largely indicate a reparative process. Some scholars favour the term osteoarthrosis, as the suffix "-itis" in osteoarthritis suggests inflammation, which was initially believed not to be a prominent feature of the condition. However, it is now acknowledged that inflammation is a characteristic of this condition. Given the absence of a consensus on the most suitable terminology, based on the prevalent usage of the term, we opt to use "osteoarthritis" in this book.

DOI: 10.4324/9781003475026-9

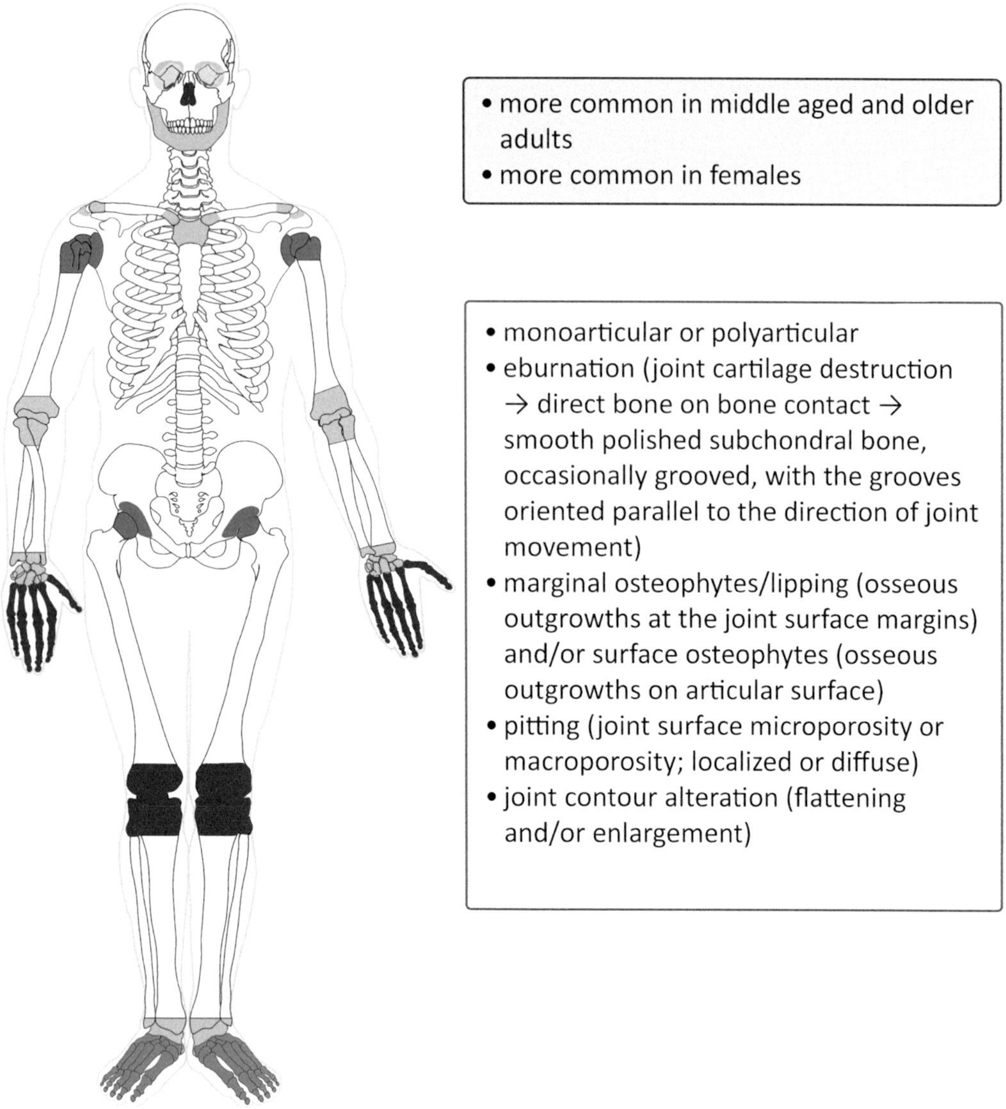

Figure 9.1 Skeletal manifestation of osteoarthritis. (Data from Burt et al. 2013; Dieppe 1995, 2008; Jurmain and Kilgore 1995; Rogers and Waldron 1995; Rogers et al. 1987; Scott et al. 2021; Turkiewicz et al. 2014; Waldron 1997, 2020a)

Note: The spine (zygapophyseal joints) is also often affected by osteoarthritis, especially in the cervical and lumbar regions, but this is covered below in the *Diseases of the joints of the spine*

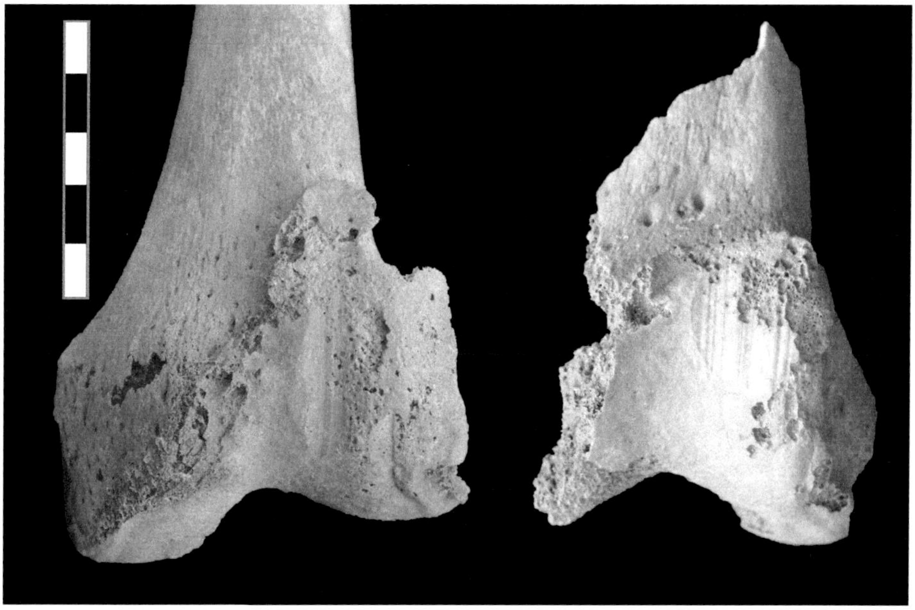

Figure 9.2 Osteoarthritis of the knee. Note the extensive lipping across the joint margin (left) and the eburnation with parallel grooves (left and right). (Philadelphia, Roman/Byzantine; photos by Efthymia Nikita, with the kind permission of Dr. Ahmet Ihsan Aytek, Burdur Mehmet Akif Ersoy University)

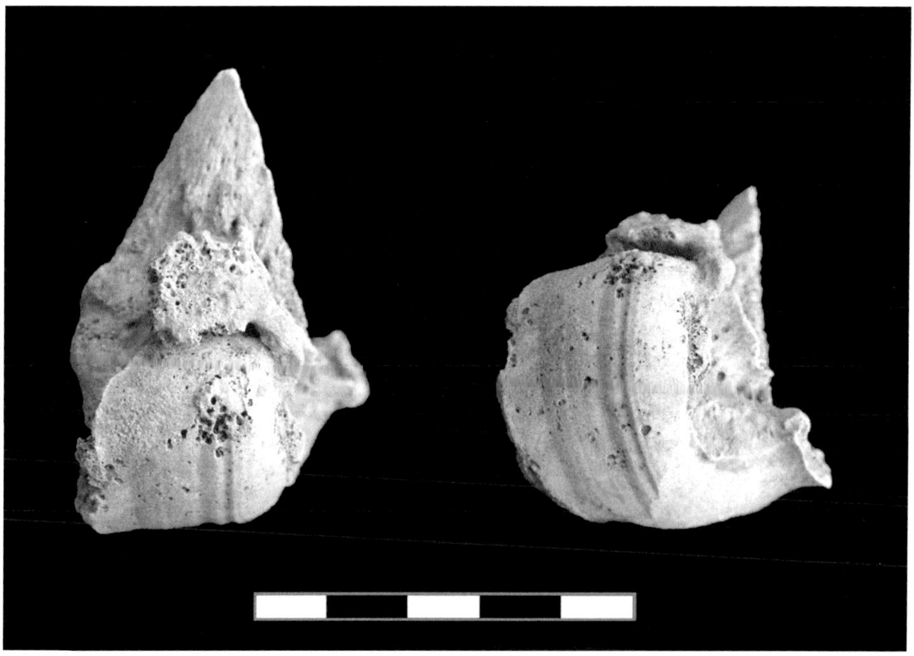

Figure 9.3 Osteoarthritis of the knee. Note the extensive eburnation with deep parallel grooves across the articular facet of the distal femur; in addition, the extensive lipping on the superior posterior part of the joint, and pitting and surface osteophytes on the joint surface. (Sbide, Roman/Byzantine; photos by Efthymia Nikita, with the kind permission of Dr. Ahmet Ihsan Aytek, Burdur Mehmet Akif Ersoy University)

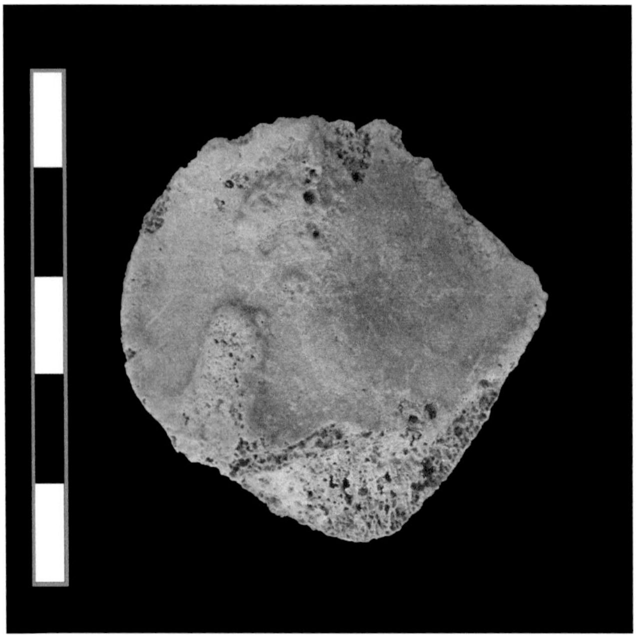

Figure 9.4 Osteoarthritis of the knee. Note the surface osteophytes and macroporosity at the patellar articular surface. (Sbide, Roman/Byzantine; photo by Efthymia Nikita, with the kind permission of Dr. Ahmet Ihsan Aytek, Burdur Mehmet Akif Ersoy University)

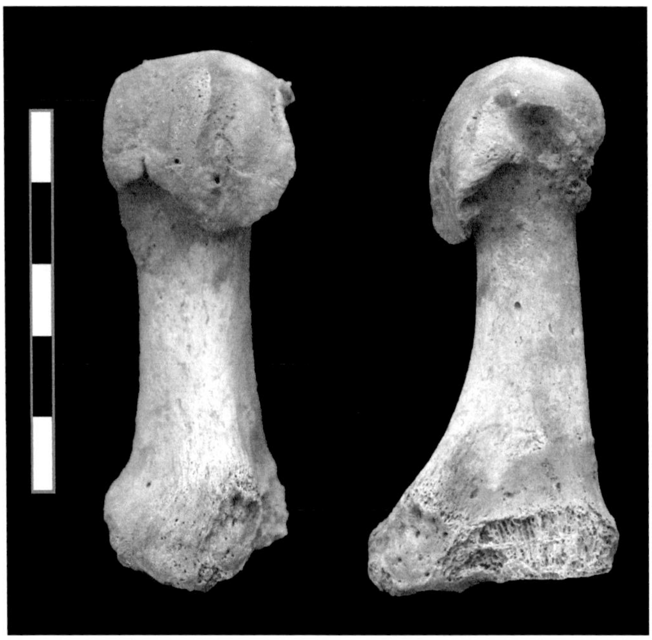

Figure 9.5 Osteoarthritis of the first metatarsophalangeal joint. Note the extensive marginal osteophyte formation, as well as the eburnation and minimal porosity on the metatarsal head. (Sbide, Roman/Byzantine; photos by Efthymia Nikita, with the kind permission of Dr. Ahmet Ihsan Aytek, Burdur Mehmet Akif Ersoy University)

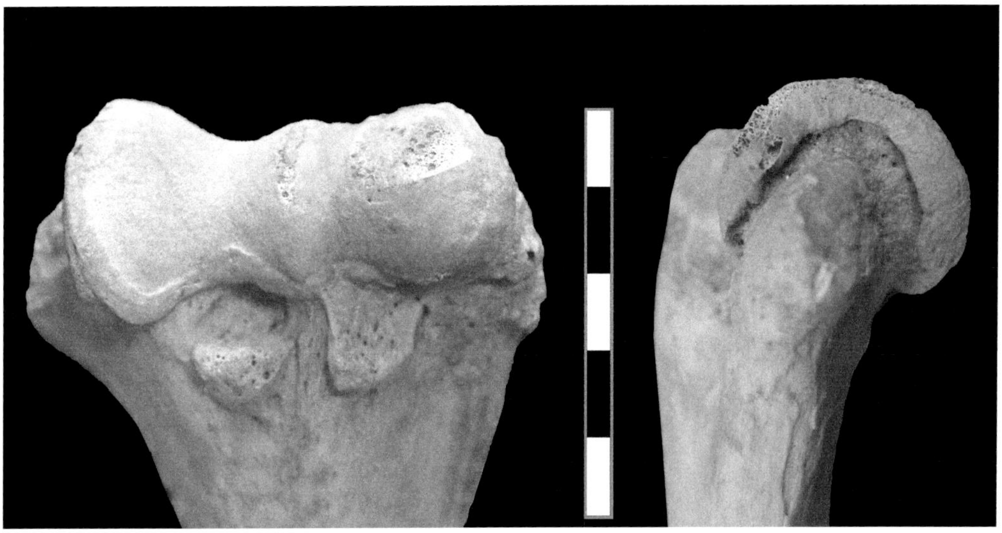

Figure 9.6 Osteoarthritis of the elbow. Note the extensive marginal osteophyte formation and eburnation on the capitulum. (Sbide, Roman/Byzantine; photos by Efthymia Nikita, with the kind permission of Dr. Ahmet Ihsan Aytek, Burdur Mehmet Akif Ersoy University)

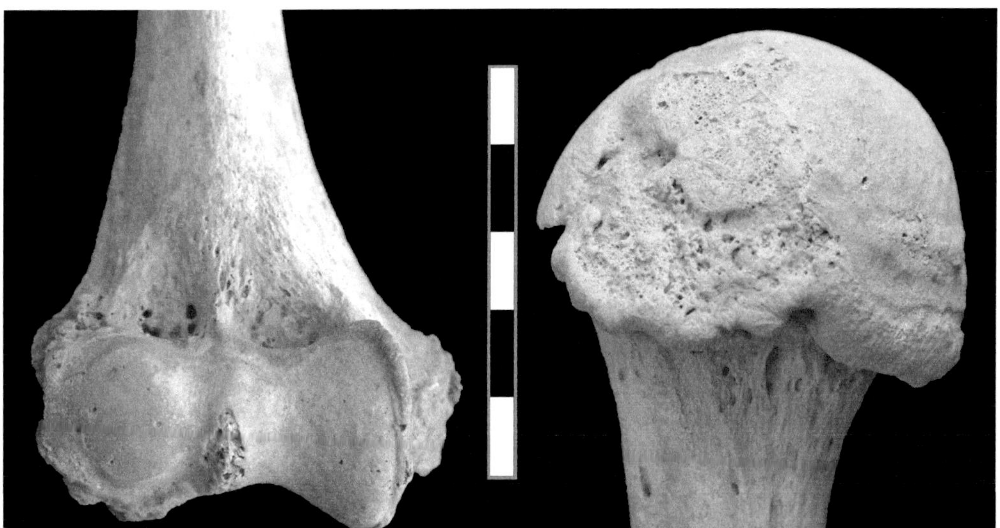

Figure 9.7 Osteoarthritis of the elbow (left). Note the extensive marginal osteophyte formation, eburnation on the capitulum, and porosity on the trochlea. Osteoarthritis of the shoulder (right). Note the extensive marginal osteophyte formation, as well as porosity on the humeral head. (Left: Sbide, right: Philadelphia, Roman/Byzantine; photos by Efthymia Nikita, with the kind permission of Dr. Ahmet Ihsan Aytek, Burdur Mehmet Akif Ersoy University)

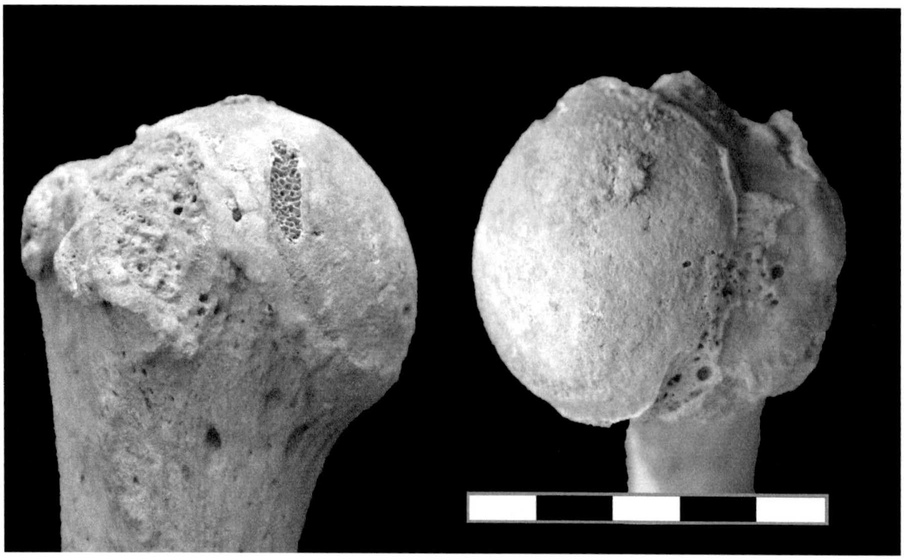

Figure 9.8 Osteoarthritis of the shoulder. Note the mild marginal lipping and a surface osteophyte on the humeral head. Note also the extensive porosity and lipping on the lesser and greater tubercles, adjacent to the articular surface. (Sbide, Roman/Byzantine; photos by Efthymia Nikita, with the kind permission of Dr. Ahmet Ihsan Aytek, Burdur Mehmet Akif Ersoy University)

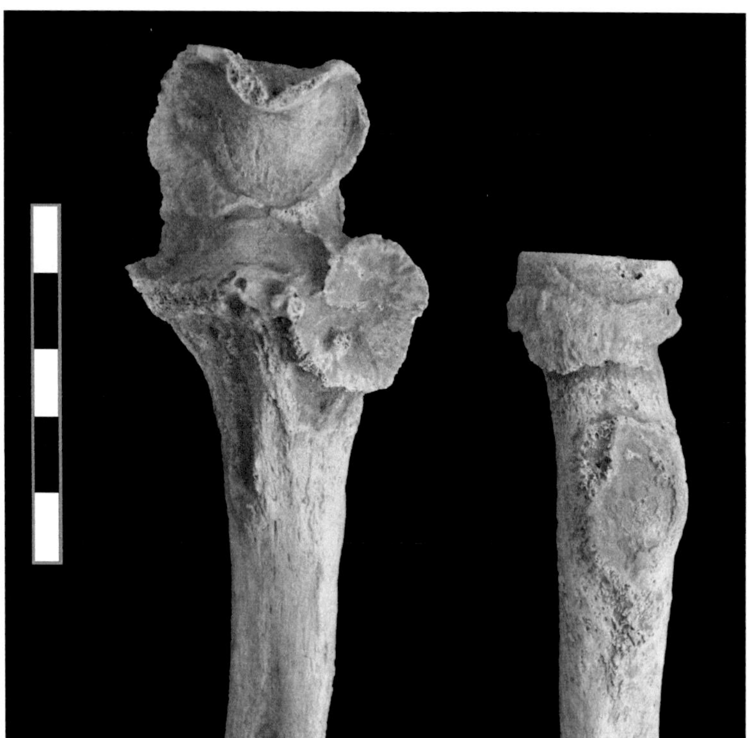

Figure 9.9 Osteoarthritis of the elbow. Note the extensive marginal lipping on the proximal radius and ulna. (Başköy, Roman/Byzantine; photos by Efthymia Nikita, with the kind permission of Dr. Ahmet Ihsan Aytek, Burdur Mehmet Akif Ersoy University)

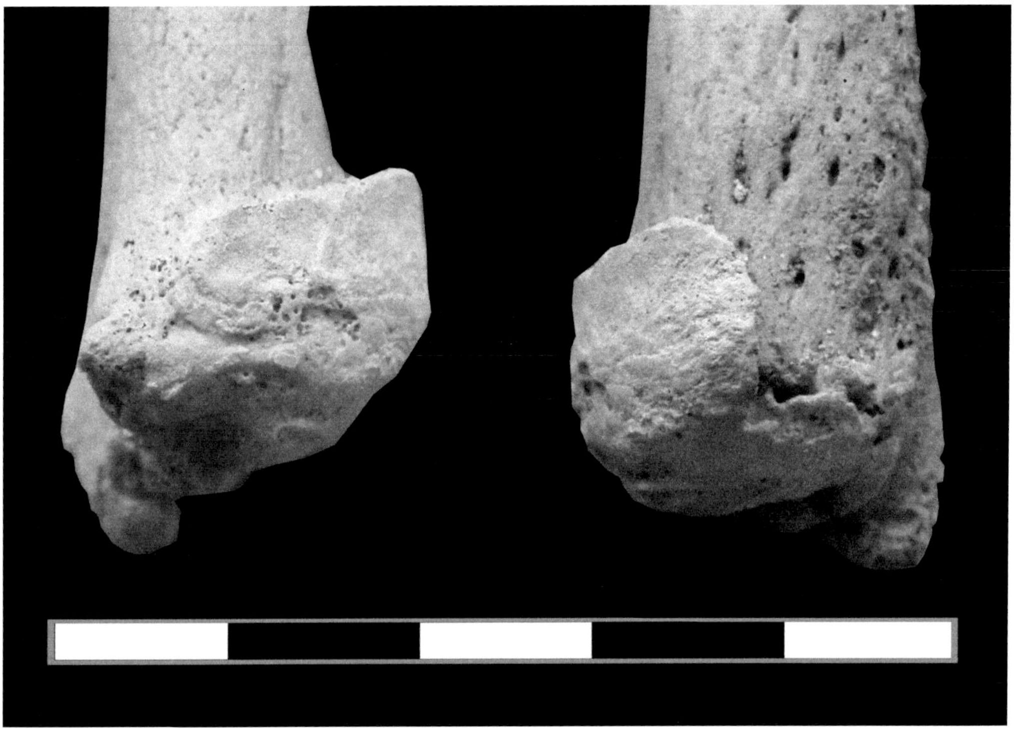

Figure 9.10 Osteoarthritis of the wrist. Note the extensive marginal lipping on the distal ulna. (Female, Collection NAD Nuis inv. Nr. F 2008-XII-101 (4); photos by Efthymia Nikita, with permission from the Noordelijk Archeologisch Depot)

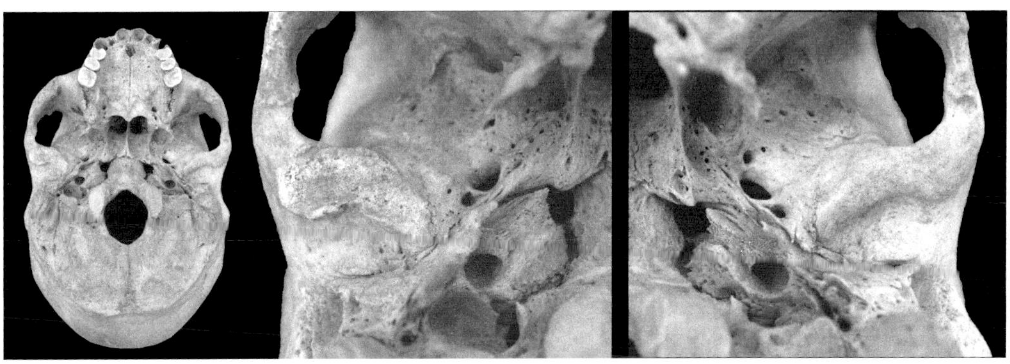

Figure 9.11 Temporomandibular joint arthritis. Note that the left articular eminence is unaffected, whereas the right one shows marginal lipping, porosity, and an alteration of the bone contour. (Sbide, Roman/Byzantine; photos by Efthymia Nikita, with the kind permission of Dr. Ahmet Ihsan Aytek, Burdur Mehmet Akif Ersoy University)

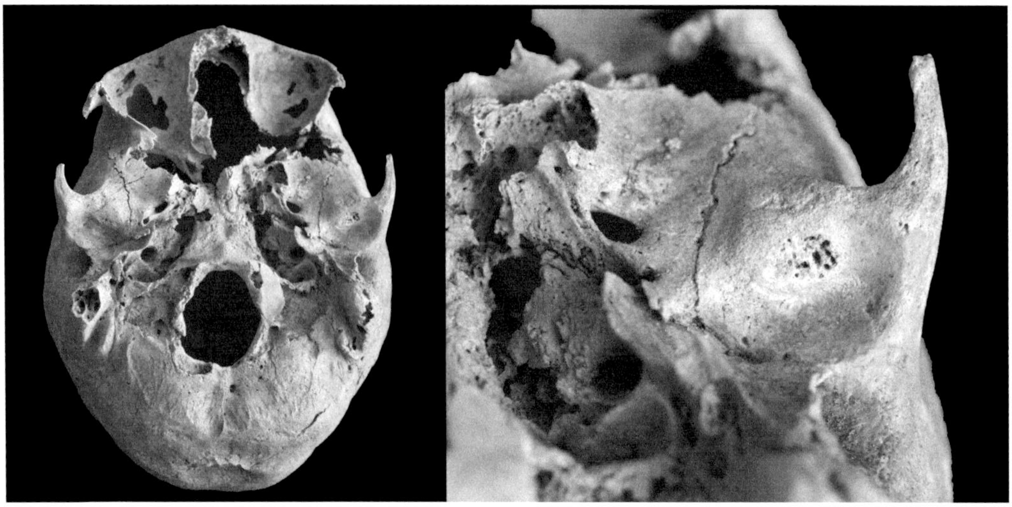

Figure 9.12 Temporomandibular joint arthritis. Both articular eminences show porosity but it is more pronounced on the left side (right image). (Kibyra, Byzantine; photos by Efthymia Nikita, with the kind permission of Dr. Ahmet Ihsan Aytek, Burdur Mehmet Akif Ersoy University)

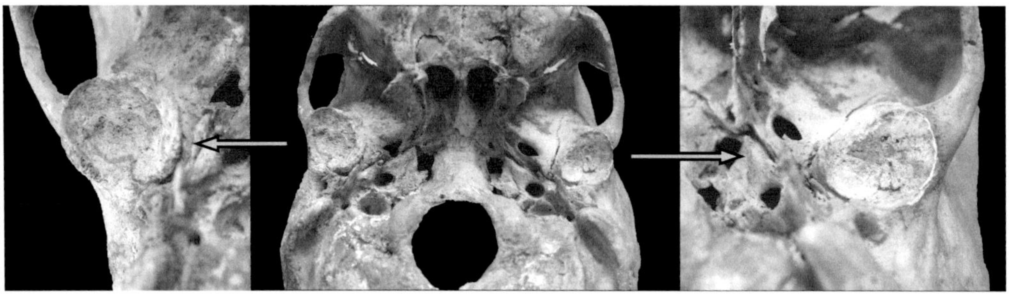

Figure 9.13 Temporomandibular joint arthritis. Note that both articular eminences show marginal lipping, porosity, surface osteophytes as well as an alteration of the bone contour. (Probable female, over 46 years old, Diever, Reformed Church graveyard, Collection NAD Nuis inv. Nr. D 2019-III.469; photos by Efthymia Nikita, with permission from the Noordelijk Archeologisch Depot)

to cartilage destruction. Over time, new bone forms in order to compensate for joint damage; this process results in the appearance of osteophytes. Osteophytes are osseous projections at the margins of the joint or on the joint surface. They increase the area available for load bearing and can improve joint stability, but they may also limit the functionality of the joint. In addition, pitting may form on the surface of the joint, appearing as multiple perforations, some of which may be connected with subchondral cysts. Alterations in the normal joint contour are also possible, and often result in widening and flattening of this contour. If cartilage degradation is severe, the articulating bones can come into direct contact, causing abrasion of the subchondral surfaces. This phenomenon leads to eburnation, which appears as a dense, shiny surface on the subchondral bone (Box 9.2).

Box 9.2 Diagnosing osteoarthritis

Eburnation is considered pathognomonic of OA; however, in its absence, a diagnosis of OA may be established with the presence of at least two of the following: marginal osteophytes, pitting, surface osteophytes, or joint contour alteration (Rogers and Waldron 1995, Waldron 2020a). Nonetheless, Rothschild et al. (2023 and references cited therein) argue that pitting is not associated with osteoarthritis, eburnation can occur in various other joint disorders, while osteophytes are seen as the diagnostic indicator for osteoarthritis.

Osteoarthritis may be primary or secondary. In primary osteoarthritis, the underlying cause is not clear. In contrast, secondary osteoarthritis arises as a consequence of trauma, infection, circulatory disorders, or other pathological conditions, as well as due to mechanical stress or anatomical variation/deformity in the joint.

The aetiology of osteoarthritis is complex; age, sex, genetic predisposition, anatomical variation, mechanical stress, obesity, bone density, pre-existing joint conditions, and trauma can affect its expression.

Age is a major factor in the progression of osteoarthritis and influences the development of this condition through different mechanisms, such as inflammation, oxidative stress, cellular senescence, mitochondrial dysfunction, impaired energy metabolism, and alterations in the cellular signalling pathways. These mechanisms contribute to the degradation of joint tissues and inhibit their repair.

Osteoarthritis is generally more common in females compared to males. This pattern has been attributed to various factors, including anatomical differences in joint structure, hormonal effects, obesity, and genetics. Moreover, females experience more severe pain compared to males, potentially due to differences in the biological pain pathways and the central pain activation mechanisms, but also due to differences in the perception of pain and the strategies employed to manage it. Finally, in females, osteoarthritis causes more severe limitations to physical functions compared to males, irrespective of any differences in the severity of osteoarthritis, history of injury, and levels of weekly physical activity.

With regard to genetic predisposition, twin and family studies show that the heritability of osteoarthritis ranges from 0.4 to 0.7. However, heritability estimates show considerable variability across different populations.

Concerning anatomical factors, certain individuals exhibit anatomical variations that can exert greater mechanical stress on the joints compared to the rest of the population. For example, discrepancies in leg length promote osteoarthritis in the knee. Similarly, individuals with acetabular dysplasia, which is characterised by shallow hip sockets, are more likely to develop hip osteoarthritis.

Many bioarchaeologists study osteoarthritis to reconstruct past activity patterns, assuming that the manifestation of osteoarthritis is predominantly a result of repetitive mechanical stress. However, due to its multifactorial aetiology, osteoarthritis may not be a reliable indicator of general activity levels and is certainly not a predictor of specific activities. Importantly, a certain level of physical activity can promote healthy joints by stimulating the synthesis of synovial fluid, facilitating nutrient circulation to the joints through improved blood flow, strengthening the muscles surrounding the joints, suppressing chronic inflammation, and activating autophagy, a process that breaks down and eliminates damaged cells within the joint.

Body size is another important contributing factor in the aetiology of osteoarthritis. Overweight or obese individuals usually experience more severe manifestations of the disease. The relationship between body mass index and osteoarthritis involves mechanical and systemic effects. With regard to mechanical effects, joints subjected to excessive loads experience mechanical stress, leading to cartilage degeneration, particularly in the knee and hip. On the other hand, systemic effects relate to obesity-induced inflammation and fibrosis.

In what concerns bone density, there is a complex relationship between osteoarthritis and osteoporosis. Both conditions are prevalent among older individuals and share various risk factors, including advancing age and genetic predisposition. Mechanical loading, oxidative stress, and inflammation are among the key mechanisms underlying the relationship between osteoarthritis and osteoporosis. Mechanical loading promotes subchondral bone sclerosis in osteoarthritis and influences the loss of trabecular bone in osteoporosis. Oxidative stress is implicated in the degradation of articular cartilage in osteoarthritis and in the process of bone loss associated with osteoporosis. Finally, chronic low-grade inflammation contributes to cartilage damage in osteoarthritis, whereas systemic inflammation triggers bone loss in osteoporosis. Nonetheless, several studies have also supported a negative correlation between osteoarthritis and osteoporosis because elevated bone mineral density (BMD) has been found in individuals with osteoarthritis.

Osteoarthritis may also arise as a result of traumatic injury. For example, osteoarthritis will almost certainly appear when a fracture has healed improperly, particularly if the fracture directly involves the joint or when it results in asymmetry of the affected bones. In addition, unresolved joint dislocation can result in abnormal joint use or the formation of a secondary joint. Finally, surgical procedures such as meniscectomy increase the risk of developing osteoarthritis, as do soft tissue injuries, such as damage to the anterior cruciate ligament.

Before closing the discussion on OA and moving on to erosive arthropathies, mention should be made of a special type of osteoarthritis, called erosive OA (EOA). This is an inflammatory condition that principally affects the interphalangeal joints of the hands. EOA is most commonly observed in postmenopausal women, who experience symptoms including pain, swelling, redness, warmth, and decreased functionality of the hand joints.

Erosive arthropathies

Erosive arthropathies lead to the destruction of the articular surfaces. Most erosive arthropathies can be categorised into two groups: rheumatoid arthritis and the seronegative spondyloarthritides (i.e. ankylosing spondylitis, psoriatic arthritis, reactive arthritis, and enteropathic arthritis).

Rheumatoid arthritis

Rheumatoid arthritis (RA) is a chronic autoimmune disorder (Figures 9.14 and 9.15). In most cases, it is a seropositive condition, that is, a large number of patients have an antibody called rheumatoid factor in their blood. Moreover, patients with RA often have anti-citrullinated

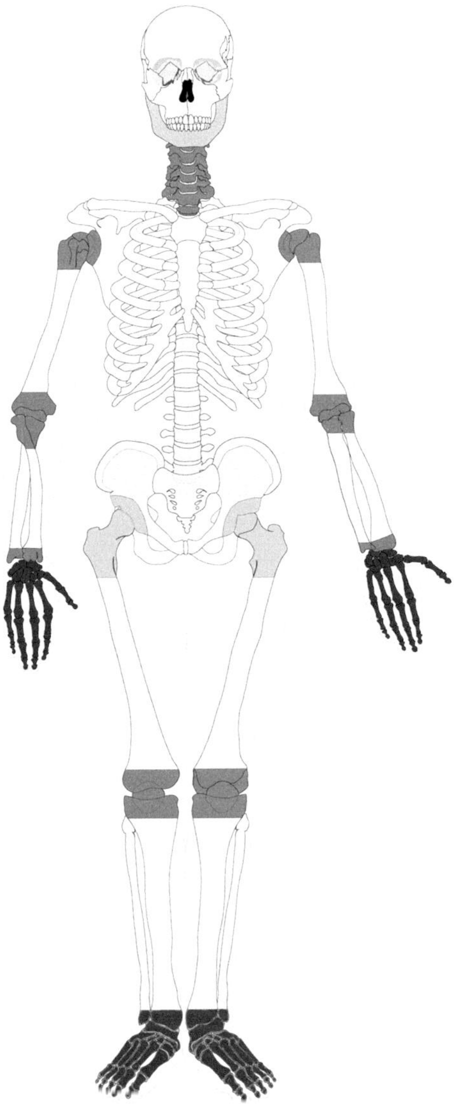

- age of onset 30-50 years
- more common in females

General
- erosive lesions with smooth margins
- several joints affected bilaterally and symmetrically
- periarticular bone erosion, which later spreads to subchondral bone surface
- extensive joint destruction
- eburnation in severe cases
- minimal, if any, new bone formation; rare joint fusion and seen only in small joints
- osteopenia

Skull
- temporomandibular joint involvement

Vertebrae
- cervical vertebrae erosion (mostly in C1-C2); very rare involvement of thoracic and lumbar vertebrae
- odontoid peg erosion may lead to atlantoaxial joint subluxation, spinal cord compression and death
- no ankylosis

Pelvic girdle
- very rare sacroiliitis (if present, bilateral, symmetric and mild)

Figure 9.14 Skeletal manifestation of rheumatoid arthritis. (Data from Arriaza 1993; Bouysset et al. 2006; Burt et al. 2013; Leden et al. 2009, 2012; Rogers 2000; Rogers and Waldron 1995; Rogers et al. 1987; Rothschild et al. 1990; Sweeney et al. 2013; Waldron 2012, 2019, 2020b)

Note: Diagnosing rheumatoid arthritis in archaeological skeletal remains is impossible if there are no osseous lesions in the hands or feet (Rogers et al. 1987).

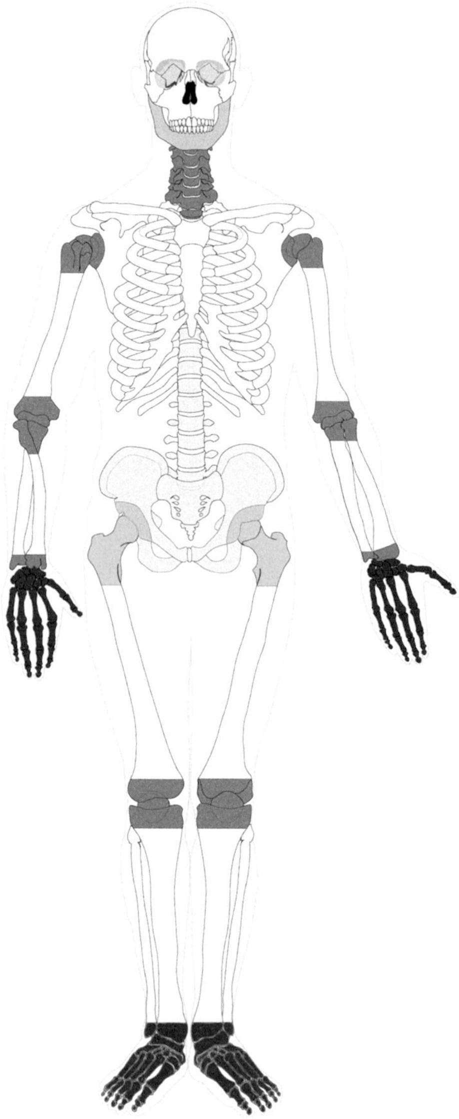

Hand/foot

- mostly in metacarpophalangeal and proximal interphalangeal joints, rare in distal interphalangeal joints
- carpal and interphalangeal ankylosis in severe cases
- tarsal ankylosis (rarer than carpal) in severe cases
- small joint subluxation → lateral extension of metacarpal or metatarsal articular surface with marginal lipping on corresponding phalangeal articular surface
- "cup and pencil" interphalangeal appearance
- symmetric lesions

Arm/leg

- involvement of wrist, elbow, knee, ankle, hip, and shoulder in advanced stages of the condition

Figure 9.14 (Continued)

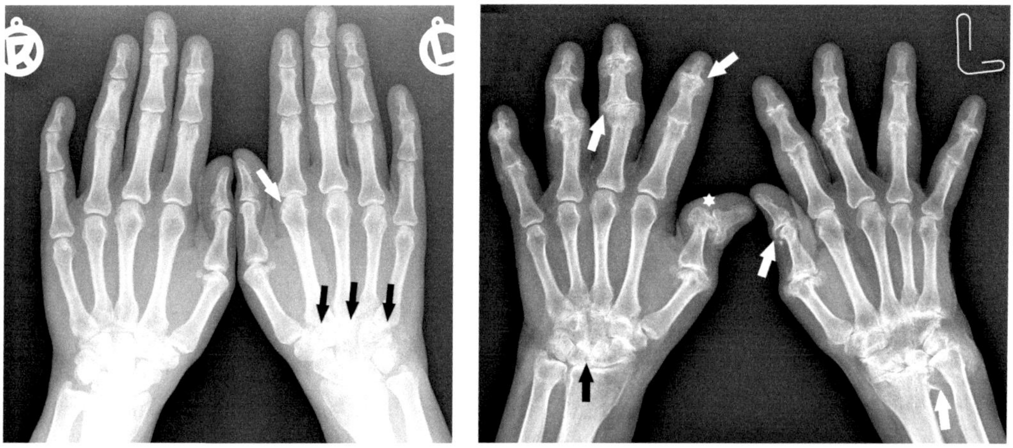

Figure 9.15 Radiograph of individual with asymmetric seropositive rheumatoid arthritis; note the bone cyst in the left second metacarpal head (a). Radiograph of the same individual taken 13 years later; note the severe progression of the joint changes (b). (Figure 1 in Żelnio et al. 2023; article licensed under a Creative Commons Attribution 4.0 International License)

protein antibodies, which are actually more specific for RA than the rheumatoid factor. The exact aetiology of RA remains unclear, but potential risk factors include smoking, obesity, and exposure to infections and toxins. Furthermore, females and older individuals are more likely to develop RA. In addition, a genetic susceptibility to RA has been identified.

Regarding its progression, chronic inflammation of the synovial membrane results in the formation of pannus, a thick, hypertrophied synovial membrane that invades the adjacent tissues, causing degradation of the cartilage and erosion of the bone. Erosive bone lesions are initially located at the joint margin, but they can later expand to the subchondral bone, forming cyst-like lesions. Smaller joints may deform. In severe cases, eburnation can develop, while ankylosis is also possible. In addition to localised joint destruction, RA patients may develop osteoporosis at anatomical locations far from the affected joint.

RA causes pain, tenderness, stiffness, and swelling of the joints. Individuals with this condition may also feel fatigue, malaise, and depression. The expression of symptoms can vary throughout the day and from one day to another. At later stages, the hands and feet may become severely deformed. Beyond the joints, the disease can affect the skin, eyes, kidneys, lungs, heart, and other tissues and organs.

Spondyloarthritides

Spondyloarthritides are inflammatory disorders that cause spinal fusion, sacroiliitis, and enthesitis. The conditions classified in this group include ankylosing spondylitis, psoriatic arthritis, reactive arthritis, and enteropathic arthritis. They are classified as seronegative arthropathies because individuals afflicted with them do not have rheumatoid factor in their blood. In contrast, these conditions are characterised by the frequent presence of the HLA-B27 antigen in affected individuals, an antigen that is rarely found in patients with RA.

Ankylosing spondylitis

Ankylosing spondylitis (AS) has unclear aetiology, but likely arises from the interaction between genetic and environmental factors (Box 9.3, Figures 9.16–9.19). Genetic background, microbial agents, and endocrine abnormalities have been associated with the development of AS. Importantly, a direct association has been established between AS and the human leukocyte antigen (HLA)-B27, as this antigen is much more prevalent among individuals with AS than in the general population. However, this association varies across different populations.

Patients diagnosed with AS often feel chronic pain and stiffness, especially in the pelvis and lower back. Additional symptoms include inflammation of other joints of the body, enthesitis (inflammation at the tendon or ligament attachment sites on bone), fatigue, weight loss, skin rashes, and potential damage to organs beyond the skeleton, such as the heart, lungs, and eyes. Furthermore, an association has been found between AS and inflammatory bowel disease.

Box 9.3 Diagnosing ankylosing spondylitis

Waldron (2019) supports that the combined presence of fused sacroiliac joint, fused vertebrae without skip lesions, and syndesmophytes should be sufficient for a secure diagnosis of AS.

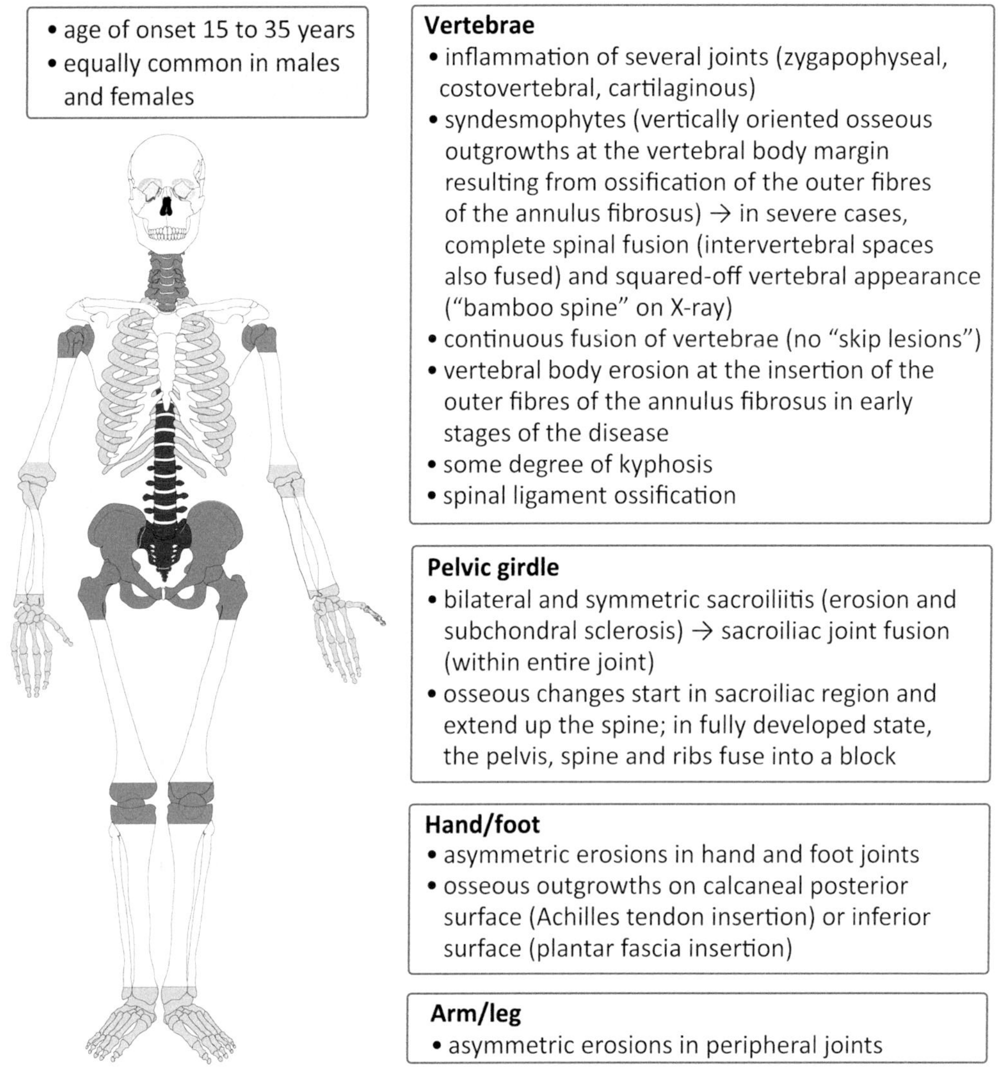

Figure 9.16 Skeletal manifestation of ankylosing spondylitis. (Data from Arriaza 1993; Horváth et al. 1994; Kataria and Brent 2001; McEwan et al. 1971; Nelson et al. 2023; Reynolds and Rankin 1974; Rogers and Waldron 1995; Tersigni-Tarrant and Zachow 2012; Ventades et al. 2018; Waldron 2012, 2020b)

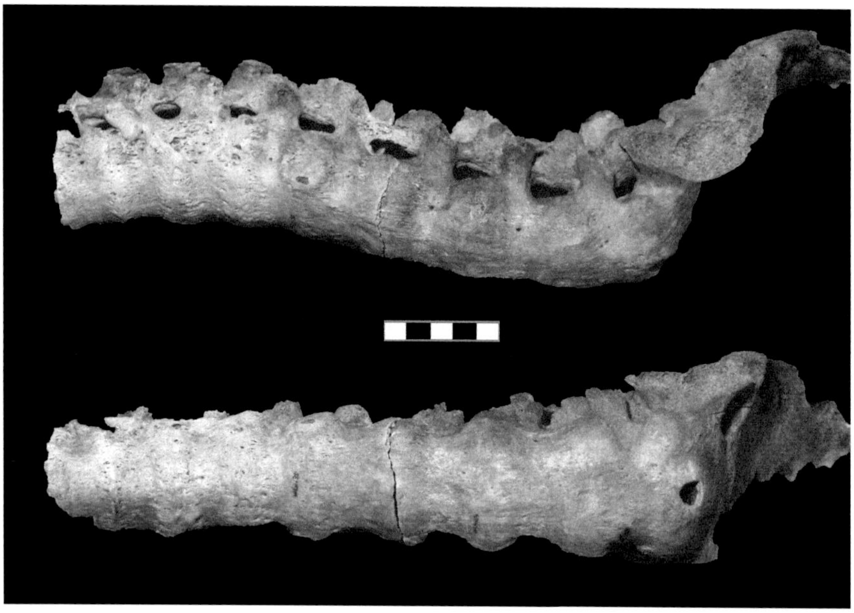

Figure 9.17 Ankylosing spondylitis. Continuous fusion of lower thoracic and lumbar vertebrae, as well as the lumbo-sacral joint. The sacroiliac joints were also fused, but this is not visible in the photo because they have broken. The fusion involves the entire spine with no skip lesions (see also Figures 9.18 and 9.19). (Male, Athens Collection, WLH35; photos by Efthymia Nikita; copyright: Athens Collection, Department of Animal and Human Physiology of the National and Kapodistrian University of Athens)

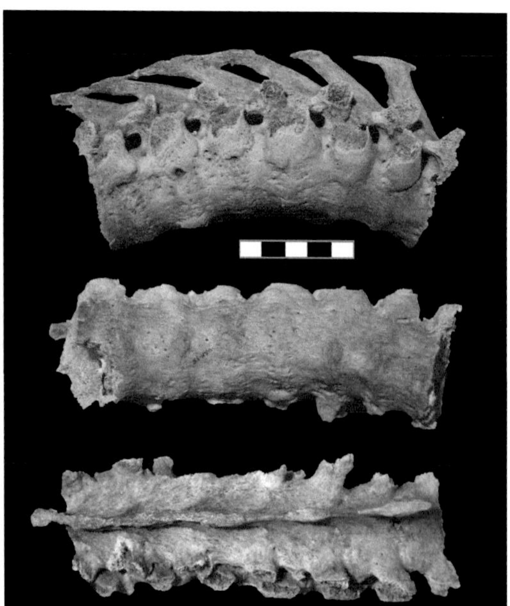

Figure 9.18 Ankylosing spondylitis. Continuous fusion of thoracic vertebrae with no skip lesions. All ribs are also fused, though they broke post-mortem. (Same individual as in Figure 9.17; photos by Efthymia Nikita; copyright: Athens Collection, Department of Animal and Human Physiology of the National and Kapodistrian University of Athens)

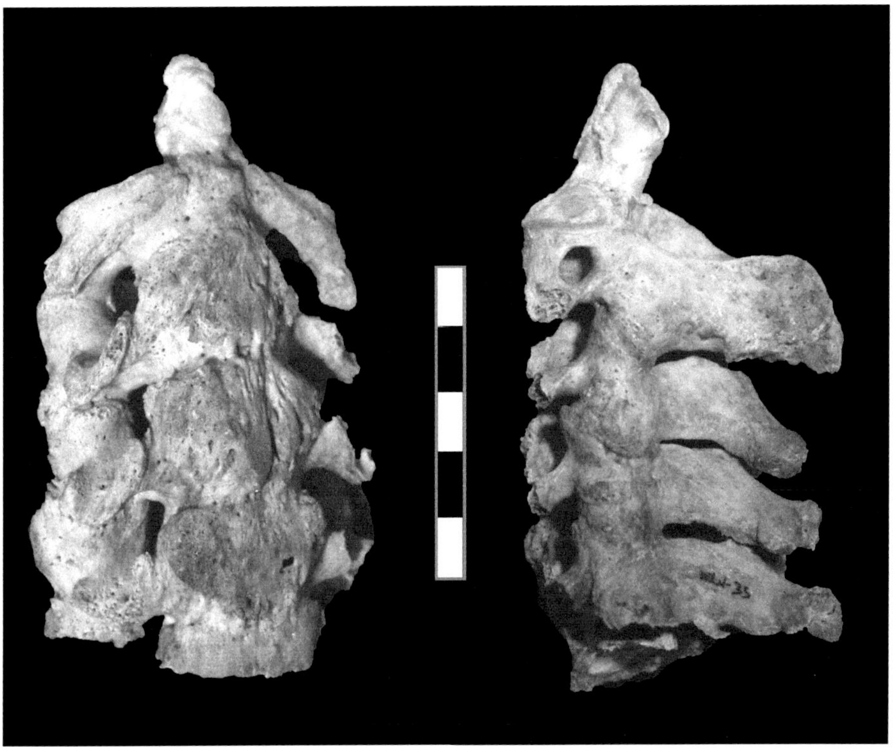

Figure 9.19 Ankylosing spondylitis. Continuous fusion of cervical vertebrae with no skip lesions. (Same individual as in Figures 9.17 and 9.18; photos by Efthymia Nikita; copyright: Athens Collection, Department of Animal and Human Physiology of the National and Kapodistrian University of Athens)

Psoriatic arthritis

Psoriatic arthritis is a form of chronic inflammatory arthropathy associated with the skin disorder psoriasis (Figures 9.20 and 9.21). It causes joint pain, stiffness, swelling, fatigue, skin rashes, enthesitis, and changes in the appearance of the fingernails and toenails. The symptoms of the disease typically appear intermittently, whereby periods of remission are interrupted by flares. In the absence of treatment, psoriatic arthritis can result in significant disability.

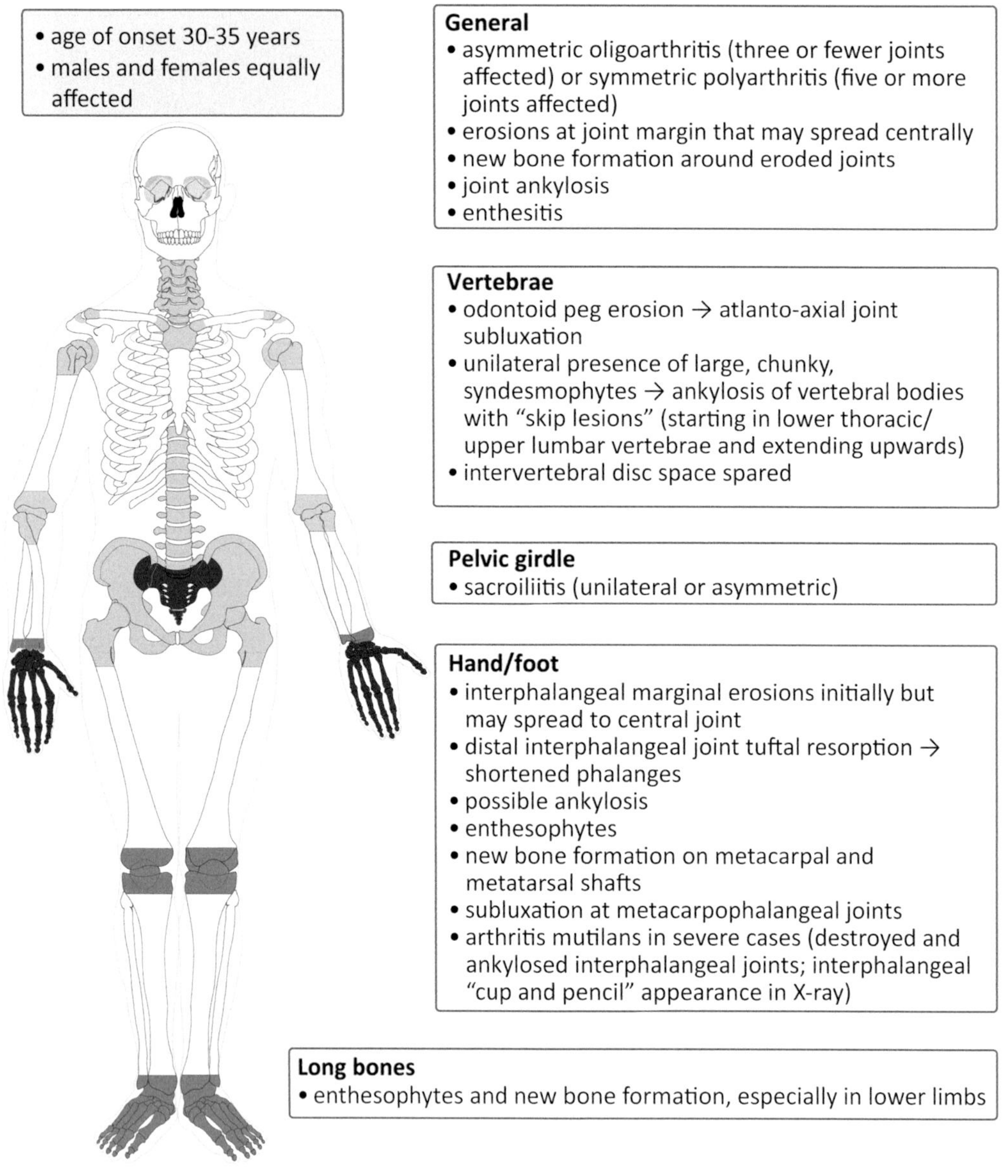

Figure 9.20 Skeletal manifestation of psoriatic arthritis. (Data from Arnett 1985; Arriaza 1993; Cawley and Paine 2015; Helliwell and Taylor 2005; Helliwell et al. 2000; Khan 2002; Queiro et al. 2002; Rogers and Waldron 1995; Rogers et al. 1987; Veale et al. 1994; Waldron 2012, 2019, 2020b; Zabotti et al. 2024)

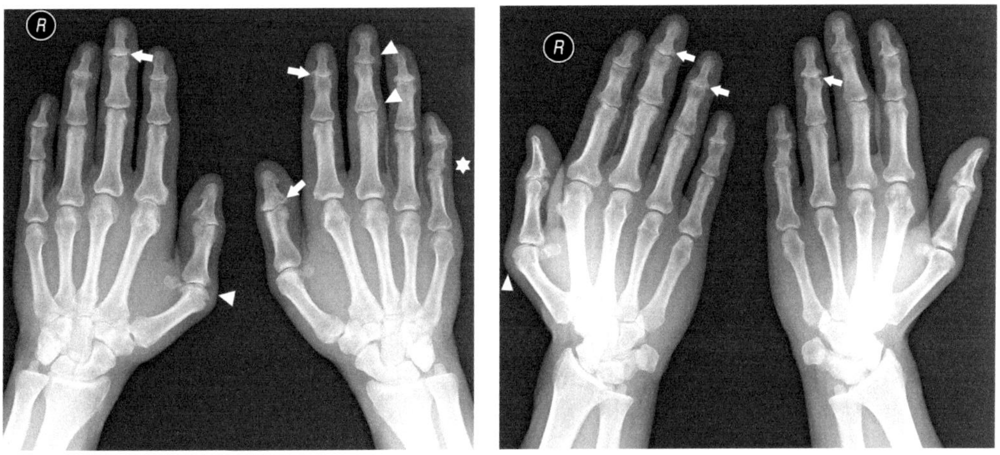

(a) (b)

Figure 9.21 Radiograph of the hands of individual with psoriatic arthritis. Note the swan neck deformity (star), and scattered bone cysts, erosions, and bone formation (arrows). (Figure 2 in Żelnio et al. 2023; article licensed under a Creative Commons Attribution 4.0 International License)

Reactive arthritis

Reactive arthritis is triggered by an infection located in a different part of the body; the gastrointestinal, genital, and urinary tract are the most common sites of primary infection (Figure 9.22). A wide range of pathogens can trigger the onset of the condition; some of these are sexually transmitted, while others are transmitted through contaminated food. Symptoms typically appear within one to three weeks following exposure to infection; they may include joint pain, swelling, stiffness, gut inflammation, eye lesions, urinary complications, enthesitis, and skin lesions. In most cases, the symptoms resolve within 6 months. If they last longer, the condition becomes chronic.

Enteropathic arthritis

Enteropathic arthritis is a chronic inflammatory arthritis that appears in about 10–20% of individuals with inflammatory bowel disease, and it is more common in cases of Crohn's disease. The symptoms of enteropathic arthritis include joint pain, redness, stiffness, swelling, tenderness, and warmth. Beyond the skeleton, enteropathic arthritis can cause skin lesions and eye inflammation. Importantly, the symptoms of enteropathic arthritis may precede the gastrointestinal ones.

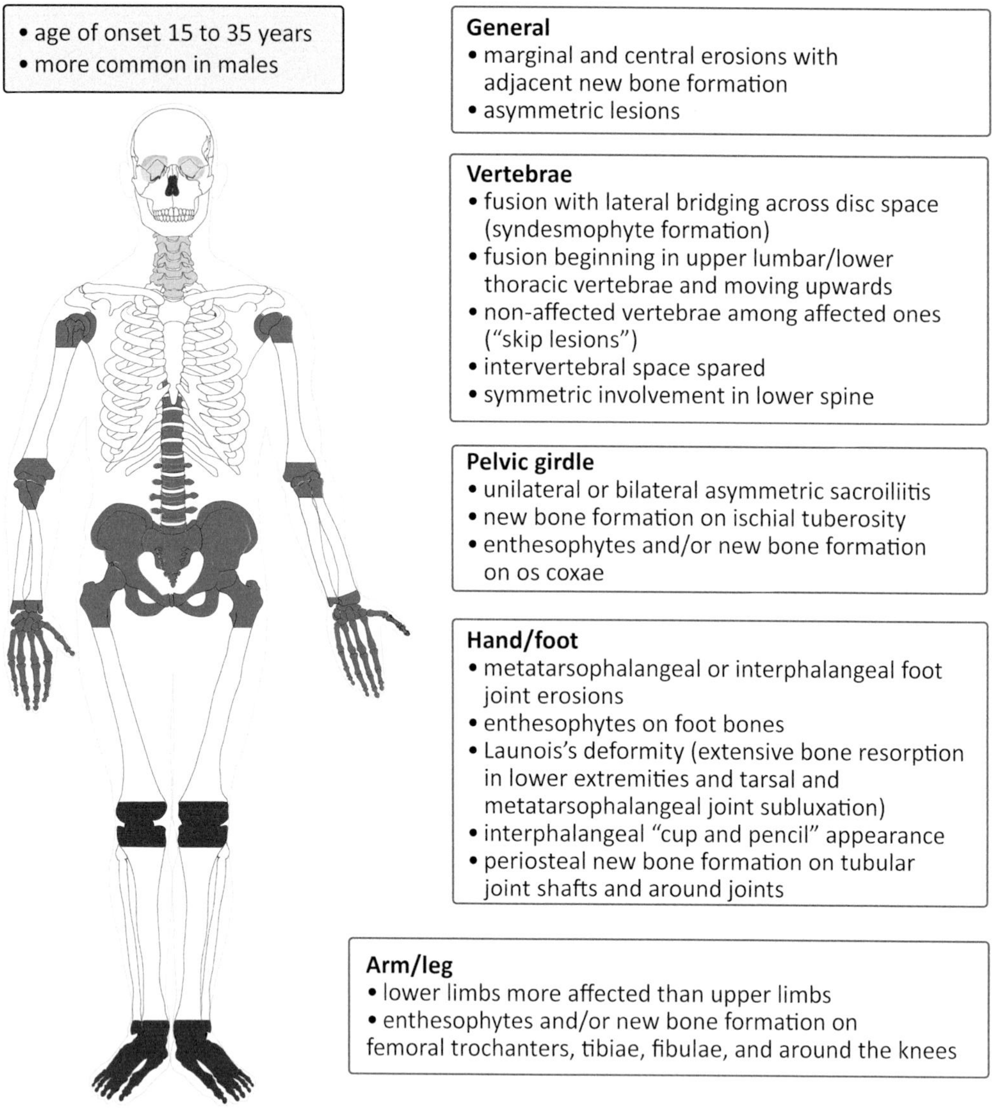

Figure 9.22 Skeletal manifestation of reactive arthritis. (Data from Arriaza 1993; Carter and Hudson 2009; Cawley and Paine 2015; Kataria and Brent 2004; Khan 2002; Rogers and Waldron 1995; Tersigni-Tarrant and Zachow 2012; Waldron 2020b; Wilkins et al. 1981)

Less common forms of synovial joint disease

Gout

Gout is an inflammatory type of arthritis, characterised by high uric acid levels in the blood (hyperuricemia) and the presence of monosodium urate crystals within the joints and adjacent tissues. The first metatarsophalangeal joint is the most frequently affected site; however, gout can appear in any joint of the body. Gouty attacks are initially acute; they have a rapid onset and cause severe pain, swelling, and redness. Most of these acute attacks affect a single joint (especially the first metatarsophalangeal joint, as mentioned above). Joint pain typically peaks within 24 hours after onset, and then it gradually subsides, often without requiring treatment. The acute attack is followed by an asymptomatic phase, called intercritical gout. Subsequent acute gouty attacks generally increase in frequency over time and affect more joints. Most individuals experience a second attack within one or two years, but a few may not have another attack for over a decade. The final phase of the disease is chronic gout, and it is characterised by the formation of uric acid tophi, deposits of monosodium urate crystals located in the articular and periarticular tissues. Although the tophi rarely survive in archaeological contexts, their effects on bone are evident and appear as erosive lesions (Figures 9.23 and 9.24).

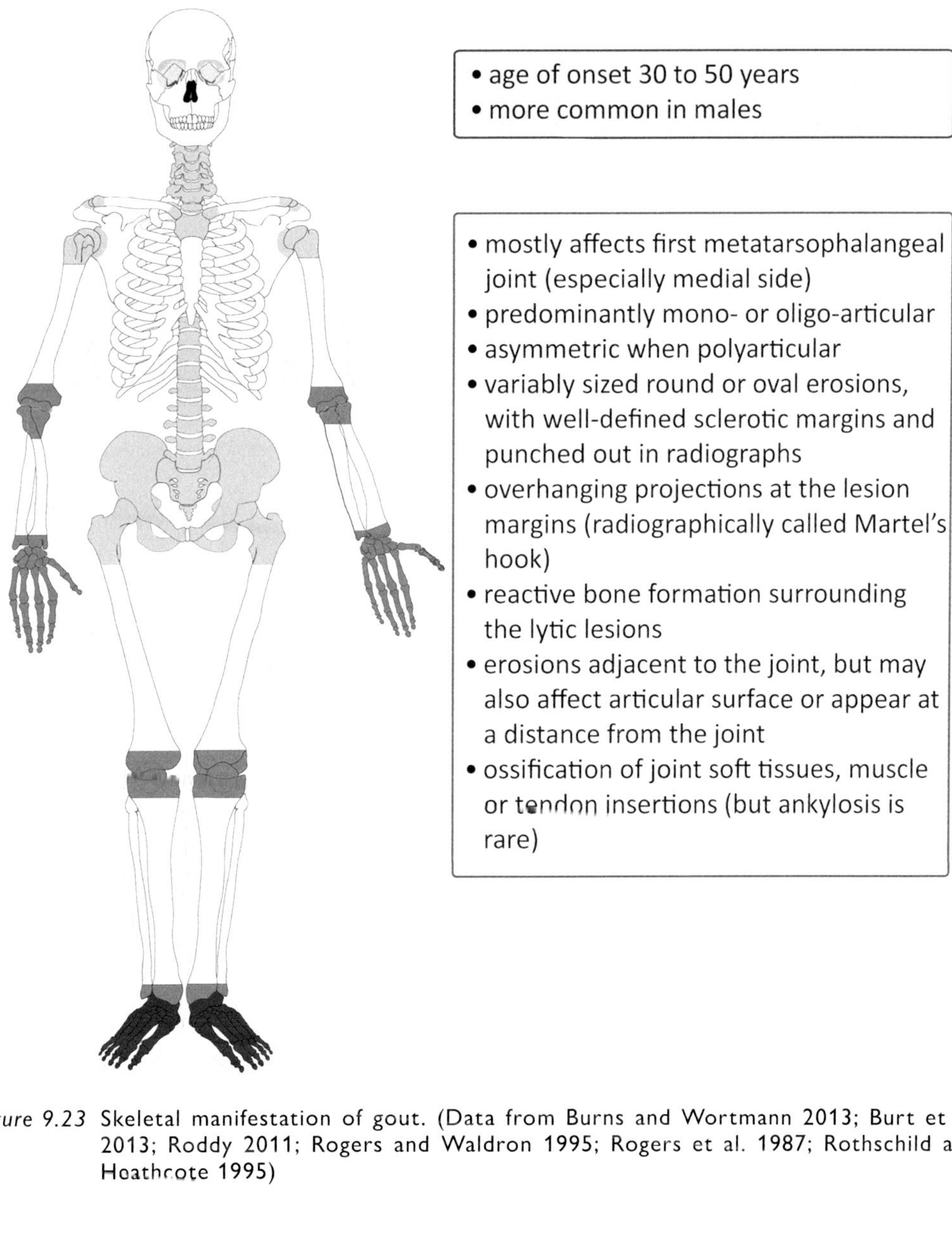

Figure 9.23 Skeletal manifestation of gout. (Data from Burns and Wortmann 2013; Burt et al. 2013; Roddy 2011; Rogers and Waldron 1995; Rogers et al. 1987; Rothschild and Heathcote 1995)

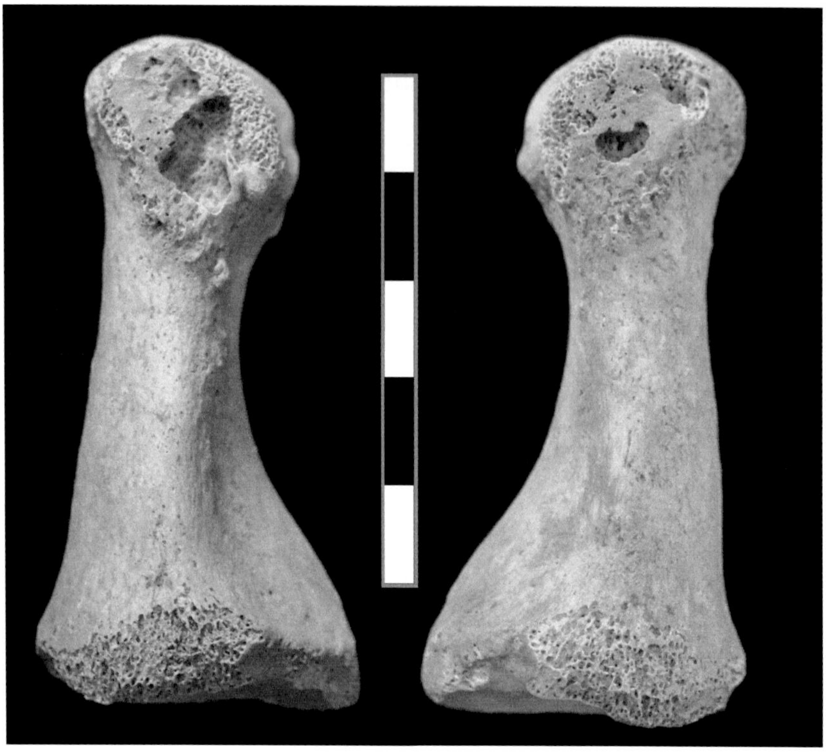

Figure 9.24 Probable gout. Note the lytic lesions adjacent to the metatarsophalangeal joint on the first metatarsals. (London Road, Grantham, 12th-15th c. CE, GLR91-036; photos by Efthymia Nikita; copyright: Human Skeletal Collection, University of Sheffield)

Obesity, high consumption of red meat, shellfish, alcohol, and fructose-sweetened beverages promote the accumulation of excess uric acid in the blood. A familial predisposition to gout has also been observed. Importantly, hyperuricemia has been found to be associated with an elevated risk of hypertension, kidney disease, and diabetes.

Gout may be confused for hallux valgus in certain contexts, so a brief description of the latter is given in Box 9.4.

Box 9.4 Hallux valgus

Hallux valgus is characterised by the lateral deviation of the hallux (great toe) in relation to the first metatarsal (Figures 9.25 and 9.26). The development of hallux valgus has been associated with genetic predisposition, congenital anatomical variation in metatarsal alignment, abnormal foot mechanics, muscle imbalance in abductor and adductor muscles, and body mass index. The condition is primarily associated with wearing narrow, high-heeled, or pointed footwear.

- more common in older adults
- more common in females

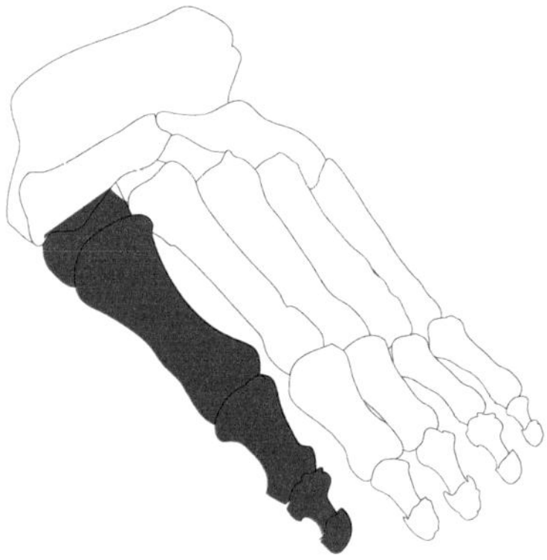

- lateral deviation of first metatarso-phalangeal joint
- basal phalanx subluxation → roughened medial part of first metatarsal head articular surface, which no longer articulates with displaced phalanx; possible separation of this part from functioning articular surface by a sagittal groove
- lateral subluxation of sesamoids → intersesamoid ridge erosion and lipping → eventual smoothing out of ridge
- erosion and exostoses on medial part of metatarsal head
- osteoarthritis on metatarso-phalangeal joint surface
- medially deviated first metatarsal facet on medial cuneiform
- abnormal angulation of basal hallucial phalanges proximal joint surfaces

Figure 9.25 Skeletal manifestation of hallux valgus. (Data compiled from Cai et al. 2023; Mays 2005; Trujillo-Mederos et al. 2014)

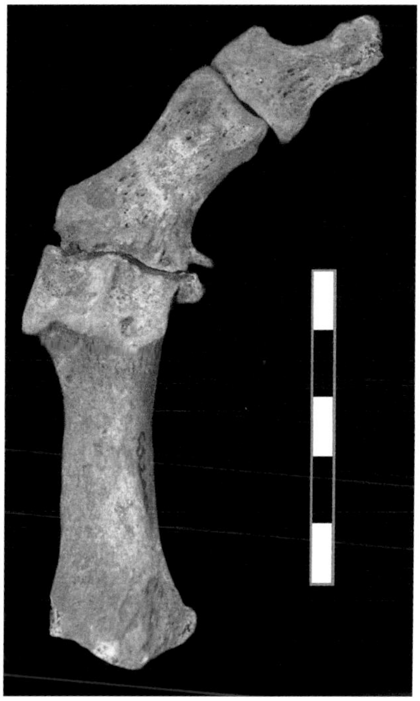

Figure 9.26 Hallux valgus. Note the pronounced lateral deviation of the first metatarsophalangeal joint. (Male, 25–35 years old, St Hilda's Church, Coronation Street, South Shields, Newcastle, 19th c., CS06 268; photo by Efthymia Nikita; copyright: Human Skeletal Collection, University of Sheffield)

Juvenile idiopathic arthritis

The term juvenile idiopathic arthritis (JIA) is used here to denote any form of arthritis that appears before an individual's sixteenth birthday and lasts for more than six weeks (Box 9.5). This group of arthropathies includes systemic arthritis, seronegative idiopathic arthritis, seropositive juvenile-onset adult-type RA, juvenile-onset AS, and psoriatic arthritis. Differential diagnosis of a particular type of JIA through macroscopic skeletal analysis can be challenging. In any case, JIA manifests in early childhood, and there is a subsequent peak just before puberty. It is mostly a benign condition, but it can cause serious complications, such as damage to joint cartilage and bone, and abnormal growth. The severity of JIA depends on the sex and age at onset; individuals afflicted before the age of five are at higher risk of death. Females are more frequently affected by these disorders and also tend to experience more severe forms of the disease. Many children diagnosed with JIA make a full recovery with time; however, in several cases, the condition remains active into adulthood.

Box 9.5 Skeletal manifestation of juvenile idiopathic arthritis

General

- marginal and subchondral erosions
- osteopenia
- if affected in young childhood, chronic inflammation causes overgrowth of affected bones; if affected towards the end of maturity, early epiphyseal closure may make the affected bones shorter

Skull

- short mandibular ascending rami with underdeveloped condyles → micrognathia
- temporomandibular joint erosion and condyle collapse; TMJ fusion in severe cases → disuse atrophy and receding chin
- maxilla reduced in height → smaller face
- malocclusion

Ribs

- subchondral erosions and new bone formation on costal facets

Vertebrae

- mostly in cervical vertebrae
- fused zygapophyseal joints and vertebral bodies in severe cases
- zygapophyseal erosions (including at odontoid process)
- thoracic and lumbar spine compression fractures → scoliosis
- atlantoaxial subluxation

Pelvic girdle

- hypoplastic ilium
- protruding acetabulum
- sacroiliac joint erosions

Arm/leg

- early epiphyseal closure → enlargement of epiphyses
- growth retardation → short and over-tubulated long bones
- osteoarthritis
- coxa valga
- subperiosteal new bone formation
- ankylosis
- epiphyseal compression fractures
- joint dislocation/subluxation
- squared patella

Hand/foot

- short and wide metacarpals, metatarsals, and phalanges
- flexion deformities
- articular marginal and subchondral erosions
- subperiosteal new bone formation
- ankylosis of metacarpophalangeal, metatarsophalangeal, and interphalangeal joints
- carpal and tarsal erosion or ankylosis

(Data from Bernstein et al. 1977; Burgos-Vargas 1993; Hu et al. 2009; Lewis 2017; Lovell 2008; Rothschild et al. 1997; Wedderburn and Nistala 2013)

Diseases of the joints of the spine

Spinal osteophytosis

The spinal joints show anatomical variation and, therefore, they are not affected by joint disease in a uniform manner. Similar processes as the ones observed in osteoarthritis of the synovial joints of the appendicular skeleton can affect the spinal zygapophyseal joints, which are the synovial joints between the articular processes of adjacent vertebrae (Figures 9.27 and 9.28). The joints between vertebral bodies are fibrocartilaginous; however, the arthritic changes found here resemble those found in true synovial joints. In the literature, the terms used to describe arthritic changes in the vertebral bodies are spondylosis deformans or spinal osteophytosis (Figures 9.29 and 9.30).

Spinal osteophytosis arises from damage to the annulus fibrosus of the intervertebral discs. As a result, the annulus is anteriorly displaced, exerting traction on the Sharpey's fibres, and resulting in the formation of osteophytes. Initially, osteophytes develop horizontally, but they can later extend vertically, occasionally leading to fusion of adjacent vertebrae while

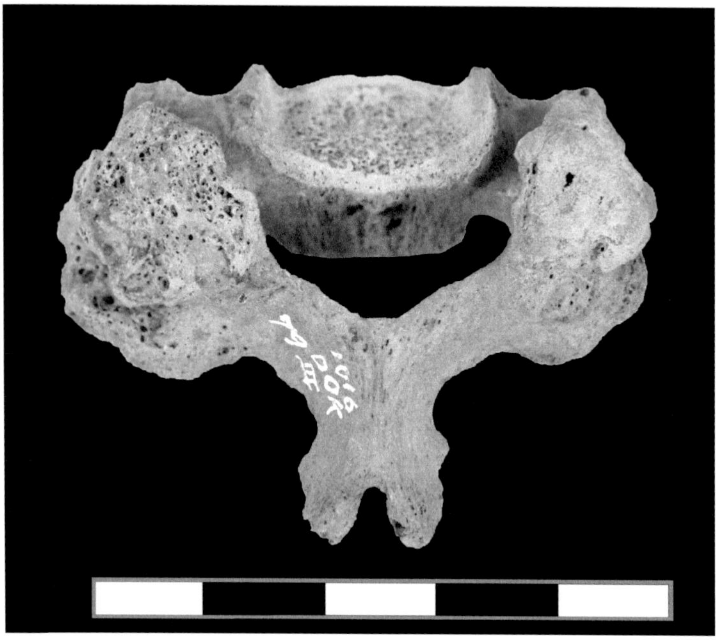

Figure 9.27 Extensive marginal lipping and porosity on the left superior articular facet of a cervical vertebra. A milder expression of lipping and porosity is visible on the right facet. (Female, over 46 years old, Dokkum Marktplein, Collection NAD Nuis inv. Nr. F 2021-X-79; photo by Efthymia Nikita, with permission from the Noordelijk Archeologisch Depot)

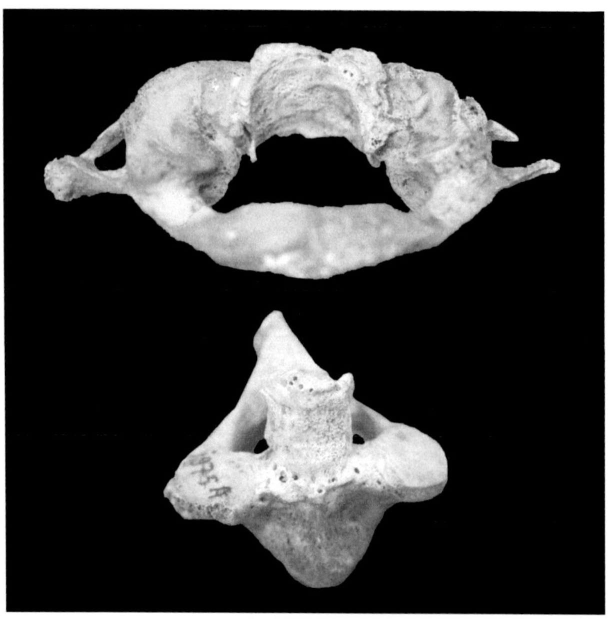

Figure 9.28 Extensive marginal lipping at the atlanto-axial joint. (Probable female, over 46 years old, Diever, Reformed Church graveyard, Collection NAD Nuis inv. Nr. D 2019-III.469; photos by Efthymia Nikita, with permission from the Noordelijk Archeologisch Depot)

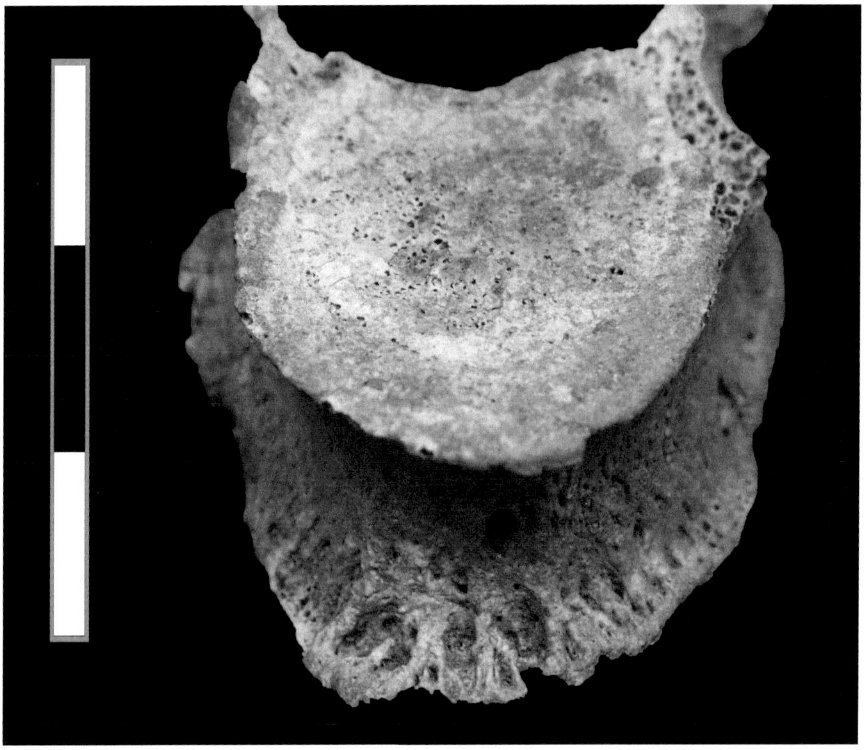

Figure 9.29 Marginal lipping on the body of a thoracic vertebra. (Male, Adult, Linou Tomb 9, Cyprus; photo by Gkampriella Selempa; permission to use this image has been granted by the Director of the Department of Antiquities, Cyprus)

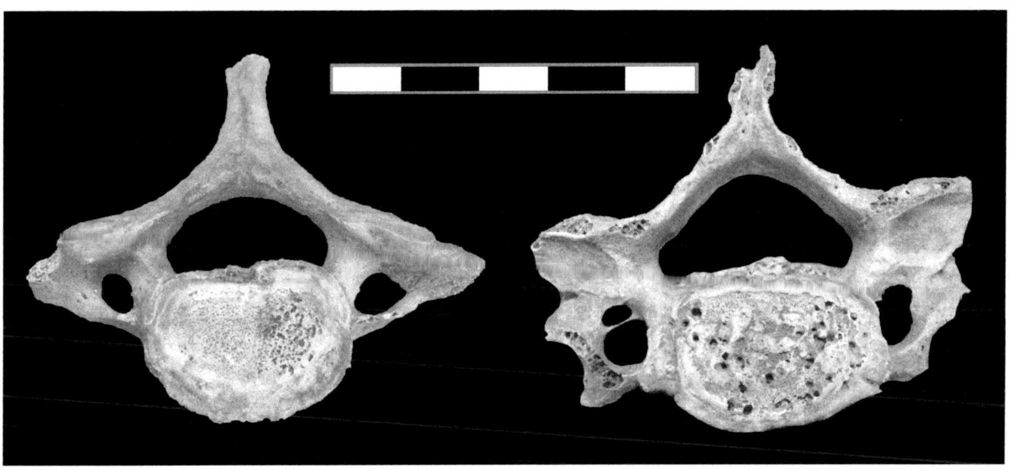

Figure 9.30 Porosity on the body of two cervical vertebrae and minimal marginal lipping. (Diever, Reformed Church graveyard, Collection NAD Nuis inv. Nr. D 2019-III.468 (left) and D 2019-III.470 (right); photos by Efthymia Nikita, with permission from the Noordelijk Archeologisch Depot)

maintaining the integrity of the disc space. In many cases, along with the formation of marginal osteophytes, pitting develops on the superior/inferior vertebral body surface. Such lesions are particularly prevalent in the cervical and lower lumbar parts of the spine.

Spinal osteophytosis has been linked to mechanical stress applied to the vertebral bodies as a result of weight-bearing, coupled with the physical demands of bipedal posture and locomotion. Age is another significant factor in the aetiology of spinal osteophytosis, as this condition is rather rare among individuals younger than 40 years but increases markedly in frequency over the age of 70. In addition, genetic predisposition can also contribute to the development of spinal osteophytosis.

Schmorl's nodes

The term Schmorl's node refers to the herniation of the nucleus pulposus into the adjacent vertebral bodies. However, this term has been extended to express the final manifestation of the herniated material, that is, a cavity on the vertebral body surfaces (Figures 9.31–9.33).

Schmorl's nodes arise from processes that compromise the integrity of the cartilaginous endplate, thus allowing the herniation of the nucleus pulposus. Key factors linked to the development of these lesions include (1) defects or weak areas in the cartilaginous endplate or vertebral body subchondral bone (due to developmental defects, Scheuermann's disease,

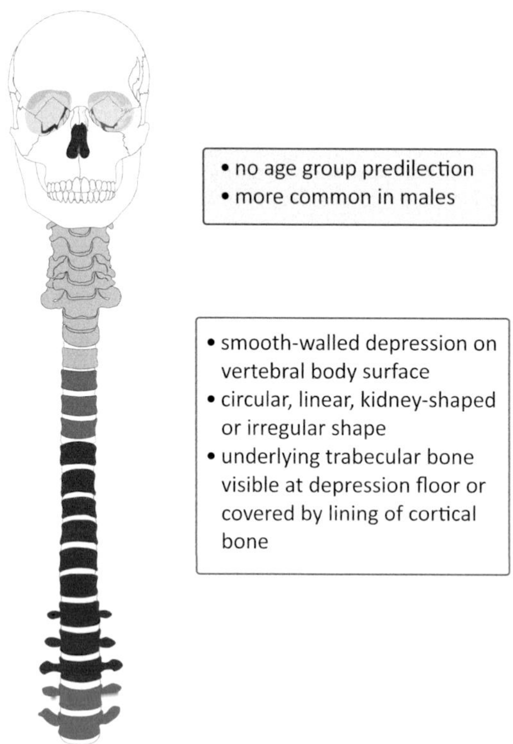

Figure 9.31 Skeletal manifestation of Schmorl's nodes. (Data from Brito and Santos 2024; Burt et al. 2013; Hilton et al. 1976; Rogers and Waldron 1995; Schmorl and Junghanns 1971)

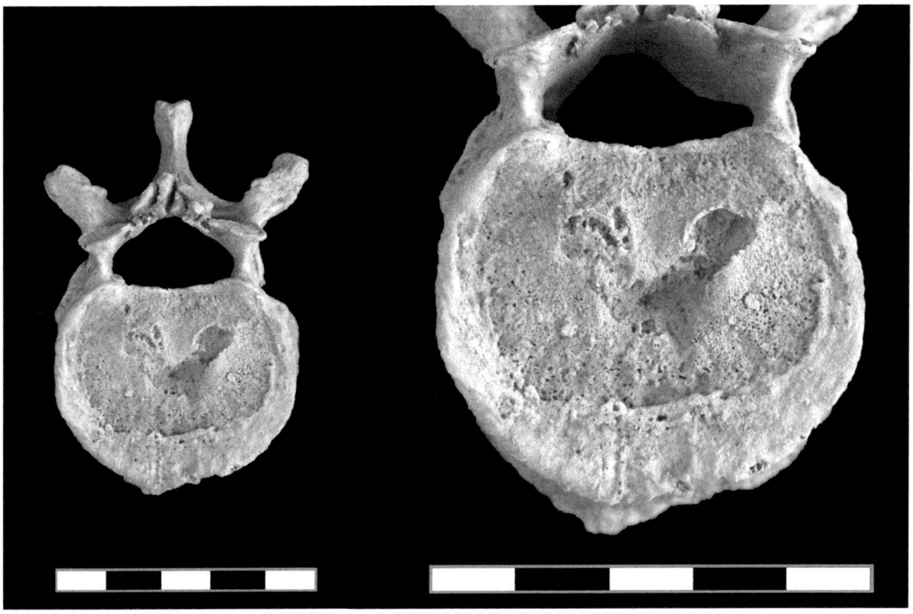

Figure 9.32 Schmorl's nodes at the centre of a thoracic vertebral body. (Sbide, Roman/Byzantine; photo by Efthymia Nikita, with the kind permission of Dr. Ahmet Ihsan Aytek, Burdur Mehmet Akif Ersoy University)

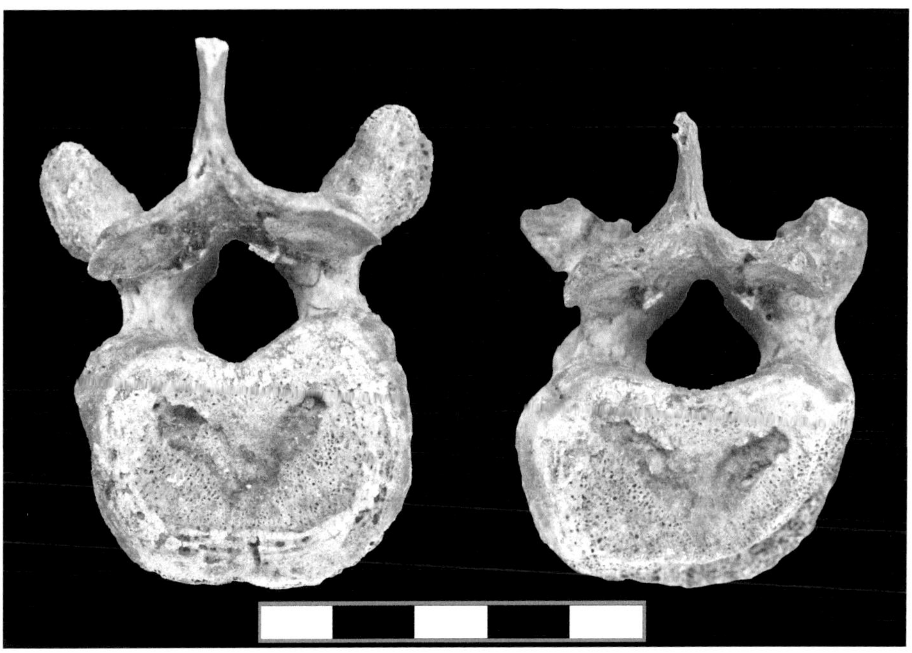

Figure 9.33 Schmorl's nodes at the centre of two thoracic vertebral bodies. (Male, 18–25 years old, Diever, Reformed Church graveyard, Collection NAD Nuis inv. Nr. D 2019-III.471; photos by Efthymia Nikita, with permission from the Noordelijk Archeologisch Depot)

Paget's disease, degenerative changes, osteoporosis, neoplasm, infection etc.); (2) trauma (acute injuries or repetitive stress); and (3) ageing (due to progressive dehydration of the nucleus pulposus accompanied by disorganisation and weakening of the annulus fibrosus; however, several studies have found no association between age and Schmorl's nodes).

Diffuse idiopathic skeletal hyperostosis (DISH)

Diffuse idiopathic skeletal hyperostosis (DISH) is characterised by the ossification of spinal and extra-spinal soft tissues (Box 9.6, Figures 9.34–9.39). The key manifestation of this condition is the ossification of the anterior longitudinal ligament (ALL). As the disease progresses, it creates a distinctive pattern that resembles melted candle wax. In the thoracic spine, ossification occurs on the right side, because the descending aorta lies on the left. In contrast, in the cervical and lumbar vertebrae, ossification is more symmetrical. DISH may also affect bones beyond the spine, such as the ulna, patella, calcaneus, and os coxa, resulting in the ossification of tendon and ligament attachment sites.

DISH aetiology is unclear, but it is likely to be multifactorial. The clinical literature frequently links DISH with the metabolic syndrome (MetS), suggesting that DISH may represent a broader manifestation of metabolic dysfunction. Moreover, evidence supporting a genetic predisposition to DISH comes from the presence of the condition in multiple family members, while several genes implicated in bone remodelling have been associated with DISH. DISH is also strongly linked to ageing, as it mostly affects individuals aged 40 years and older. Furthermore, a higher prevalence of DISH in males has been documented in numerous clinical studies.

DISH may be asymptomatic or cause symptoms such as stiffness, muscle weakness, and pain in the back and/or neck. In addition, individuals may experience restricted mobility in the spine and other joints, including the shoulders, elbows, knees, and ankles. In cases where DISH affects the cervical spine, individuals may also experience dysphagia or hoarseness.

Box 9.6 Diagnosing DISH

Different authors have proposed different DISH diagnostic criteria. Below, we present the ones by Foster et al. (2018) and references therein.

Definite: flowing ALL ossification and ankylosis of four or more adjacent thoracic vertebrae, and at least moderately developed enthesophytes bilaterally at the olecranon process, patella, tibial tuberosity, or posterior part of the calcaneus.

Probable: ALL ossification or ankylosis of two or more thoracic or lumbar vertebrae, and at least moderately developed enthesophytes bilaterally at the olecranon process, patella, tibial tuberosity, or posterior part of the calcaneus.

Possible: ALL ossification, ankylosis *or* at least moderately developed enthesophytes bilaterally at the olecranon process, patella, tibial tuberosity, or posterior part of the calcaneus.

- no exclusion of individuals with sacroiliac joint fusion
- no exclusion of individuals with intervertebral disc degeneration or zygapophyseal joint ankyloses

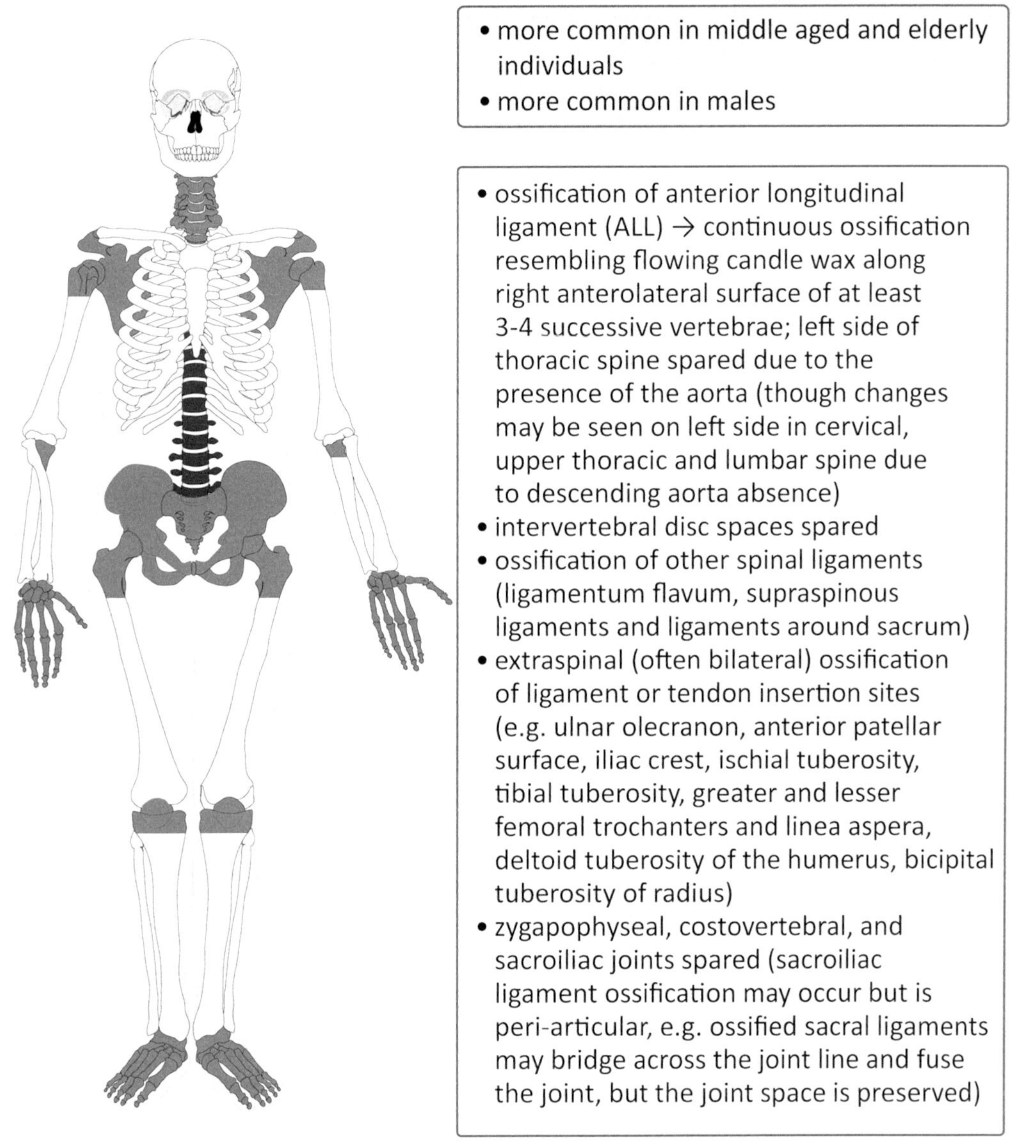

Figure 9.34 Skeletal manifestation of DISH. (Data from Arriaza 1993; Cammisa et al. 1998; Forestier and Lagier 1971; Haller et al. 1989; Nascimento et al. 2014; Navarro and Buckberry 2020; Resnick and Niwayama 1976; Rogers and Waldron 1995, 2001; Rogers et al. 1997; Rotés-Querol 1996; Utsinger 1985)

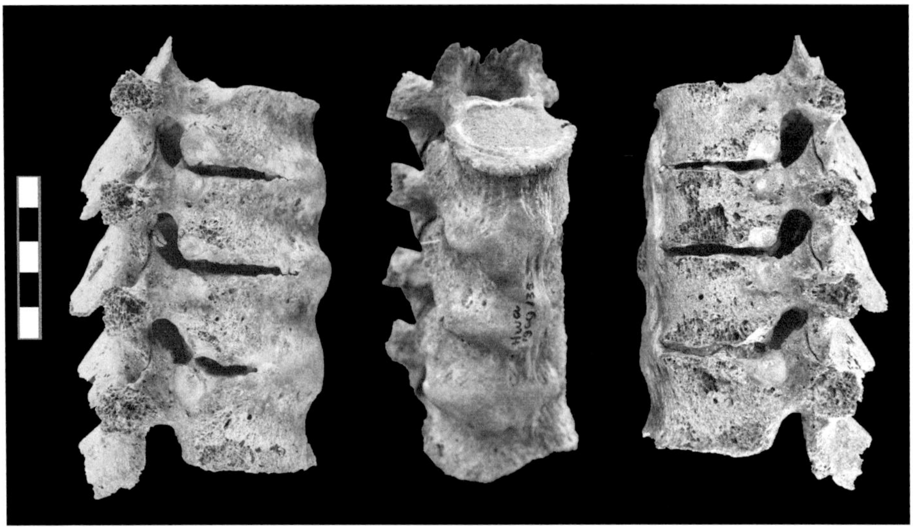

Figure 9.35 DISH on four thoracic vertebrae. Note the continuous ossification of the anterior longitudinal ligament resembling flowing candle wax. (Eemsdelta-Hoogwatum, Collection NAD Nuis inv. Nr. G 2018-IX.268; photos by Efthymia Nikita, with permission from the Noordelijk Archeologisch Depot)

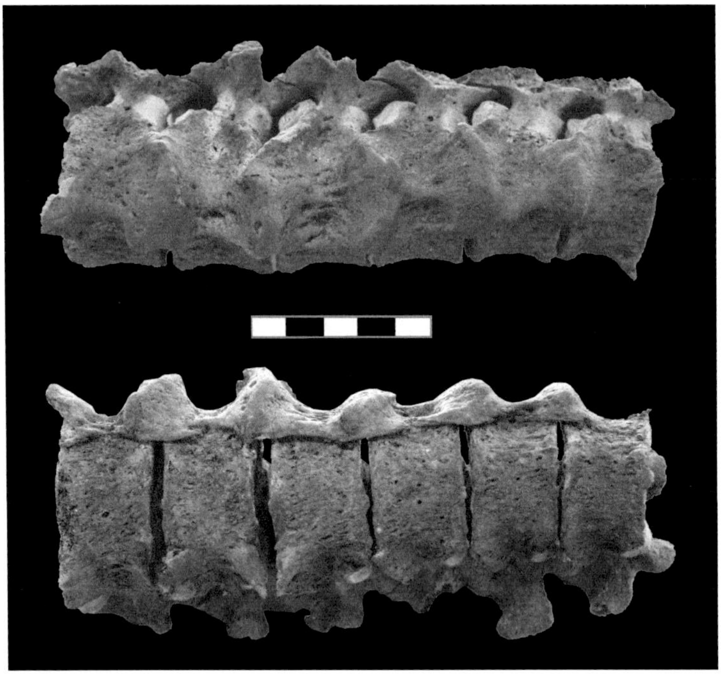

Figure 9.36 DISH on six thoracic vertebrae. Note the continuous ossification of the anterior longitudinal ligament resembling flowing candle wax, and the sparing of the intervertebral disc spaces. (Male, Young/Middle adult, Westerveld-Diever, Collection NAD Nuis inv. Nr. D 2019-III.326; photos by Efthymia Nikita, with permission from the Noordelijk Archeologisch Depot)

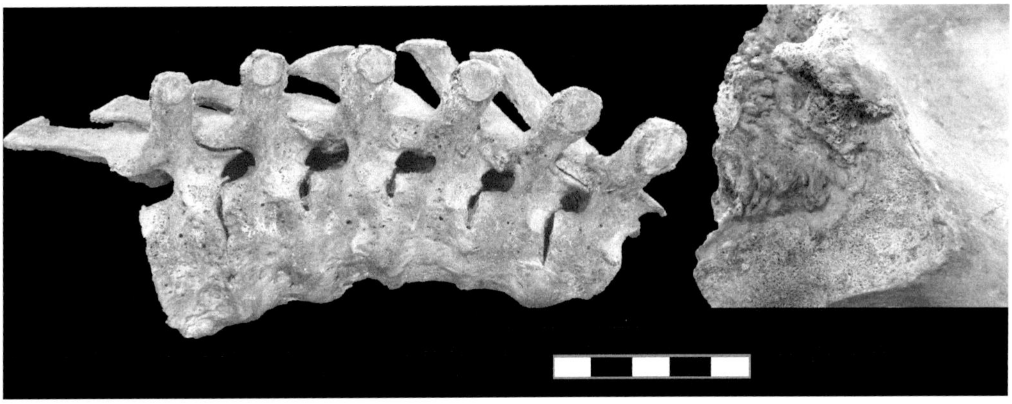

Figure 9.37 DISH on six thoracic vertebrae and sacroiliac ligament ossification. (Female, Adult, Veendam-Veendam, Collection NAD Nuis inv. Nr. G 2008-XII.69; photos by Efthymia Nikita, with permission from the Noordelijk Archeologisch Depot)

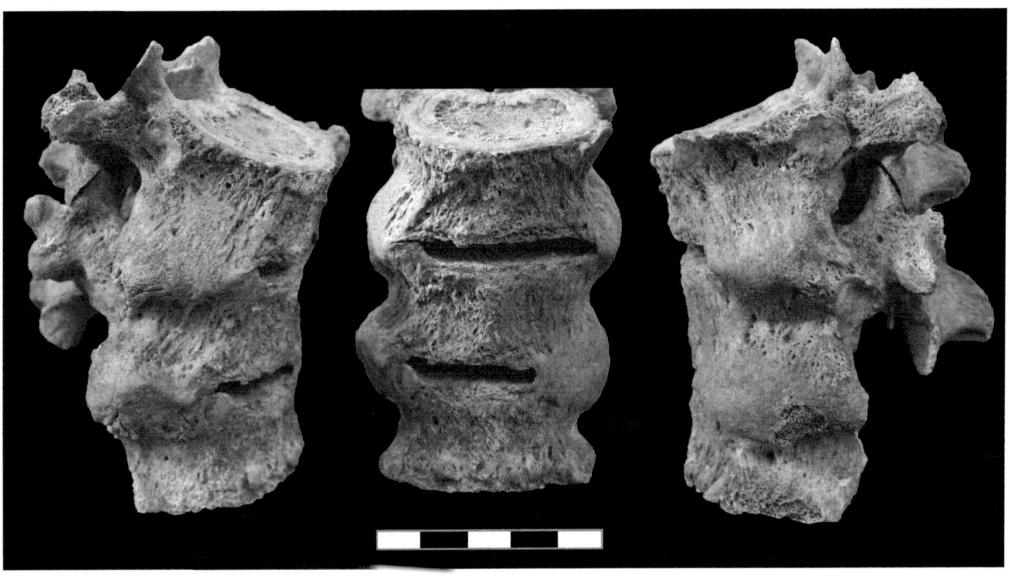

Figure 9.38 DISH on lower thoracic-upper lumbar vertebrae. Note the bilateral ossification, contrary to the right side preference typically seen in the upper thoracic spine. (Male, 22–35 years old, All Saints Church, Fishergate, York, Medieval, Y-2705; photo by Efthymia Nikita; copyright: Human Skeletal Collection, University of Sheffield)

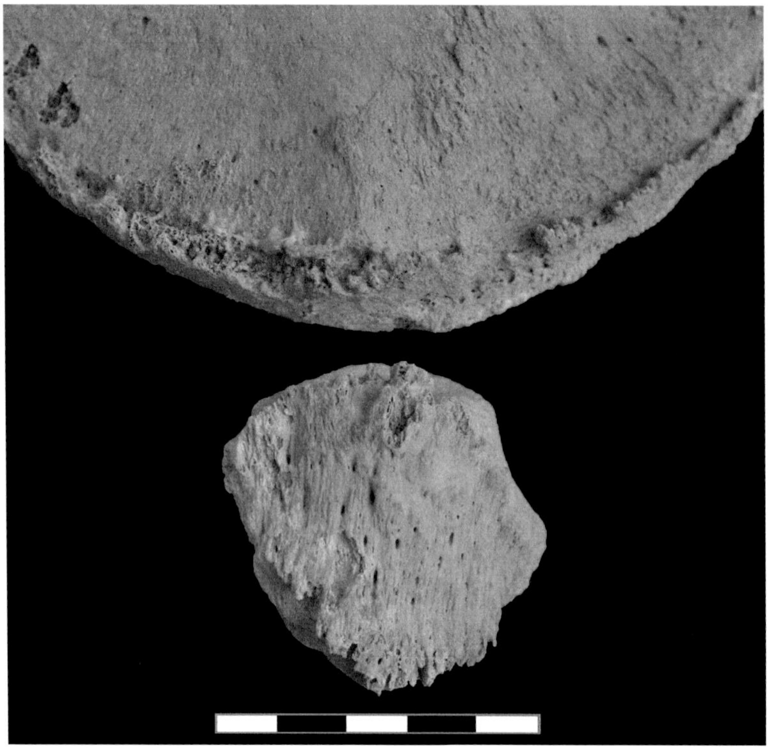

Figure 9.39 Patellar tufting and osteophytes along the iliac crest. A diagnosis of DISH cannot be reached based on these lesions alone but they can complement spinal and other extraspinal changes. (Sbide, Roman/Byzantine; photos by Efthymia Nikita, with the kind permission of Dr. Ahmet Ihsan Aytek, Burdur Mehmet Akif Ersoy University)

References and suggested readings

Arnett, F.C. (1985). Psoriatic arthritis: Relationship to other spondyloarthropathies. In *Psoriatic Arthritis*, edited by Gerber, L., Espinoza, L., pp. 95–108. New York: Grune and Stratton, Inc.

Arriaza, B.T. (1993). Seronegative spondyloarthropathies and diffuse idiopathic skeletal hyperostosis in ancient Northern Chile. *American Journal of Physical Anthropology* 91:263–278. https://doi.org/10.1002/ajpa.1330910302

Arruda, A.L., Katsoula, G., Chen, S., Reimann, E., Kreitmaier, P., Zeggini, E. (2024). The genetics and functional genomics of osteoarthritis. *Annual Review of Genomics and Human Genetics* 25:239–257. https://doi.org/10.1146/annurev-genom-010423-095636

Bernstein, B., Stobie, D., Singsen, B., Koster-King, K., Kornreich, H., Hanson, V. (1977). Growth retardation in juvenile rheumatoid arthritis (JRA). *Arthritis and Rheumatism* 20:212–216.

Biehler-Gomez, L., Cattaneo, C. (2018). The diagnostic implications of two cases of known rheumatoid arthritis from the CAL milano cemetery skeletal collection. *Journal of Forensic Sciences* 63:1880–1887. https://doi.org/10.1111/1556-4029.13799

Bouysset, M., Tourné, Y., Tillmann, K. (2006). *Foot and Ankle in Rheumatoid Arthritis*. Berlin: Springer Verlag.

Brito, J.T., Santos, A.L. (2024). Schmorl's nodes in a historic adult skeletal sample (19th to 20th centuries): An analysis of age, sex and occupation. *International Journal of Paleopathology* 46:1–8. https://doi.org/10.1016/j.ijpp.2024.05.002

Buckley, H.R. (2011). Epidemiology of gout: Perspectives from the past. *Current Rheumatology Reviews* 7:106–113.

Burgos-Vargas, R. (1993). Spondyloarthropathies and psoriatic arthritis in children. *Current Opinion in Rheumatology* 5:634–643. https://doi.org/10.1097/00002281-199305050-00012

Burns, C.M., Wortmann, R. (2013). Clinical features and treatment of gout. In *Kelley's Textbook of Rheumatology*, edited by Firestein, F., Budd, R., Gabriel, S.E., Mclnnes, I.B., O'Dell, J.R., 9th edition, pp. 1554–1575. Philadelphia: Saunders.

Burt, N.M., Semple, D., Waterhouse, K., Lovell, N.C. (2013). *Identification and Interpretation of Joint Disease in Paleopathology and Forensic Anthropology*. Springfield, IL: Charles C. Thomas.

Cai, Y., Song, Y., He, M., He, W., Zhong, X., Wen, H., Wei, Q. (2023). Global prevalence and incidence of hallux valgus: A systematic review and meta-analysis. *Journal of Foot and Ankle Research* 16:63. https://doi.org/10.1186/s13047-023-00661-9

Calce, S.E., Kurki, H.K., Weston, D.A., Gould, L. (2018). The relationship of age, activity, and body size on osteoarthritis in weight-bearing skeletal regions. *International Journal of Paleopathology* 22:45–53. https://doi.org/10.1016/j.ijpp.2018.04.001

Cammisa, M., De Serio, A., Gugliemi, G. (1998). Diffuse idiopathic skeletal hyperostosis. *European Journal of Radiology* 27:S7–S11. https://doi.org/10.1016/S0720-048X(98)00036-9

Carter, J.D., Hudson, A.P. (2009). Reactive arthritis: Clinical aspects and medical management. *Rheumatic Disease Clinics of North America* 35:21–44. https://doi.org/10.1016/j.rdc.2009.03.010

Cawley, W.D., Paine, R.R. (2015). Skeletal indicators of reactive arthritis: A case study comparison of other skeletal conditions, such as rheumatoid arthritis, ankylosing spondylitis, ankylosing sero-negative SpA, and DISH. *International Journal of Paleopathology* 11:70–74. https://doi.org/10.1016/j.ijpp.2015.10.001

Craps, D.D., Gowland, R. (2015). The proximal ulna as an additional diagnostic feature of advanced rheumatoid arthritis. *International Journal of Paleopathology* 10:26–30. https://doi.org/10.1016/j.ijpp.2015.04.002

Dar, G., Masharawi, Y., Peleg, S., Steinberg, N., May, H., Medlej, B., Peled, N., Hershkovitz, I. (2010). Schmorl's nodes distribution in the human spine and its possible etiology. *European Spine Journal* 19:670–675. https://doi.org/10.1007/s00586-009-1238-8

Dieppe, P. (1995). The classification and diagnosis of osteoarthritis. In *Osteoarthritic Disorders*, edited by Kuettner, K.E., Goldberg, V., pp. 5–12. Rosemont, IL: American Academy of Orthopaedic Surgeons.

Dieppe, P. (2008). Osteoarthritis: Clinical features. In *Primer on the Rheumatic Diseases*, edited by Klippel, J.H., Stone, J.H., Crofford, I.J. White, P.H., 13th edition, pp. 224–228. New York: Springer.

Ehrlich, G.E. (2001). Erosive osteoarthritis: Presentation, clinical pearls, and therapy. *Current Rheumatology Reports* 3:484–488. https://doi.org/10.1007/s11926-001-0062-x

Faccia, K.J., Williams, R.C. (2008). Schmorl's nodes: Clinical significance and implications for the bioarchaeological record. *International Journal of Osteoarchaeology* 18:28–44. https://doi.org/10.1002/oa.924

Forestier, J., Lagier, R. (1971). Ankylosing hyperostosis of the spine. *Clinical Orthopaedics and Related Research* 74:65–83.

Foster, A., Kinaston, R., Spriggs, M., Bedford, S., Gray, A., Buckley, H. (2018). Possible diffuse idiopathic skeletal hyperostosis (DISH) in a 3000-year-old Pacific Island skeletal assemblage. *Journal of Archaeological Science: Reports* 18:408–419. https://doi.org/10.1016/j.jasrep.2018.01.002

Giancane, G., Alongi, A., Ravelli, A. (2016). Update on the pathogenesis and treatment of juvenile idiopathic arthritis. *Current Opinion in Rheumatology* 5:523–529. https://doi.org/10.1097/bor.0000000000000417

Haller, J., Resnick, D., Miller, C.W., Schils, J.P., Kerr, R., Bielecki, D., Sartoris, D.J., Gundry, C.R. (1989). Diffuse idiopathic skeletal hyperostosis: Diagnostic significance of radiographic abnormalities of the pelvis. *Radiology* 172:835–839. https://doi.org/10.1148/radiology.172.3.2788894

Helliwell, P.S., Taylor, W.J. (2005). Classification and diagnostic criteria for psoriatic arthritis. *Annals of the Rheumatic Diseases* 64:ii3–ii8.

Helliwell, P.S., Hetthen, J., Sokoll, K., Green, M., Marchesoni, A., Lubrano, E., Veale, D., Emery, P. (2000). Joint symmetry in early and late rheumatoid and psoriatic arthritis: Comparison with a mathematical model. *Arthritis & Rheumatism* 43:865–871. https://doi.org/10.1002/1529-0131(200004)43:4%3C865::aid-anr18%3E3.0.co;2-w

Henriques, J., Berenbaum, F., Mobasheri, A. (2024). Obesity-induced fibrosis in osteoarthritis: Pathogenesis, consequences and novel therapeutic opportunities. *Osteoarthritis and Cartilage Open* 6:100511. https://doi.org/10.1016/j.ocarto.2024.100511

Hilton, F.C., Ball, J., Benn, R.T. (1976). Vertebral end-plate lesions (Schmorl's nodes) in the dorsolumbar spine. *Annals of the Rheumatic Diseases* 35:127–132.

Holgate, R.L., Steyn, M. (2016). Diffuse idiopathic skeletal hyperostosis: Diagnostic, clinical, and paleopathological considerations. *Clinical Anatomy* 29: 870–877. https://doi.org/10.1002/ca.22716

Horváth, G., Molnár, E., Kovács, J., Wicker, E., Bérato, J., Pálfi, G.Y. (1994). Paleopathological diagnosis and interpretation of seronegative spondylarthropathies from the 17th century. *Acta Biologica Szegediensis* 40:103–115.

Hu, Y., Billiau, A., Verdonck, A., Wouers, C., Carels, C. (2009). Variation in dentofacial morphology and occlusion in juvenile idiopathic arthritis subjects: A case-control study. *European Journal of Orthodontics* 31:51–58. https://doi.org/10.1093/ejo/cjn085

Huang, K., Cai, H. (2024). The interplay between osteoarthritis and osteoporosis: Mechanisms, implications, and treatment considerations–A narrative review. *Experimental Gerontology* 197:112614. https://doi.org/10.1016/j.exger.2024.112614

Jurmain, R.D., Kilgore, L. (1995). Skeletal evidence of osteoarthritis: A palaeopathological perspective. *Annals of the Rheumatic Diseases* 54:443–450. https://doi.org/10.1136/ard.54.6.443

Kataria, R.K., Brent, L.H. (2004). Spondyloarthropathies. *American Family Physician* 69:2853–2860.

Khan, M. (2002). Update on spondyloarthropathies. *Annals of Internal Medicine* 136:896–907. https://doi.org/10.7326/0003-4819-136-12-200206180-00011

Leden, I., Svensson, B., Götherström, A., Daskalaki, E., Arcini, C., Drenzel, L., Hårding, B., Molnar, P., Bennike, P. (2009). Criteria for the paleopathological diagnosis of rheumatoid arthritis (RA): A proposal for an updating. *Paleopathology Newsletter* 145:22–24.

Leden, I., Forslind, K., Svensson, B., BARFOT Study Group. (2012). Ankylosis of wrist and small joints of the hand occurs in rheumatoid arthritis: Diagnostic implication in paleopathology. *International Journal of Paleopathology* 2:249–251. https://doi.org/10.1016/j.ijpp.2012.09.001

Lewis, M. (2017). Juvenile arthropathies, circulatory, and endocrine disorders. In: *Paleopathology of Children: Identification of Pathological Conditions in the Human Skeletal Remains of Non-Adults*, edited by Lewis, M. pp. 245–265. San Diego: Academic Press.

Loeser, R.F., Collins, J.A., Diekman, B.O. (2016). Ageing and the pathogenesis of osteoarthritis. *Nature Reviews Rheumatology* 12:412–420. https://doi.org/10.1038/nrrheum.2016.65

Lovell, D. (2008). Juvenile idiopathic arthritis. In *Primer on the Rheumatic Diseases*, edited by Klippel J., pp. 142–149. New York: Springer.

Maat, G.J., Mastwijk, R.W., van der Velde, E.A. (1995). Skeletal distribution of degenerative changes in vertebral osteophytosis, vertebral osteoarthritis and DISH. *International Journal of Osteoarchaeology* 5:289–298. https://doi.org/10.1002/oa.1390050308

Mays, S.A. (2005). Paleopathological study of hallux valgus. *American Journal of Physical Anthropology* 126:139–149. https://doi.org/10.1002/ajpa.20114

McEwan, C., Ditata, D., Lingg, C., Porini, A., Good, A., Rankin, T. (1971). Ankylosing spondylitis and spondylitis accompanying ulcerative colitis, regional enteritis, psoriasis and Reiter's disease: A comparative study. *Arthritis & Rheumatology* 14:291–318. https://doi.org/10.1002/art.1780140302

Mobasheri, A., Batt, M. (2016). An update on the pathophysiology of osteoarthritis. *Annals of Physical and Rehabilitation Medicine* 59:333–339. https://doi.org/10.1016/j.rehab.2016.07.004

Nascimento, F.A., Gatto, L.A.M., Lages, R.O., Neto, H.M., Demartini, Z. (2014). Diffuse idiopathic skeletal hyperostosis: A review. *Surgery Neurology International* 5:S122–S125.

Navarro, L.C., Buckberry, J. (2020). Back to the beginning: Identifying lesions of diffuse idiopathic skeletal hyperostosis prior to vertebral ankylosis. *International Journal of Paleopathology* 28:59–68. https://doi.org/10.1016/j.ijpp.2019.12.004

Nelson, D.A., Kaplan, R.M., Kurina, L.M., Weisman, M.H. (2023). Incidence of ankylosing spondylitis among male and female United States Army personnel. *Arthritis Care & Research* 75:332–339. https://doi.org/10.1002/acr.24774

Plomp, K.A., Roberts, C.A., Viðarsdóttir, U.S. (2012). Vertebral morphology influences the development of Schmorl's nodes in the lower thoracic vertebrae. *American Journal of Physical Anthropology* 149:572–582. https://doi.org/10.1002/ajpa.22168

Queiro, R., Sarasqueta, C., Belzunegui, J., Gonzalez, C., Figueros, M., Torre-Alonso, J.C. (2002). Psoriatic spondyloarthropathy: A comparative study between HLA-B27 positive and HLA-B27 negative disease. *Seminars in Arthritis and Rheumatism* 31:413–418. https://doi.org/10.1053/sarh.2002.33470

Resnick, D.J. (2002). *Diagnosis of Bone and Joint Disorders*, 4th edition. Philadelphia: Saunders.

Resnick, D., Niwayama, G. (1976). Radiographic and pathologic features of spinal involvement in diffuse idiopathic skeletal hyperostosis (DISH). *Radiology* 119:559–568. https://doi.org/10.1148/119.3.559

Resnick, M., Jacobson, J.A., Chung, C.B., Kransdorf, M.J., Pathria, M.N. (2024). *Resnick's Bone and Joint Imaging*, 4th edition. Philadelphia: Saunders.

Reynolds, M.D., Rankin, T.J. (1974). Diagnosis of "rheumatoid variants": Ankylosing spondylitis, the arthritides of gastrointestinal diseases and psoriasis, and Reiter's Syndrome. *Western Journal of Medicine* 120:441–447.

Roddy, E. (2011). Revisiting the pathogenesis of podagra: Why does gout target the foot? *Journal of Foot and Ankle Research* 4:13. https://doi.org/10.1186/1757-1146-4-13

Rogers, J. (2000). The paleopathology of joint disease. In *Human Osteology in Archaeology and Forensic Science*, edited by Cox, M., Mays, S., pp. 163–182. London: Greenwich Medical.

Rogers, J., Dieppe, P. (1990). Skeletal palaeopathology and rheumatic diseases: Where are we now? *Annals of the Rheumatic Diseases* 49:885–886.

Rogers, J., Waldron, T. (1995). *A Field Guide to Joint Disease in Archaeology*. Chichester: Wiley.

Rogers, J., Waldron, T. (2001). DISH and the monastic way of life. *International Journal of Osteoarchaeology* 11:357–365. https://doi.org/10.1002/oa.574

Rogers, J., Watt, I., Dieppe, P. (1985). Palaeopathology of spinal osteophytosis, vertebral ankylosis, ankylosing spondylitis and vertebral hyperostosis. *Annals of the Rheumatic Diseases* 44:113–120.

Rogers, J., Waldron, T., Dieppe, P., Watt, I. (1987). Arthropathies in palaeopathology: The basis of classification according to most probable cause. *Journal of Archaeological Science* 14:179–193. https://doi.org/10.1016/0305-4403(87)90005-7

Rogers, J., Shepstone, L., Dieppe, P. (1997). Bone formers: Osteophyte and enthesophyte formation are positively associated. *Annals of the Rheumatic Diseases* 56:85–90.

Rotés-Querol, J. (1996). Clinical manifestations of diffuse idiopathic skeletal hyperostosis. *British Journal of Rheumatology* 35:1193–1196.

Rothschild, B.M. (1995). Paleopathology, its character and contribution to understanding and distinguishing among rheumatologic diseases: Perspectives on rheumatoid arthritis and spondyloarthroplasty. *Clinical and Experimental Rheumatology* 13:657–662.

Rothschild, B.M., Woods, J.R. (1991). Spondyloarthropathy: Erosive arthritis in representative defleshed bones. *American Journal of Physical Anthropology* 85:125–134. https://doi.org/10.1002/ajpa.1330850202

Rothschild, B.M., Heathcote, G.M. (1995). Characterization of gout in a skeletal population sample: Presumptive diagnosis in a micronesian population. *American Journal of Physical Anthropology* 98:519–525. https://doi.org/10.1002/ajpa.1330980411

Rothschild, B.M., Woods, R.J., Ortel, W. (1990). Rheumatoid arthritis "in the buff": Erosive arthritis in defleshed bones. *American Journal of Physical Anthropology* 82:441–449. https://doi.org/10.1002/ajpa.1330820406

Rothschild, B.M., Hershkovitz, I., Bedford, L., Latimer, B., Dutour, O., Rothschild, C., Jellema, L.M. (1997) Identification of childhood arthritis in archaeological material: Juvenile rheumatoid arthritis versus juvenile spondyloarthropathy. *American Journal of Physical Anthropology* 102:249–264. https://doi.org/10.1002/(SICI)1096-8644(199702)102:2%3C249::AID-AJPA7%3E3.0.CO;2-T

Rothschild, B.M., Surmik, D., Bertozzo, F. (2023). *Modern Paleopathology, The Study of Diagnostic Approach to Ancient Diseases, their Pathology and Epidemiology*. London: Springer.

Samsel, M., Kacki, S., Villotte, S. (2014). Palaeopathological diagnosis of spondyloarthropathies: Insights from the biomedical literature. *International Journal of Paleopathology* 7:70–75. https://doi.org/10.1016/j.ijpp.2014.07.002

Sanchez-Lopez, E., Coras, R., Torres, A. Lane, N.E., Guma, M. (2022). Synovial inflammation in osteoarthritis progression. *Nature Reviews Rheumatology* 18:258–275. https://doi.org/10.1038/s41584-022-00749-9

Schmorl, G., Junghanns, H. (1971). *The Human Spine in Health and Disease*. New York: Grune & Stratton.

Scott, M.E., Dust, W.N., Cooper, D.M., Walker, E.G., Lieverse, A.R. (2021). The physiopathology of osteoarthritis: Paleopathological implications of non-articular lesions from a modern surgical sample. *International Journal of Paleopathology* 32:31–40. https://doi.org/10.1016/j.ijpp.2020.11.001

Segal, N.A., Nilges, J.M., Oo, W.M. (2024). Sex differences in osteoarthritis prevalence, pain perception, physical function and therapeutics. *Osteoarthritis and Cartilage* 32:1045–1053. https://doi.org/10.1016/j.joca.2024.04.002

Sweeney, S.E., Harris, E.D., Jr., Firestein, G.S. (2013). Clinical features of rheumatoid arthritis. In *Kelley's Textbook of Rheumatology*, edited by Firestein, G., Budd, R.C., Gabriel, S.E., McInnes, I.B., O'Dell, J.R., 9th edition, pp. 1109–1136. Philadelphia: Saunders.

Tersigni-Tarrant, M.A., Zachow, R. (2012). Antemortem pathological changes suggestive of reactive and degenerative arthritic disorders. *International Journal of Osteoarchaeology* 22:718–730. https://doi.org/10.1002/oa.1233

Trujillo-Mederos, A., Arnay-de-la-Rosa, M., González-Reimers, E., Ordóñez, A.C. (2014). Hallux valgus among an 18th century population of the Canary Islands. *International Journal of Osteoarchaeology* 24:590–601. https://doi.org/10.1002/oa.2244

Turkiewicz, A., Petersson, I. F., Björk, J., Hawker, G., Dahlberg, L.E., Lohmander, L.S., Englund, M. (2014). Current and future impact of osteoarthritis on health care: A population-based study with projections to year 2032. *Osteoarthritis and Cartilage* 22:1826–1832. https://doi.org/10.1016/j.joca.2014.07.015

Utsinger, P.D. (1985). Diffuse idiopathic skeletal hyperostosis. *Clinics in Rheumatic Diseases* 11:325–351. https://doi.org/10.1016/S0307-742X(21)00544-0

Veale, D., Rogers, S., Fitzgerald, O. (1994). Classification of clinical subsets in psoriatic arthritis. *British Journal of Rheumatology* 33:133–138. https://doi.org/10.1093/rheumatology/33.2.133

Ventades, N.G., Laza, I.M., Hervella, M., de-la-Rúa, C. (2018). A recording form for differential diagnosis of arthropathies. *International Journal of Paleopathology* 20:45–49. https://doi.org/10.1016/j.ijpp.2018.01.004

Vina, E.R., Kwoh, C.K. (2018). Epidemiology of osteoarthritis: Literature update. *Current Opinion in Rheumatology* 30:160–167. https://doi.org/10.1097/bor.0000000000000479

Waldron, T. (1997). Osteoarthritis of the hip in past populations. *International Journal of Osteoarchaeology* 7:186–189. https://doi.org/10.1002/(SICI)1099-1212(199703)7:2%3C186::AID-OA328%3E3.0.CO;2-H

Waldron, T. (2012). Joint disease. In *A Companion to Paleopathology*, edited by Grauer, A.L., pp. 513–530. Hoboken, NJ: Wiley-Blackwell.

Waldron, T. (2019). Joint disease. In *Ortner's Identification of Pathological Conditions in Human Skeletal Remains*, edited by Buikstra, J., pp. 719–748. San Diego: Academic Press.

Waldron, T. (2020a). Joint diseases 1. In *Paleopathology*, edited by Waldron D., 2nd edition, pp. 73–95. Cambridge: Cambridge University Press.

Waldron, T. (2020b). Joint diseases 2. In *Paleopathology*, edited by Waldron D., 2nd edition, pp. 97–124. Cambridge: Cambridge University Press.

Waldron, T. (2020c). Spinal pathology. In *Paleopathology*, edited by Waldron D., 2nd edition, pp. 125–146. Cambridge: Cambridge University Press.

Wedderburn, L.R., Nistala, K. (2013). Juvenile idiopathic arthritis. In *Kelley's Textbook of Rheumatology*, edited by Firestein, F., Budd, R., Gabriel, S.E., Mclnnes, I.B., O'Dell, J.R., 9th edition, pp. 1741–1751. Toronto: W.B. Saunders.

Weiss, E., Jurmain, R. (2007). Osteoarthritis revisited: A contemporary review of aetiology. *International Journal of Osteoarchaeology* 17:437–450. https://doi.org/10.1002/oa.889

Wilkins, R.F., Arnett, F.C., Bitter, T., Calin, A., Fisher, L., Ford, D.K., Good, A.E., Masi, A.T. (1981). Reiter's syndrome. Evaluation of preliminary criteria for definite disease. *Arthritis and Rheumatology* 24:844–849. https://doi.org/10.1002/art.1780240612

Zabotti, A., Fagni, F., Gossec, L., Giovannini, I., Sticherling, M., Tullio, A., Baraliakos, X., De Marco, G., De Vita, S., Errichetti, E., Quartuccio, L., Silvagni, E., Smolen, J.S., Tinazzi, I., Watad, A., Schett, G., McGnonagle, D.G., Simon, D. (2024). Risk of developing psoriatic arthritis in psoriasis cohorts with arthralgia: Exploring the subclinical psoriatic arthritis stage. *RMD Open* 10:e004314. https://doi.org/10.1136/rmdopen-2024-004314

Żelnio, E., Taljanovic, M., Mańczak, M., Sudoł-Szopińska, I. (2023). Hand and wrist involvement in seropositive rheumatoid arthritis, seronegative rheumatoid arthritis, and psoriatic arthritis—the value of classic radiography. *Journal of Clinical Medicine* 12:2622. https://doi.org/10.3390/jcm12072622

Zhu, W., He, X., Cheng, K., Zhang, L., Chen, D., Wang, X., Qiu, G., Cao, X., Weng, X. (2019). Ankylosing spondylitis: Etiology, pathogenesis, and treatments. *Bone Research* 7:22. https://doi.org/10.1038/s41413-019-0057-8

Chapter 10

Trauma

Skeletal trauma covers the changes that may happen to the skeleton due to bone fracture, joint dislocation, surgical procedures, punitive or violent practices, or artificial alteration in bone morphology. The analysis of trauma in human skeletal remains from archaeological contexts provides important information regarding the prevalence and nature of violence, as well as the risks associated with occupational and environmental factors.[1] When cultural and historical contextual information is available, it may also be possible to identify the implements responsible for various wounds, as well as care practices adopted by members of the society for the well-being of those injured.

Various classification systems have been developed for traumatic injuries. Here, we first categorise injuries into fractures (any disruption in bone continuity) and dislocations (the displacement of the bones comprising a joint). Within the group of fractures, we include a separate discussion on blunt force trauma, sharp force trauma, and projectile trauma, as these categories appear frequently in the bioarchaeological and forensic literature. At the end of the chapter, separate sections are dedicated to surgical procedures (e.g. trepanation, amputation), punitive or violent practices (e.g. scalping, decapitation, strangulation), as well as to cultural practices that result in abnormal bone morphology (cranial modification and foot binding). This chapter excludes trauma associated with vehicular collisions or blast injuries, and only provides minimal mention of gunshot wounds, as these are rather recent phenomena.

Fractures

A fracture disrupts bone continuity. The characteristics of a bone fracture depend on several factors, such as the direction of the force applied, the energy associated with the impact, the loading rate, and the duration for which the load is applied. In addition, the health and maturity of bone tissue are important in fracture dynamics. For the interpretation of bone fractures, it is critical to understand basic biomechanical principles, as briefly outlined below.

Biomechanics and key terminology

Two critical parameters that relate to bone response to external forces are strain and stress. Strain is the deformation experienced by an object when external forces are applied to it, while stress is the force applied per unit area. The modulus of elasticity, defined as the slope of the stress-strain curve for a particular material, such as bone, in the elastic region (see below), expresses the material's ability to resist deformation when subjected to external forces. When stress is applied to bones, the latter first exhibit elastic deformation, that is, they may deform,

DOI: 10.4324/9781003475026-10

but they can resume their original shape once the applied stress is removed. However, beyond a certain point, called the elastic limit, bones will exhibit plastic deformation, which is a permanent alteration in their shape. When the applied stress exceeds the bone's strength, the bone will cross its failure point and fracture. Two important concepts in this context are strength and stiffness. Strength is the maximum stress a material can withstand before failing, while stiffness is a material's resistance to deformation when exposed to an external force. The forces that can lead to bone fractures include tension, compression, shear, bending, torsion, or various combinations of these (Figure 10.1). Tension arises when opposing forces are applied to a bone, pulling it apart. In contrast, compression occurs when opposing forces are applied to the bone, pushing it together. Shear forces are applied in a direction parallel to the surface of the bone. Bending induces tensile forces on one side of the bone and compressive forces on the opposing side. Finally, torsion twists the bones about their longitudinal axis.

Classification of fractures

Fractures may be classified in different categories using various criteria (Figure 10.2). Here we present the most common classifications according to the degree of continuity between the fractured bone segments, the extent of soft tissue involvement, the direction of the fracture, the number of resultant bone fragments, the injury mechanism, and the underlying aetiology of the fracture.

In incomplete fractures, partial continuity between the segments of the fractured bone is preserved. Such fractures are more common in children because immature bone is more plastic. In addition, these fractures may arise from low-impact forces or when the area of impact is wide and allows the dissipation of the applied force. In contrast, complete fractures result in a discontinuity among two or more bone fragments (Figures 10.3–10.9). Clinically, these fractures are categorised based on the degree of soft tissue involvement. In closed fractures,

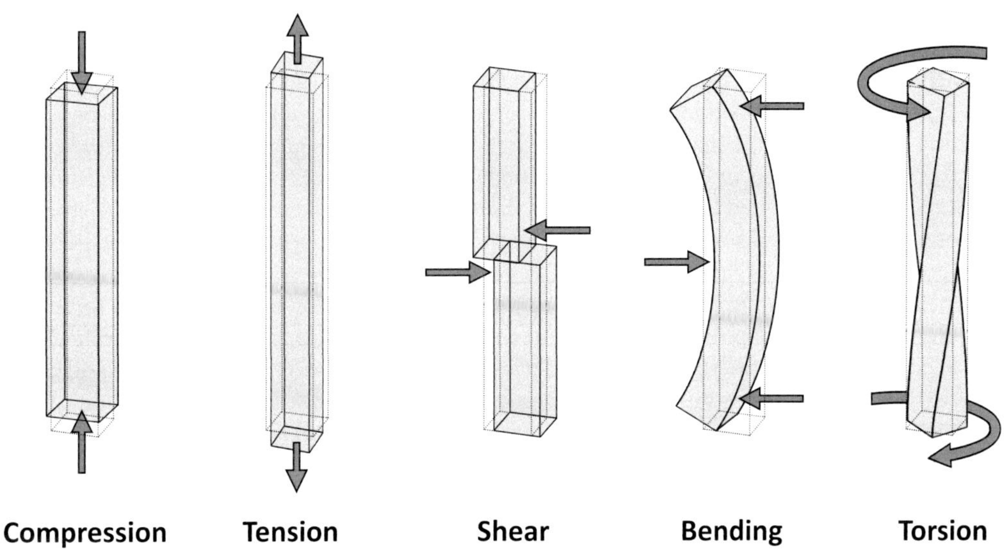

Figure 10.1 Different forces that may be imposed on bones. (Image created by the authors, inspired by a different image shared through Wikimedia Commons - https://commons.wikimedia.org/wiki/File:Different-types-of-mechanical-stress_EN.svg - and licensed under a Creative Commons Attribution-Share Alike 4.0 license)

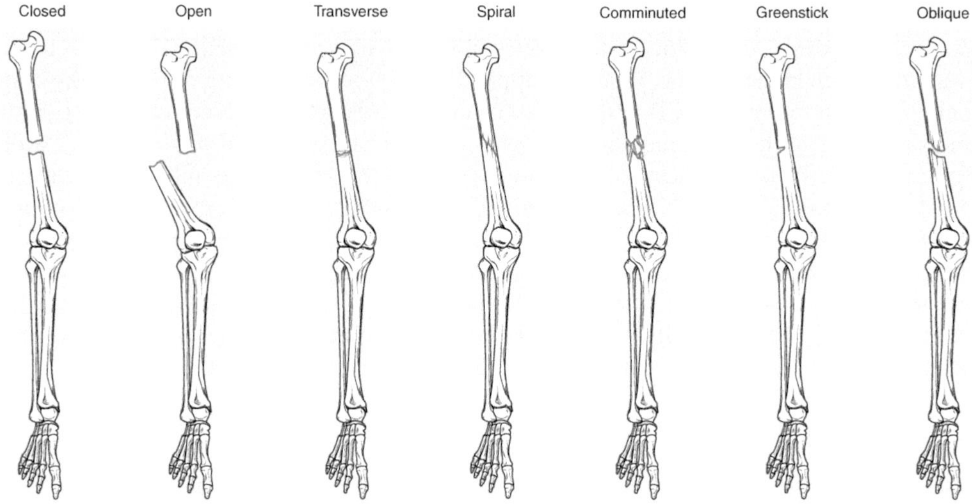

Figure 10.2 Different types of fractures. (Adapted from an image by OpenStax College, shared through Wikimedia Commons and licensed under a Creative Commons Attribution 4.0 International license)

there is no disruption to the overlying skin at the fracture site, which reduces the risk of infection. In contrast, in open or compound fractures, the overlying skin is compromised and allows external organisms and contaminants to access the injury site.

Based on direction, fractures are categorised as transverse, oblique, and spiral. In transverse fractures, the fracture line intersects the long axis of the bone at approximately right angles (Figure 10.10). In cases of transverse fracturing, the bone experiences significant tensile stress on the convex side, while the concave side is subjected to compressive forces. Oblique fractures usually arise from combined moderate bending and compressive forces, or torsional and bending forces; they show a diagonal fracture line across the diaphysis (Figure 10.11). Finally, spiral fractures are induced by torsional forces or combined torsion and bending, resulting in a fracture line that encircles the shaft of the bone (Figure 10.12).

A fracture that results in the bone being divided into two pieces is called a simple fracture. In contrast, a comminuted fracture produces multiple bone fragments. Finally, in a segmental fracture, the bone breaks at two different points at least, and the part of the bone between them gets displaced.

Depending on the injury mechanism, trauma can be direct or indirect. Direct force will fracture the bone at the point of impact and can cause transverse, oblique, comminuted (see above), but also crush fractures. Crush fractures belong to two types: depression and compression. A depression fracture occurs when a crushing force is applied to one side of the bone, a phenomenon frequently seen in the cranium. Compression fractures are characterised by a force that acts upon both sides of the bone, and are common in the vertebrae. Direct trauma also includes the penetration of the bone, during processes such as cutting, piercing, drilling, or scraping.

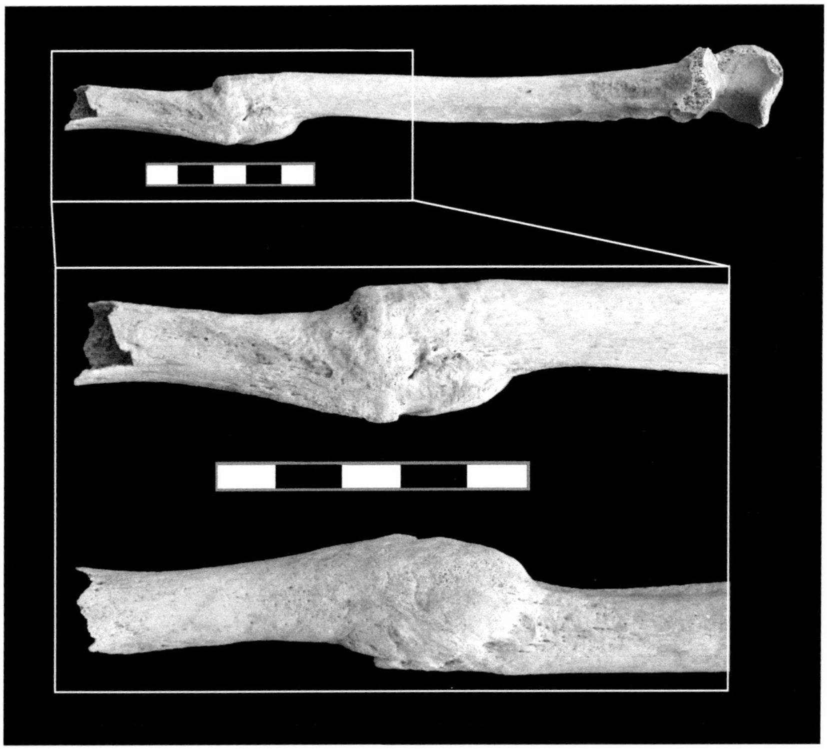

Figure 10.3 Healed complete ulnar fracture. Note the large callus formation and the displacement of the distal part of the fractured bone compared to the proximal one. (Sbide, Roman/Byzantine; photos by Efthymia Nikita, with the kind permission of Dr. Ahmet Ihsan Aytek, Burdur Mehmet Akif Ersoy University)

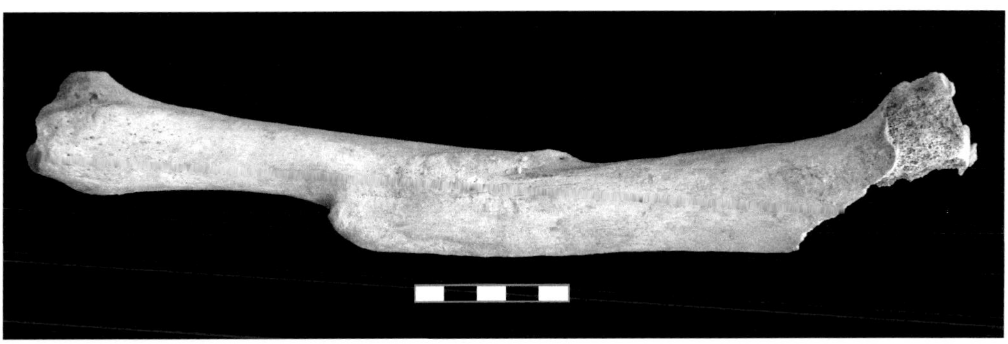

Figure 10.4 Healed complete fracture of the tibia with substantial overlap of the fractured ends. (Sbide, Roman/Byzantine; photo by Efthymia Nikita, with the kind permission of Dr. Ahmet Ihsan Aytek, Burdur Mehmet Akif Ersoy University)

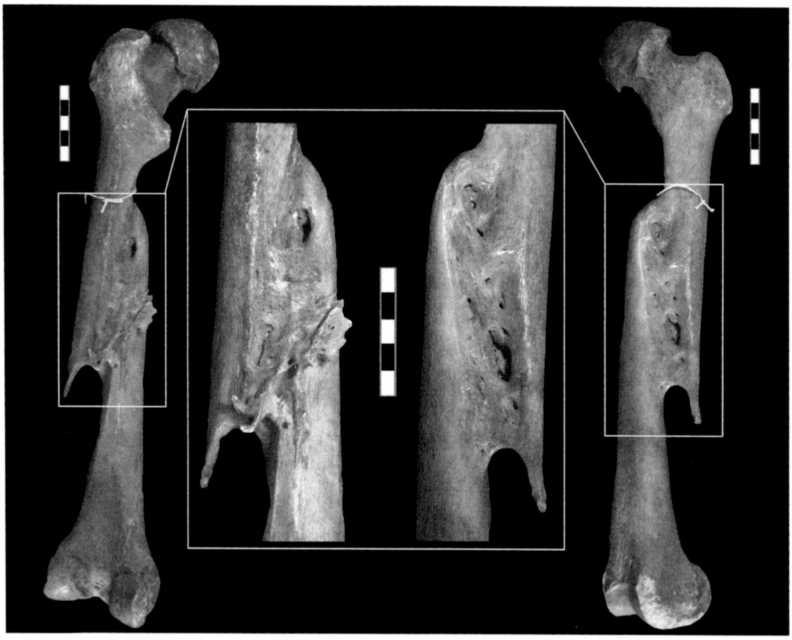

Figure 10.5 Healed complete fracture of the midshaft of a left femur. Note the major overlap of the fractured ends. (Kerma IVB YA (ETC) PTO; photos by Efthymia Nikita; copyright: Duckworth Laboratory, University of Cambridge)

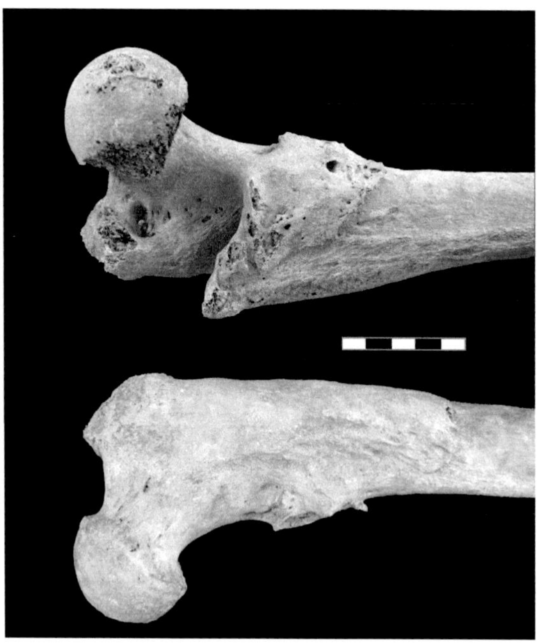

Figure 10.6 Healed complete fracture of a left femur. Note the overlap and misalignment of the fractured ends. (Male, Young adult, Eemsdelta-Hoogwatum, Collection NAD Nuis inv. Nr. G 2018-IX.319; photos by Efthymia Nikita, with permission from the Noordelijk Archeologisch Depot)

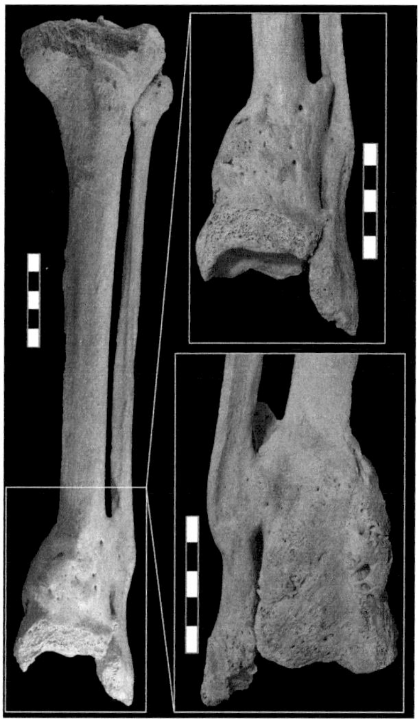

Figure 10.7 Healed complete fracture of the distal left tibia and fibula, resulting in the fusion of these two elements. (Photos by Efthymia Nikita; copyright: Duckworth Laboratory, University of Cambridge)

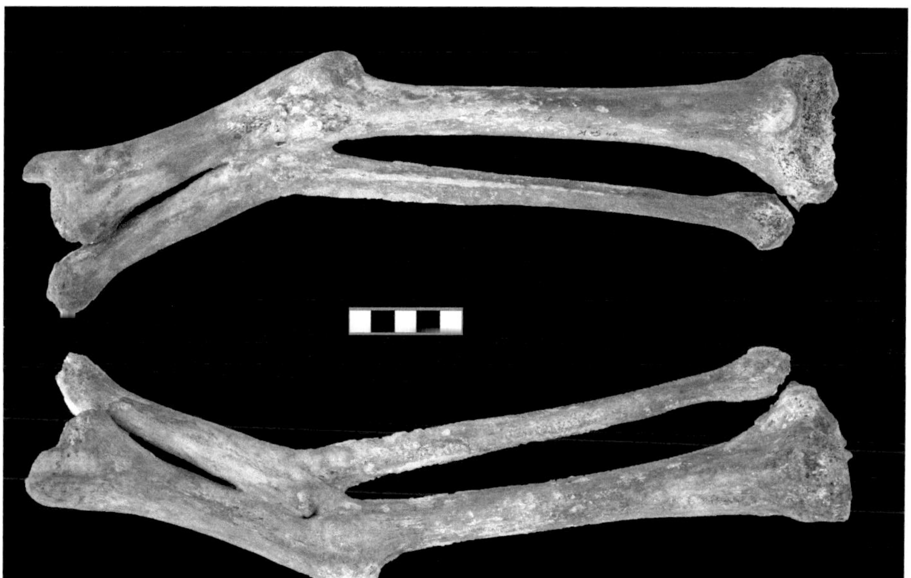

Figure 10.8 Complete fracture of a left tibia and fibula. Note the pronounced angulation of these elements due to malunion. (Female, Adult, Alkmaar-Grote Kerk, Medieval-Modern, 5079; photos by Efthymia Nikita, from the reference collection of the Cultural Heritage Agency of the Netherlands)

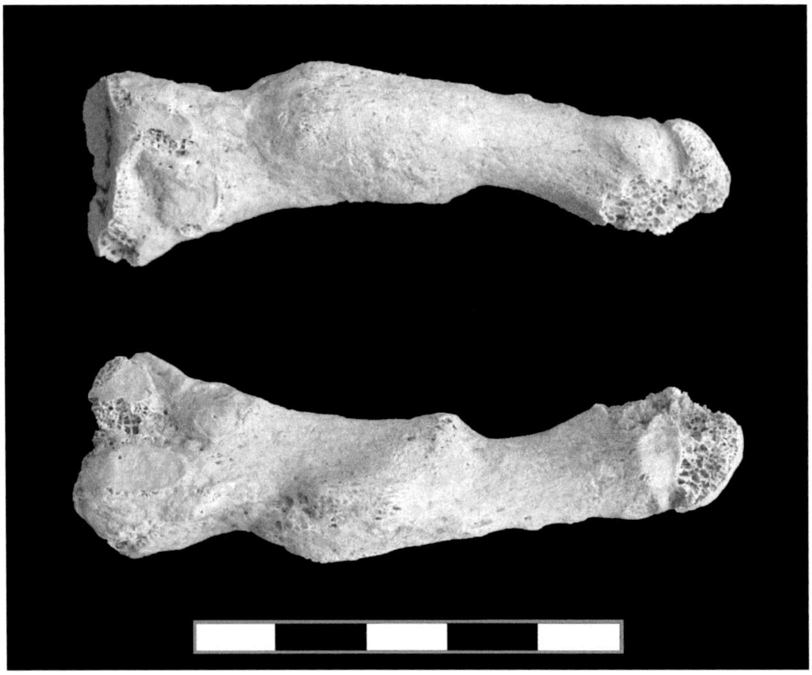

Figure 10.9 Healed complete metatarsal fracture with overlap of the fractured ends. (Samantaş, Byzantine; photos by Efthymia Nikita, with the kind permission of Dr. Ahmet Ihsan Aytek, Burdur Mehmet Akif Ersoy University)

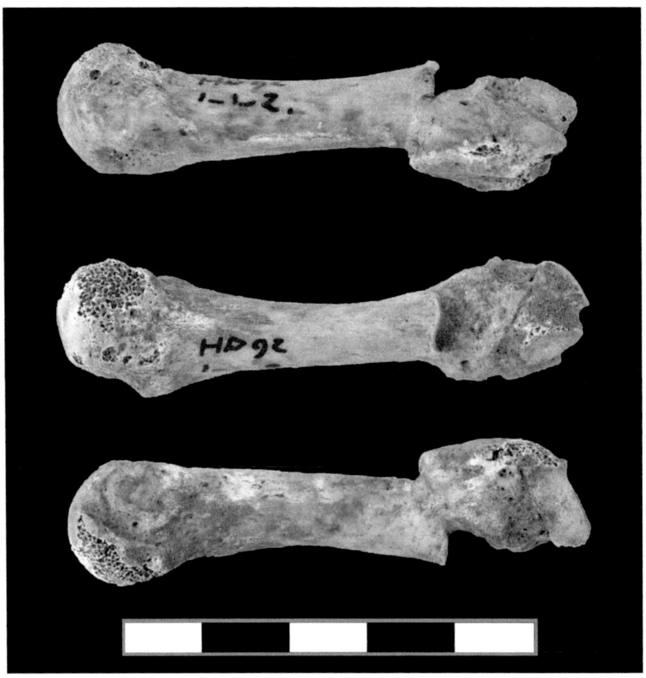

Figure 10.10 Transverse fracture of a metacarpal; note the marked misalignment of the fractured ends. (Male, Adult, Harderwijk, 1450–1600 CE, 5053; photos by Efthymia Nikita, from the reference collection of the Cultural Heritage Agency of the Netherlands)

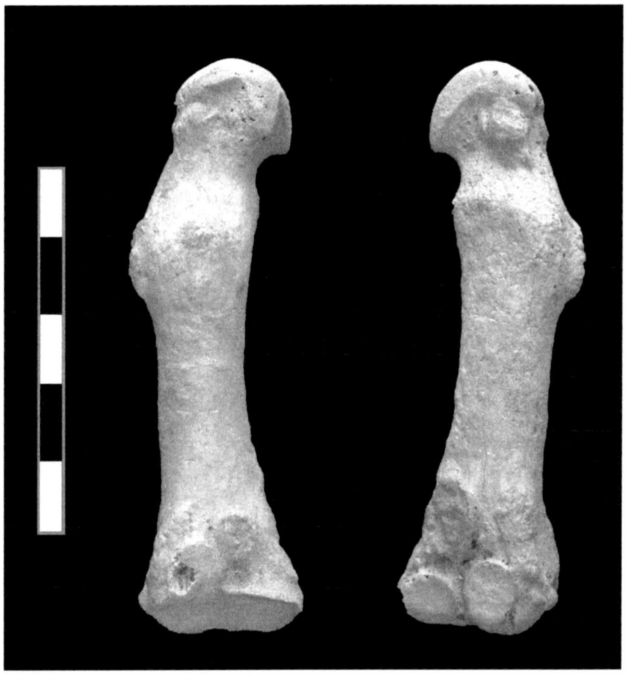

Figure 10.11 Healed oblique metatarsal fracture. Note the callus and slight angulation. (Sbide, Roman/Byzantine; photos by Efthymia Nikita, with the kind permission of Dr. Ahmet Ihsan Aytek, Burdur Mehmet Akif Ersoy University)

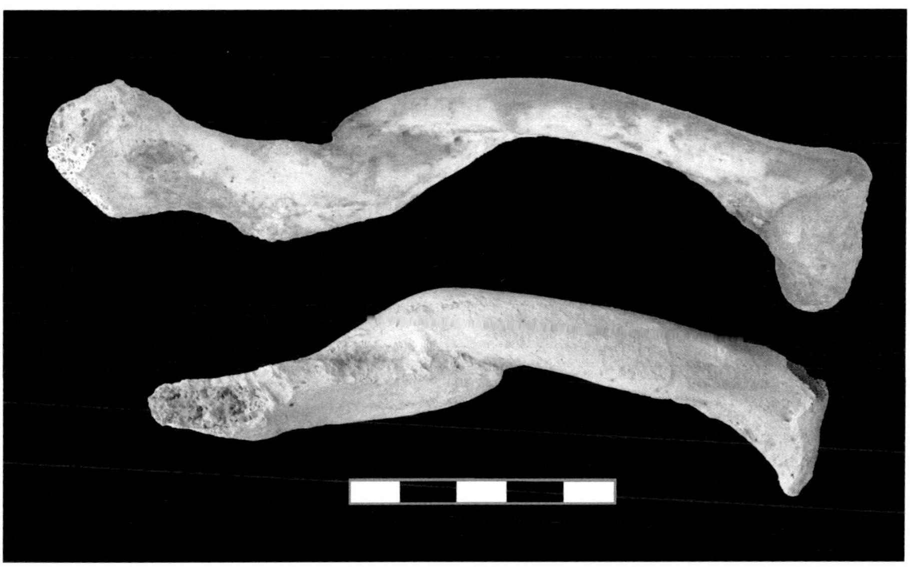

Figure 10.12 Healed spiral clavicular fractures. Both fractures are near the midshaft, and they have healed with visible malunion. (Top: Male, 35–45 years old, Diever, Reformed Church graveyard, Collection NAD Nuis inv. Nr. D 2019-III.472; photo by Efthymia Nikita, with permission from the Noordelijk Archeologisch Depot; bottom: Sbide, Roman/Byzantine; photo by Efthymia Nikita, with the kind permission of Dr. Ahmet Ihsan Aytek, Burdur Mehmet Akif Ersoy University)

Indirect trauma produces fractures far from the site of direct impact. For example, linear fractures may appear in the skull as a result of the out-bending of bone segments following a high-velocity direct blow. In addition, avulsion fractures occur when small bone fragments detach from bony prominences due to forces exerted by the attached ligaments or tendons. Such fractures frequently appear in the patella, the ulnar olecranon process, and the tibial medial malleolus. Other fracture types, such as oblique and spiral fractures, can also result from indirect trauma. Impacted fractures, which occur when the force of injury drives the fractured bone ends into one another, may also arise from indirect trauma. Finally, comminuted fractures can result from both indirect and direct trauma.

Based on their aetiology, fractures can be classified as traumatic, stress or fatigue, and pathological. Traumatic fractures result from trauma (e.g. from falls); stress or fatigue fractures arise from repetitive loading, while pathological fractures are associated with underlying pathological conditions that have compromised bone integrity (e.g. osteoporosis).

Fracture timing

Antemortem trauma refers to injuries sustained before the individual's death. Such trauma can be skeletally identified through evidence of bone remodelling. Evidence of remodelling may include porosity near the fracture site, rounding of the fracture edges, the formation of bony bridges, but also potential signs of infection.

If there is no observable bone healing, the injury may be macroscopically classified as either a perimortem or postmortem fracture. Perimortem fractures either occurred shortly before death, before any visible healing had time to develop, or they occurred shortly after death when the bone was still rather fresh. The interpretation of perimortem fractures is, thus, challenging because bone tissue requires a few weeks to show signs of healing macroscopically, yet it retains some degree of plasticity for a short period following death.

Several criteria have been proposed to distinguish perimortem from postmortem fractures macroscopically. First, bone surfaces that are exposed to the burial environment get stained from the soil and other elements in that environment. Therefore, fracture surfaces that are stained in a similar manner to the rest of the bone surface are likely to have formed at the time of burial. In contrast, bone surfaces that have fractured at a later stage should exhibit a different colour compared to the rest of the exposed bone surfaces. In practice, colouration is useful in distinguishing excavation-induced damage from pre-existing fractures. However, it is challenging to use this approach for other post-mortem events, especially for remains with complex taphonomic histories.

Besides discolouration, perimortem trauma is likely to result in bone deformation before failure, leading to bending deformities and/or greenstick fractures. This pattern is because living or recently deceased bone has high moisture content and elasticity. Furthermore, perimortem injuries typically show oblique angles at the fracture margins, smooth fracture margins, and small bone fragments adhering to these margins (hinging). In addition, these injuries may display radiating fracture lines that are either linear or concentric.

As the process of body decomposition advances, there is a gradual loss of moisture from the bone, the collagen fibres degrade, and bone flexibility is reduced. As a result, when a force is applied to dry bone, it can easily fracture as its ability for plastic deformation is limited. Fractures that occur postmortem typically do not show bending deformities; rather, the fracture surfaces have right angles and a more irregular, jagged appearance. The resulting bone fragments tend to be smaller, and the bone is more likely to shatter. In addition, in cases of postmortem bone fractures, it is rare to have hinging and radiating fractures.

Despite the above criteria, experimental studies have shown that it can be challenging to distinguish perimortem from postmortem fractures macroscopically. Furthermore, there are cases where a single skeleton may have trauma that occurred at various stages (ante-, peri-, and post-mortem), thereby, interpretations should be cautious.

Fracture healing

Healing begins immediately after an injury, if the individual has survived. The process of bone healing has three distinct phases: inflammatory, repair, and remodelling. During the inflammatory phase, a haematoma forms and immune cells such as neutrophils, macrophages, and lymphocytes remove necrotic tissue. These immune cells also stimulate angiogenesis and recruit progenitor cells that undergo chondrogenic and osteogenic differentiation, contributing to fracture callus formation. During the repair phase, cartilaginous tissue bridges the fracture gap. The cartilage is then converted into bone. Finally, at the remodelling phase, osteoclasts remodel the bony callus to restore the bone's original geometry and replace the previously formed woven bone with mature lamellar bone.

The above repair process pertains to cortical bone; in contrast, cancellous bone has a trabecular structure that offers a larger contact area between fractured fragments, as well as ample vasculature. These factors promote the healing process. Bone healing in the case of trabecular bone involves the direct deposition of new bone trabeculae between the fracture ends, promoting direct union between bone fragments, bypassing the need for callus formation. Therefore, the healing process in trabecular bone is faster.

The duration of fracture healing is controlled by several factors, including the specific bone fractured, the fracture's severity, the apposition and stability of the fracture ends, the individual's age, and nutritional status. The potential complications associated with the healing process are classified into three broad groups: a) Delayed union, which may arise from inadequate apposition (i.e. limited contact of the fracture surfaces) as well as insufficient stabilisation, advanced age, nutritional deficiencies, and pre-existing medical conditions; b) Nonunion, which can result from inadequate stabilisation, infection, other medical issues, or severe initial trauma; and c) Malunion, where the fractured ends overlap, form an abnormal angle or are rotated (Figures 10.13–10.21). Additional complications include infection, which typically arises in cases of open or compound fractures; osteonecrosis, resulting from the traumatic disruption of the blood supply to the fractured segments; and myositis ossificans (see Box 10.1). Pseudarthrosis, that is, the formation of a false joint, ankylosis, neuropathy, and traumatic arthritis may also appear after a fracture. Fractures in children may cause complications such as growth arrest or joint deformities, if they result in premature closure of the growth plate, or conversely, excessive growth due to increased blood flow in the injured area.

Fractures in juveniles

Fractures in juveniles may differ from those seen in adult skeletons. The juvenile skeleton is more plastic than that of adults; thus, incomplete fractures are more common. Moreover,

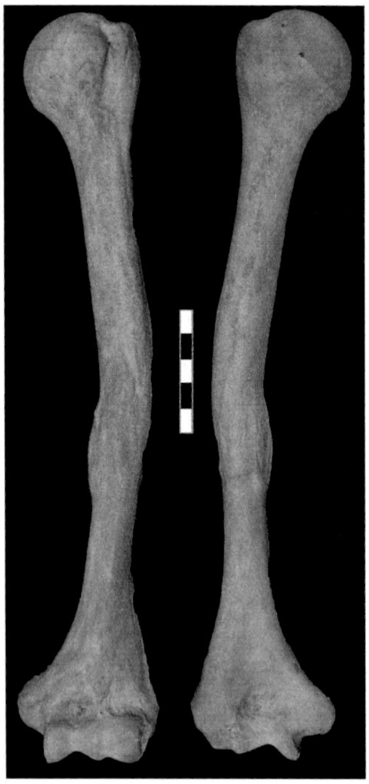

Figure 10.13 Healed fracture of the midshaft of a left humerus with slight misalignment. (Photos by Efthymia Nikita; copyright: Duckworth Laboratory, University of Cambridge)

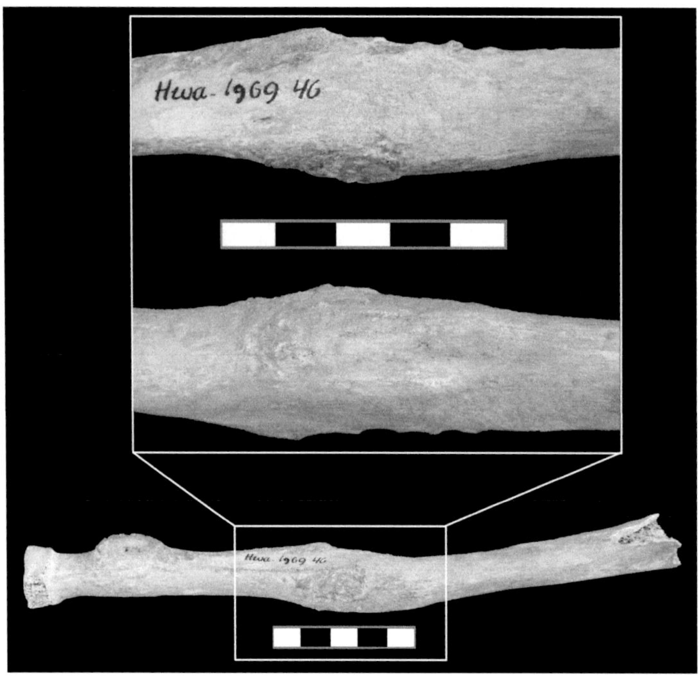

Figure 10.14 Healed fracture of the midshaft of a right radius. Note the abnormal angulation of the bone. (Male, Adult, Eemsdelta-Hoogwatum, Collection NAD Nuis inv. Nr. G 2018-IX.270; photos by Efthymia Nikita, with permission from the Noordelijk Archeologisch Depot)

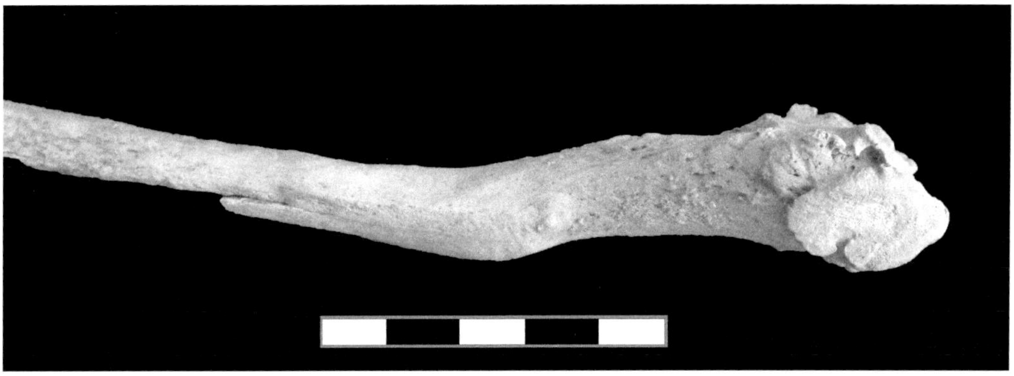

Figure 10.15 Healed fibular fracture. Note that there is no remnant callus, but the bone has not healed properly as there is angulation. (Philadelphia, Roman/Byzantine; photo by Efthymia Nikita, with the kind permission of Dr. Ahmet Ihsan Aytek, Burdur Mehmet Akif Ersoy University)

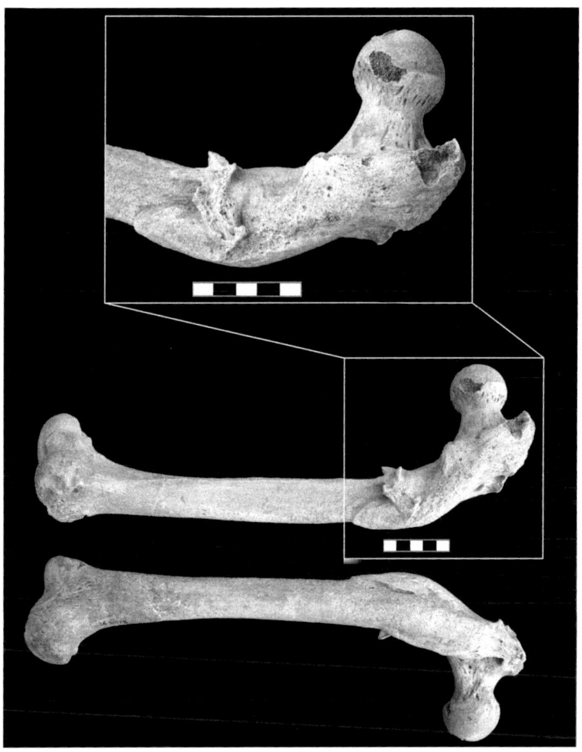

Figure 10.16 Healed fracture of the proximal right femur. Note the angulation of the bone and the new bone formation, probably associated with myositis ossificans traumatica at the fracture site. (Samantaş, Byzantine; photos by Efthymia Nikita, with the kind permission of Dr. Ahmet Ihsan Aytek, Burdur Mehmet Akif Ersoy University)

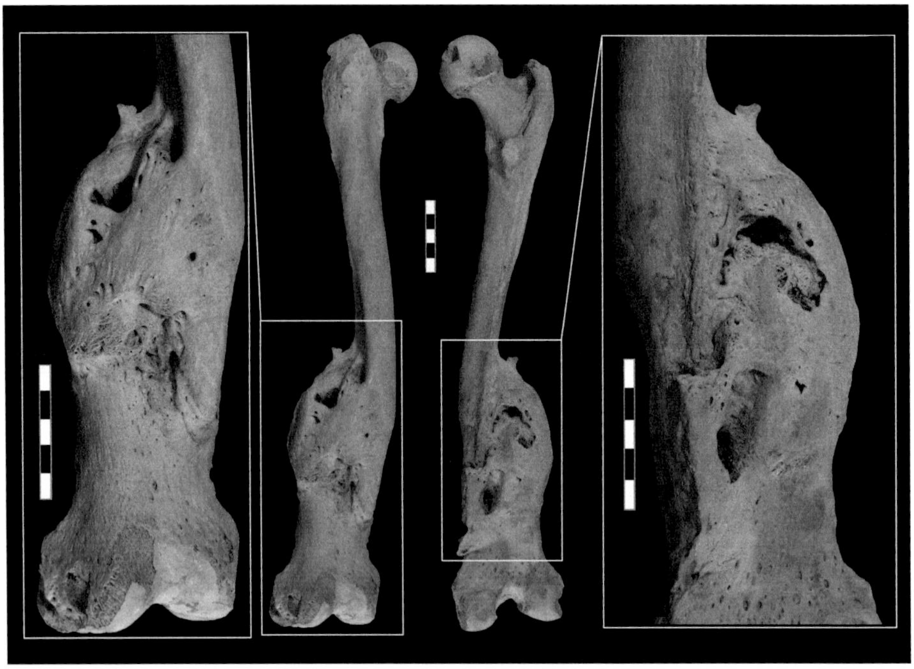

Figure 10.17 Healed fracture of the distal diaphysis of a right femur. Note the major overlap of the fractured ends and associated new bone formation and myositis ossificans traumatica. (Photos by Efthymia Nikita; copyright: Duckworth Laboratory, University of Cambridge)

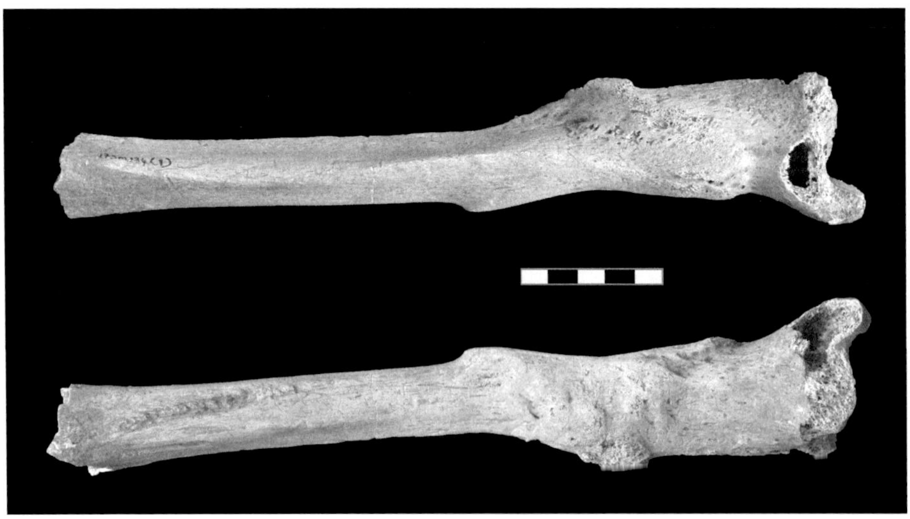

Figure 10.18 Healed fracture of the distal left tibia. Note the new bone formation at the fracture site and misalignment of the healed bone. (Samantaş, Byzantine; photos by Efthymia Nikita, with the kind permission of Dr. Ahmet Ihsan Aytek, Burdur Mehmet Akif Ersoy University)

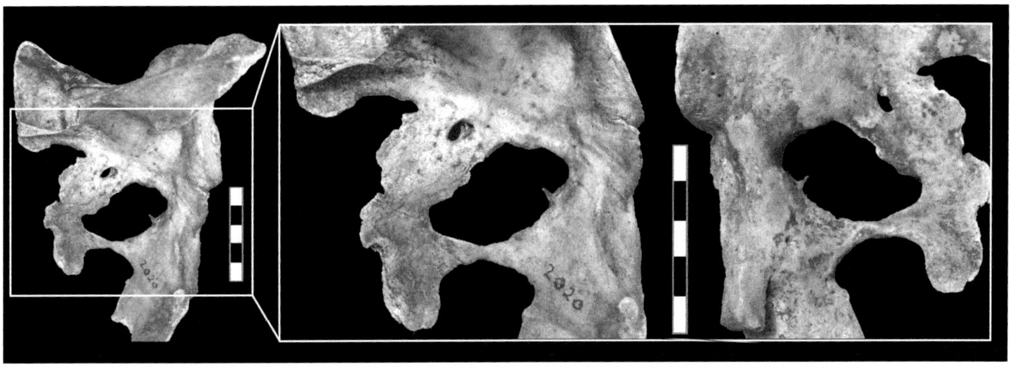

Figure 10.19 Fractured right scapula with major lytic lesions in the infraspinatus fossa and involvement of the lateral border. (Male, 35–45 years old, Diever, Reformed Church graveyard, Collection NAD Nuis inv. Nr. D 2019-III.472; photo by Efthymia Nikita, with permission from the Noordelijk Archeologisch Depot)

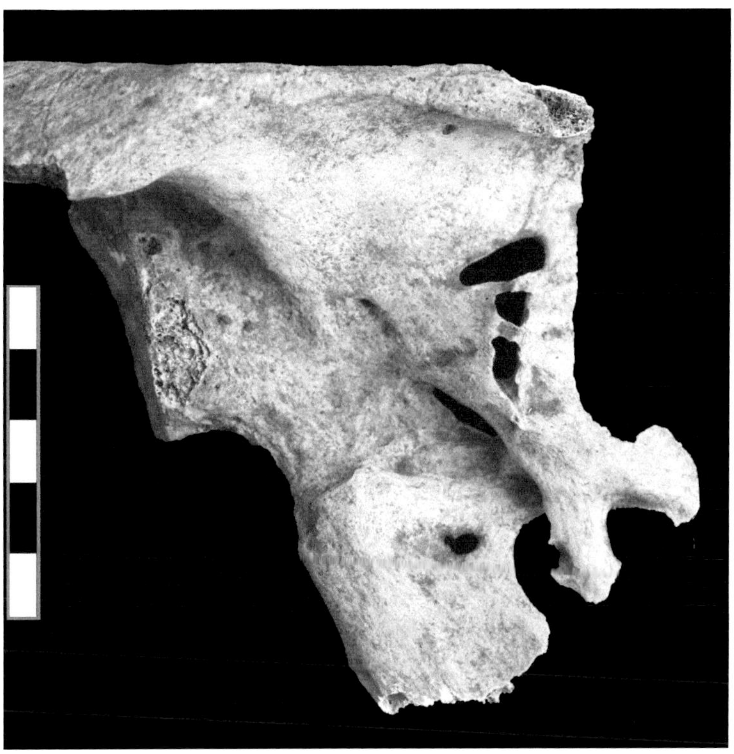

Figure 10.20 Fractured left scapula. Note the transverse healed fracture under the glenoid cavity, the displacement of the scapular spine, and the overall deformity of the bone. (Samantaş, Byzantine; photo by Efthymia Nikita, with the kind permission of Dr. Ahmet Ihsan Aytek, Burdur Mehmet Akif Ersoy University)

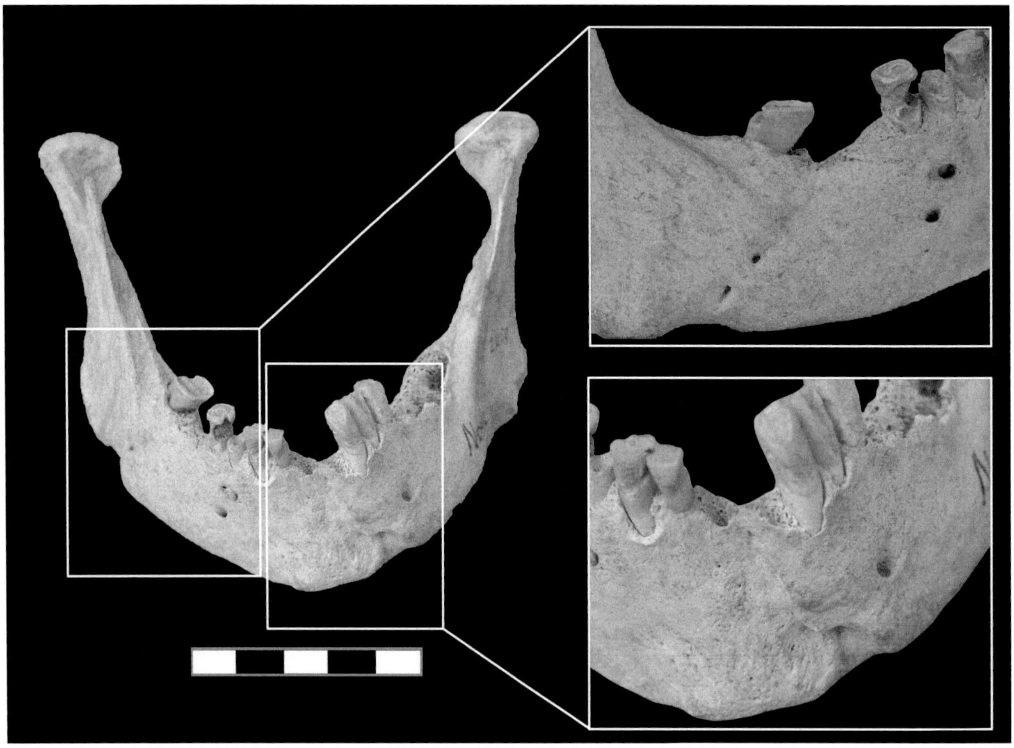

Figure 10.21 Multiple healed fractures in a mandibular corpus. Note that despite the complex anatomy of the mandible and the multiple injuries, the fractures have healed with minimal deformity. (Male, Adult, Nes (Ameland), 5066; photos by Efthymia Nikita, from the reference collection of the Cultural Heritage Agency of the Netherlands)

Box 10.1 Myositis ossificans traumatica

Myositis ossificans traumatica is characterised by the formation of bone tissue within soft tissues as a result of traumatic injury (Figure 10.22, see also below Figure 10.42). It mostly occurs in the large muscles of the extremities. This condition is generally localised, self-limiting, and benign. Although trauma is its primary etiological factor, myositis ossificans can also arise secondary to burns and neurological damage. The condition is more common in adolescent or young adult males; however, it has been documented in individuals from infancy to old age.

fractures often heal without deformities, which complicates their identification in palaeopathological contexts. Furthermore, new bone deposits indicative of callus formation can resemble several pathological conditions, including infections, and any observed bowing may be wrongly attributed to rickets. In juvenile bones, the periosteum is more loosely attached to the underlying bone; thus, it is less prone to rupture after a fracture and more likely to detach

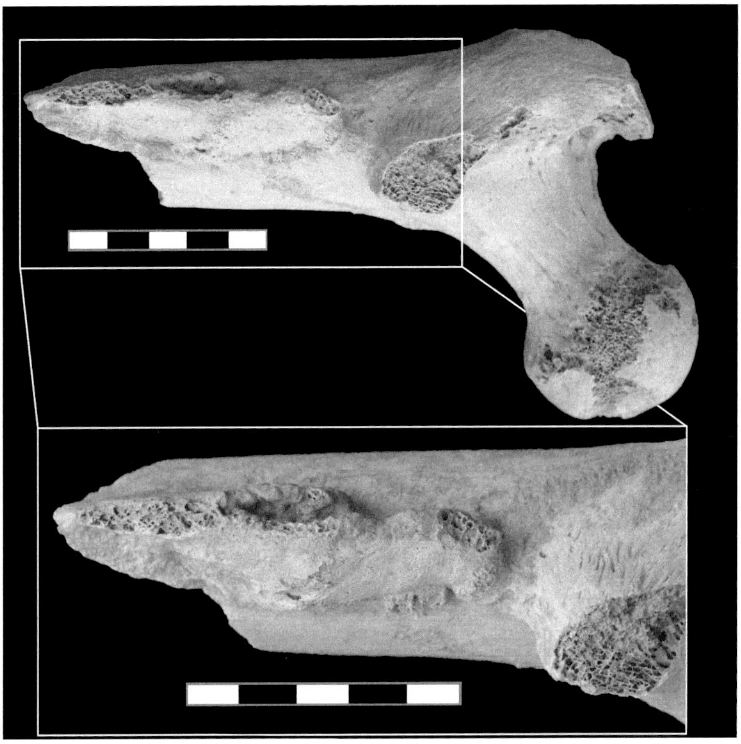

Figure 10.22 Extensive new bone formation at the posterior part of the left proximal femur, suggesting ossification of the soft tissues, though no evidence of trauma is visible to confirm the traumatic origin of the ossification. (Sbide, Roman/Byzantine; photos by Efthymia Nikita, with the kind permission of Dr. Ahmet Ihsan Aytek, Burdur Mehmet Akif Ersoy University)

from the bone while remaining intact. This phenomenon reduces deformity and enhances stability during healing. Similarly, the cranium in infants and young children is elastic, with bones loosely connected by sutures and fontanelles. As a result, trauma may cause inward depression but no fracturing; alternatively, the sutures may separate (diastatic fractures). Nevertheless, infants are more likely to develop subdural haematomas, even following relatively minor head injuries.

The aetiology of fractures varies based on the individual's developmental stage. From birth until two years of age, children depend on their caregivers for their overall wellbeing; therefore, fractures in this age group may be linked to abuse and neglect, or to injury during childbirth. In children older than two years, fractures are often the result of their engagement in physical activities such as walking and climbing, as they become increasingly independent. Moreover, when analysing fracture patterns, one should take into account anatomical differences between adults and juveniles. For example, when adults fall, they usually land on their feet, fracturing their lower extremities. In contrast, children tend to land head-first during a fall because their cranium is relatively large and heavy.

Fracture mechanisms

Blunt force trauma

Blunt force trauma results when force is applied over a rather large surface area (Box 10.2, Figures 10.23 and 10.24). This type of trauma can be caused by various mechanisms, including the impact of a solid object (e.g. hammer), an explosion that propels an individual into a stationary object, motor vehicle collisions, falls from heights, and others. Blunt force trauma to bone can lead to diverse fracture types, depending on the biomechanical properties of the affected bone, the dimensions and shape of the object/weapon, the individual's age, the magnitude and direction of the applied force, and others.

Low-velocity trauma to the cranium can produce simple linear fractures, while high-velocity trauma usually creates depressed fractures. Upon impact, the bone bends inward; compressive stresses develop ectocranially and tensile stresses endocranially. Given that bone is more prone to fracture under tensile forces compared to compressive forces, the inner table is the first to fracture. As the applied force persists, the fracture expands and extends toward the outer table. The bone around the impact area bends outward, and radiating fractures may appear. These fractures propagate along the path of least resistance; thus, they follow predictable patterns determined by bone curvature and thickness, the presence of sinus cavities and sutures, or pre-existing fractures. In addition, concentric fractures also form perpendicular to the radiating ones. Coup-contrecoup injuries are also commonly found in cases of cranial injuries and represent a combination of direct and indirect trauma. They are characterised by

Box 10.2 Skeletal manifestation of blunt force trauma

Skull

- depressed fractures
- radiating fractures from impact point
- concentric fractures perpendicular to radiating ones
- delamination at entrance wound
- contrecoup fracture when the blow force propagates towards the opposite side of the cranium from the impact area
- comminuted fractures from heavy-impact forces
- linear fractures from forces of large mass (often due to direct impact with an object or forces from other areas of the body or other parts of the skull)

Postcranial skeleton

- different types of blunt-force trauma (e.g. fractured ribs due to beating, parry fractures, butterfly fractures, fractures of the scapular body, vertebral compression fractures, etc.)

(Data from Berryman and Haun 1996; Berryman and Symes 1998; Boylston 2000; Galloway and Wedel 2014a; Gurdjian 1975; Kimmerle and Baraybar 2008a; Komar and Buikstra 2008; Lovell 1997)

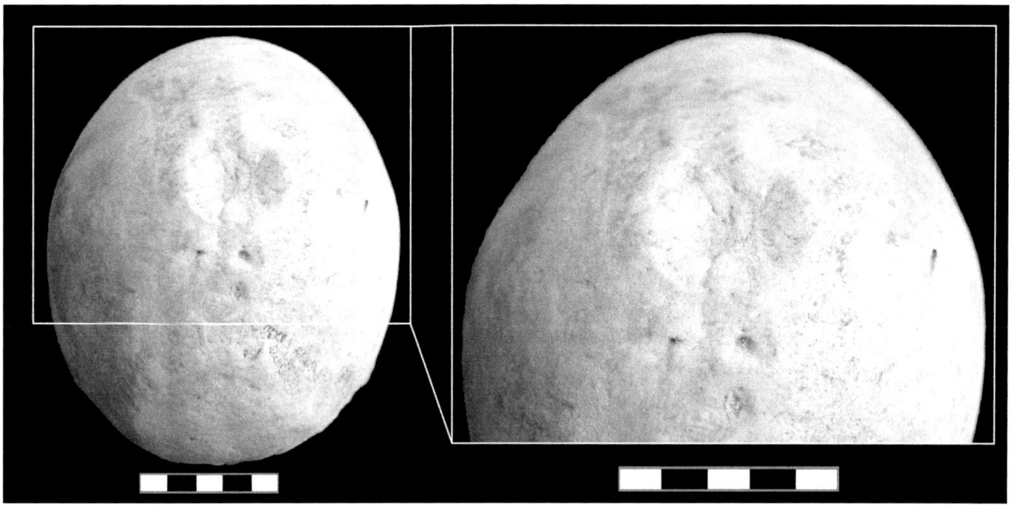

Figure 10.23 Healed blunt force trauma (circular depressed area) on the sagittal suture. (Sbide, Roman/Byzantine; photos by Efthymia Nikita, with the kind permission of Dr. Ahmet Ihsan Aytek, Burdur Mehmet Akif Ersoy University)

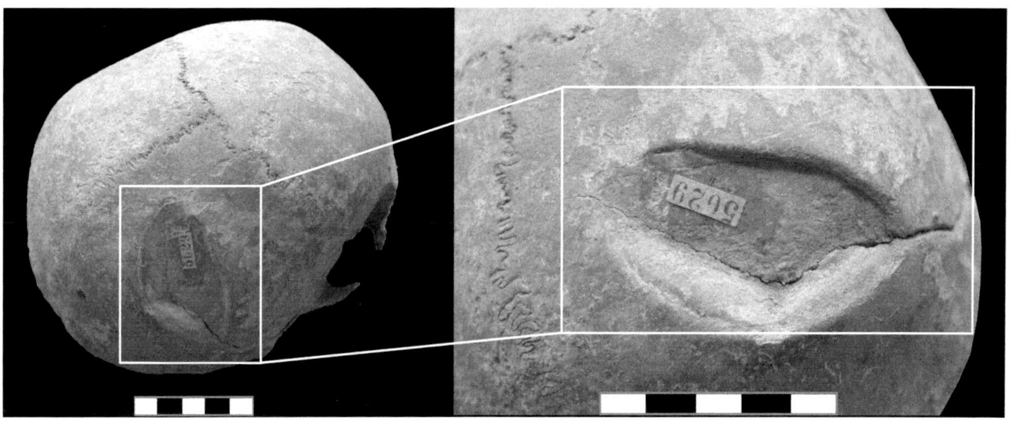

Figure 10.24 Healed blunt force trauma (distinct oval depression) of the right parietal bone. (Male, Young adult, Waadhoeke-Ritsumazijl, Collection NAD Nuis inv. Nr. F 2010-IV-2155; photos by Efthymia Nikita, with permission from the Noordelijk Archeologisch Depot)

the coup injury at the point of impact, while the contrecoup injury appears opposite or distal to the impact site.

Indirect cranial blunt force trauma may result from various mechanisms, for example, vertical loading forces generated during a fall from a height and transmitted to the cranium from the feet or buttocks can cause a "ring" fracture that encircles the foramen magnum. Another example is fractures of the petrous bones and mandibular condyles resulting from blows to the chin.

Sharp force trauma

Sharp force injuries are caused by weapons with a sharp, pointed, or bevelled edge (Box 10.3, Figures 10.25–10.31). Such weapons may cut, chop, or crush bone. Puncture (or stab) and chop marks are typically produced by knives, swords, axes, and machetes, which exert compressive forces perpendicularly on narrow bone surfaces. In contrast, incisions arise from slashing motions, resulting in lesions where the length exceeds the depth (as seen with knives and swords).

The type of wounds and the extent of bone involvement are influenced by several variables, such as the condition of the instrument or weapon used, the nature and amount of soft tissue surrounding the bone, and the clothes worn by the affected individual. Furthermore, attacks with sharp instruments often involve two individuals moving and struggling; thus, the resulting injury will be larger or more irregular than expected based on the type of blade itself. In general, sharp force injuries are linear and have well-defined, sharp edges. Their cross-section may be V, semi-V, or U-shaped, with flat, smooth, and polished walls and floor. The tool

Box 10.3 Skeletal manifestation of sharp force trauma

Cuts

- linear wounds that are longer than deep
- well-defined cut marks with clean edges
- flat and smooth cut surfaces, with possible polishing and parallel scratch marks
- V-shaped cross-section (perpendicular impacts produce horizontal V-shaped defects; in nonperpendicular impacts well defined edges and flat and smooth surfaces characterise the wall of the lesion that is at an obtuse angle, while flakes and/or cracks occur on the opposite wall)
- stone knives produce wider and shallower marks compared to metal ones, with irregular walls and ill-defined apex

Stabs

- linear wounds that are deeper than long
- triangular or V-shaped cross section
- exit defect caused during weapon extraction
- mark left behind by blade back may reflect blade size

Chop wounds

- lesions with almost equal width and depth
- smooth surface along impact point, rough opposing surface due to bone flaking
- linear fractures extending from the defect (due to blow force and damage when removing the weapon from the bone)

(Data from Boylston 2000; Houck 1998; Humphrey and Hutchinson 2001; Kimmerle and Baraybar 2008b; Lewis 2008; Polson et al. 1985; Rodríguez-Martín 2006; Spitz 1993; Walker and Long 1977)

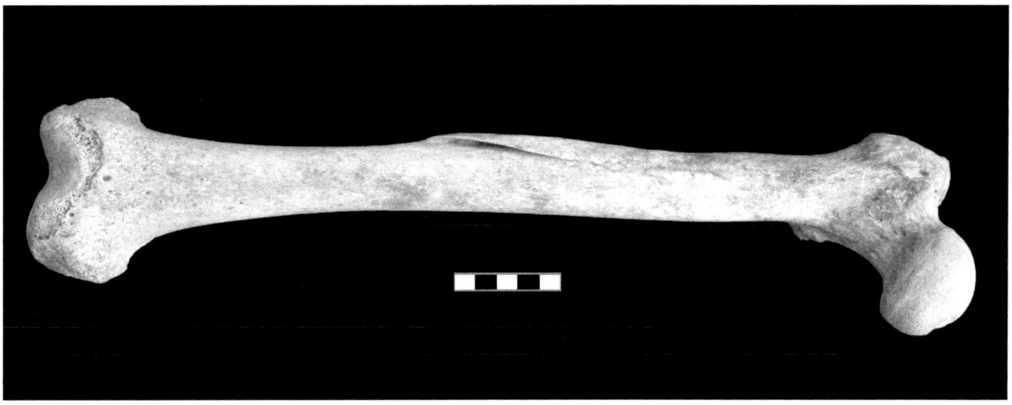

Figure 10.25 Sharp force trauma of a right femur. Note the linear wound at the midshaft and proximal part of the diaphysis. (Patara, Byzantine; photo by Efthymia Nikita, with the kind permission of Dr. Ahmet Ihsan Aytek, Burdur Mehmet Akif Ersoy University)

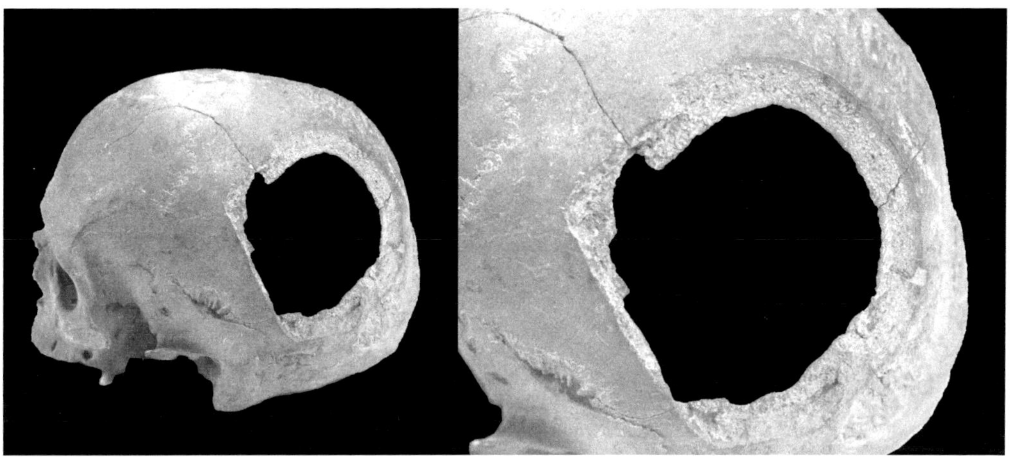

Figure 10.26 Major sharp force trauma of the left parietal and occipital bones, probably inflicted using a sword. The injury was inflicted perimortem as there is no evidence of healing. (From unknown location in Friesland, Collection NAD Nuis inv. Nr. F 2021-X-236 (4); photos by Efthymia Nikita, with permission from the Noordelijk Archeologisch Depot)

employed may leave smaller parallel cuts or scratch marks along the smooth margins of the wound. These features will be present on both wound facets when the weapon impacts the bone perpendicularly. However, if the strike occurs at an angle other than perpendicular, such markings will be visible on the wall that forms an obtuse angle, while flaking, feathering, and cracking may be found on the opposite wall of the wound.

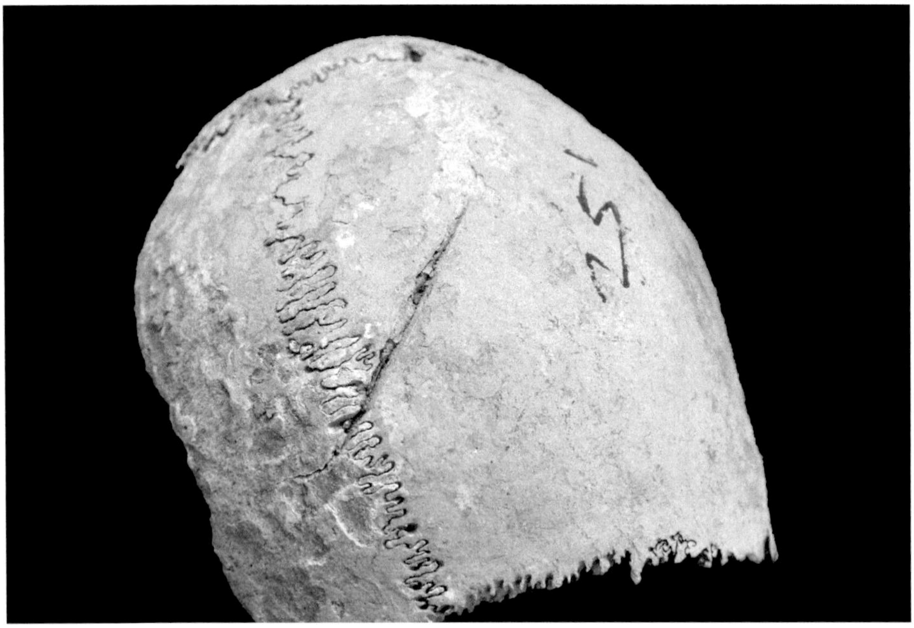

Figure 10.27 Cut mark on a left parietal bone. The injury was inflicted perimortem as there is no evidence of healing. (Aduard, Cistersian Monastery of St. Bernardus, Collection NAD Nuis inv. Nr. G 2013-IV.251; photo by Efthymia Nikita, with permission from the Noordelijk Archeologisch Depot)

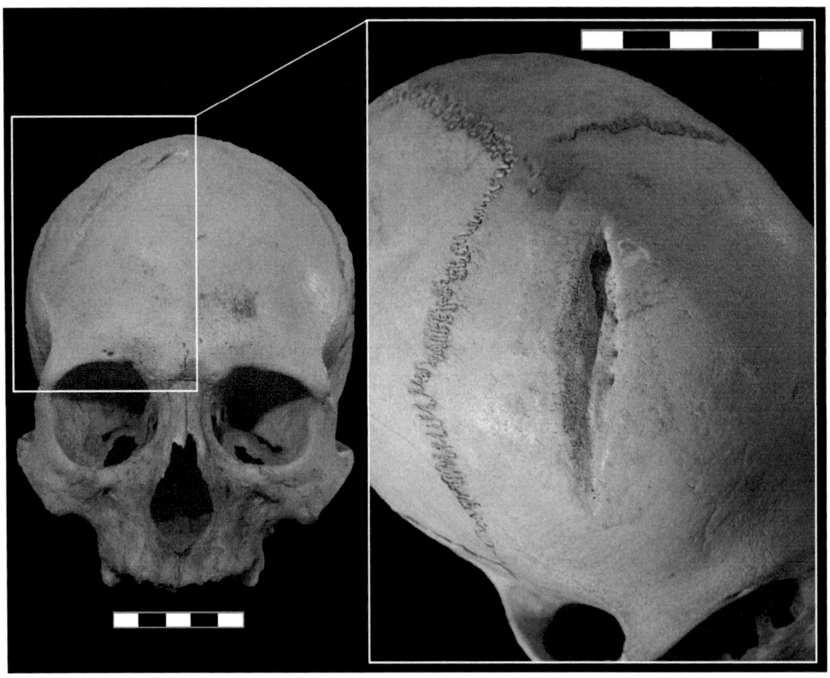

Figure 10.28 Sharp force trauma of the frontal bone, potentially inflicted using an axe or similar instrument. Note that the lesion had largely healed. (Gizeh E492; photos by Efthymia Nikita; copyright: Duckworth Laboratory, University of Cambridge)

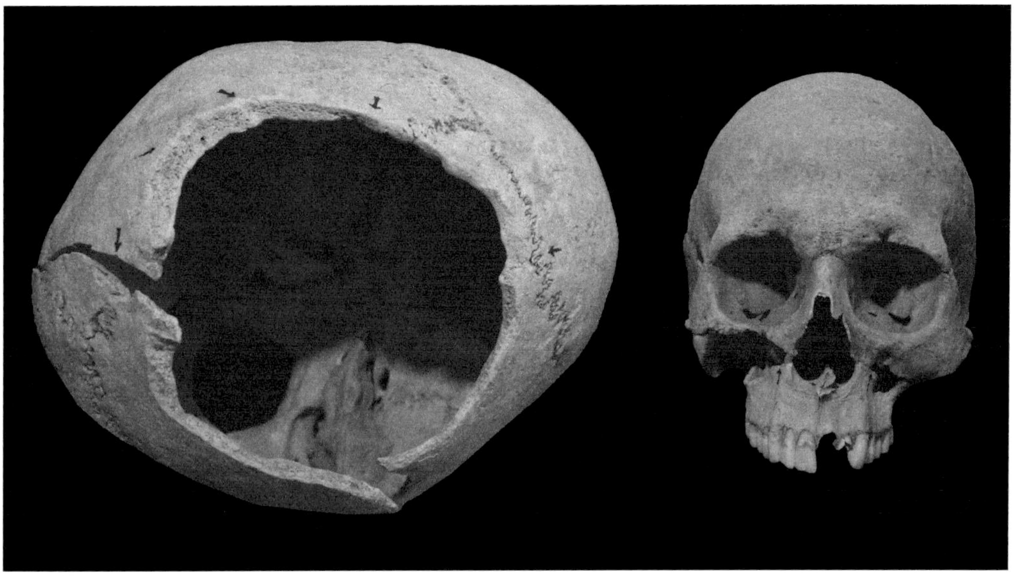

Figure 10.29 Major sharp force trauma that has removed a large part of the left parietal bone. (Huntingdon Roman Villa Saxon Cemetery site; photos by Efthymia Nikita; copyright: Duckworth Laboratory, University of Cambridge)

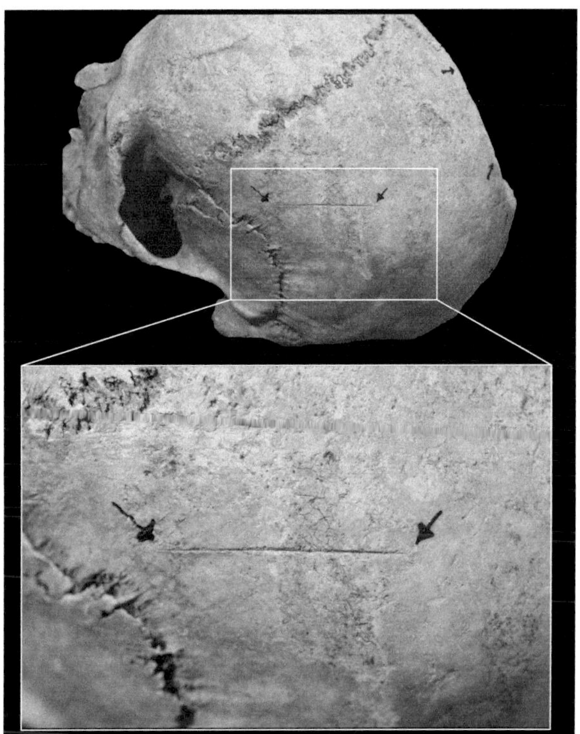

Figure 10.30 Cut mark on the left parietal bone. (Same individual as in Figure 10.29; photos by Efthymia Nikita; copyright: Duckworth Laboratory, University of Cambridge)

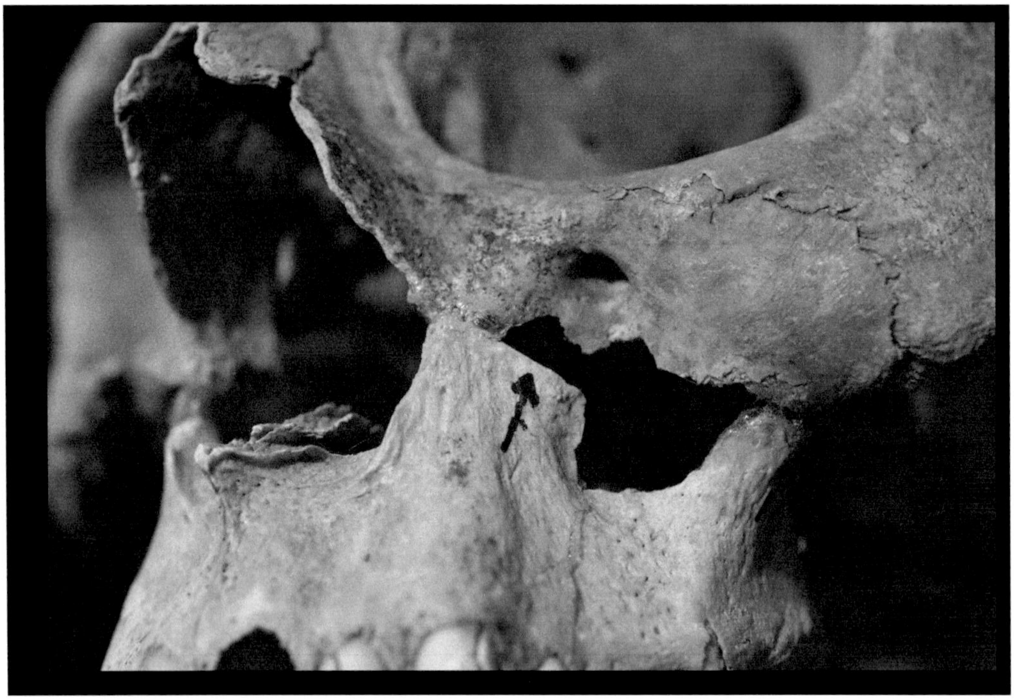

Figure 10.31 Linear cut on the left maxilla. (Same individual as in Figures 10.29 and 10.30; photo by Efthymia Nikita; copyright: Duckworth Laboratory, University of Cambridge)

Sharp force trauma may be divided into several categories, the most common being cuts, stabs, and chop wounds.

Cuts result from a slashing action. Several factors affect wound morphology, such as the blade's properties, the angle at which the blade contacts the bone, the number of strikes delivered, the type of bone involved (e.g. cortical, trabecular), as well as the quantity and nature of the soft tissues and clothing that the blade encounters before reaching the bone.

Stabs occur when the tip of a penetrating instrument breaches the surface of the bone. The characteristics of the resulting lesion, including its shape and depth, are influenced by the properties of the blade and the biomechanical properties of the bone. Moreover, it is important to consider that during the penetration, but also the withdrawal of the weapon, the blade may move in different directions, leading to the formation of exit defects.

Chop wounds are inflicted by heavy implements that have at least one cutting edge (e.g. machetes, axes, or cleavers). These instruments result in both cutting and crushing of the tissues (sharp-blunt trauma). Skeletal injuries can occur during the initial impact of the weapon on the bone, but also during its removal. In comparison to cutting injuries, chop wounds generally involve greater force, leading to a complete disruption of bone continuity, often accompanied by the fragmentation of the bone into multiple pieces.

Projectile trauma

Projectile trauma results from a high-velocity projectile that penetrates bone (Box 10.4). In archaeological contexts, such injuries are mostly associated with weapons such as arrows

Box 10.4 Skeletal manifestation of projectile trauma

- projectile points may remain imbedded in bone or not
- hole in bone surface at point of impact
- V/semi-V/U-shaped cross section
- cranium: internal bevelling at entrance defects, and external bevelling at exit defects; radiating and concentric heaving fractures; delamination at entry wound
- vertebrae: comminution of vertebral bodies, linear fractures across neighbouring vertebrae
- thorax: fracturing or perforation of single or multiple adjacent ribs; exit wounds larger than entry defects, with comminuted fracturing; radiating fractures extending from entrance and/or exit wound; if point of impact is on superior or inferior rib edge, defect with two radiating fractures, mimicking butterfly fracture

(Data from Byers and Juarez 2023; Galloway et al. 2014; Milner et al. 1991; Smith et al. 2007)

and crossbow bolts. For more recent periods, projectile trauma primarily includes gunshot wounds and wounds from shrapnel. Unlike blunt force injuries, which generally have a broad impact area, projectile wounds have a narrow point of impact. High-velocity projectiles release significant amounts of energy within the body, with this energy propagating from the interior to the exterior.

Projectile trauma can be considered present when projectile points are still embedded within the skeleton, and can be assumed to have been present based on the size and overall morphology of the lesions when the points are missing. Nonetheless, it can be difficult to differentiate between blunt force trauma and projectile trauma due to the variability that exists in weapon size, calibre, and the magnitude of force applied. In addition, the potential presence of intermediate targets can affect the characteristics of the projectile, such as its trajectory and fragmentation patterns.

A gunshot wound is a form of high-velocity projectile trauma, characterised by the application of significant force and rapid loading over a small surface area. In cases of gunshot injury, bone behaves as a brittle material, that is, it fails almost instantly with considerable fracturing and minimal or no plastic deformation. The skeletal lesions caused by bullets can be variable, as they depend on intrinsic factors (e.g. elastic modulus of the affected bone), extrinsic factors (e.g. type of weapon used, mass and velocity of the bullet, distance from which it was fired, presence of intermediate targets), and additional contextual variables (e.g. location and positioning of the victim).

Non-accidental versus accidental trauma

Injuries caused by interpersonal violence are usually found in the cranium and thorax, as well as in the distal ulna. While other types of injuries, such as dislocations or fractures of the extremities, may also occur during violent encounters, they can also arise from several other actions.

The head is a key target in violent interpersonal confrontations. Injuries above the hat brim line – an area parallel to the Frankfort horizontal plane, with its upper margin intersecting the glabella and its lower margin crossing the centre of the external auditory meatus – are primarily linked to intentional blunt force trauma rather than accidental falls. Assault-related injuries are mostly found on the left side of the skull, which is likely related to the fact that most individuals (thus, the potential assailants) are right-handed. In addition, fractures sustained from intentional blows are predominantly comminuted or depressed, contrary to fractures resulting from falls, which are usually linear or radial. Facial fractures are also often the result of intentional blunt force trauma and are frequently associated with fractures and avulsion of the teeth. Finally, injuries on the posterior of the skull may have been sustained while trying to run away from the attacker.

In the postcranial skeleton, a parry fracture is often interpreted as a defensive injury, occurring when an individual raises their forearm to protect the head. This injury is a transverse or slightly oblique fracture in the distal one-third part of the ulnar diaphysis (Figure 10.32). While parry fractures are regarded as a sign of deliberate trauma, the ulna can also be injured accidentally. Because parry fractures are, by definition, associated with defensive wounds, and because it is impossible to know with certainty the mechanism that produced ulnar fractures in archaeological contexts, it is more accurate to speak of "possible parry fractures."

Rib fractures frequently result from interpersonal violence, as blows are often directed towards the torso during violent confrontations (Figure 10.33). Similarly, metacarpal fractures (e.g. "boxer's fractures" in the fifth metacarpal) may arise when the hands are used as weapons. Although injuries resulting from violence can be diverse, a pattern involving the cranium, ulnae, ribs, and hands can indicate interpersonal violence. Fractures resulting from weapons (e.g. swords and firearms), as well as embedded projectiles, also indicate cases of intentional violence.

Long bone fractures, except for parry fractures, are generally associated with accidents. In addition, accidental head injuries are very common in juveniles and older adults. It is important to acknowledge, however, that many fractures typically associated with accidents can also result from deliberate actions; for example, fractures sustained from falling onto an outstretched arm may be the outcome of an intentional push rather than an accidental fall.

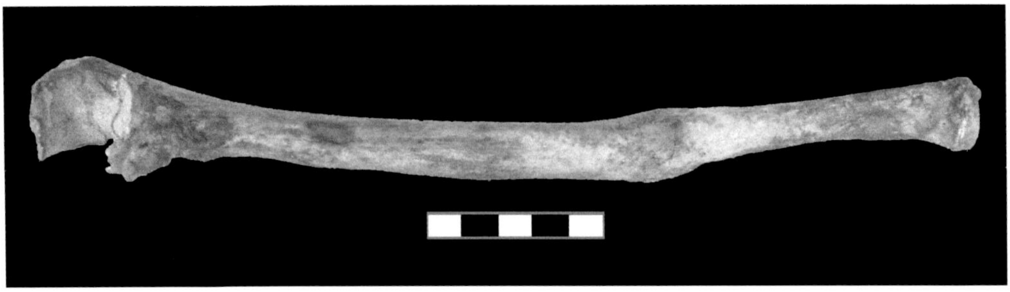

Figure 10.32 Possible Parry fracture of the right ulna, with slight misalignment at the distal diaphysis. (Male, 35–45 years old, Diever, Reformed Church graveyard, Collection NAD Nuis inv. Nr. D 2019-III.472; photo by Efthymia Nikita, with permission from the Noordelijk Archeologisch Depot)

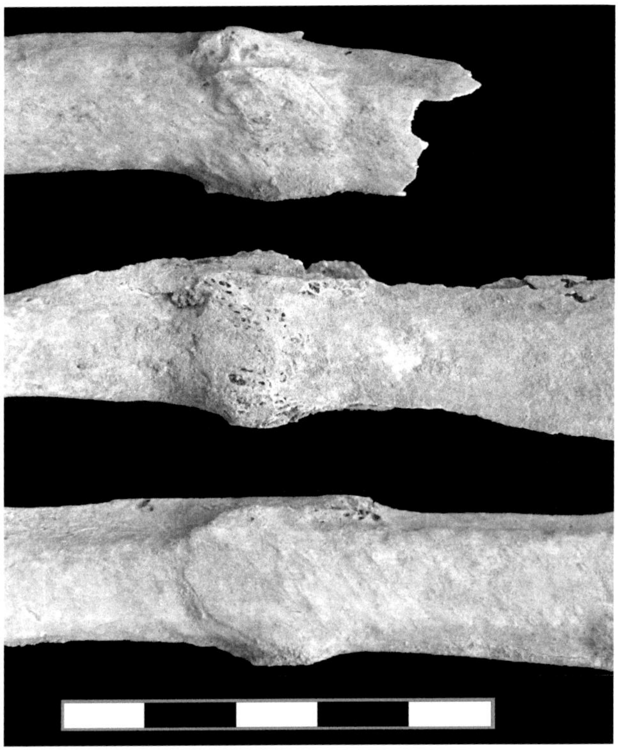

Figure 10.33 Healed rib fractures. (Samantaş, Byzantine; photos by Efthymia Nikita, with the kind permission of Dr. Ahmet Ihsan Aytek, Burdur Mehmet Akif Ersoy University)

Spondylolysis

Spondylolysis is an osseous defect that appears as a separation of the dorsal part of the neural arch from the rest of the vertebra (Box 10.5, Figures 10.34 and 10.35). This separation is due to a fracture in the region of the neural arch located between the superior and inferior articular facets, known as the pars interarticularis.

The aetiology of spondylolysis is unclear. The predominant theory supports that spondylolysis is a fatigue fracture resulting from repetitive stress and microtrauma to the lower vertebral column. Bipedal locomotion has been suggested as a significant mechanical stressor associated with spondylolysis, given that this defect is primarily found in the lumbosacral region, and it is absent in infants who have not begun to walk yet, as well as in adults who have never walked.

Spondylolysis may also have a hereditary component, given its high prevalence among siblings and offspring of individuals with the condition compared to the general population. This genetic predisposition may be associated with reduced cortical bone density at the pars interarticularis. In addition, normal anatomical variation, which may also be inherited, has been associated with spondylolysis (e.g. there is a correlation between spondylolysis and the sacral base angle). Spondylolysis is often found in association with other defects, such as spina bifida occulta. Its prevalence varies among different populations,

Box 10.5 Skeletal manifestation of spondylolysis

- cleft at pars interarticularis, separating the vertebra into two parts
- more common in the fifth lumbar vertebra, occurring with decreasing frequency from L5 to L1 or in other parts of the spine
- incomplete or complete separation
  - incomplete separations look like a crack at the pars interarticularis
  - complete separations may show irregular edges, giving the appearance of a recent fracture, or may have undergone significant modification
- mostly bilateral
- instead of occurring at the pars interarticularis, separation may occur through a lamina, pedicle, or between the superior articular and transverse processes

(Data from Fredrickson et al. 1984; Mays 2006; Merbs 1989, 1996, 2002; Nathan 1959; Peng 2016; Więckowski 2021)

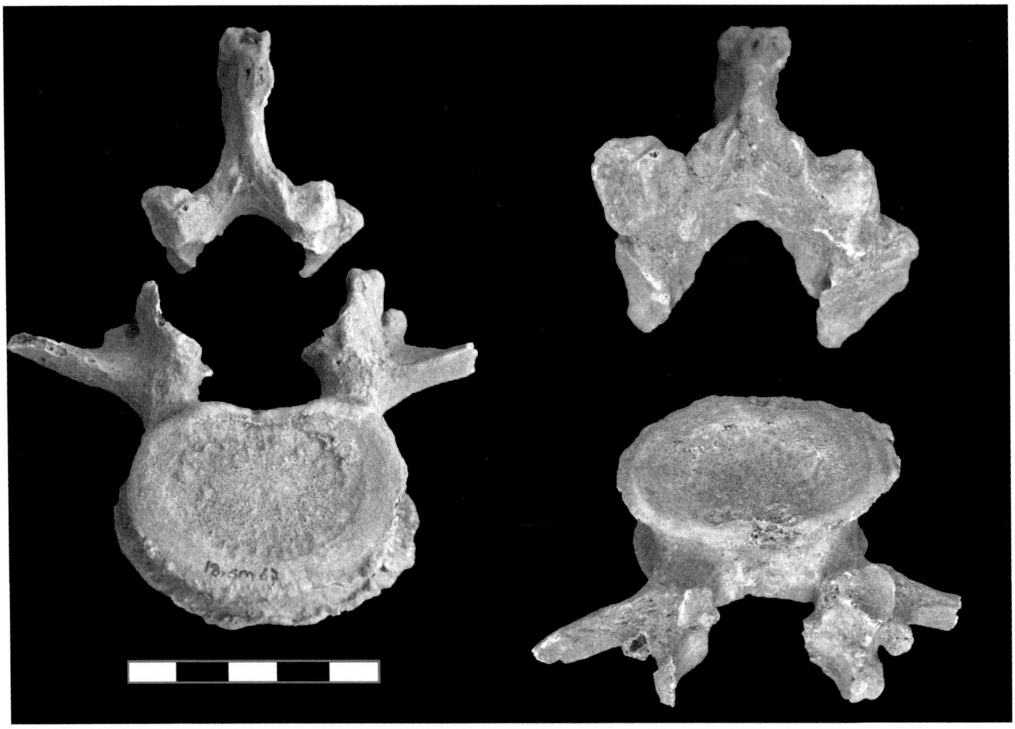

Figure 10.34 Spondylolysis of lumbar vertebra. Note the bilateral separation of the posterior part of the neural arch from the rest of the vertebra at the pars interarticularis. (Samantaş, Byzantine; photos by Efthymia Nikita, with the kind permission of Dr. Ahmet Ihsan Aytek, Burdur Mehmet Akif Ersoy University)

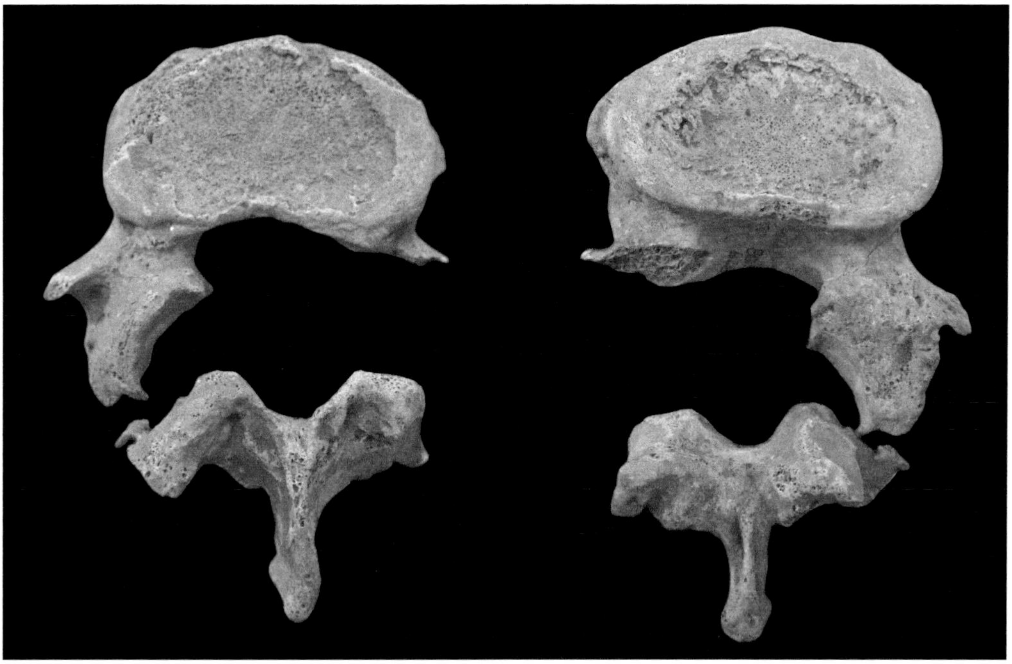

Figure 10.35 Spondylolysis of lumbar vertebra. (Male, 35–45 years old, Black Gate cemetery, Newcastle-Upon-Tyne, 8th-12th c. CE, BG-628; photos by Efthymia Nikita; copyright: Human Skeletal Collection, University of Sheffield)

being around 7% in the average population but approaching 50% in various Alaskan groups; this pattern may be due to differences in physical activity levels, genetic predisposition, or a combination of the two.

Bilateral spondylolysis may result in spondylolisthesis, where a vertebral body is anteriorly displaced in relation to the vertebra beneath it. Anterior slippage is more pronounced in the lower lumbosacral region, where the vertebral bodies are oriented ventrally and are thus subjected to gravitational forces. The degree of spondylolisthesis can range from minimal displacement to complete slippage. The variability in the degree of olisthesis can be linked to the degree of laxity in the intervertebral discs and ligaments, the orientation of the affected vertebral body, and the mechanical stresses applied to the region. Spondylolisthesis can develop in the absence of spondylolysis; such cases of spondylolisthesis are associated with degenerative disc disease and changes in the facet joints (e.g. anterior displacement of the zygapophyses due to osteoarthritic remodelling), subluxation of the facet joints, or facet joint dysplasia.

Dislocation

A dislocation, also called luxation, is the complete displacement of the articulating bones within a joint (i.e. there is no articulation anymore between the bones forming a joint), whereas a subluxation represents a partial displacement. While dislocations and subluxations may arise from congenital conditions or occur spontaneously, they are mostly linked to traumatic events. In cases of traumatic dislocation, the joint displacement is often accompanied by a

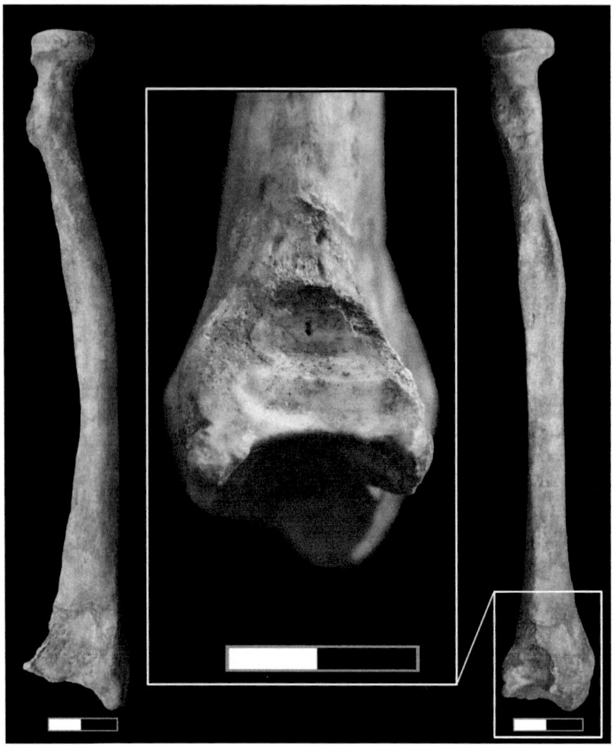

Figure 10.36 Dislocation of the distal radioulnar joint. Note the eburnation at the ulnar notch but also the superior extension of the articular surface due to the dislocation. (Male, Young-Middle adult, St Hilda's Church, Coronation Street, South Shields, Newcastle, 19th c., CS06-346; photos by Efthymia Nikita; copyright: Human Skeletal Collection, University of Sheffield)

fracture. The glenohumeral joint is prone to dislocation because the shoulder joint is rather shallow, which increases its susceptibility to displacement.

Dislocations are identifiable in skeletal remains only if they remained unreduced (i.e. not properly realigned) for a sufficient amount of time to allow for osseous changes to develop (Figure 10.36). Some dislocations are easy to reduce (e.g. those affecting the digits), while others may result in immediate death (e.g. atlanto-axial dislocations). In such cases, the dislocation will not be identifiable in archaeological skeletal remains.

Surgical procedures

Trepanation

Trepanation is the intentional perforation of the cranial vault and has been performed across the world (Figures 10.37–10.39). The parietal bone is the site most involved, followed by the frontal bone. Multiple trepanations could also be performed on a single cranium. The high survival rates associated with this procedure suggest that ancient surgeons were skilful and could minimise the risks of infection.

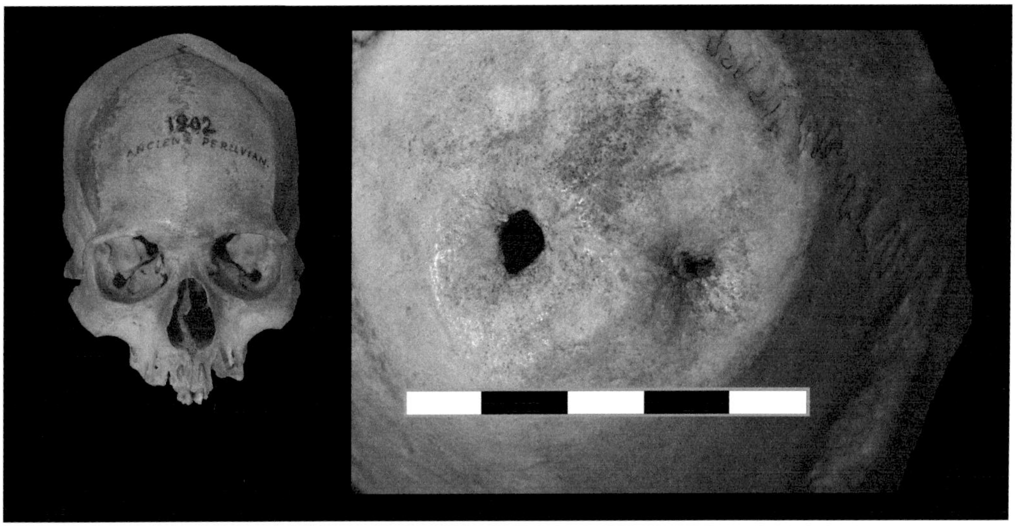

Figure 10.37 Two trepanations of a left parietal bone at different stages of healing. (Peru, SA 131; photos by Efthymia Nikita; copyright: Duckworth Laboratory, University of Cambridge)

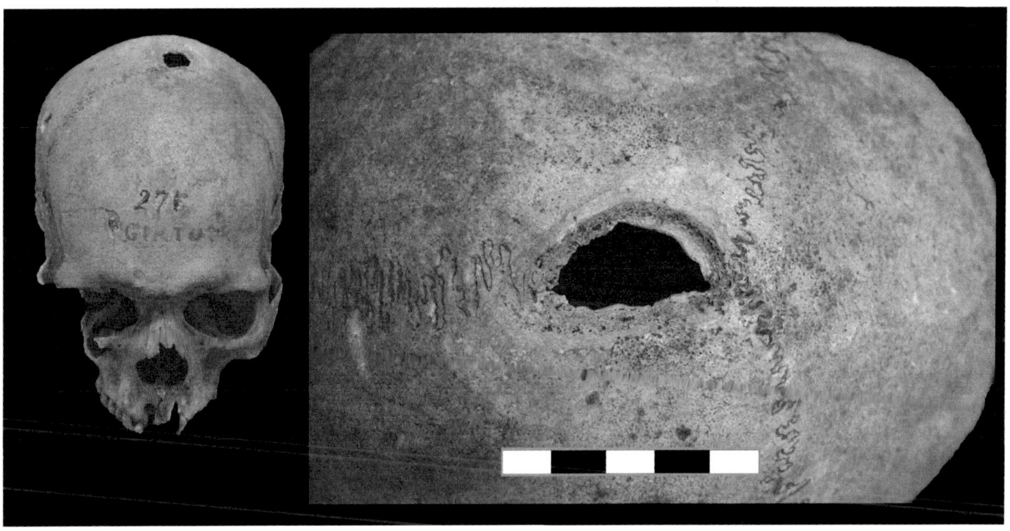

Figure 10.38 Trepanation of a left parietal bone. (Girton, Cambridge, Romano British 271; photos by Efthymia Nikita; copyright: Duckworth Laboratory, University of Cambridge)

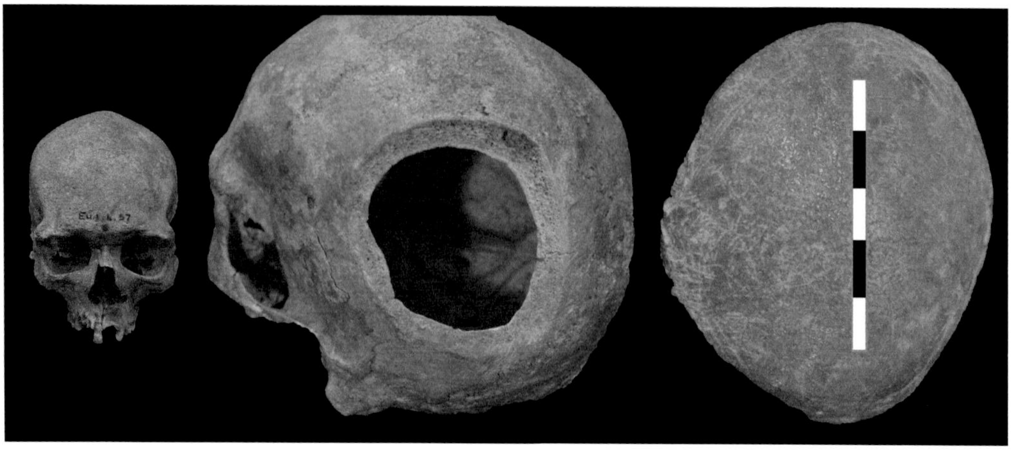

Figure 10.39 Trepanation that has removed a large part of the left parietal bone and a smaller part of the occipital bone; the removed bone piece is also preserved. The individual did not survive the procedure as attested by the lack of any evidence of healing. (Crichel Down, Dorsetshire, Bronze Age Eu.1.4.57; photos by Efthymia Nikita; copyright: Duckworth Laboratory, University of Cambridge)

Trepanation has been associated with therapeutic and magical-ritual practices. As a therapeutic practice, trepanation was used as a surgical procedure to manage cranial fractures, intracranial pressure, headaches, brain tumours, and other conditions. Trepanation has also been used as a magico-therapeutic practice, reflecting the belief that headaches, seizures, and similar issues were due to spirits. Finally, trepanation may have served as a magico-ritual procedure, for example, when the excised bone fragment was used to create amulets.

Trepanations can be performed using different methods. Among the most frequently used methods is scraping, which involves the gradual abrasion of the outer table and diploë in order to reveal the inner table. This inner layer may then be scraped through or broken out. The resultant lesions are usually ellipsoidal in shape and encircled by a crater-like depression. Another common method is linear cutting, which is characterised by the creation of intersecting incisions that produce a rectangular piece of bone. Circular grooving or circular cutting, on the other hand, consists of dislodging a circular bone segment from the cranium. In addition, the technique of boring and cutting involves drilling a series of small holes around a perimeter and then extracting the central piece of bone. Finally, drilling could be used for the creation of a single hole.

Amputation

Amputation is the surgical removal of part of the body (Figures 10.40–10.42). In contemporary Western societies, this procedure is often associated with complications due to diabetes mellitus, atherosclerosis, severe trauma, infection, or due to the presence of malignant tumours. Evidence of amputation in past skeletal remains is rather rare, complicating the interpretation of its underlying motivations. In different contexts, amputations were performed as medical treatments, forms of punishment, part of ritual practices, or outcomes of accidental injuries or acts of violence. Skeletal evidence of amputation may be confused with cases of nonunion fractures.

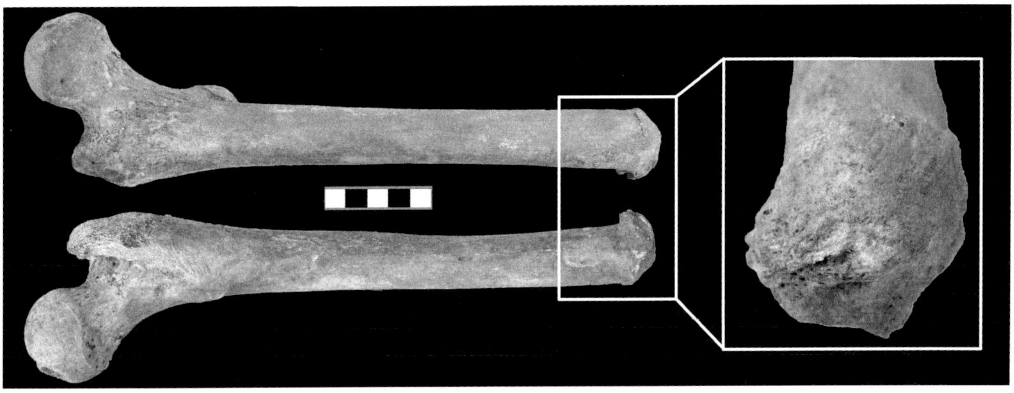

Figure 10.40 Amputation of a right femur. Note the complete healing with bone formation that has sealed the medullary cavity at the distal end of the bone. (Probable female, 35 years old, Alkmaar-Grote Kerk, 5591; photos by Efthymia Nikita, from the reference collection of the Cultural Heritage Agency of the Netherlands)

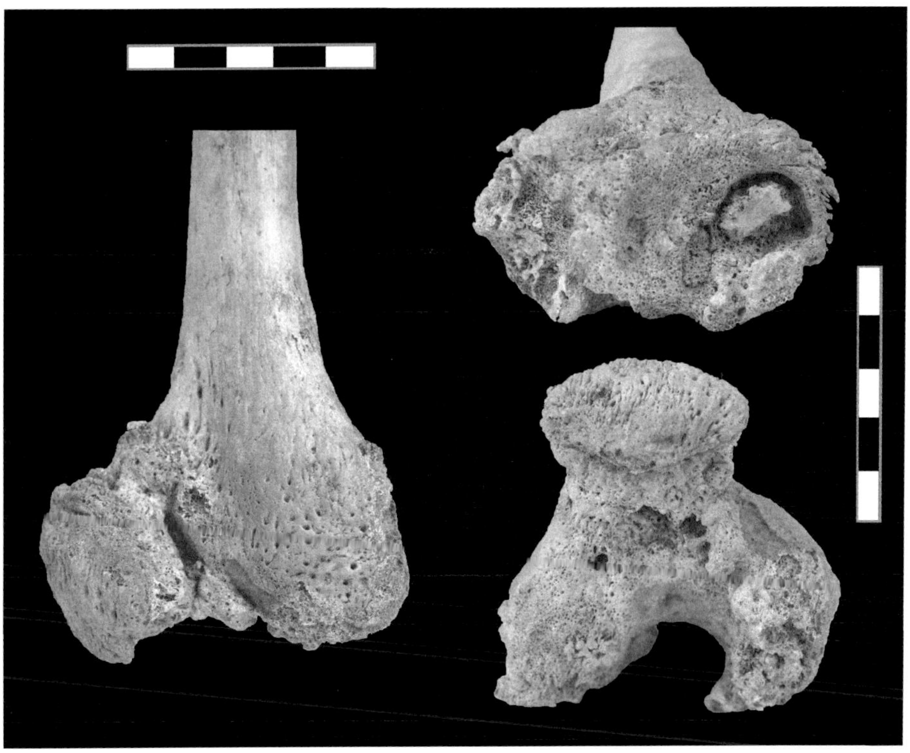

Figure 10.41 Amputated femur (left and bottom right) and associated tibia (top right). This is the part of the femur that has been removed through amputation from the individual of Figure 10.40. The distal part of the femur has fused with the patella and shows extensive new bone formation and resorption, supporting that an infection affecting the knee joint was the reason for the amputation. Similar lesions are seen on the proximal tibia. (Photos by Efthymia Nikita, from the reference collection of the Cultural Heritage Agency of the Netherlands)

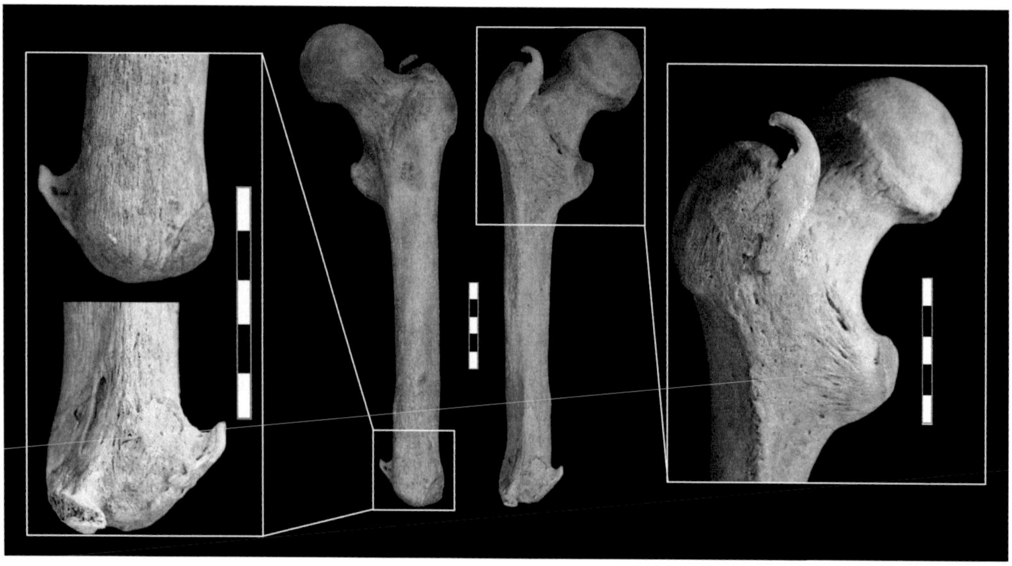

Figure 10.42 Amputation of a left femur, approximately at the midshaft. Note the complete healing with bone formation that has sealed the medullary cavity at the distal end. Note also the formation of myositis ossificans. (Charnel 980, St Hilda's Church, Coronation Street, South Shields, Newcastle, 19th c., CS06-980; photos by Efthymia Nikita; copyright: Human Skeletal Collection, University of Sheffield)

Punitive or violent practices

Scalping

Scalping is the removal of the scalp, that is, the skin and other soft tissues that cover the skull. This procedure typically involves the use of a sharp instrument to make incisions around the skin that overlays the skull, facilitating the removal of soft tissue. This practice is seen in various cultures across the world, often as a means of acquiring trophies that symbolise success in combat. Scalping may also have been performed as part of magico-religious rituals. Finally, there are also documented cases of accidental scalping. Scalping may appear on skeletal remains as necrosis of the affected cranial surface, secondary osteomyelitis, and cut marks encircling the crown of the skull or only on the frontal bone.

Decapitation

Decapitation is the act of severing the head from the body; it can occur as part of mortuary practices, during armed conflict, as a means of trophy-taking, as an act of sacrifice, or as part of judicial executions. Regardless of its motivation, decapitation leads to distinct bone changes. In addition, the burial context can provide valuable insights regarding past decapitation, particularly by observing the positioning of dismembered remains, such as the placement of a skull between the legs of the deceased individual. On skeletal remains, decapitation may be visible as cut marks on the cervical vertebrae, mandible, mastoid processes, occipital condyles or first rib, as well as crush fractures when an axe rather than a sword has been used (Figures 10.43–10.44).

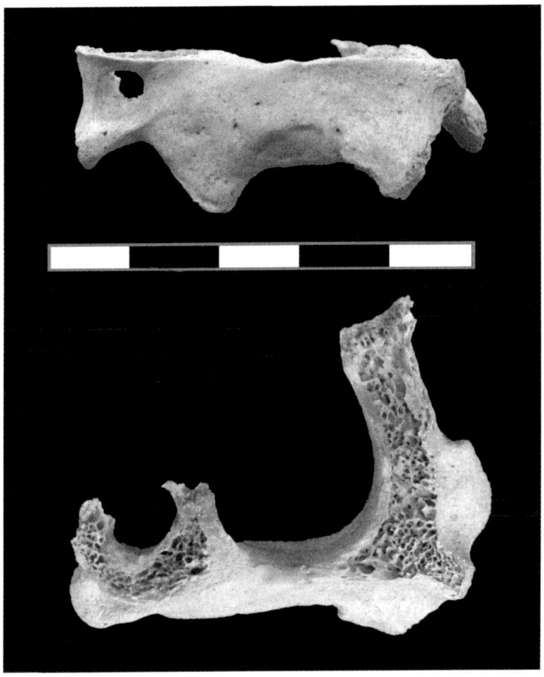

Figure 10.43 Decapitation. Note the linear cut across the axis. (Male, 14–25 years old, Ten Boer-Stederwalde, Collection NAD Nuis inv. Nr. G 2008-IX.92; photos by Efthymia Nikita, with permission from the Noordelijk Archeologisch Depot)

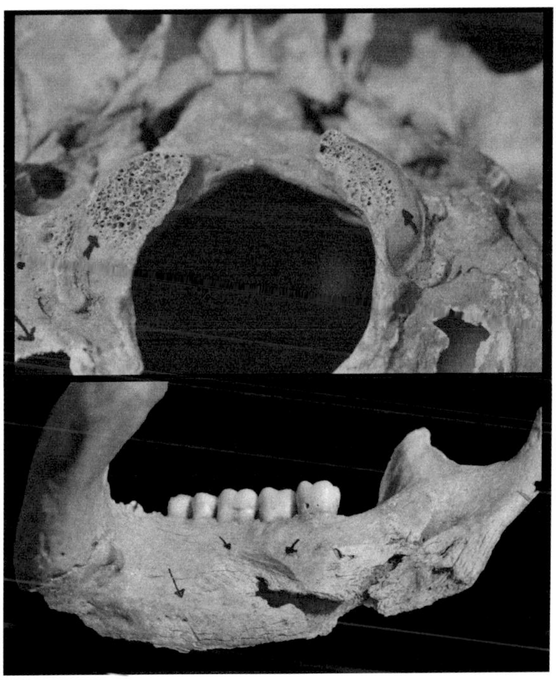

Figure 10.44 Decapitation. Note the linear cut of the occipital condyles (top) as well as the multiple cut marks on the inferior part of the mandibular corpus (bottom). (Huntingdon Roman Villa Saxon Cemetery site; photos by Efthymia Nikita; copyright: Duckworth Laboratory, University of Cambridge)

Strangulation

Strangulation can be caused by different methods, which result in similar skeletal lesions, though they may also leave no skeletal evidence:

- *Hanging*: traumatic spondylolysis of the axis or fractures of the pedicles or laminae of the third or fourth cervical vertebrae, fractures of the hyoid bone, and thyroid cartilage
- *Ligature strangulation*: fracture of the hyoid bone, mandible, and cervical vertebrae laminae
- *Manual strangulation*: fracture of the hyoid bone and thyroid cartilage

Bone shape modification

Cranial modification

Cranial modification has been included in this chapter because it may be seen as a form of "chronic, low-grade trauma" (Ortner and Putschar 1981:90). This practice alters the normal growth of the infant neurocranium in specific directions, promoting compensatory growth in other directions, and has a widespread occurrence across the world (Figure 10.45). Cranial deformation may arise either unintentionally or intentionally. Unintentional deformation usually results from the use of cradleboards or from infants resting for long periods on hard

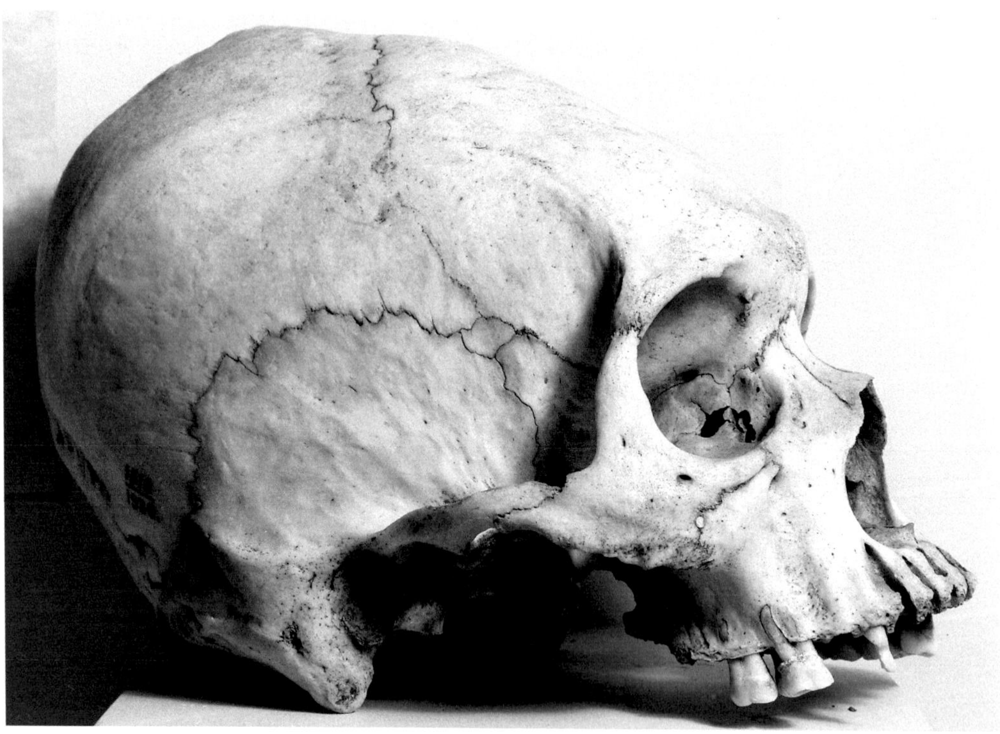

Figure 10.45 Elongated skull from Vanuatu

surfaces. In contrast, intentional deformation (headshaping) aims at altering the natural shape of the skull to achieve a culturally preferable form. The latter often functions as a marker of specific cultural identity, while individuals with modified crania may also be perceived as more attractive or healthy. Therefore, when encountering cases of cranial modification, it is important to be aware of the cultural and historical context in order to interpret its function.

Artificial cranial modification can take many forms, but the two most frequently documented types are annular (circumferential) and tabular (fronto-occipital) deformation. Annular deformation is produced by the encirclement of the cranial vault with materials such as bands, threads, or cords. Tabular deformation involves applying pressure on the anterior and posterior parts of the skull using pads, boards, or other means.

Foot binding

Foot binding was a cultural tradition in China, which involved the intentional alteration of female feet in order to decrease their size and modify the natural gait. This practice started in the 10th century CE, or even earlier, and was abolished with the founding of the People's Republic of China in 1949. Foot binding typically began between the ages of five and eight, when the bones of the foot are still pliable. This practice caused several issues, including chronic pain, oedema, infections, skin ulcers, muscle atrophy, diminished sensation in the lower extremities, and compromised blood flow. The skeletal effects of foot binding varied, but generally included a significant reduction in bone size, changes in bone shape and proportions, and degenerative lesions.

Note

1 More recently, bioarchaeology has increasingly focused on a different form of violence – structural violence. This concept encompasses the social structures that hold back individuals and societies from reaching their potential.

References and suggested readings

Allington, N. (2003). Child abuse. In *Trauma*, edited by Sherry, E., Trieu, L., Templeton, J., pp. 583–588. Oxford: Oxford University Press.

Antón, S.C. (1989). Intentional cranial vault deformation and induced changes of the cranial base and face. *American Journal of Physical Anthropology* 79:253–267. https://doi.org/10.1002/ajpa.1330790213

Ardagna, Y., Richier, A., Vernet, C., Dutour, O. (2005). A case of beheading dating from the celtic period (la Tène B, Sarliève-Grande Halle, France). *International Journal of Osteoarchaeology* 15:73–76. https://doi.org/10.1002/oa.776

Arnott, R., Finger, S., Smith, C.U.M. (2003). *Trepanation: History, Discovery, Theory*. Lisse: Swets & Zeitlinger.

Baiker-Sørensen, M., Herlaar, K. (2022). Variability and specificity of bone cutting mark properties in cases involving stabbing with knives. *International Journal of Legal Medicine* 136:603–621. https://doi.org/10.1007/s00414-021-02752-3

Bennike, P. (2008). Trauma. In *Advances in Human Paleopathology*, edited by Pinhasi, R., Mays, S., pp. 309–328. Hoboken, NJ: John Wiley & Sons.

Berger, R.G., Doyle, S.M. (2019). Spondylolysis 2019 update. *Current Opinion in Paediatrics* 31:61–68. https://doi.org/10.1097/MOP.0000000000000706

Berryman, H.E., Haun, S.J. (1996). Applying forensic techniques to interpret cranial fracture patterns in an archaeological specimen. *International Journal of Osteoarchaeology* 6:2–9. https://doi.org/10.1002/(SICI)1099-1212(199601)6:1<2::AID-OA244>3.0.CO;2-R

Berryman, H.E., Symes, S.A. (1998). Recognizing gunshot and blunt cranial trauma through fracture interpretation. In *Forensic Osteology: Advances in the Identification of Human Remains*, edited by Reichs K.J., pp. 333–352. Springfield, IL: Charles C. Thomas.

Boylston, A. (2000). Evidence for weapon-related trauma in British archaeological samples. In *Human Osteology in Archaeology and Forensic Science*, edited by Cox, M., Mays, S., pp. 357–380. Cambridge: Cambridge University Press.

Bueschgen, W.D., Case, D.T. (1996). Evidence of prehistoric scalping at Vosberg, Central Arizona. *International Journal of Osteoarchaeology* 16:230–248. https://doi.org/10.1002/(SICI)1099-1212(199606)6:3<230::AID-OA268>3.0.CO;2-Y

Byers, S.N., Juarez, C.A. (2023). *Introduction to Forensic Anthropology*, 6th edition. London: Routledge.

Byrnes, J.F., Gaddis, K. (2022). "Sticks and stones may break my bones": Traumatic injuries in paleopathology. In *The Routledge Handbook of Paleopathology*, edited by Grauer, A.L., pp. 231–249. London: Routledge.

Canavese, F., Samba, A., Rousset, M. (2016). Pathological fractures in children: Diagnosis and treatment options. *Orthopaedics & Traumatology: Surgery & Research* 102:S149–S159. https://doi.org/10.1016/j.otsr.2015.05.010

Cappella, A., Amadasi, A., Castoldi, E., Mazzarelli, D., Gaudio, D., Cattaneo, C. (2014). The difficult task of assessing perimortem and postmortem fractures on the skeleton: A blind test on 210 fractures of known origin. *Journal of Forensic Sciences* 59:1498–1601. https://doi.org/10.1111/1556-4029.12539

Cheverud, J.M., Kohn, L.A.P., Konigsberg, L.W., Leigh, S.R. (1992). Effects of fronto-occipital artificial cranial vault modification on the cranial base and face. *American Journal of Physical Anthropology* 88:323–345. https://doi.org/10.1002/ajpa.1330880307

Claes, L., Recknagel, S., Ignatius, A. (2012). Fracture healing under healthy inflammatory conditions. *National Review of Rheumatology* 8:133–143. https://doi.org/10.1038/nrrheum.2012.1

Currey, J.D. (2013). *Bones: Structure and Mechanics*. Princeton: Princeton University Press.

De Boer, H., Merwe, A., Hammer, S., Steyn, M., Maat, G. (2015). Assessing post-traumatic time interval in human dry bone. *International Journal of Osteoarchaeology* 25:98–109. https://doi.org/10.1002/oa.2267

Flaherty, E.G., Perez-Rossello, J.M., Levine, M.A., Hennrikus, W.L. (2014). Evaluating children with fractures for child physical abuse. *Pediatrics* 133:e477–489. https://doi.org/10.1542/peds.2013-3793

Fredrickson, B.E., Baker, D., McHolick, W.J., Yuan, H.A., Lubicky, J.P. (1984). The natural history of spondylolysis, and spondylolisthesis in children and adolescents. *The Journal of Bone & Joint Surgery* 66:699–707.

Galloway, A., Wedel, V.L. (2014a). Bones of the skulls, the dentition, and osseous structures of the throat. In *Broken Bones: An Anthropological Analysis of Blunt Force Trauma*, edited by Wedel, V.L., Galloway, A., 2nd edition, pp. 133–160. Springfield, IL: Charles C. Thomas.

Galloway, A., Wedel, V.L. (2014b). Common circumstances of blunt force trauma. In *Broken Bones: Anthropological Analysis of Blunt Force Trauma*, edited by Wedel, V.L., Galloway, A., 2nd edition, pp. 91–132. Springfield, IL: Charles C. Thomas.

Galloway, A., Zephro, L., Wedel, V.L. (2014). Diagnostic criteria for the determination of timing and fracture mechanism. In *Broken Bones: Anthropological Analysis of Blunt Force Trauma*, edited by Wedel, V.L., Galloway, A., 2nd edition, pp. 47–58. Springfield, IL: Charles C. Thomas.

Gerszten, P.C., Gerszten, E. (1995). Intentional cranial deformation: A disappearing form of self-mutilation. *Neurosurgery* 37:374–382.

Gowland, R.L. (2016). Elder abuse: Evaluating the potentials and problems of diagnosis in the archaeological record. *International Journal of Osteoarchaeology* 26:514–523. https://doi.org/10.1002/oa.2442

Gurdjian, E.D. (1975). *Impact Head Injury*. Springfield, IL: Charles C. Thomas.

Hoskote, A.U., Martin, K., Hormbrey, P., Burns, C.E. (2003). Fractures in infants: One in four is non-accidental. *Child Abuse Review* 12:384–391. https://doi.org/10.1002/car.806

Houck, M.H. (1998). Skeletal trauma and the individualization of knife marks in bone. In *Forensic Osteology: Advances in the Identification of Human Remains*, edited by Reichs, K.J., pp. 410–424. Springfield, IL: Charles C. Thomas.

Humphrey, J.H., Hutchinson, D.L. (2001). Macroscopic characteristics of hacking trauma. *Journal of Forensic Sciences* 46:228–233.

Ikata, T., Miyake, R., Katoh, S., Morita, T., Murase, M. (1996). Pathogenesis of sports-related spondylolisthesis in adolescents. *The American Journal of Sports Medicine* 24:94–98.

Judd, M.A. (2008). The parry problem. *Journal of Archaeological Science* 35:1658–1666. https://doi.org/10.1016/j.jas.2007.11.005

Judd, M.A., Redfern, R. (2012). Trauma. In *A Companion to Paleopathology*, edited by Grauer, A.L., pp. 359–379. Hoboken, NJ: John Wiley & Sons.

Kimmerle, E.H., Baraybar, J.P. (2008a). Blunt force trauma. In *Skeletal Trauma: Identification of Injuries Resulting from Human Rights Abuse and Armed Conflict*, edited by Kimmerle, E.H., Baraybar, J.P., pp. 151–200. Boca Raton, FL: CRC Press.

Kimmerle, E.H., Baraybar, J.P. (2008b). Sharp force trauma. In *Skeletal Trauma: Identification of Injuries Resulting from Human Rights Abuse and Armed Conflict*, edited by Kimmerle, E.H., Baraybar, J.P., pp. 263–320. Boca Raton, FL: CRC Press.

King, A.I. (2018). *The Biomechanics of Impact Injury: Biomechanical Response, Mechanisms of Injury, Human Tolerance and Simulation*. Cham: Springer.

Komar, D.A., Buikstra, J.E. (2008). *Forensic Anthropology: Contemporary Theory and Practice*. New York: Oxford University Press.

Kozakaitė, J., Ryčkov, A., Ramonaitė, M., Brindzaitė, R., Jankauskas, R., Piombino-Mascali, D. (2022). On some paleopathological examples of amputation and the implications for healthcare in 13th–17th century Lithuania. *International Journal of Paleopathology* 37:68–76. https://doi.org/10.1016/j.ijpp.2022.04.005

Krakowka, K. (2017). Patterns and prevalence of violence-related skull trauma in medieval London. *American Journal of Physical Anthropology* 164:488–504. https://doi.org/10.1002/ajpa.23288

Kranioti, E.F. (2015). Forensic investigation of cranial injuries due to blunt force trauma: Current best practice. *Research and Reports in Forensic Medical Science* 2015:25–37. https://doi.org/10.2147/RRFMS.S70423

Lewis, J.E. (2008). Identifying sword marks on bone: Criteria for distinguishing between cut marks made by different classes of bladed weapons. *Journal of Archaeological Science* 35:2001–2008. https://doi.org/10.1016/j.jas.2008.01.016

Lewis, M. (2013). Sticks and stones: Exploring the nature and significance of child trauma in the past. In *The Routledge Handbook of the Bioarchaeology of Human Conflict*, edited by Knüsel, C., Smith, M., pp. 39–62. London: Routledge.

Lewis, M. (2017). Trauma and treatment. In *Paleopathology of Children: Identification of Pathological Conditions in the Human Skeletal Remains of Non-Adults*, edited by Lewis, M, pp. 91–129. San Diego: Academic Press.

Lovell, N.C. (1997). Trauma analysis in paleopathology. *Yearbook of Physical Anthropology* 40:139–170 https://doi.org/10.1002/(SICI)1096-8644(1997)25+%3C139::AID-AJPA6%3E3.0.CO;2-%23

Lovell, N.C., Grauer, A.L. (2018). Analysis and interpretation of trauma in skeletal remains. In *Biological Anthropology of the Human Skeleton*, edited by Katzenberg, M.A., Grauer, A.L., 3rd edition, pp. 335–383. Hoboken, NJ: John Wiley & Sons.

Matcuk, G.R., Mahanty, S.R., Skalski, M.R., Patel, D.B., White, E.A. Gottsegen, C.J. (2016). Stress fractures: Pathophysiology, clinical presentation, imaging features, and treatment options. *Emergency Radiology* 23:365–375. https://doi.org/10.1007/s10140-016-1390-5

Mays, S. (2006). Spondylolysis, spondylolisthesis, and lumbo-sacral morphology in a medieval English skeletal population. *American Journal of Physical Anthropology* 131:352–362. https://doi.org/10.1002/ajpa.20447

Merbs, C.F. (1989). Spondylolysis: Its nature and anthropological significance. *International Journal of Anthropology* 4:163–169. https://doi.org/10.1007/BF02446238

Merbs, C.F. (1996). Spondylolysis and spondylolisthesis: A cost of being an erect biped or a clever adaptation? *American Journal of Physical Anthropology* 101:201–228. https://doi.org/10.1002/(SICI)1096-8644(1996)23+<201::AID-AJPA8>3.0.CO;2-7

Merbs, C.F. (2002). Asymmetrical spondylolysis. *American Journal of Physical Anthropology* 119:156–174. https://doi.org/10.1002/ajpa.10100

Milner, G.R., Anderson, E., Smith, V.G. (1991). Warfare in late prehistoric west-central Illinois. *American Antiquity* 56:581–603. https://doi.org/10.2307/281538

Nabian, M.H., Zadegan, S.A., Zanjani, L.O. Mehrpour, S.R. (2017). Epidemiology of joint dislocations and ligamentous/tendinous injuries among 2,700 patients: Five-year trend of a tertiary center in Iran. *The Archives of Bone and Joint Surgery* 5:426–434.

Nathan, H. (1959). Spondylolysis. Its anatomy and mechanism of development. *The Journal of Bone & Joint Surgery* 41:303–320.

O'Driscoll, C.A., Thompson, J.C. (2014). Experimental projectile impact marks on bone: Implications for identifying the origins of projectile technology. *Journal of Archaeological Science* 49:398–413. https://doi.org/10.1016/j.jas.2014.05.036

Okaluk, T.R., Greenfield, H.J. (2022). Macroscopic chop mark identification on archaeological bone: An experimental study of chipped stone, ground stone, copper, and bronze axe heads on bone. *Quaternary* 5:15. https://doi.org/10.3390/quat5010015

Ortner, D.J., Putschar, W.G.J. (1981). *Identification of Pathological Conditions in Human Skeletal Remains*. Washington, DC: Smithsonian Institution Press.

Pankowská, A., Galeta, P., Uhlík Spěváčková, P., Nováček, K. (2019). Violence in European medieval monasteries: Skeletal trauma in Teplá monastery (Czech Republic). *International Journal of Osteoarchaeology* 29:908–921. https://doi.org/10.1002/oa.2804

Passalacqua, N.V., Rainwater, C.W. (2015). *Skeletal Trauma Analysis: Case Studies in Context*. Chichester: Wiley-Blackwell.

Peng, B. (2016). Natural history of lumbar spondylolysis—Advances and concerns. *International Journal of Orthopaedics* 3:591–594.

Polson, C., Gee, D., Knight, B. (1985). *The Essentials of Forensic Medicine*, 4th edition. Oxford: Pergamon Press.

Redfern, R.C., Roberts, C.A. (2019). Trauma. In *Ortner's Identification of Pathological Conditions in Human Skeletal Remains*, edited by Buikstra, J.E., pp. 211–284. San Diego: Academic Press.

Ribeiro, P., Jordana, X., Scheirs, S., Ortega-Sánchez, M., Rodriguez-Baeza, A., McGlynn, H., Galtés, I. (2020). Distinction between perimortem and postmortem fractures in human cranial bone. *International Journal of Legal Medicine* 134:1765–1774. https://doi.org/10.1007/s00414-020-02356-3

Rodríguez-Martín, C. (2006). Identification and differential diagnosis of traumatic lesions of the skeleton. In *Forensic Anthropology and Medicine: Complementary Sciences from Recovery to Cause of Death*, edited by Schmitt, A., Cunha, E., Pinheiro, J., pp. 197–221. Totowa, NJ: Humana Press.

Sauer, N. (1998). The timing of injuries and manner of death: Distinguishing among antemortem, perimortem, and postmortem trauma. In *Forensic Osteology: Advances in the Identification of Human Remains*, 2nd edition, edited by Reichs, K.J., pp. 321–332. Springfield, IL: Charles C. Thomas.

Smith, M.J., Brickley, M.B., Leach, S.L. (2007). Experimental evidence for lithic projectile injuries: Improving identification of an under-recognised phenomenon. *Journal of Archaeological Science* 34:540–553. https://doi.org/10.1016/j.jas.2006.06.008

Spitz, W.U. (1993). Sharp force injury. In *Spitz and Fisher's Medicolegal Investigation of Death: Guidelines for the Application of Pathology to Crime Investigation*, edited by Spitz, W.U., 3rd edition, pp. 252–310. Springfield, IL: Charles C. Thomas.

Steppe, L., Megafu, M., Tschaffon-Müller, M.E., Ignatius, A., Haffner-Luntzer, M. (2023). Fracture healing research: Recent insights. *Bone Reports* 19:101686. https://doi.org/10.1016/j.bonr.2023.101686

Sun, X., Man, X., Liao, X., Yang, J., Cao, J., Zhu, H., Zhang, Q., Wang, Q. (2021). Footbinding and non-footbinding Han Chinese females in the Qing Dynasty (1644–1912 CE) Xifengbu cemetery: A skeletal and mortuary analysis. *Archaeological and Anthropological Sciences* 13:18. https://doi.org/10.1007/s12520-020-01241-9

Tiesler, V. (2014). *The Bioarchaeology of Artificial Cranial Modifications*. New York: Springer.

Torres-Rouff, C. (2002). Cranial vault modification and ethnicity in Middle Horizon San Pedro de Atacama, Chile. *Current Anthropology* 43:163–171. https://doi.org/10.1086/338290

Ubelaker, O.A., Adams, B.J. (1995). Differentiation of perimortem and postmortem trauma using taphonomic indicators. *Journal of Forensic Sciences* 40:509–512.

van Houten, M.E., Vloet, L.C., Pelgrim, T., Reijnders, U.J., Berben, S.A. (2021). Types, characteristics and anatomic location of physical signs in elder abuse: A systematic review: Awareness and recognition of injury patterns. *European Geriatric Medicine* 13:53–85. https://doi.org/10.1007/s41999-021-00550-z

Verano, J.W. (2016). Differential diagnosis: Trepanation. *International Journal of Paleopathology* 14:1–9. https://doi.org/10.1016/j.ijpp.2016.04.001

Walczak, B.E., Johnson, C.N., Howe, B.M. (2015). Myositis ossificans. *Journal of the American Academy of Orthopaedic Surgeons* 23:612–622. https://doi.org/10.5435/JAAOS-D-14-00269

Waldron, T. (2020). Trauma. In *Palaeopathology*, edited by Waldron, T., 2nd edition, pp. 208–234. Cambridge: Cambridge University Press.

Walker, P.L., Long, J.C. (1977). An experimental study of the morphological characteristics of toolmarks. *American Antiquity* 42:605–616. https://doi.org/10.2307/278934

Wedel, V.L., Galloway, A. (2014). *Broken Bones: Anthropological Analysis of Blunt Force Trauma*. Springfield, IL: Charles C. Thomas.

Wieberg, D.M.A., Westcott, D.J. (2008). Estimating the timing of long bone fractures: Correlation between the postmortem interval, bone moisture content, and blunt force trauma fracture characteristics. *Journal of Forensic Sciences* 53:1–7. https://doi.org/10.1111/j.1556-4029.2008.00801.x

Więckowski, W. (2021). A rare case of multilevel spondylolysis—A nineteenth century Chinese immigrant to Peru from Castillo de Huarmey archaeological site. *International Journal of Osteoarchaeology* 31:782–788. https://doi.org/10.1002/oa.2989

Chapter 11

Dental disease

This chapter examines conditions that may affect the maxilla, mandible, and dentition. We largely follow Pilloud and Fancher's (2019) recommendation on which conditions should be classified as *dental diseases* or *pathological conditions of the oral cavity*, and we include in this chapter dental caries, periodontal disease, periapical lesions, dental calculus, and antemortem tooth loss. However, we have also included enamel hypoplasia because it often appears in palaeopathological publications together with the conditions outlined above. Nonetheless, we acknowledge that enamel hypoplasia should not be considered a dental disease but rather an indicator of physiological stress.

Dental caries

Dental caries is a process that starts as localised demineralisation of the enamel, but it can gradually involve other dental tissues (Figures 11.1–11.3). This demineralisation results from the corrosive action of acids that are produced during the bacterial fermentation of dietary carbohydrates.

Several bacteria have been linked to the formation of carious lesions, such as Streptococci and Lactobacilli. Nonetheless, carious lesions may form even when bacteria commonly associated with this condition are absent. This suggests that the aetiology of dental caries may be more strongly linked to a disruption of the oral microbiota than the presence of specific pathogens. In addition, certain bacterial genera may inhibit the proliferation of cariogenic bacteria, and thus protect the teeth from caries. Note that bacteria associated with dental caries have also been linked to several other conditions, such as cardiovascular disease, rheumatoid arthritis, respiratory tract infections, and even certain cancers; though these relationships are largely correlational and not clearly causal.

Bacteria present in dental plaque metabolise dietary sugars from carbohydrates; during this process, lactic acid is produced and gradually reduces the pH of the plaque below 5.5. This reduction in pH triggers demineralisation, that is, the loss of minerals such as phosphate and calcium from the dental tissues. If equilibrium is re-established, these minerals can be restored, but if the rate of demineralisation exceeds that of remineralisation, carious lesions will form. Early carious lesions are not visible macroscopically, but over time, a small white or brown spot will appear on the enamel, which will gradually enlarge, and a cavity will form. Eventually, the lesion may involve the dentine and the pulp chamber. The exposure of the pulp to microorganisms can cause inflammation. In such cases, the pulp will eventually undergo necrosis. Inflammation can extend down the root canal, and microorganisms and inflammatory

DOI: 10.4324/9781003475026-11

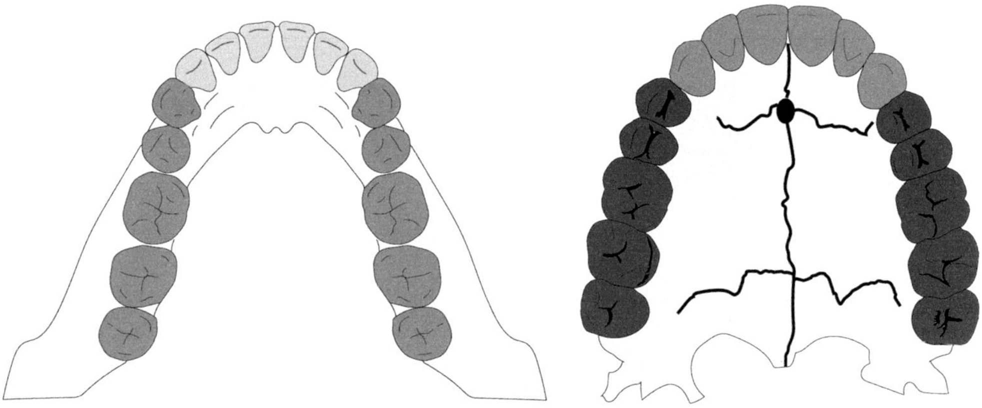

- crown: focal enamel demineralisation manifesting as discolouration → localised enamel destruction → dentine penetration → gross cavity with exposed pulp chamber or root canal

- root and/or cemento-enamel junction: focal demineralisation of enamel and/or cementum manifesting as discolouration → cavity penetrating dentine along cemento–enamel junction, or restricted to root surface → gross cavity with exposed pulp chamber or root canal

Figure 11.1 Manifestation of dental caries. The different shades of grey reflect teeth that are more or less frequently affected by caries; the lighter the shade, the less frequently a tooth is affected. (Data from Hillson 2001, 2008, 2023; Larsen et al. 1991; Lukacs 1989; Rudney et al. 1983)

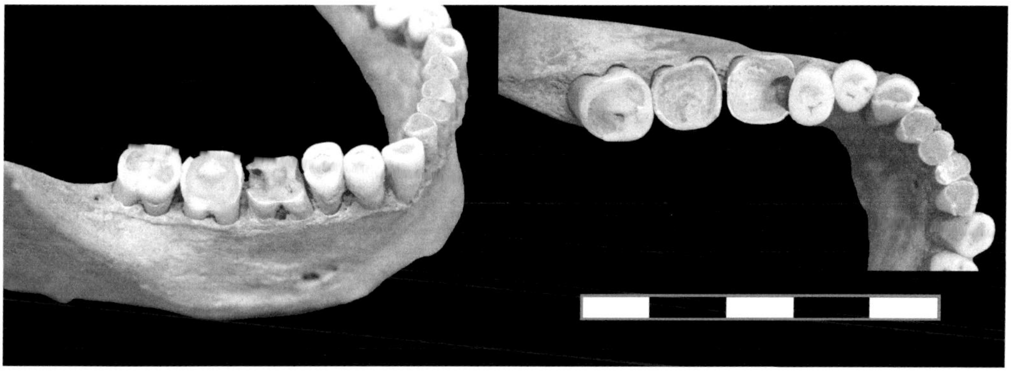

Figure 11.2 Interproximal caries of the right and left mandibular first molars; the cavities penetrate the dentine and pulp cavity. Note also the small occlusal caries of the left third molar. (Diever, Reformed Church graveyard, Collection NAD Nuis inv. Nr. D 2019-III.468; photos by Efthymia Nikita, with permission from the Noordelijk Archeologisch Depot)

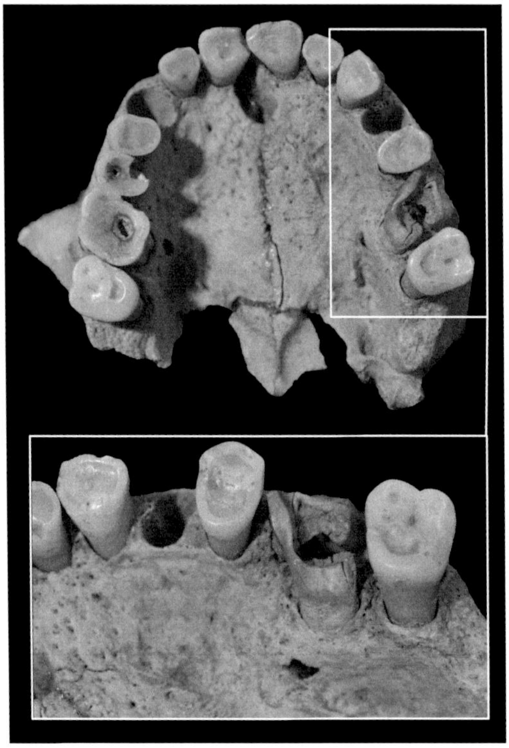

Figure 11.3 Gross caries of the left maxillary first molar, and occlusal caries of the right fourth premolar and first molar. (Photos by Efthymia Nikita; copyright: Duckworth Laboratory, University of Cambridge)

byproducts will exit the tooth through the apical foramen, triggering inflammation in the periapical tissues.

The progression of a carious lesion is not only gradual but also irregular. Even after the formation of a cavity, the lesion may remain stable for extended periods, while early lesions, before cavitation, may remineralise. Moreover, the deposition of secondary dentine can delay the involvement of the pulp chamber. Even in cases where the pulp is inflamed, the inflammation may be localised and progress slowly. However, untreated caries may lead to meningitis, chronic maxillary sinusitis, and other health problems.

Dental caries has a complex and multifactorial aetiology. Some of the key factors involved in the development of carious lesions include the consumption of dietary carbohydrates, the use of specific cooking methods, the morphology of different teeth, salivary composition and flow rate, hormonal levels, poor oral hygiene, and a genetic predisposition to caries.

A high consumption of cariogenic carbohydrates, such as sugars and starches, promotes the formation of carious lesions. The methods of food preparation also play an important role in dental caries formation, particularly when cooking enhances the refining or gelatinisation of carbohydrates. These processes promote the adhesion of carbohydrates to the tooth surfaces, thus they facilitate the proliferation of cariogenic bacterial colonies. In addition, cooking softens the food and, thus, it reduces tooth wear. Tooth wear and dental caries have a complex relationship. Wear removes food debris from the teeth and eliminates dental

> **Box 11.1 Male–female differences in dental caries**
>
> Females overall show a higher prevalence of dental caries compared to males, both in past and modern groups. This pattern has been attributed by bioarchaeologists primarily to behavioural factors, such as different food consumption patterns associated with sex-specific division of labour. In addition, teeth in females erupt earlier than in males, which is another potentially important factor in the observed male–female differences, since it implies that female teeth are exposed in the oral cavity for longer. More recently, the significance of hormonal differences that influence salivary quality and flow has been highlighted. In general, the aetiology of caries formation is complex, as briefly discussed above, and any observed differences between sexes should be interpreted as the result of the interplay of various factors.

fissures (see below); thus, it inhibits caries formation. However, excessive wear can expose the dentine or even the pulp, making the tooth more susceptible to carious damage.

The susceptibility of teeth to dental caries is also affected by tooth morphology. The grooves and fissures on the occlusal surface of the posterior teeth facilitate the development of bacterial colonies, while the large interproximal contact areas that form between these teeth are prone to dental caries.

Saliva has several important functions that contribute to the protection of teeth from dental caries (see Lukacs and Largaespada 2006), including the (1) cleaning of tooth surfaces from food particles, (2) formation of the salivary pellicle that covers and protects the enamel, (3) oral pH buffering, (4) increase of antimicrobial protein levels in the oral cavity, and (5) introduction of calcium and phosphate ions that increase enamel resistance to bacterial acids. Therefore, a reduction in salivary flow promotes dental caries. The quality and quantity of saliva may be affected by medical conditions, the masticatory demands associated with different foods, as well as daily practices such as smoking. In females, the mean salivary flow rate is lower compared to males; this pattern may be linked to sex hormones, particularly oestrogen. Therefore, life events that involve hormonal fluctuations in females (e.g. pregnancy, menopause) may affect their susceptibility to dental caries (see also Box 11.1).

Periodontal disease

Periodontal disease is the inflammation of the periodontium, that is, the gingivae, periodontal ligament, alveolar bone, and cementum. Periodontal disease is classified into gingivitis and periodontitis. Gingivitis is the inflammation of the gingivae due to the build-up of dental plaque, and it is reversible if oral hygiene practices are improved. Importantly, in gingivitis, the underlying alveolar bone is not affected; thus, this condition cannot be detected in skeletal remains (Figure 11.4). If gingivitis is not adequately treated, it progresses to periodontitis. Periodontitis is an inflammation of the periodontal tissues; it damages the periodontal ligament, causes the resorption of alveolar bone, and results in the eventual loss of teeth before death (Boxes 11.2 and 11.3, Figure 11.5). Tissue destruction associated with periodontitis is irreversible; however, the progression of this condition is not linear. Instead, periods of relative stability are interrupted by episodes of destructive activity.

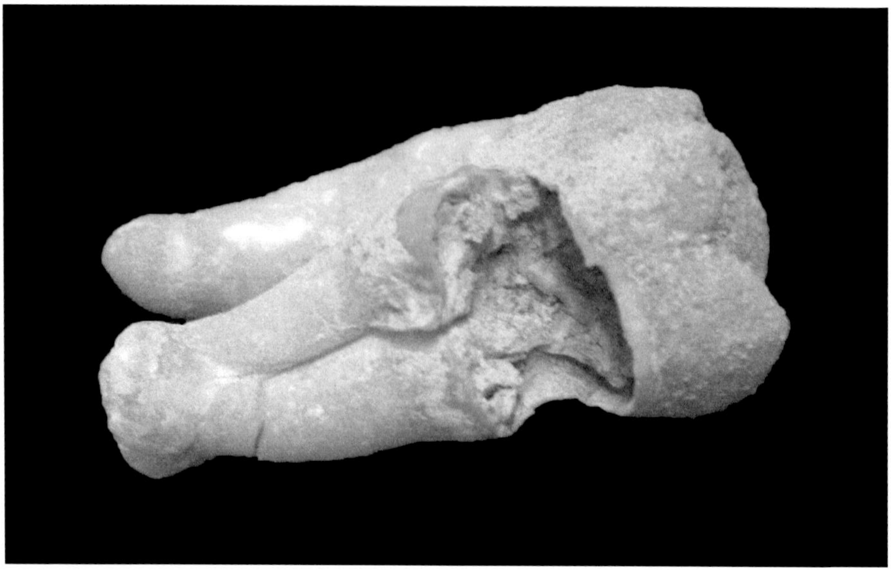

Figure 11.4 Root caries of a left maxillary third molar. (Alambra *Kato Lakkos*, Middle Bronze Age, Cyprus; Photo by Gkampriella Selempa; permission to use this image has been granted by the Director of the Department of Antiquities, Cyprus)

Individuals with periodontal disease show a change in the composition of the oral microbiota: communities primarily composed of gram-positive bacteria are found in healthy individuals, whereas communities predominantly including anaerobic gram-negative bacteria are

Box 11.2 Manifestation of periodontal disease

- alveolar bone loss → exposure of underlying trabecular bone (porosity), recession of alveolar crest relative to cemento-enamel junction
- signs of inflammation and remodelling in interdental septum

(Data from Clarke 1990; Clarke and Hirsch 1991; Clarke et al. 1986; Hildebolt and Molnar 1991; Hillson 2023; Kerr 1988, 1991; Lukacs 1989; Ogden 2008; Tal 1985)

Box 11.3 How much alveolar bone recession is enough?

Most scholars recommend that periodontitis should be classified as present in skeletal remains if the distance between the cemento-enamel junction (CEJ) and the alveolar crest (AC) is at least 3 mm. This principle aligns with clinical standards, where the threshold for attachment loss is 2 mm; in skeletal remains, an additional 1 mm is added to the calculations due to the absence of soft tissues. However, when using this approach, it is important to consider complications that may arise from the continued eruption of teeth throughout an individual's life to maintain contact between occlusal surfaces.

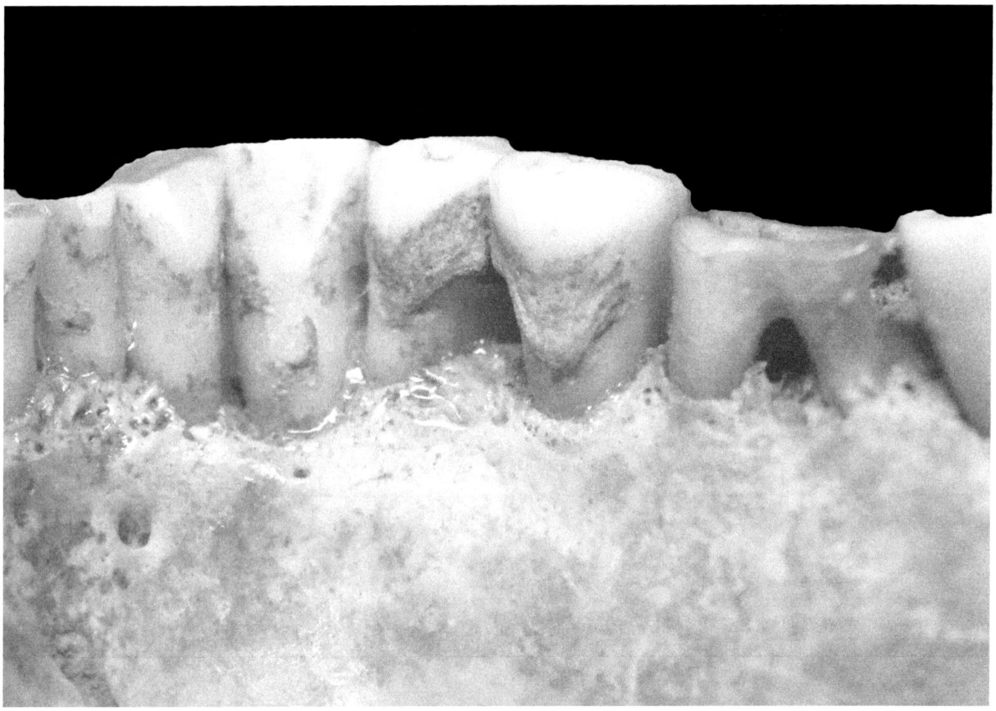

Figure 11.5 Lingual view of a right mandible with periodontal disease. Note the recession of the alveolar bone, the exposure of a large part of the tooth roots, and the distance between the cemento-enamel junction and the alveolar crest. Note also the calculus deposits on the lingual surface of the two premolars; smaller deposits are visible on the incisors and canines. (Diever, Reformed Church graveyard, Collection NAD Nuis inv. Nr. D 2019-III.468; photo by Efthymia Nikita, with permission from the Noordelijk Archeologisch Depot)

found in individuals with periodontal disease. Besides bacteria, certain viruses and fungi also contribute to this condition.

Tooth morphology, biofilm virulence, socioeconomic status, smoking, alcohol consumption, nutritional deficiencies, and obesity can also affect the appearance of periodontal disease. It is important to note that associations have been found between periodontal disease and several systemic conditions; however, these relationships are complex and not fully understood.

Periapical lesions

A periapical lesion (or periapical cavity) affects the bone around the apex of a tooth and arises when an infection reaches the pulp chamber (Table 11.1, Figures 11.6–11.8). Once the infection is established, it can spread to the periapical tissues through the apical foramen, triggering an inflammatory response. The inflammatory response depends on the host's immune system as well as the pathogenicity of the infectious agent. If the immune response is efficient, inflammation will resolve, and the tissues will heal. In contrast, if the infection persists, the inflammatory response can become chronic. In cases of low-grade infection, chronic inflammation may develop directly without an initial acute inflammatory phase.

Table 11.1 Characteristics of different types of periapical lesions

Lesion	*Characteristics*
periapical granuloma	• smooth cavity walls • circumscribed cavity margins • <3 mm in diameter
apical periodontal cyst	• smooth cavity walls • circumscribed cavity margins • >3 mm in diameter
acute abscess	• roughened cavity walls
chronic abscess	• roughened cavity walls • <3 mm in diameter • sinus extending to subperiosteal surface or into maxillary sinus
chronic osteomyelitis	• roughened cavity margins • larger irregular area • sequestrum, involucrum, and several sinuses

(Data compiled from Dias and Tayles 1997; Dias et al. 2007)

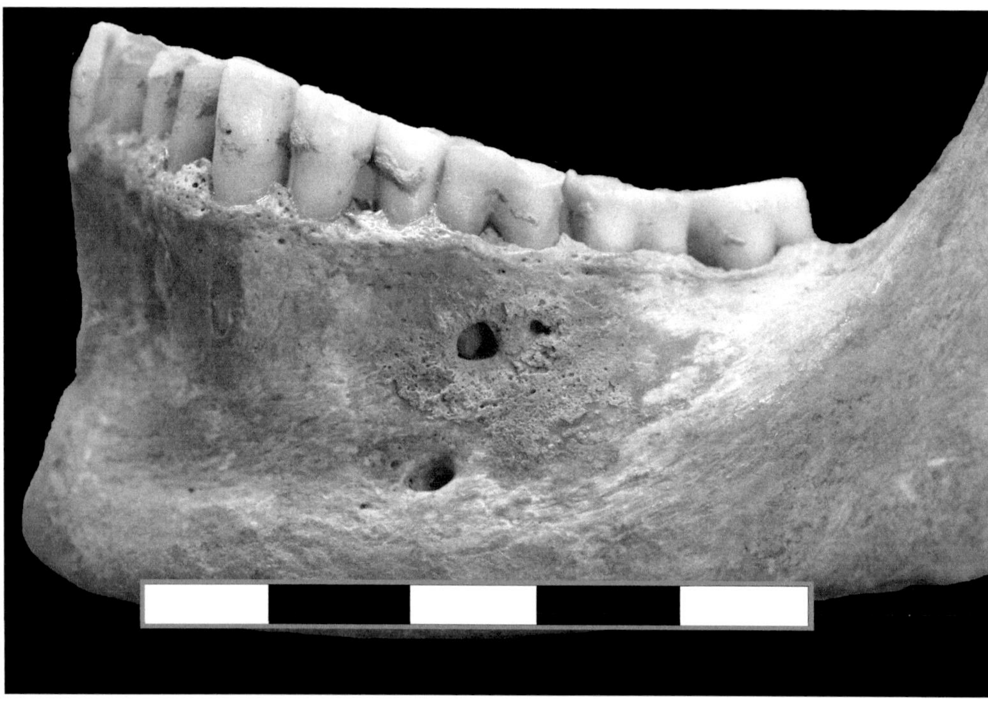

Figure 11.6 Two periapical cavities on the buccal surface of a mandible, associated with the first molar (not to be confused with the mental foramen); extensive woven new bone has formed around the two cavities. Note that the same mandible exhibits periodontal disease, as attested by the exposure of all tooth roots and the distance between the cemento-enamel junction and the alveolar crest, while small calculus deposits are visible on the buccal and interproximal surfaces of most teeth. (Diever, Reformed Church graveyard, Collection NAD Nuis inv. Nr. D 2019-III.468; photo by Efthymia Nikita, with permission from the Noordelijk Archeologisch Depot)

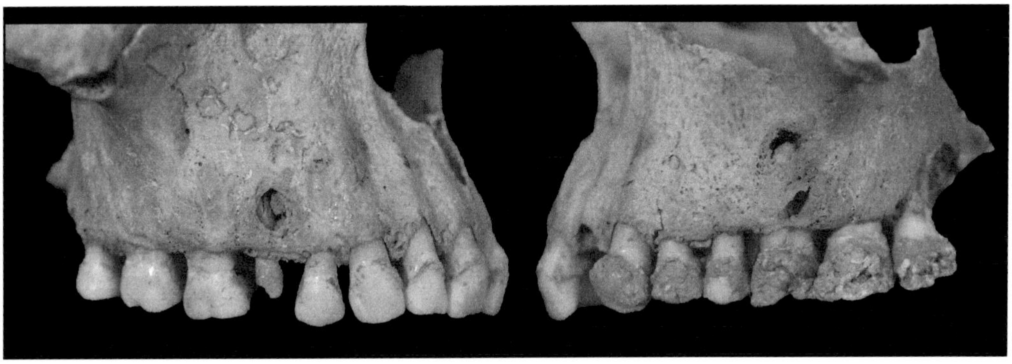

Figure 11.7 Left: Periapical cavity on the buccal surface of the maxilla, associated with the right fourth premolar, which has largely been destroyed by gross caries. Right: Two periapical cavities on the buccal maxillary surface, associated with the left first molar. Note the calculus deposits that fully cover all tooth crown surfaces (part of the deposit on P4 has fallen off). (Photos by Efthymia Nikita; copyright: Duckworth Laboratory, University of Cambridge)

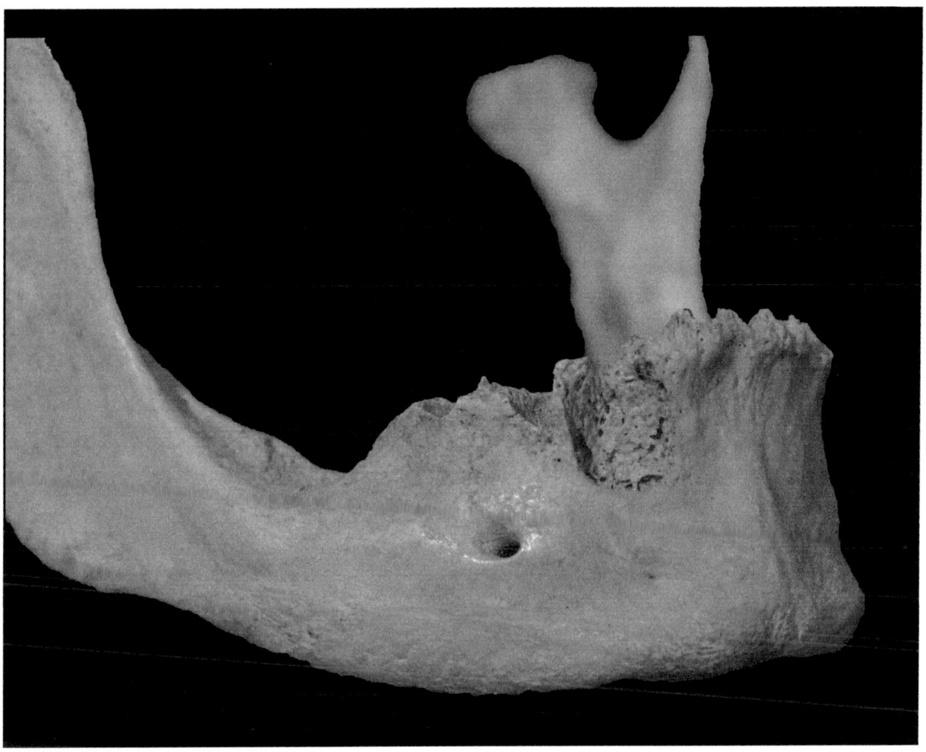

Figure 11.8 Periapical cavity on the buccal surface of the mandible, associated with the right canine. All three molars on the right side have been lost antemortem, and their sockets have been fully resorbed. (Photo by Efthymia Nikita; copyright: Duckworth Laboratory, University of Cambridge)

A periapical granuloma indicates chronic inflammation due to infection of the pulp. It consists of a mass of granulation tissue that forms in response to pulpal necrosis. A fibrous capsule, composed of bundles of collagen fibres, separates the granulation tissue from the surrounding bone. Gradually, an osseous cavity with smooth walls is formed. The detection of periapical granulomas in skeletal remains can be challenging without radiographic examination. Over a period of time, a granuloma may progress into an apical periodontal cyst.

In a periodontal cyst, fluid takes the place of granulation tissue, while epithelial tissue lines the cavity. Since periodontal cysts represent a chronic process that develops from a pre-existing granuloma, a cyst is larger than the original granuloma. If left untreated, the cyst will usually increase in size, leading to an expansion of the alveolar bone. In some cases, the cyst may eventually discharge through a sinus tract. While a periapical granuloma can resolve once the infection source is eliminated, an apical periodontal cyst will keep expanding even in the absence of the initial source of infection.

If the individual experiences severe infection involving pyogenic organisms, an acute periapical abscess can develop. Such an abscess can arise from an acute infection of the dental pulp or, more frequently, it arises secondarily and is linked to a pre-existing granuloma or cyst. An acute infection usually causes pain and fever; however, there is not enough time for an osseous cavity to form. If the infection that leads to the acute abscess does not resolve completely, but only partially, the abscess can become chronic. In such chronic infections, a channel forms through which pus is expelled (sinus or fistula).

An acute abscess may rarely progress into either acute or chronic osteomyelitis. In such cases, the infection extends into adjacent bone marrow spaces. Acute osteomyelitis does not produce osseous changes, but, if left untreated, it can cause death in immunocompromised individuals. In contrast, individuals with some degree of resistance to the infecting organism may develop chronic osteomyelitis, manifesting as sequestrum, involucrum, and cloacae (see Chapter 7).

Dental calculus

Dental calculus is mineralised plaque, a bacterial biofilm on the tooth surfaces (Figures 11.9 and 11.10). Dental plaque formation begins when salivary proteins adhere to the enamel, forming a pellicle that protects the tooth surface from demineralisation. Subsequently, oral bacteria attach to this pellicle, and additional bacteria adhere to the initial bacterial layer. The bacterial communities within dental plaque mostly include streptococci and actinomycetes. Subsequently, plaque starts mineralising as calcium phosphate crystals are deposited into its organic matrix.

Dental calculus is composed of about 80% inorganic material, primarily calcium and phosphorus, and smaller amounts of carbonate, sodium, fluoride, and magnesium. The mineral part of dental calculus consists of brushite, octacalcium phosphate, whitlockite, and hydroxyapatite. Proteins, carbohydrates, and lipids form the organic component.

Depending on its location, dental calculus can be supragingival or subgingival. Supragingival calculus lies above the gingival margin, while subgingival calculus forms within the gingival pocket and is usually seen in teeth with exposed roots due to periodontal disease. These two types of calculus deposits have a number of differences. Supragingival calculus derives its minerals primarily from saliva, whereas subgingival calculus derives them mostly from crevicular fluid. Moreover, subgingival calculus tends to be more mineralised than supragingival calculus, which has a more heterogeneous composition. Finally, supragingival calculus is covered by a layer of microorganisms that mostly consists of filaments oriented perpendicularly

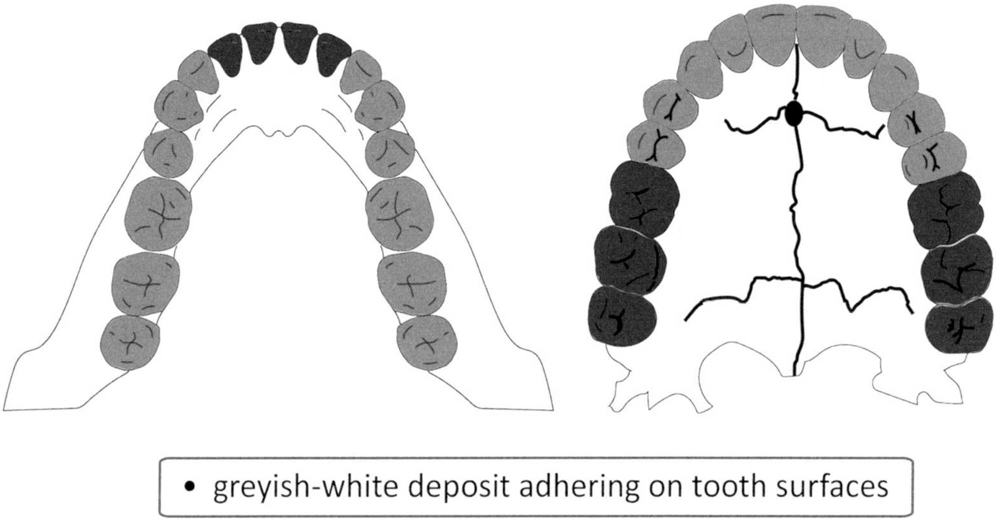

Figure 11.9 Manifestation of dental calculus. The different shades of grey reflect teeth that are more or less frequently affected by calculus; the lighter the shade, the less frequently a tooth is affected. Note that the distribution pattern shown in this figure reflects supragingival calculus; there is no distinct pattern in the distribution of subgingival calculus among teeth. (Data from Brothwell 1981; Driessens and Verbeeck 1988; Hillson 2023; Lieverse 1999)

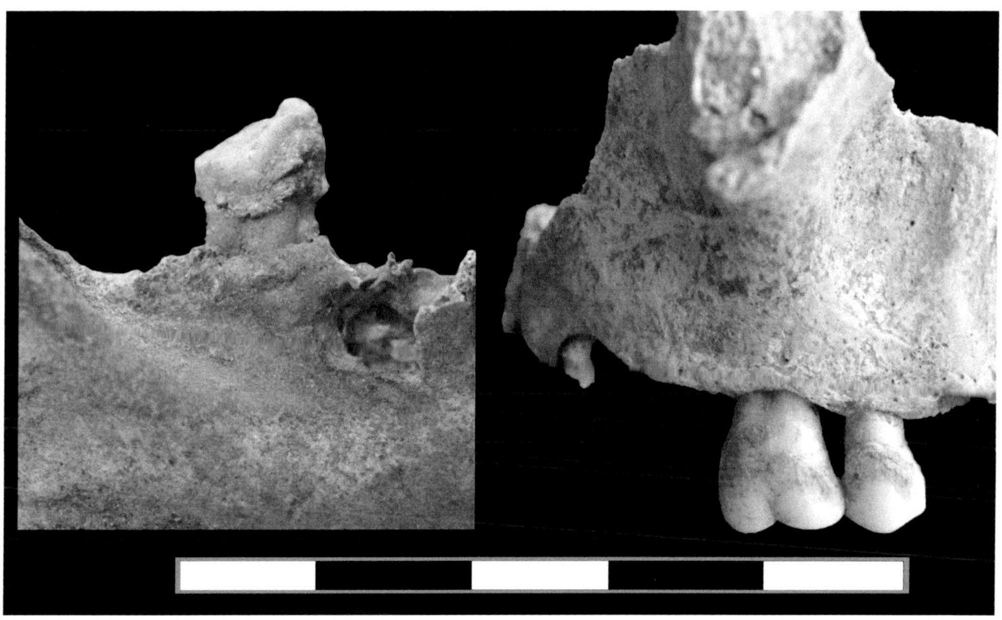

Figure 11.10 Left: Calculus deposit on the buccal and mesial surfaces of a mandibular molar. Note the periapical cavity associated with the alveolus of the missing molar anterior to the one shown in the photo. Right: Calculus deposit on the buccal surface of the right maxillary fourth premolar. Note that a similar deposit was originally present on the first molar, but it has fallen off. (Left: Probable male, Adult, Leeuwarden-Wergea, Collection NAD Nuis inv. Nr. F 1983-IX-14; photo by Efthymia Nikita, with permission from the Noordelijk Archeologisch Depot. Right: Sbide, Roman/Byzantine; photo by Efthymia Nikita, with the kind permission of Dr. Ahmet Ihsan Aytek, Burdur Mehmet Akif Ersoy University)

to the calculus surface. In contrast, subgingival calculus is covered by cocci, rods, and filaments, without a clear orientation.

Dental calculus formation is associated with diet, salivary flow rates, and oral hygiene. The formation of dental calculus is promoted in an alkaline oral environment. Thus, foods that increase oral alkalinity enhance calculus formation. Moreover, dental plaque is essential in calculus formation, as briefly discussed above. Therefore, diets that promote plaque formation (e.g. rich in carbohydrates) not only contribute to the development of dental caries but also facilitate the development of dental calculus.[1] The mineral content of drinking water may also be important in the formation of calculus deposits. Furthermore, elevated salivary flow rates lead to increased concentrations of salivary proteins and calcium, as well as increased alkalinity. Cultural practices such as chewing tobacco or gum, oral hygiene, and the use of teeth in extramasticatory activities can impact dental calculus formation. Chewing enhances the salivary flow rates, thus it promotes calculus formation; however, chewing hard materials may have the opposite effect by cleaning the teeth of calculus deposits. Similarly, oral hygiene practices and the use of teeth as tools can eliminate dental calculus.

Dental calculus is an important repository of starches, phytoliths, and other microdebris that can be entrapped in its matrix after they enter the mouth. Such microdebris can provide key information on past diet, natural environment, and occupational patterns. Furthermore, dental calculus can be used for the extraction of ancient DNA and proteins.

Antemortem tooth loss

Antemortem tooth loss (AMTL) is the loss of teeth while an individual was still alive (Figures 11.11 and 11.12). Several factors can contribute to AMTL, such as: (1) advanced periodontal disease, (2) tooth extraction due to inflammation, (3) nutritional deficiencies, (4) intentional

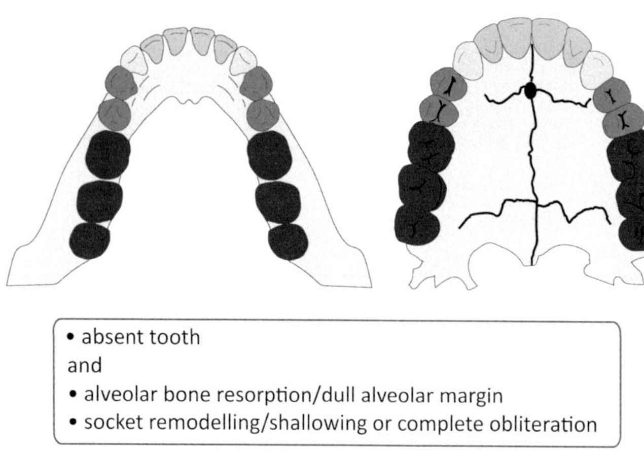

Figure 11.11 Manifestation of antemortem tooth loss. The different shades of grey reflect teeth that are more or less frequently affected by AMTL; the lighter the shade, the less frequently a tooth is affected. (Data from Delgado-Darias et al. 2006; Freeth 2000; Lukacs 1989)

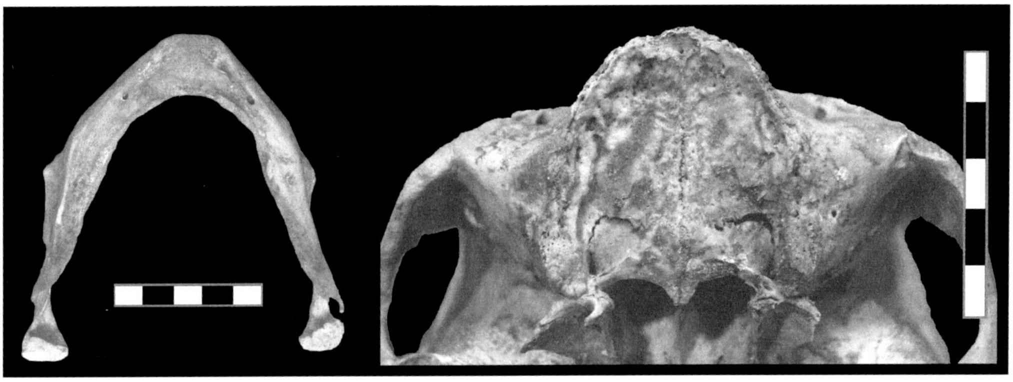

Figure 11.12 Edentulous individual; all mandibular and maxillary teeth have been lost antemortem, and the sockets have been fully remodelled. (Probable female, over 46 years old, Diever, Reformed Church graveyard, Collection NAD Nuis inv. Nr. D 2019-III.469; photos by Efthymia Nikita, with permission from the Noordelijk Archeologisch Depot)

tooth removal for cultural reasons, (5) trauma, and (6) continued eruption in order to maintain occlusion in severely worn teeth. AMTL should not be confused with dental agenesis, which may be common in the third molars or maxillary lateral incisors.

Enamel hypoplasia

Enamel hypoplasia results from a temporary disruption in normal enamel formation and appears as enamel of reduced thickness (Box 11.4, Figures 11.13–11.16). The main etiological factors associated with enamel hypoplasia include genetics, localised trauma, and physiological/systemic stressors. Defects associated with localised trauma mostly affect a single tooth, while hereditary enamel hypoplasia tends to be more severe and affects several teeth. Enamel hypoplasia linked to physiological/systemic stress generally impacts antimeric or adjacent

Box 11.4 Some basics on enamel formation

Ameloblasts are the cells responsible for enamel secretion. These cells start forming enamel from the cusp of the tooth towards the cervix; enamel formation is an incremental process that takes place in growth layers, which appear on the enamel surface as lines called perikymata. In modern humans, each perikyma corresponds to a period of enamel growth ranging from 6 to 12 days. The spacing of perikymata differs along the length of the crown; many more perikymata per mm are found towards the cervix compared to the cusp. Enamel hypoplasia occurs when there is a temporary disruption in enamel matrix formation by ameloblasts, and appears as abnormally large spacings between adjacent perikymata. In the middle of the crown, such a defect is easily observable. In contrast, when a similar disruption occurs near the cervix, it may be undetectable unless the tooth is examined histologically.

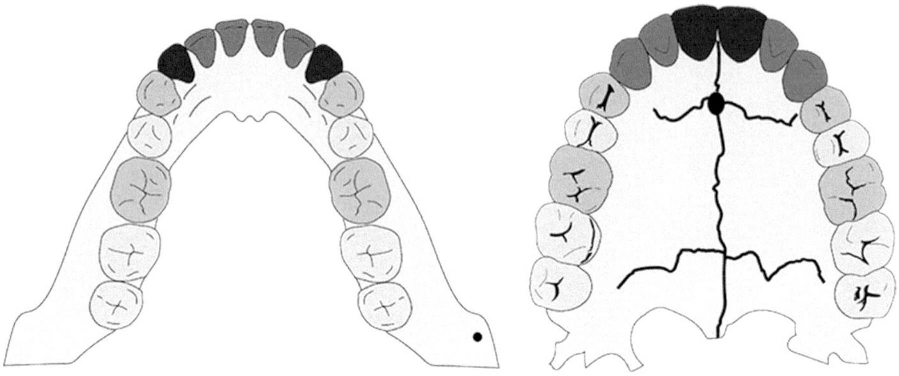

- horizontal lines/grooves (furrow-form defects)
- pits (single or multiple); multiple pits may be organised in horizontal alignment or dispersed across the tooth crown surface
- plane-form defects (large areas of deficient or missing enamel)

Figure 11.13 Manifestation of enamel hypoplasia. The different shades of grey reflect teeth that are more or less frequently affected by enamel hypoplasia; the lighter the shade, the less frequently a tooth is affected. (Data from Fédération Dentaire International 1982, 1992; Goodman and Armelagos 1985; Goodman and Rose 1990; Hassett 2014; Hillson 1992, 2023; Hillson and Bond 1997; Ogden 2008; Sarnat and Schour 1941)

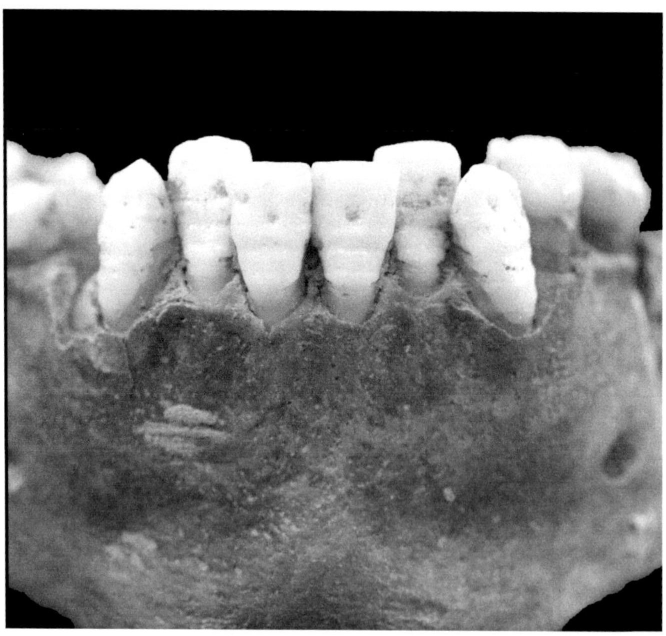

Figure 11.14 Linear enamel hypoplasia on mandibular incisors and canines. Note the multiple linear grooves visible on each tooth, suggesting successive episodes of physiological stress. The teeth also show individual distinct pits on their buccal surface. (Juvenile, Eemsdelta-Hoogwatum, Collection NAD Nuis inv. Nr. G 2018-IX.183; photo by Efthymia Nikita, with permission from the Noordelijk Archeologisch Depot)

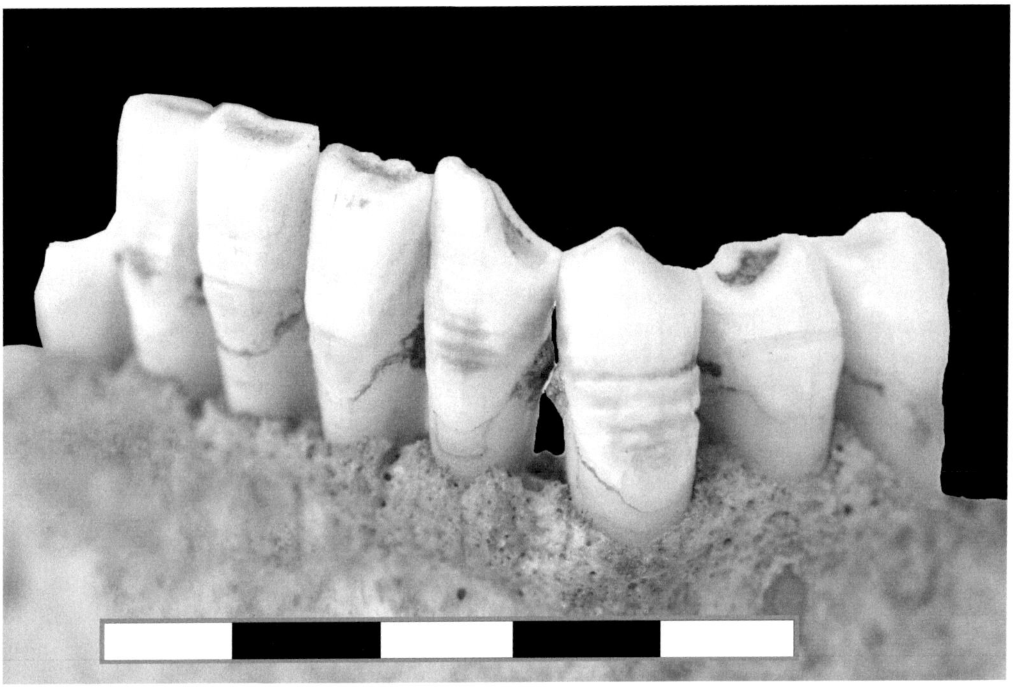

Figure 11.15 Linear enamel hypoplasia on the mandibular incisors, left canine, and third premolar. Note the multiple defects visible on the canine and incisors. Note also the distinctive occlusal wear pattern on the left lateral incisor, canine, and third premolar, which indicates some extramasticatory function of the teeth. (Male, Adult, Alkmaar-Grote Kerk, Medieval-Modern, 5062; photo by Efthymia Nikita, from the reference collection of the Cultural Heritage Agency of the Netherlands)

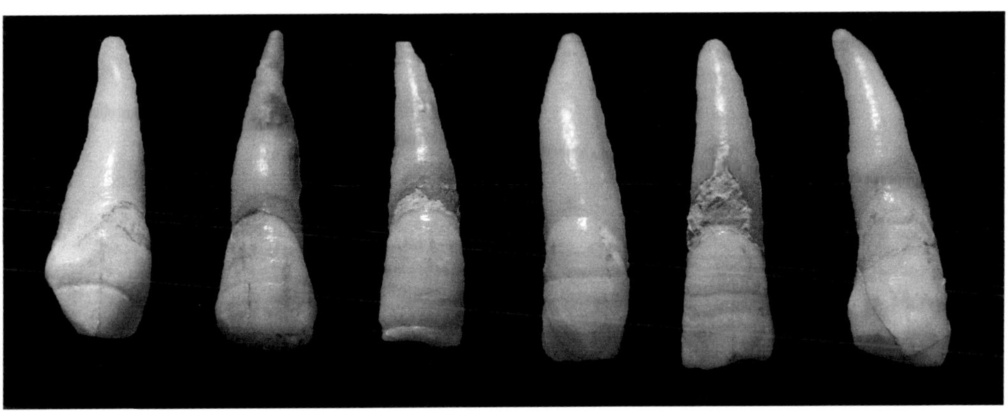

Figure 11.16 Linear enamel hypoplasia on loose maxillary and mandibular teeth. Note the multiple lines and/or grooves visible on the buccal surfaces, suggesting successive episodes of physiological stress. (Photos by Efthymia Nikita; copyright: Duckworth Laboratory, University of Cambridge)

teeth, affecting the part of the crown that was being formed at the time when stress was experienced.

Systemic stress is the main cause of enamel hypoplasia in archaeological assemblages. Malnutrition is considered a key factor contributing to enamel hypoplasia, alongside exposure to infectious diseases. Malnutrition and infections have a complex relationship as infections compromise the body's physiological functions and interfere with the effective absorption of nutrients, while malnutrition compromises an individual's immune system.

Enamel defects may have various forms, such as pits, horizontal grooves, or extensive areas of insufficient or absent enamel (plane-form defects). Pits can be single or multiple, and they range in size from tiny circular defects to large, irregular depressions. Small pits are associated with the disruption of the activity of a few ameloblasts, while larger pits involve the interruption of hundreds of ameloblasts. Horizontal defects may appear as a pronounced line, groove, or furrow on the crown surface. These hypoplastic defects are also known as linear enamel hypoplasia or furrow-form defects and are the most frequently documented in the bioarchaeological literature. Plane-form defects are regions of minimal or absent enamel deposition; they often co-occur with other significant enamel anomalies and are linked to conditions such as congenital syphilis and amelogenesis imperfecta.

Enamel defects are usually identified macroscopically; however, macroscopic methods cannot recognise all lesions, even when using a hand lens. Histological techniques and scanning electron microscopy provide more precise assessments, but require access to specialised equipment. The mandibular canines and maxillary first incisors are the teeth in which defects are most frequently observed. As a result, these teeth are often the main focus of examination in bioarchaeological research.

The physiological/systemic stress that can cause linear enamel hypoplasia affects the part of the crown that is actively being formed during the stressful episode. Thus, one can estimate how old the individual was when the defects occurred based on the lesions' spatial distribution (decile location) on the tooth crown. Charts and regression equations have been established to allow such estimates. Earlier approaches assumed a uniform rate of enamel formation throughout the crown development, but more recent methods recognise that enamel growth gradually decelerates from onset to the completion of crown formation.

Note

1 Nonetheless, calculus deposits may actually protect the teeth from the development of carious lesions by physically shielding the enamel from acid attacks.

References and suggested readings

Bocaege, E., Hillson, S. (2016). Disturbances and noise: Defining furrow-form enamel hypoplasia. *American Journal of Physical Anthropology* 161:744–751. https://doi.org/10.1002/ajpa.23070

Brothwell, D.R. (1981). *Digging Up Bones*. New York: Cornell University Press.

Cares Henriquez, A., Oxenham, M.F. (2019). New distance-based exponential regression method and equations for estimating the chronology of linear enamel hypoplasia (LEH) defects on the anterior dentition. *American Journal of Physical Anthropology* 168:510–520. https://doi.org/10.1002/ajpa.23764

Clarke, N.G. (1990). Periodontal defects of pulpal origin: Evidence in early man. *American Journal of Physical Anthropology* 82:371–376. https://doi.org/10.1002/ajpa.1330820312

Clarke, N.G., Hirsch, R.S. (1991). Physiological, pulpal, and periodontal factors influencing alveolar bone. In *Advances in Dental Anthropology*, edited by Kelly, A., Larsen, C.S., pp. 241–266. New York: Wiley-Liss.

Clarke, N.G., Carey, S.E., Srikandi, W., Hirsch, R.S., Leppard, P.I. (1986). Periodontal disease in ancient populations. *American Journal of Physical Anthropology* 71:173–183. https://doi.org/10.1002/ajpa.1330710205

Dawes, C. (2008). Salivary flow patterns and the health of hard and soft oral tissues. *The Journal of the American Dental Association* 139:18S–24S. https://doi.org/10.14219/jada.archive.2008.0351

Delgado-Darias, T., Velasco-Vázquez, J., Arnay-de-la-Rosa, M., Martín-Rodríguez, E., González-Reimers, E. (2006). Calculus, periodontal disease and tooth decay among the prehispanic population from Gran Canaria. *Journal of Archaeological Science* 33:663–670. https://doi.org/10.1016/j.jas.2005.09.018

Dias, G., Tayles, N. (1997). 'Abscess cavity' – a misnomer. *International Journal of Osteoarchaeology* 7:548–554. https://doi.org/10.1002/(SICI)1099-1212(199709/10)7:5%3C548::AID-OA369%3E3.0.CO;2-I

Dias, G.J., Prasad, K., Santos, A.L. (2007). Pathogenesis of apical periodontal cysts: Guidelines for diagnosis in palaeopathology. *International Journal of Osteoarchaeology* 17:619–626. https://doi.org/10.1002/oa.902

Dobney, K., Brothwell, D. (1987). A method for evaluating the amount of dental calculus on teeth from archaeological sites. *Journal of Archaeological Science* 14:343–351. https://doi.org/10.1016/0305-4403(87)90024-0

Driessens, F.C.M., Verbeeck, R.M.H. (1988). Possible pathways of mineralization of dental plaque. In *Recent Advances in the Study of Dental Calculus*, edited by ten Cate, J.M., pp. 7–17. Oxford: Oxford University Press.

Fédération Dentaire International. (1982). An epidemiological index of developmental defects of dental enamel (DDE Index). *International Dental Journal* 32:159–167.

Fédération Dentaire International. (1992). A review of the developmental defects of enamel index (DDE index). *International Dental Journal* 42:411–426.

Freeth, C. (2000). Dental health in British antiquity. In *Human Osteology in Archaeology and Forensic Science*, edited by Cox, M., Mays, S., pp. 227–237. London: Greenwich Medical Media.

Goodman, A.H., Armelagos, G. (1985). Factors affecting the distribution of enamel hypoplasias within the human permanent dentition. *American Journal of Physical Anthropology* 68:479–493. https://doi.org/10.1002/ajpa.1330680404

Goodman, A.H., Rose, J.C. (1990). Assessment of systemic physiological perturbations from dental enamel hypoplasia and associated histological structures. *Yearbook of Physical Anthropology* 33:59–110. https://doi.org/10.1002/ajpa.1330330506

Goodman, A.H., Armelagos, G.J., Rose, J.C. (1980). Enamel hypoplasias as indicators of stress in three prehistoric populations from Illinois. *Human Biology* 52:515–528.

Guatelli-Steinberg, D., Lukacs, J.R. (1999). Interpreting sex differences in enamel hypoplasia in human and non-human primates: Developmental, environmental, and cultural considerations. *American Journal of Physical Anthropology* 110:73–126. https://doi.org/10.1002/(SICI)1096-8644(1999)110:29+%3C73::AID-AJPA4%3E3.0.CO;2-K

Hassett, B.R. (2014). Missing defects? A comparison of microscopic and macroscopic approaches to identifying linear enamel hypoplasia. *American Journal of Physical Anthropology* 153:463–472. https://doi.org/10.1002/ajpa.22445

Hildebolt, C.F., Molnar, S. (1991). Measurement and description of periodontal disease in anthropological studies. In *Advances in Dental Anthropology*, edited by Kelley, M.A., Larsen, C.S., pp. 225–240. New York: Wiley-Liss.

Hillson, S. (1979). Diet and dental disease. *World Archaeology* 2:147–162. https://doi.org/10.1080/00438243.1979.9979758

Hillson, S. (1992). Dental enamel growth, perikymata and hypoplasia in ancient tooth crowns. *Journal of the Royal Society of Medicine* 85:460–466. https://doi.org/10.1177/014107689208500813

Hillson, S. (2001). Recording dental caries in archaeological human remains. *International Journal of Osteoarchaeology* 11:249–289. https://doi.org/10.1002/oa.538

Hillson, S. (2008). The current state of dental decay. In *Technique, and Application in Dental Anthropology*, edited by Irish, J.D., Nelson, G.C., pp. 111–135. Cambridge: Cambridge University Press.
Hillson, S. (2014). *Tooth Development in Human Evolution and Bioarchaeology*. Cambridge: Cambridge University Press.
Hillson, S. (2023). *Dental Anthropology*, 2nd edition. Cambridge: Cambridge University Press.
Hillson, S., Bond, S. (1997). Relationship of enamel hypoplasia to the pattern of tooth crown growth: A discussion. *American Journal of Physical Anthropology* 104:89–103. https://doi.org/10.1002/(SICI)1096-8644(199709)104:1%3C89::AID-AJPA6%3E3.0.CO;2-8
Hubbard, A., Guatelli-Steinberg, D., Sciulli, P.W. (2009). Under restrictive conditions, can the widths of linear enamel hypoplasias be used as relative indicators of stress episode duration? *American Journal of Physical Anthropology* 138:177–189. https://doi.org/10.1002/ajpa.20917
Irish, J.D., Scott, G.R. (2015). *A Companion to Dental Anthropology*. Hoboken, NJ: John Wiley & Sons.
Jin, Y., Yip, H.K. (2002). Supragingival calculus: Formation and control. *Critical Reviews in Oral Biology & Medicine* 13:426–441. https://doi.org/10.1177/154411130201300506
Kerr, N.W. (1988). A method of assessing periodontal status in archaeologically derived skeletal material. *Journal of Paleopathology* 2:67–78.
Kerr, N.W. (1991). Prevalence and natural history of periodontal disease in Scotland – the mediaeval period (900–1600 A.D.). *Journal of Periodontal Research* 26:346–354. https://doi.org/10.1111/j.1600-0765.1991.tb02073.x
King, T., Humphrey, L., Hillson, S.W. (2005). Linear enamel hypoplasias as indicators of systemic physiological stress: Evidence from two known age-at-death and sex populations from Post-medieval London. *American Journal of Physical Anthropology* 128:547–559. https://doi.org/10.1002/ajpa.20232
Kubehl, K., Temple, D.H. (2020). Reproductive life histories influence cariogenesis: Exploring sex-specific variation in dental caries and survivorship in the human past. *American Journal of Physical Anthropology* 172:376–385. https://doi.org/10.1002/ajpa.24034
Larsen, C.S., Shavit, R., Griffin, M.C., Kelley, M.A. (1991). Dental caries evidence for dietary change: An archaeological context. In *Advances in Dental Anthropology*, edited by Kelly, A., Larsen, C.S., pp. 179–202. New York: Wiley-Liss.
Lewis, M. (2017). Dental disease, defects, and variations in dental morphology. In *Paleopathology of Children: Identification of Pathological Conditions in the Human Skeletal Remains of Non-Adults*, edited by Lewis, M. pp. 67–89. San Diego: Academic Press.
Lieverse, A.R. (1999). Diet and the aetiology of dental calculus. *International Journal of Osteoarchaeology* 9:219–232. https://doi.org/10.1002/(SICI)1099-1212(199907/08)9:4%3C219::AID-OA475%3E3.0.CO;2-V
Lingström, P., van Houte, J., Kashket, S. (2000a). Food starches and dental caries. *Critical Reviews in Oral Biology & Medicine* 11:366–380.
Lingström, P., Van Ruyven, F.O.J., Van Houte, J., Kent, R. (2000b). The pH of dental plaque in its relation to early enamel caries and dental plaque flora in humans. *Journal of Dental Research* 79:770–777. https://doi.org/10.1177/00220345000790021101
Lukacs, J.R. (1989). Dental paleopathology: Methods for reconstructing dietary patterns. In *Reconstruction of Life from the Skeleton*, edited by İşcan, M.Y., Kennedy, K.A.R., pp. 261–286. New York: Alan R. Liss.
Lukacs, J.R. (2012). Oral health in past populations: Context, concepts and controversy. In *A Companion to Paleopathology*, edited by Grauer, A.L., pp. 553–581. Hoboken, NJ: John Wiley & Sons.
Lukacs, J.R., Largaespada, L.L. (2006). Explaining sex differences in dental caries prevalence: Saliva, hormones, and "life-history" etiologies. *American Journal of Human Biology* 18:540–555. https://doi.org/10.1002/ajhb.20530
Martin, S.A., Guatelli-Steinberg, D., Sciulli, P.W., Walker, P.L. (2008). Brief communication: Comparison of methods for estimating chronological age at linear enamel formation on anterior dentition. *American Journal of Physical Anthropology* 135:362–365. https://doi.org/10.1002/ajpa.20725

Ogden, A. (2008). Advances in the palaeopathology of teeth and jaws. In *Advances in Human Palaeopathology*, edited by Pinhasi, R., Mays, S., pp. 283–307. Hoboken, NJ: John Wiley & Sons.
Pilloud, M.A., Fancher, J.P. (2019). Outlining a definition of oral health within the study of human skeletal remains. *Dental Anthropology* 32. https://doi.org/10.26575/daj.v32i2.297
Radini, A., Nikita, E., Buckley, S., Copeland, L., Hardy, K. (2017). Beyond food: The multiple pathways for inclusion of materials into ancient dental calculus. *American Journal of Physical Anthropology* 162:71–83. https://doi.org/10.1002/ajpa.23147
Reid, D.J., Dean, M.C. (2006). Variation in modern human enamel formation times. *Journal of Human Evolution* 50:329–346. https://doi.org/10.1016/j.jhevol.2005.09.003
Rudney, J.D., Katz, R.V., Brand, J.W. (1983). Interobserver reliability of methods for paleopathological diagnosis of dental caries. *American Journal of Physical Anthropology* 62:243–248. https://doi.org/10.1002/ajpa.1330620303
Sarnat, B.G., Schour, I. (1941). Enamel hypoplasia (chronologic enamel aplasia) in relation to systemic disease: A chronologic, morphologic and etiologic classification. *The Journal of the American Dental Association* 28:1989–2000. https://doi.org/10.14219/jada.archive.1942.0381
Selwitz, R.H., Ismail, A.I., Pitts, N.B. (2007). Dental caries. *The Lancet* 369:51–59. https://doi.org/10.1016/s0140-6736(07)60031-2
Skinner, M.F. (2023). Meaningful measures of enamel hypoplasia: Prevalence and comparative intensity of developmental stress. *American Journal of Biological Anthropology* 180:761–767. https://doi.org/10.1002/ajpa.24699
Skinner, M.F., Hung, J.T.W. (1989). Social and biological correlates of localized enamel hypoplasia of the human deciduous canine tooth. *American Journal of Physical Anthropology* 79:159–175. https://doi.org/10.1002/ajpa.1330790204
Strohm, T.F., Alt, K.W. (1998). Periodontal disease—etiology, classification and diagnosis. In *Dental Anthropology: Fundamentals, Limits, and Perspectives*, edited by Alt, K.W., Rosing, F.W., Teschler-Nicola, M., pp. 247–276. New York: Springer.
Tal, H. (1985). Periodontal bone loss in dry mandibles of South African blacks: A biometric study. *Journal of Dental Research* 64:925–929. https://doi.org/10.1177/00220345850640061401
Temple, D.H. (2015). Caries: The ancient scourge. In *A Companion to Dental Anthropology*, edited by Irish, J.D., Scott, G.R., pp. 433–449. New York: Wiley.
Touger-Decker, R., van Louveren, C. (2003). Sugars and dental caries. *The American Journal of Clinical Nutrition* 78:881S–882S. https://doi.org/10.1093/ajcn/78.4.881S
Towle, I., Irish, J.D. (2020). Recording and interpreting enamel hypoplasia in samples from archaeological and palaeoanthropological contexts. *Journal of Archaeological Science* 114:105077. https://doi.org/10.1016/j.jas.2020.105077
Ullinger, J., Loewen, T. (2023). Dental disease. In *The Routledge Handbook of Paleopathology*, edited by Grauer, A.L., pp. 360–377. London: Routledge.
van Houte, J. (1994). Role of micro organisms in caries etiology. *Journal of Dental Research* 73:672–681. https://doi.org/10.1177/00220345940730031301
Watson, J.T., Tuggle, A. (2019). Periodontal health and the life-course approach in bioarchaeology. *Dental Anthropology Journal* 32:12–21. https://doi.org/10.26575/daj.v32i2.289
White, D.J. (1997). Dental calculus: Recent insights into occurrence, formation, prevention, removal and oral health effects of supragingival and subgingival deposits. *European Journal of Oral Sciences* 105:508–522. https://doi.org/10.1111/j.1600-0722.1997.tb00238.x

Index

Pages in *italics* refer to figures, pages in **bold** refer to tables, and pages followed by "n" refer to notes.